Cambridge History of Medicine

EDITORS: CHARLES WEBSTER AND CHARLES ROSENBERG

Professional and popular medicine in
France, 1770–1830

Charles Webster, ed.   *Health, medicine, and mortality in the sixteenth century*

Ian Maclean   *The Renaissance notion of woman*

Michael MacDonald   *Mystical Bedlam*

Robert E. Kohler   *From medical chemistry to biochemistry*

Walter Pagel   *Joan Baptista Van Helmont*

Nancy Tomes   *A generous confidence*

Roger Cooter   *The cultural meaning of popular science*

Anne Digby   *Madness, morality and medicine*

Guenter B. Risse   *Hospital life in Enlightenment Scotland*

Roy Porter, ed.   *Patients and practitioners*

Ann G. Carmichael   *Plague and the poor in Renaissance Florence*

S. E. D. Shortt   *Victorian lunacy*

Hilary Marland   *Medicine and society in Wakefield and Huddersfield 1780–1870*

Susan Reverby   *Ordered to care*

Russell C. Maulitz   *Morbid appearances*

Professional and popular medicine in France, 1770–1830

THE SOCIAL WORLD OF MEDICAL PRACTICE

MATTHEW RAMSEY

Department of History, Vanderbilt University

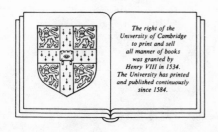

The right of the
University of Cambridge
to print and sell
all manner of books
was granted by
Henry VIII in 1534.
The University has printed
and published continuously
since 1584.

CAMBRIDGE UNIVERSITY PRESS

CAMBRIDGE

NEW YORK   NEW ROCHELLE   MELBOURNE   SYDNEY

Published by the Press Syndicate of the University of Cambridge
The Pitt Building, Trumpington Street, Cambridge CB2 1RP
32 East 57th Street, New York, NY 10022, USA
10 Stamford Road, Oakleigh, Melbourne 3166, Australia

First published 1988

Printed in the United States of America

Library of Congress Cataloging-in-Publication Data
Ramsey, Matthew, 1948–
Professional and popular medicine in France, 1770–1830.
(Cambridge history of medicine)
Includes index.
1. Medicine – France – History – 18th century.
2. Medicine – France – History – 19th century.   3. Medicine,
Magic, mystic, and spagyric – France – History – 18th
century.   4. Medicine, Magic, mystic, and spagyric –
France – History – 19th century.   5. Social medicine –
France – History – 18th century.   6. Social medicine –
France – History – 19th century.   I. Title.   II. Title:
Social world of medical practice. [DNLM: 1. History
of Medicine, 18th Cent. – France.   2. History of Medicine,
19th Cent. – France.   WZ 70 GF7 R18p]
R504.R36   1988   610'.944   87–15882
ISBN 0 521 30517 9

British Library Cataloguing in Publication applied for

To the memory of my parents

CONTENTS

List of tables, maps, and illustrations   *page* ix
Preface   xi
Acknowledgments   xiv

Introduction: Professionalization and popular culture –
approach and methods   1

PART I. PROFESSIONAL MEDICINE

1 The regular medical network at the end of the Old Regime   17
     The traditional structure of the regular network   18
     Professional institutions   38
     Medical and surgical practice   45
     Access to a medical career   49
     Social and economic status   54
     Density and distribution of personnel   58
     Costs of professional services   62
     Attitudes toward the medical profession   65
2 The medical profession in the early nineteenth century   71
     The revolutionary decade   71
     The medical profession and the laws of Ventôse
     and Germinal   77
     Who was coopted into the new sytem?   84
     Professional institutions   105
     Access to a medical career   108
     Social and economic status   110
     Access to a practitioner   115
     Attitudes toward the medical profession   122

PART II. POPULAR MEDICINE

3   Irregulars: itinerants   129
    The old-style mountebank and other charlatans   132
    Varieties of itinerancy: peddlers, marginals, and inspired
    healers   164
4   Irregulars: sedentary empirics   176
    Remedy vendors   177
    Varieties of empiricism   182
    The population of empirics: numbers, density,
    distribution   204
    Sedentary empiricism: a social and economic analysis   213
5   Folk healers: *maiges* and witches   229
    The folk practitioner: concepts and approaches   230
    Maiges   239
    Witches and *devins-guérisseurs*   264

PART III. TOWARD A SOCIAL INTERPRETATION

6   The structure of medical practice: an overview   279
    Rivalry and cooperation   279
    The market for medical services   284
    Medical practitioners and society   291
    Medical practice and social change   296

    Afterword: medicalization and social theory   299

    Appendix A: Density of French medical personnel in the
    nineteenth century   302
    Appendix B: Some itinerant empirics, 1802–1844   306
    Appendix C: Some French remedy sellers, 1773–1830   309
    Appendix D: Some empirics and their occupations,
    1775–1838   311
    Notes   313
    Glossary and note on French money   387
    Index   391

TABLES, MAPS, AND ILLUSTRATIONS

TABLES

1	Regional densities of practitioners in 1786	*page*	59
2	Disparities in urban/rural densities of practitioners, 1786		60
3	Unauthorized medical practitioners in the Bas-Rhin, 1813		212
4	Types of practitioners		253
5	Densities of practitioners in the 1830's		304

MAPS

1	Hué's itinerary, 1803–08	172
2	*Rebouteurs* around Ancenis (Loire-Inférieure), 1827	188
3	Milfort case, 1822: Origins of patients traveling to Charleville	201

ILLUSTRATIONS

The physician: morning visits	112
The physician in search of subscribers	120
The orvietan vendor, 1817	134
The German charlatan, 1776	141
The conjuror	143
The "great charlatan" harangues the crowd, 1816	144
The boastful itinerant on his cabriolet with drum and trumpet	148
Charlatan showing the skin of a man he has cured	149
The French charlatan, 1776	151
"Without effort": M. Mâchoire, dentist of the great mogul	152

Surgery without a surgeon: a quack peddles his self-help
book.   162
Vendor of Swiss vulnerary   165
A Breton *rebouteur*: popular medicine captured by
photography   186
The urine doctor   193
"The rustic pharmacy": Michel Schuppach,
urinoscopist, 1774   194
The *metze* Chazal (blacksmith-healer)   250

This book is the first part of a larger and ongoing study of the history of popular and official medicine in France. The project began as an attempt to make sense of the medical ideas and practices of a culture very different from our own. In eighteenth-century France, as in much of preindustrial Europe, saints were thought to kill as well as cure; healers raised "fallen" stomachs or dispelled disease with their touch, saliva, breath, and voice; and even an educated man might accept that one way to treat a fever was to steep an egg in the patient's urine and feed it to a dog.[1] I also hoped to understand how, over the course of generations, people ceased to believe in these things, gradually adopting the conceptions of the body and disease developed by medical science and relegating the medical lore of their forebears – an object of derision for some, of curiosity for others – to the domain of popular superstition.

As the work progressed and the curious receipts and charms accumulated, another related story began to emerge, just as absorbing and more congenial to historical analysis[2] – the evolution of France from a society in which only a narrow elite consulted physicians to one in which nearly everyone does. Two centuries ago, most Frenchmen and Frenchwomen saw "healers" as familiar figures and doctors as exotic ones; since then these roles have been reversed. This secular trend changed what it meant to the average patient to be sick. More than that, it radically transformed what it meant to practice medicine. As I explored this problem, my attention shifted from patients' beliefs and behavior to the practitioners who ministered to them; from medicine as a cultural system to medicine as an occupation.

The investigation now centered on the evolving relationship between popular and official practice in the era that saw the emergence of the modern medical profession. These things, it seemed to me, had to be understood together; they formed two aspects of the same story. But such an approach also created peculiar difficulties, for popular and official medicine moved according to different rhythms. The first, seemingly the product of what

Claude Lévi-Strauss, in a famous metaphor, called a "cold" society, changed only slowly, lending itself more readily to anthropological interpretation than to a historical narrative. The profession, in contrast, clearly belonged to the world of history, of "hot" societies: its changes could be measured in years and decades, rather than centuries, and it left behind an abundant documentation that invites research monographs with a sharper chronological focus. The only solution seemed to be an awkward compromise: to join the two accounts, but to concentrate on a crucial period of several decades in the history of the profession – preferably one in which official medicine significantly transformed its relationship with its rivals. Although this project began as an exploration of popular *mentalités*, its present framework therefore reflects the history of the profession and its institutions.

The choice of dates reflects both the priorities of this project and its French emphasis. In most histories of Western medicine, particularly those written from an American perspective, the late nineteenth and early twentieth centuries stand out as the critical epoch in the formation of a strong modern profession. Advances in medical science, such as the discoveries in bacteriology associated with the names of Robert Koch and Louis Pasteur, promised physicians a superiority over their unqualified rivals that they had never before enjoyed. Physicians' social and economic status rose; their services became more widely available, thanks in part to expanding schemes of health insurance, social security, and other forms of third-party payment. In the United States, medical education was reformed and standardized, and the profession won for the first time a rigorous system of licensure. All these developments seemed to be interrelated, and many scholars have since argued that the profession owed to its new technical prowess both its enhanced prestige and its dominance over unqualified rivals.[3]

France largely shared this experience. But French medicine had also known another heroic age, in the late eighteenth and early nineteenth centuries, long familiar to medical historians for having produced the highly influential Paris clinical school. Three other considerations made this period exceptionally interesting for the purposes of this study. In the last decade of the eighteenth century and the first decade of the nineteenth, the French medical occupations were completely reorganized. Medicine and surgery were formally joined, and medical education was standardized for the first time. In addition, the late eighteenth and early nineteenth centuries saw the opening and conclusion of a major debate on the practice of medicine, which pitted one against the other two radically divergent Enlightenment visions. In the first, the old restrictions on teaching and practice would be lifted and medical knowledge diffused so widely that, in some versions, physicians would become superfluous. In the second, the authority of the physician, whose expertise no layman could hope to challenge, would be greatly reinforced, and all forms of popular medical practice would be extirpated. The latter view decisively prevailed in the nineteenth century.

Finally, between the last years of the Old Regime and the first years of the new century, France passed through not only a succession of political regimes but also – as a result of these larger upheavals – three basic legislative regimes in the medical field, the last of which (in 1803) imposed the tightest de jure monopoly the West had ever seen. More than any other period, then, the late eighteenth and early nineteenth centuries defined the French medical profession and its relationship with outsiders. The advances that the profession made during this era, moreover, preceded by decades the Pasteurian revolution of the late nineteenth century, and this experience raises questions about the extent to which the profession's success can be ascribed to the triumphs of medical science in France or anywhere else.

Hence the chronological emphasis of this study. Although it occasionally glances back to the late seventeenth or forward to the early twentieth century (particularly in its discussion of popular medicine), it centers on the sixty years from 1770 to 1830. During this period, popular medicine remained very much alive; indeed, one of the aims of this book is to show the great diversity of practitioners who still made up the French medical network of a century and a half ago. The profession, however, was consolidated, and the border between qualified and unqualified practice more sharply defined. A new consensus began to emerge among educated Frenchmen that medical care for the entire population should be in the hands of qualified professionals. The profession and the state, finally, embarked on a drive against unauthorized medical practice. Although police measures predictably failed to eliminate popular medicine (whose long-term decline owed more to schooling, improved transportation, higher living standards, and third-party systems of payment), this campaign of repression did influence its form and scope and turned unqualified practice, once widely tolerated, into an act of defiance.

The central problem, then, of the larger project is the emergence in French medicine of what was arguably the first modern professional monopoly. The present volume begins by examining the social world of medical practice in the eighteenth and nineteenth centuries: the diverse network of medical practitioners, qualified and unqualified; the creation of a unified medical profession and its differentiation from unqualified practice; and the social and economic constraints that helped shape the great variety of medical and paramedical occupations. A future study will turn to ideas and politics: the developing ideology of professional power; the new legislation on professional monopoly and the institutions charged with enforcing it; and the actual struggle for control of the medical domain.

ACKNOWLEDGMENTS

During the long gestation of this project, I have incurred more than the usual number of obligations. It is a pleasant duty to express my appreciation here, although it is not possible, in the space available, either to thank by name all the individuals who have assisted me or to convey the extent of my indebtedness.

I am grateful, first of all, to Patrice Higonnet, who, since my undergraduate years, has done more than anyone else to inspire my love of French history and who directed the (very different) doctoral dissertation on popular medicine from which this study emerged. I was also fortunate to receive advice and encouragement from many other specialists on French history or the history of medicine, among them Keith Baker, Robert Darnton, Natalie Davis, Elizabeth Eisenstein, Robert Forster, Louis Greenbaum, Arthur Imhof, Harvey Mitchell, and Dora Weiner. Caroline Hannaway helped sharpen my perception of medical institutions in eighteenth-century France. Toby Gelfand, in numerous letters and conversations over the years, has proved a congenial and unfailing source of advice, information, and constructive criticism. In France, I profited from the hospitality and counsel of numerous scholars, among them Jean-Paul Aron, Jeanne Favret-Saada, François Lebrun, Robert Mandrou, and Jean Meyer. Jean-Pierre Peter introduced me to the then uncatalogued archives of the Société Royale de Médecine; my understanding of the social history of medicine owes much to his seminar at the VIe Section of the École Pratique des Hautes Études (the present École des Hautes Études en Sciences Sociales), in which I took part in 1974–75. Jacques Léonard guided my explorations of the sources of nineteenth-century French medical history, generously furnishing bibliographical and archival references. Françoise Loux shared her vast knowledge of medical ethnography, welcomed me at the Musée National des Arts et Traditions Populaires, and helped locate some of the illustrations that appear in this volume. Claire Ambroselli, director of the Centre de Documentation et d'Information d'Éthique des Sciences de la Vie et de la Santé, has proved an inexhaustible source of ideas and information on all branches of the history and philosophy of medicine. Above all, I owe a special debt of gratitude to Jean-Pierre Goubert, mentor and friend, who has followed this study almost from its inception and unstintingly shared with me his knowledge of French medical and social history.

In addition, my work has benefitted over the years from exchanges with other researchers in Paris; with teachers (later colleagues) and students in the Departments of History and History of Science at Harvard University; with fellow participants in the seminar on the history of the professions held in 1979–80 at the Shelby Cullom Davis Center for Historical Studies at Princeton University under the direction of Lawrence Stone; and with present colleagues in the Department of History at Vanderbilt University. At Harvard, I particularly valued the counsel and support of Barbara Rosenkrantz, who read nearly every piece of writing related to this project and from whom I learned much as co-instructor of a course on health, disease, and society in Europe and America. I also profited from teaching a version of that course with Allan Brandt and from discussions with graduate students who shared an interest in the social history of medicine, notably Jo Gladstone, Leonard Groopman, Joy Harvey, and Margaret Warner. Thanks also to other friends and colleagues, in the United States and abroad, who shared insights and information, especially Marc Alexander, Harold Cook, François Delaporte, Lynn Hunt, Thomas Kaiser, Alison Klairmont Lingo (who also supplied copies of documents from the municipal archives of Lyons), Jeremy Popkin, Michael Sibalis, George Sussman, and George Weisz. Michel Boyer, Olivier Faure, and Jacques Idoux graciously furnished copies of their unpublished theses. Evelyn Ackerman, Gerald Geison, Robert Isherwood, and Paul Conkin, among others, read and commented on one of the several versions of the manuscript, as did Ted Margadant (who suggested the subtitle of this volume); I am particularly grateful to Harry Marks, who wrote a searching and detailed critique of each chapter – though the end product still falls short of his high standards. (I of course remain responsible for any errors of fact or interpretation.) A number of able assistants at Harvard University helped lighten the burden of research: graduate students James Donato and Benjamin Kaplan, and undergraduates Marjorie Beale, Sheila Crowley, Aguia Heath, Wanda Kim, Rani Kronick, Lisa Mihaly, and Andres Reyes. The generous hospitality of Claude Debru, Thomas and Helen Kaiser, Henri Roy, and Jean-Claude Schmitt greatly facilitated three stays in Paris. Most recently, Charles Rosenberg, as editor of the series in which this book appears, provided advice and encouragement in therapeutic doses; and Helen Wheeler and her colleagues at Cambridge University Press have eased the painful transition from manuscript to book.

The research for this study was assisted by the librarians, archivists, and curators of numerous institutions, including the Countway Library of Medicine at Harvard (especially its rare books collection in Holmes Hall, presided over by the omniscient Richard Wolfe), the libraries of the New York Academy of Medicine and the College of Physicians of Philadelphia, the National Library of Medicine (especially the History of Medicine Division), the Firestone Library of Princeton University, and the central and medical libraries of Vanderbilt University; in London, the Wellcome Institute for the History of Medicine; in Paris, the Archives Nationales, the Bibliothèque Nationale, the Académie Nationale de Médecine, the libraries of the faculties of medicine and pharmacy, the Musée National des Arts et Traditions Populaires, and the archives of the Préfecture de Police; the *archives départementales* of the Aube, Ille-et-Vilaine, Maine-et-Loire, and Loire-Atlantique; the municipal libraries of Angers and Nantes; and the Cité des Archives Contemporaines in Avon (where, thanks to the *conservateur* Jacques d'Orléans, I was able to consult the nineteenth-century archives of the Académie Royale de Médecine, then in the process of being inventoried). I am especially grateful to Michel Roussier, librarian of the Bibliothèque Administrative de la Préfecture de la Seine, who allowed me into the cramped but well-furnished stacks at the Hôtel de Ville and was always ready with a word of advice when I emerged; and to the *conservateur en mission* Marie-Antoinette Fleury, who in the later stages of this project made available to me her manuscript inventory of the archives of the Société Royale de Médecine. During the main phase of research in France, the École Normale Supérieure generously offered a former *pensionnaire étranger* both office space and access to that rare thing in Paris, a good circulating open-stack library. At a later stage, the Bureau d'Accueil des Professeurs d'Universités Étrangères provided some secretarial assistance and a variety of helpful practical services.

The initial research for this project was supported by a foreign area fellowship from the Social Science Research Council and American Council of Learned Societies and a Sheldon Travelling Fellowship from Harvard University; much of the remaining research was completed during a postdoctoral year at the Davis Center at Princeton, funded by a fellowship from the National Endowment for the Humanities (with an additional research allowance from the Davis Center). I would also like to acknowledge smaller grants to defray the costs of research trips to France from the American Council of Learned Societies and the American Philosophical Society, and two faculty research grants from the Clark Fund at Harvard University. Funding for student assistants was provided by the Faculty Aide Program and the Junior Faculty Research Assistant/College Work-Study Program at Harvard. The Vanderbilt History Department subsidized the typing of the final manuscript.

Some of the material in this study has appeared earlier in article form. I would like to thank the *Journal of Social History* for permission to use portions of "Medical Power and Popular Medicine: Illegal Healers in Nineteenth-Century France," vol. 10 (1976–77), pp. 560–87, and "Review Essay: History of a Profession, *Annales* Style: The Work of Jacques Léonard," vol. 17 (1983–84), pp. 319–38; and *Eighteenth-Century Life*, for permission to draw on "The Repression of Unauthorized Medical Practice in Eighteenth-Century France," n.s. vol. 7 (1982), pp. 118–35. Jean-Pierre Goubert kindly allowed me to include data from his article "The Extent of Medical Practice in France around 1780," *Journal of Social History*, vol. 10, p. 421, table 2, "Regional Disparities in Medical Activity." The illustrations in this book come from prints or photographs in the collections of the Bibliothèque Nationale, the Musée Carnavalet, and the Musée National des Arts et Traditions Populaires; the source in each case is indicated in the caption.

Especial thanks, finally, to Linda Burcher Ramsey and David Burcher Ramsey, who patiently endured a protracted enterprise that impinged on their lives almost as much as it did on mine. Linda read and astutely criticized numerous parts and versions of this study and in countless other ways offered loyal support. They have my deepest gratitude.

INTRODUCTION:
PROFESSIONALIZATION AND
POPULAR CULTURE – APPROACH AND
METHODS

This enterprise deliberately joins two major lines of inquiry that have attracted growing attention in recent years but have generally been pursued separately: the history of popular culture and of the professions. Over the last decade and a half, several prominent studies have charted the shifting relationship between popular and elite culture in Europe between the sixteenth and the nineteenth centuries. Perhaps their most salient theme has been what Max Weber called *die Entzauberung der Welt* (the disenchantment of the world), that is, the rise and spread of modern scientific rationalism. In a wide-ranging and learned work on the decline of magic (1971), Keith Thomas showed how in seventeenth-century England, "magic was ceasing to be intellectually acceptable."[1] Later in the decade, in a broad overview of popular culture in early modern Europe (1978), Peter Burke argued that between the Renaissance and the Enlightenment, learned culture evolved rapidly, absorbing in particular the unsettling influence of the Scientific Revolution, while popular culture lagged behind; the result, he suggested, was that the elites withdrew from a shared traditional culture.[2] Two years earlier, Eugen Weber, in a richly detailed account of the modernization of rural France in the years between the founding of the Third Republic and World War I, had described how the rational-scientific world view eventually reached the peasantry, shattered the old beliefs and customs, and narrowed once again the gap between popular and elite culture.[3]

The last decade has also witnessed new stirrings of interest in one influential fraction of the elite, the professions (although until recently the French case has suffered from relative neglect).[4] Whereas the appeal of popular culture owed something to nostalgia for a world we have lost, the study of the professions derives much of its impetus from the commonplace observation that professionals have become a dominant force in contemporary society, a group whose numbers exceed what anyone would have predicted a century ago and whose influence reaches far beyond what their numbers alone would indicate.[5] In recent years, a diverse group of historians have emphasized the role in nineteenth- and twentieth-century history of the noncapitalist middle classes, of which professionals are perhaps the most conspicuous members.[6] In addition, a growing literature, often highly polemical, deals more specifically with the contemporary phenomenon of professional success. On one side, observers of industrial and prophets of postindustrial society point, usually with approval, to what they see as the rising importance of possessors of human capital and the declining importance of the industrial proletariat and the old capitalist elites.[7] On the other, critics of professional power look askance at what seems to them the excessive authority enjoyed by professionals, particularly members of the helping professions, whose work directly affects the well-being of individual clients.[8] Like many another debate on contemporary social issues, this one has helped shape historical research. It has also contributed a certain pungency to a number of recent studies in the field.

The marriage of the history of popular culture to the history of the professions has something to offer each partner. On the one hand, recent scholarship suggests that the radical separation of popular and elite culture between 1500 and 1800 has perhaps been overdrawn.[9] Our understanding of the problem may profit from considering another disjunction, the growing rift between layman and professional, consumer and specialized producer of services, in science, religion, or even (by the nineteenth century) the world of public entertainment, where more and more rigorously trained artists performed before increasingly passive audiences. The early modern campaign against popular error was led by two professional groups, the post-Tridentine clergy[10] and enlightened physicians; in their eyes, anyone who clung to traditional superstitions, whatever his social background, belonged to the people. This study attempts to sort out the various meanings of "popular" medical practice, from folk healing to charlatanism, and to understand them from the point of view both of the profession and of laymen from divergent social backgrounds.

In the history of the professions, on the other hand, a consideration of popular beliefs and behavior will take us beyond the sort of genealogical account that explores the past in search of the premodern antecedents of contemporary occupations. If we wish to see what medicine as an occupation looked like two hundred years ago, we must consider not only university-trained physicians but also authorized practitioners without university training and the great variety of unauthorized practitioners, from itinerant mountebanks and local empirics to village *maiges* (folk healers) and witches. They are important in their own right, for they provided most of the health care that preindustrial populations received; they are important, too, for our understanding of the development of the medical profession. Modern medicine did not arise in a vacuum; it established itself by denying legitimacy to competing medical practitioners and cultures. This project, then, examines the professionalization of French medicine from the bottom up.

The concept of "professionalization" requires a further word of explanation. The introduction to a standard collection of essays by sociologists defines professionalization as "the dynamic process whereby many occupations can be observed to change certain crucial characteristics in the direction of a 'profession.' "[11] What is a profession? Students of the sociology of the professions, who have labored mightily to determine exactly what a profession is, have never reached perfect agreement on the subject, beyond recognizing in common that professions involve the application of specialized intellectual skills. But most accept that the ideal type of the profession includes certain characteristics associated with the traditional liberal callings, such as a body of theory taught at institutions of higher learning; uniform standards for training and performance; a system of certification for qualified practitioners; and so on – though no two actual professions possess the same characteristics (and indeed, some sociologists have abandoned the effort to distinguish rigidly between professions and nonprofessions).[12] "Professionalization," then, denotes the acquisition by any occupation of the traits of the ideal type. In common usage, the term refers to the process (typically, the result of a deliberate strategy) by which a lower-status occupation, such as police work, takes on some of the attributes of the traditional liberal professions. Historians have also used the term to characterize the emergence of the same traits in the traditional professions that have come to serve as models for upwardly mobile occupations.

Like all process nouns ("modernization," "democratization," and so forth), "professionalization" carries teleological implications. The ideal type (constructed from the not entirely consistent features of a small number of present-day occupations) becomes the timeless model toward which certain other fields tend to evolve; by this ahistorical standard, probably no occupation before the last century would qualify as a profession at all. It might perhaps be preferable, then, for the historian to ask, not how an occupation "professionalizes," but how the conception and reality of professionalism have changed over time, or how they have varied from place to place.[13]

On balance, though, the convenience of "professionalization" as a shorthand description for a set of related changes in the medical occupation (or any other occupation) seems to outweigh the disadvantages. It need not be an anachronism. Although they did not use the term itself, the conception of professionalization would have been familiar to Frenchmen of the late eighteenth and early nineteenth centuries. (*Professionalisation* in French is a recent borrowing from Anglo-American sociology; *une profession*, then as now, could be any occupation, and *profession libérale* is the closest we can come to rendering the special, narrower meaning of "profession" in French.)

Eighteenth-century Frenchmen readily distinguished between a simple *métier* and a liberal profession. Athough their fundamental criteria – based on a hierarchy that ran from mere labor through the mechanical arts to the more intellectual and spiritual arts[14] – are not the same as ours, the idea of the profession shared by Enlightenment physicians stressed rigorous application of specialized learning in the interests of the public weal, and many of their proposals for reform in the medical field correspond to our own notions of professionalization. In this study, moreover, the term refers less to the ways in which eighteenth-century physicians came to resemble their twentieth-century counterparts than to the ways in which the profession achieved a clear identity and came to encompass the practice of medicine in its various forms.

The first sense of professionalization as used here is the reorganization or consolidation of practitioners in an occupational field (in this case, medicine) into a recognized and self-conscious profession. When the historian Toby Gelfand, for example, wrote of "professionalizing modern medicine," his subject was the coming together in eighteenth-century France of medicine (traditionally a liberal calling) and surgery (traditionally a mechanical art), which resulted, at the century's end, in a unified occupation with a standardized system of education.[15] At the same time that uniform standards make professionals more like each other, they make them less like people who perform similar types of work but do not meet the new standards: a sharper boundary is defined between professional and nonprofessional. In the case of medicine, the new profession excluded the lower-level surgeons who served the great majority of the French population; Gelfand has distinguished between professionals and what he calls "ordinary practitioners."[16]

A second, related meaning of professionalization follows from the first. A profession that has established a sharp boundary between its members and nonprofessional practitioners seeks to expand control over the practice of its occupation, simultaneously increasing the volume of services it provides and decreasing that of its rivals. Medicine is professionalized in this sense as nonphysicians cease to practice it. For the sociologist Magali Larson, professionalization is "the process by which producers of special services [seek] to constitute *and control* a market for their expertise."[17] One may dispute the notion that control over a nominally free market defines the profession. Eliot Freidson, for example, points to the case of medicine in the Soviet Union.[18] But a profession without a monopoly, or at least the pretense of a monopoly, is almost a contradiction in terms; and all the discussions of professional power that have appeared in recent years assume that the profession enjoys privileged access to some field of practice.

This book primarily addresses professionalization in the first sense, the organization of the occupation; professionalization in the second sense will be the subject of a future work.

In preparing this study, I have tried to draw on as wide a range as possible of both published and unpublished materials. The original sources include local, regional, and national government archives; the archives of medical faculties and societies; and manuscripts and printed ephemera from Parisian and provincial public libraries and libraries of medicine. Medical and law theses, the published work of physicians and jurists, and part of the voluminous general periodical literature of the day have been scoured for references to popular medicine and medical practitioners. Much of this material has not been used before; in other cases, I have taken previously exploited documentation and tried to present it in a new light. But this book is also a work of synthesis, and my debt to other scholars will be obvious throughout. I have made extensive use of older studies by practitioners of local history, *les érudits locaux*; though they are sometimes dismissed as antiquarians, their niggling positivism drove them to give extensive and faithful summaries or transcriptions of the documents, some of which subsequently succumbed to wartime destruction or to the other, less glamorous, mishaps that can befall old paper. For details on peasant beliefs and customs, I have relied heavily on the fieldwork of the pioneering ethnographers of the late nineteenth and early twentieth centuries, as well as the research of some of their epigoni. The use of these materials is fraught with difficulties, even for the study of contemporary France. Without them, however, it would be virtually impossible to construct a picture of the most obscure forms of popular practice. Finally, I have drawn freely on the work of the current generation of historians of France – above all Jacques Léonard, whose publications on the nineteenth-century medical profession have become an indispensable resource for anyone working in the field, but also Jean-Pierre Goubert (on provincial doctors and patients in the Old Regime), Toby Gelfand (on eighteenth-century surgeons); Caroline Hannaway (on the Société Royale de Médecine), and many others too numerous to mention here. The full extent of my debt will be apparent from the notes.

Integrating this material, particularly the disparate, scattered, and often fragmentary primary sources on irregular medical practice, raises special problems of method and presentation. For many observers, popular medicine hovered at the edge of the field of vision; it was viewed out of the corner of the eye, mentioned en passant. Few coherent bodies of documentation exist, and as a result, most of the evidence consists of isolated cases. I have given statistics where they can be found or compiled from the sources, but in the main I have had to rely on the more traditional and now unfashionable use of illustrative examples. In doing so, I have, of course, sought to support an argument about the relations between popular and official medicine. Above all, though, I have tried to convey something of the lives of mostly quite ordinary men and women, who inhabited a world that is now remote from ours and seems, at times, almost unimaginably strange. Where, as in a classic mountebank's harangue, *copia* may have become *luxuria*, I would ask the reader, in the words of a seventeenth-century writer who had long meditated on the sins of charlatans,

qu'il m'excuse en ceste digression, & qu'il pardonne à la curiosité du subiect; voire mesmes ie recognois que ce mestier des Ciarlatans est si attrayant & si babillard, qu'il s'attache mesme à moy . . . , me faisant cõme participant de son caquet & de son babil, c'est pourquoy i'appelleray à bon droit ceste digression discours babillard, non pas qu'il ne contienne verité, mais pource qu'il est plus curieux que necessaire.[19]

that he excuse me for this digression, and that he forgive me in view of the curiosity of the subject: indeed, I recognize that this charlatans' trade is so alluring and so garrulous, that it has even rubbed off on me . . . , making me as it were a participant in its chatter and its babbling; this is why, with good reason, I shall call this digression garrulous discourse – not that it does not contain the truth, but because it is more curious than necessary.

What will emerge, I hope, is not just an interpretation but also a sense of the extraordinary vitality and diversity of the premodern medical network.

The subject is a vast one, and I am aware of many omissions and limitations, some more deliberate than others. A few major topics have been deemphasized because they are the subjects of more specialized studies by other scholars – the work of Jacques Gélis on midwifery; Pierre Darmon's history of smallpox, variolation, and vaccination in France; or Yves-Marie Bercé's recent volume on the vaccination campaign of the early nineteenth century.[20] I did not use the vast and often poorly inventoried ecclesiastical archives, which could probably form the basis for another, very different, study; the records of pastoral visits are particularly rich in information on popular medical superstitions and may contain additional information on the medical profession as well.[21] Regional differences do not receive the prominence here that they deserve. Nor was it possible to give as much attention as I would have liked to the field in which this project began, the history of medical ideas and techniques. In recent years, the growth of the literature in the subdiscipline social history of medicine has provoked a sharp reaction from some medical historians who deplore what they see as a declining interest in the history of medical science, clinical practice, and the lives and work of the great physicians. The editor of one of the two leading American journals of medical history accused social historians of writing medical history without medicine, and the editor of the other leading journal complained in a wry but sometimes testy review article that social historians "simply find medicine, except as a social phenomenon, uninteresting and unimportant."[22] The debate over the competing claims of "internalist" and "externalist" approaches seems to have originated in what the French would call *une question mal posée*; ideally one would like to have both, for each can illuminate the other. But most of my material on the content of popular and official medicine, however interesting or important, will have to await a future study. Finally, I am acutely aware that this analysis of practice is not the work of a practitioner, and that all the information it contains derives from the revelatory but ultimately inadequate act of reading. I am not a physician; nor have I lived in rural France (as the historian Jean-Pierre Peter once suggested when this project was still taking shape) or even met a *guérisseur* (healer) face-to-face. (The illustrations in this volume are, at best, an inadequate compensation for the poverty of the written word.) No doubt readers will find other lacunae. But the social history of medicine is a rapidly expanding field, and in the next several years, new work can be expected to fill the gaps and modify or supplant the tentative generalizations offered here. If this book provides a useful point of departure, it will have fulfilled its purpose.

The quarrel of externalists and internalists points to a more general question about the audience for a study that crosses disciplinary lines. Much scholarly literature in the humanities and social sciences is written by and for specialists, and this book, which comes out of that tradition, visibly bears its imprint. But the topic seemed to me one that might attract readers from a variety of backgrounds with a serious interest in the professions, popular culture, French social history, or the history of medicine, and I opted in the end, despite the obvious difficulties, to try to write for all of them. Inevitably, specialists will find the treatment of parts of their own field oversimplified and misleading, and the treatment of some other topics overtechnical and obscure. But I have tried to make the whole accessible. Although a general background in French history and geography and some acquaintance with medical concepts and terminology would be helpful, it is not indispensable. Essential technical terms, especially archaic ones, have been explained, and French quotations in the text have been rendered into English or are accompanied by a translation – though it should be remembered that not all specialized terms and concepts have a precise English equivalent. (Unless otherwise indicated in the notes, all translations are by the author.) The reader may also wish to refer to the glossary of French terms on pages 387–89.

A study such as this also invites questions about the writer's point of view, for the subject of professionalization, particularly in medicine, has given rise to provocative and sometimes highly controversial interpretations. In their different idioms, Ivan Illich and the late Michel Foucault have questioned the pervasive influence of medicine in modern life. For Illich, medicine is one example, perhaps the best, of the dysfunctional and even self-destructive tendencies of technological society. We are falling prey, he suggests, to iatrogenesis, or doctor-caused disease, and to what he calls "social iatrogenesis," by which he means a loss of human autonomy resulting from dependence on the medical system. In response, he has proposed "a political programme aimed at the limitation of professional medicine."[23] Foucault, in his studies of psychiatry, medicine, and penology, has presented a more oblique but still penetrating indictment of "normalizing" forces in post-Enlightenment society. One reviewer called his approach a kind of Whig history in reverse, tracing how repression has developed pari passu with modern civilization and politics, from the first faint glimmerings in the Middle Ages to the fully realized disciplinary apparatus of the modern state.[24] And indeed, the new history of "medical power" does mirror the older celebratory histories of professionalization. If the latter tended to exalt the process through which a certified elite gained the right to apply technical solutions to human problems, the more recent writings have traced the growth of the coercive and repressive aspects of professionalism with unconcealed distaste. "There is a real danger," Eliot Freidson writes in his study of American medicine, "of a new tyranny which sincerely expresses itself in the language of humanitarianism and which imposes its own values on others for what it sees to be their own good."[25]

This project was begun in the midst of this debate over the limits of medicine and the excesses of medical power, not long before the publication of Illich's *Medical Nemesis* and Foucault's elevation to the Collège de France. In their writings, and even more in person, both Foucault and Illich were commanding presences; one could not escape their influence. Two images from student days linger with particular vividness. The first is of a smoke-filled and badly overcrowded amphitheater of the Collège de France. The dim light faintly glinting from his totally bald scalp, the master holds forth with incomparable rigor, wit, and eloquence; the disciples strain to listen, strain to understand, convinced that if only they pay close enough attention, all will fall into place – in the next line, the next quotation, or maybe the next lecture. At intervals there is a silence, punctuated by a ragged clacking noise as the disciples flip the cassettes on their portable tape recorders. The setting of the second scene is a dining room in Mather House at Harvard University. The guest, fiercely intelligent, seemingly as contemptuous of agreement as of disagreement, denounces the evils wrought by industrialization and the reign of the experts. Rousseau's mantle has fallen on his shoulders: civilization, he tells his increasingly uncomfortable listeners, has cost man his freedom. You have surrendered your health to the experts. You have surrendered the right to die. In this society, he concludes triumphantly, you do not even have the right to be stupid.

Yet it is the peculiar experience of anyone who has ever undertaken a long-term project, what the French call *un ouvrage de longue haleine*, that through some trick of relativity, as he nears his destination and looks back, he can no longer recognize his departure point as the place from which he began; its significance has altered with time. *Medical Nemesis* faded rather quickly from view. The work of Foucault, already established before his death as a French national treasure, promises to sustain a vast scholarly industry for years to come, but the initial blush of enthusiasm among practicing historians has given way to caution and an awareness of the radical differences that separate his enterprise from theirs. There is almost nothing of Illich in this study. There is something of Foucault; anyone who works on French medicine in the late eighteenth and early nineteenth centuries must try to come to terms with him and winds up, almost inevitably, appropriating some of his insights. But this is not the work of advocacy that it might possibly have been ten years ago.

Above all, this study is not an attack on the medical profession. Having lived off and on for some years with the eighteenth-century "enlightened physicians" (as they liked to call themselves) and their nineteenth-century successors, I have come to appreciate the genuine philanthropy of many of them and the basis for their claim to intellectual superiority. Although they took a lively interest in politics and hoped to exercise a moral influence over the community in which they lived, it is important to remember that the primary activity of their not particularly comfortable existence was caring for the sick. On the claim of medicine as a discipline, one can argue up hill and down dale over the relative efficacy of official and popular therapeutics in this period or the strengths and weaknesses of medical education; but it seems to me an error to suggest, as some historians have done, that "quacks" and the medical elite were simply interchangeable.[26] Knowledge of the human body and skill in diagnosis count for something, and the enlightened physicians at least cleared the armamentarium of much that was worthless in the old materia medica. As for the exercise of social control, the profession's actual influence over popular behavior was far more limited than the literature on medical power would imply.

Conversely, this book is not a defense of popular healers or a call for industrial societies to return to the natural ways of the preindustrial village. My personal preference, when seriously ill, would be to have the services of a competent and compassionate physician; to write an apologetic for unqualified practice would be disingenuous. What I do wish to argue is that the history of empirics deserves to be approached with the same imaginative sympathy that ethnographers have brought to their studies of folk healing in the field. The people we call "quacks" are somehow fundamentally *other*; they have been written about from the physician's or possibly the patient's point of view, but rarely from their own, as I have tried to do here.[27] This is not to say that empirics practiced good medicine; the following pages contain abundant evidence to the contrary. But to understand empiricism as an occupation, we must ask why people took it up and what they got out of it. To understand it as a cultural phenomenon, we must ask how it fulfilled its clients' needs and expectations. It is not enough to dismiss it as one more manifestation of human irrationality, or of the eternal commerce of knaves and fools.

Some words of explanation, finally, on the organization and major themes of this volume:

Part I deals with professional medicine, tracing the transition from what I call a "diffuse" medical network, which included a great many different sorts of practitioners, and whose boundaries were notoriously unclear, to a "tight" network, which consolidated the various certified practitioners into what was recognizably a single medical profession and in which qualified and unqualified practice were sharply distinguished. Chapter 1 outlines the situation prevailing in the Old Regime, when a patchwork of local corporations governed the three distinct orders of physicians, surgeons, and apothecaries, and numerous practitioners, particularly in the countryside, operated in the gray area between licit and illicit healing. Chapter 2 examines the reforms of the revolutionary and Napoleonic era and the experience of the first generations to live under the new medical regime of 1803. Henceforth candidates who had satisfied certain basic educational requirements would receive the license to practice; all others would not, whatever their skill, record of success, devotion to charity, or other personal qualities. Anyone who treated patients without a license was ipso facto guilty of illegal medical practice. Although the medical corps was still far from homogeneous – practitioners admitted under the Old Regime continued to work, and the new profession was divided into an elite (the doctors) and a lower tier (*officiers de santé*, or health officers) – it began to make sense to think of the continuing struggle with unauthorized practitioners as a contest between professional and popular medicine. This professional revolution, it will be argued, cannot be understood in isolation from the political history of the period; this aspect of the French experience carries important implications for theories of professionalization.

After considering the evolving structure of the old medical network as a whole, each of the first two chapters examines the emergent medical profession itself and some of the factors that helped or hindered what the French like to call the "medicalization" of society. They look first at professional institutions and at standards of practice in medicine and surgery, two indices of the profession's success in differentiating itself from the larger network of practitioners. A lack of effective national institutions and major variations in levels of training and competence (some practitioners were barely distinguishable from empirics) limited the medical men's ability to act as a coherent pressure group. The discussion turns next to the place of the profession in French society. Here the analysis takes two angles of approach. From the practitioner's point of view, it examines medicine as a career, considering the various avenues of entry into the profession and the social and economic status of its members. The difficulty of access to the higher reaches of official medicine, together with its marked social and economic stratification, continued to divide the profession and weaken it in its struggle with its popular rivals; but at the same time, the persisting economic insecurity of most medical men intensified their hostility toward unqualified practice and helped sustain the campaign against empiricism. From the patient's point of view, the discussion next considers professional medicine as a resource – the density and distribution of practitioners and the cost of their services, as well as popular attitudes toward the official personnel and their methods. Most Frenchmen were now physically within reach of a physician, surgeon, or health officer (though gaps remained in rural areas); but high fees and a lingering prejudice against the medical men continued to discourage patients from consulting them. The increased presence of licensed personnel in the countryside, in conjunction with limited professional opportunities, exacerbated the tensions between qualified and unqualified practitioners.

Part II develops a taxonomy of the great variety of irregular practitioners who served the French population. The approach is necessarily synchronic. Popular practice changed, but far more slowly than its official counterpart; to depict its evolution would require the equivalent, not of the motion picture, but of time-lapse photography. Chapter 3 is devoted to the itinerant irregulars, from classic mountebanks to the wandering peddlers and drifters who dabbled in remedy selling and medical practice. Traveling empirics reached areas that might not have been able to support a resident practitioner; they served as an economic link between the hinterland and the marketplace. The wandering life, moreover, set these practitioners apart from the local healer whose work depended on close ties to the surrounding community; and like all vagabonds, they attracted particularly close scrutiny from the police. Chapter 4 deals with the great variety of sedentary empirics: proprietors of secret remedies, bonesetters, *uromantes* (who purportedly divined the patient's illness by scanning his urine), religious and inspired healers, and the rest. Only a minority actually set themselves up as full-time physicians (the official personnel outnumbered them). But almost anyone could practice a little medicine or sell a few remedies; many occasional practitioners, most typically craftsmen, dabbled in the healing art to supplement an inadequate income from their regular trade. Chapter 5 turns to the shadowy world of *maiges* (folk healers) and witch-healers. In the ethnographic literature, the typical folk healer belongs to a village community;

relies not just on natural remedies derived from plants and animals but also on religious and magical practices and on his personal healing "gift"; and does not ask for fees. The witch–healer specializes in countersorcery, treating patients whose illness is attributed to evil spells. The surviving evidence for the late eighteenth and early nineteenth centuries suggests, however, that we may need to draw a less sharp distinction between so-called charlatanism and folk healing in this period; a surprising number of *maige*-like healers and counterwitches, for example, depended on their medical work as a source of income.

Throughout Part II, the interpretation emphasizes the social and economic position of the various practitioners. Most of the existing literature on quacks, healers, and witches has accentuated the picturesque at the expense of social analysis. (The literature on witchcraft is an important exception, but it has usually focused on accusations of black witchcraft rather than on the witch as healer.) Why did people become empirics, and what were their careers like? Why did quackery flourish in the early modern period? These and related questions have not received systematic consideration from historians.

Part III, finally, consists of a single chapter that brings together some of the major themes raised in the separate discussions of the different types of practitioners and seeks to develop a tentative social interpretation of medical practice. Doctors and healers did not inhabit two distinct universes; their territories overlapped, and the French medical network therefore needs to be considered as a whole. The discussion concentrates on two major themes: the complex relationship of the various practitioners to the marketplace, on the one hand, and to local communities and French society, on the other.

Though in principle the physician was somehow above, and the *maige* outside, the cash nexus, it is important, first of all, to consider medicine as an economic activity. Regulars and irregulars competed for a limited and relatively inelastic market for medical services. Some licensed personnel prospered, but only a restricted elite of physicians truly enjoyed financial security at a level appropriate to their station as they understood it; most medical men had to struggle. Similarly, although a minority of charlatans and remedy vendors reaped huge profits, empiricism barely supported – or failed to support – many less fortunate practitioners, including numerous women and a variety of marginals with no clear niche as peasants, craftsmen, or tradesmen. (By choice or by necessity, unauthorized practitioners stepped outside inherited roles in the traditional economy.) Medical practice, paradoxically, brought together the beneficiaries and the victims of economic change; the same forces that promoted the growth of the medical profession and enabled a handful of practitioners, qualified and unqualified, to grow wealthy made other Frenchmen and Frenchwomen increasingly insecure and drove some of them to medicine (among other activities) as a way of getting by.

Many medical practitioners endured not only economic uncertainty but also the psychological discomfort of the interloper or misfit. The city-trained physician who settled in the countryside characteristically remained a distrusted outsider (though many modest practitioners, often natives of the region in which they established their practice, resembled or came to resemble their peasant clientele). The case of irregular practitioners is more complex. Clearly, the practices of some healers depended on their integral membership in a village community; others, such as shepherds, tramps, and recognized eccentrics, lived on the margins of local society. All, however, found themselves increasingly isolated from the dominant national culture, branded as deviants by the physicians, the authorities, and the enlightened elites. Their delinquency in many cases extended beyond unauthorized practice of medicine. The reports of educated observers associated the world of popular medicine with petty criminality, alcoholism, prostitution, mental illness, and draft dodging (which the healers abetted) and other political offenses. Even allowing for exaggeration by unfriendly witnesses, the ranks of popular practitioners appear to have included a disproportionate number of what the authorities liked to call *mauvais sujets* (bad lots). Many had suffered cruelly from poverty and isolation; social and economic dislocation went hand in hand. Though they were typically portrayed (with some justice) as victimizers, closer examination suggests that they were often victims as well.

The chapter concludes with some broader observations on the social interpretation of medical practice. Though the distinction between learned and popular medicine is ancient and seemingly timeless, and although it is no doubt true, as the old literature on charlatanism insisted, that the quacks are always with us, the structure of medicine as an occupation is the product of specific social and economic conditions. A clearer sense of their influence would emerge from a comparison of the French experience with that of other Western or indeed non-Western societies. But any historical model must be dynamic. It was the growth of mercantile capitalism that made the early modern period in Europe the golden age of empiricism. Charlatans flourished in what we now perceive as a transition stage between an older agricultural society in which the medical market was virtually nonexistent and a late industrial society whose medical marketplace includes practically everyone. The ambitious physicians and administrators of the Enlightenment and the early nineteenth century had to confront this reality. The disjunction between their "modern" politics and ideology and the more traditional society they inhabited should warn against the temptation to treat the changes in the medical field as simply one manifestation of a global process of modernization; it is also what makes the relations between popular and professional medicine interesting as a historical problem.

PART I

Professional medicine

1

The regular medical network at the end of the Old Regime

"Every man is a physician" runs the old adage, meaning that everyone thinks he knows enough about health and disease to offer medical advice. Not everyone, of course, practiced medicine as a livelihood; and yet in the Old Regime it was difficult to say who was truly a medical professional, *un homme de l'art*. The occupation was so diverse and its characteristics so different from those that we take for granted today that any discussion of the field in the eighteenth century must begin by defining and explaining its subject.

It is a commonplace that the professions as we know them are a relatively recent phenomenon. In the case of medicine, the modern profession, with its extensive power and prestige, dates from barely a hundred years ago. Only in the last third of the nineteenth century (it is said) did physicians develop an adequate cognitive foundation for their work, evince technical superiority over their unqualified rivals, and begin to establish an effective monopoly over medical practice. Until then, they lacked a market for their services, and theirs was essentially a learned calling, not (in the words of the sociologist Eliot Freidson) "a consulting occupation of true professional status." The great bulk of the population relied on irregular practitioners. University-trained physicians did find patrons and clients among the nobility and the wealthy, but more because of their social standing than because of any claim to special expertise; in sickness, even the elites often turned elsewhere for medical attention.[1]

Accounts of the rise of professionalism characteristically look to the period before the later nineteenth century mainly to find the premodern antecedents of the contemporary professions, which they trace back to the three medieval faculties of theology, law, and medicine; they may mention in passing a separate group of ordinary practitioners who were not graduates (surgeons in medicine, solicitors or notaries in law), only to add that they had few of the attributes of a profession, and that they were so sharply distinguished from university-educated specialists that they practiced totally distinct occupations.[2] Work of this sort, though it has undoubtedly contributed to our understanding of the historical roots of the contemporary professions, does not provide a useful conceptual framework for talking about the medical world of two centuries ago. It is first of all ahistorical, using as its central model an ideal type derived from recent experience; too often, it lures the historian into the sterile theoretical debate over the characteristics of the "true" profession. It is also too narrow. The societies of early modern Europe, to be sure, identified medicine as a liberal profession and a learned calling, suitable for a gentleman, together with law, theology, and the liberal arts. But they also saw physicians as consultants – as one group, indeed, among a highly diverse body of recognized medical practitioners.[3] And even as an account of professionalization, the genealogical approach is incomplete. The contemporary profession did not descend in isolation from its early modern ancestors. It emerged from a transformation of the entire medical field, eliminating or denying legitimacy to a wide range of competitors. The context is an essential part of the story.

Rather than focus exclusively, then, on the premodern ancestry of the modern profession, this chapter adopts a looser descriptive category more consonant with the complex reality of the Old Regime: the regular medical network. By "regular practitioners," I mean those who enjoyed both social legitimacy and some form of legal sanction through statute, custom, or judicial decision; in other respects – training, methods, social and economic status, and occupational organization – they were highly heterogeneous. This broad classification into regulars and irregulars is obviously not the only possible one. Many contemporary observers would have drawn a different boundary line, between skilled physicians and master surgeons and the great mass of approved or tolerated practitioners, whose *impéritie* (incapacity) made them akin to charlatans and popular healers. Some historians of medicine have shared this concern with standards of training and levels of expertise, or have distinguished between practitioners of high social status, who treated the elites, and their more modest brethren, who shared a popular clientele with the quacks.[4] But the larger project of which this volume is a part deals with one crucial aspect of professionalization in medicine, the development and consolidation of a monopoly, and for that purpose it is most important to ask how the Old Regime distinguished between authorized and unauthorized practice.

THE TRADITIONAL STRUCTURE OF THE REGULAR NETWORK

The regular medical network of eighteenth-century France was characteristically diffuse: it included many different sorts of practitioners, and its boundaries, both internal and external, were notoriously unclear. Not only was the official medical field divided among the three main *corps* of physicians, surgeons, and apothecaries (in theory, collaborators; in practice, often rivals), but these *corps* were organized as municipal corporations, with purely local or regional monopolies, and were further subdivided into various grades, each with its own requirements for certification and its own special privileges. In addition, members of a distinct group of ancillary occupations, from midwives to herbalists, practiced special branches of surgery or the remedy trade, which often spilled over into the practice of medicine. Nor did belonging to one of these occupations suffice to distinguish between authorized and unauthorized practitioners. On the one hand, an official practitioner might be guilty of *empiétement* (encroachment) if he overstepped the boundaries of his occupation: technically, in such a case, he was practicing illegally. On the other hand, persons without formal training and certification might receive a special privilege, issued by authorities ranging from the Crown down to municipal officials and local nobles, to distribute a proprietary remedy or even to practice some branch of medicine or surgery. Such persons arguably practiced legally, though their rights were a subject of much dispute. What is more, the Old Regime tolerated and even encouraged the work of the clergy and charitable laymen who distributed remedies to the poor; indeed, the government relied on them to provide assistance during epidemics.

The three *corps*

France in the eighteenth century was legally a society of orders, of which the three medical *corps* formed an integral part, together with the corporations of the various urban crafts and trades.[5] Physicians were traditionally considered to form the apex of a health-care pyramid; theirs was a liberal profession, versed in medical theory and devoted to the practice of "internal" medicine. Subordinated to their oversight were the craft of surgery, one of the "mechanical arts," and the apothecary's trade. Surgeons concerned themselves with manual operations, which at this time were generally "external": bleeding, lancing, treating fractures and dislocations, and caring for wounds; they also applied topical remedies, mainly for skin diseases, and by tradition treated venereal disease. Apothecaries prepared and dispensed remedies, following the prescription of a physician or surgeon; they might also administer them (by giving a clyster, for example), but only under a physician's direction.

The actual structure of the medical network was not this simple, however; nor did it form a neat pyramid.

Physicians
Medicine itself was highly stratified.[6] Not all physicians possessed the same credentials or occupied the same rank. Under the legislation on

medical education and practice of 1707, known (after the royal chateau at which Louis XIV promulgated it) as the Edict of Marly, the minimum requirement for medical practice was the first postbaccalaureate degree, or *licence*, from a French medical faculty. *Licenciés* could legally practice in the countryside and in towns that lacked a medical corporation with a local monopoly; in the jurisdiction of the Faculty of Douai (where a doctorate required only an additional three-hour examination but cost substantially more), *licenciés* actually outnumbered doctors. Concentrations of them survived at the beginning of the nineteenth century in the Nord and the Pyrénées-Orientales.[7] Above the *licenciés* stood the doctors, who had received the highest degree in the field. A further distinction divided doctors into two basic categories. Outside Paris (which awarded only one type of doctorate) an elite trained as *internes* (residents) in order to become doctor-regents of the various faculties; only they could practice in a faculty's urban seat. The majority of students followed a less demanding and less expensive program as *externes* (nonresidents), which prepared them for careers as *docteurs forains* (literally, "outsiders") in the lesser towns. In Brittany, these "lesser" doctors (*docteurs de la petite manière*) made up 80 to 90 percent of physicians practicing at the end of the Old Regime.[8] The average medical man was hardly a learned mandarin.

All the grades of physician put together still accounted for only a small fraction of the medical practitioners in eighteenth-century France. In a cranky but often perceptive book on French "medical anarchy," the physician Jean-Emmanuel Gilibert (future anti-Jacobin mayor of Lyons), complained:

> The greater branch of practical medicine is in the hands of people born outside the precincts of the healing art; silly women, charitable ladies, charlatans, folk healers (*ma[i]ges*), bonesetters, hospital nurses, monks, nuns, druggists, herbalists, surgeons, apothecaries, treat many more illnesses, administer many more remedies, than physicians.[9]

Gilibert viewed all nonphysicians as a collective Antimedicine. Though his depiction of the range of practitioners was essentially accurate, lumping all of them together distorts the picture; above all, it misrepresents the special status of surgery.

Surgeons

That surgeons, who greatly outnumbered physicians, routinely practiced internal medicine was a widely accepted fact in the Old Regime. Their status as medical practitioners remained ambiguous, however, not only because of their traditional identity as members of a mechanical craft responsible for manual operations but also because of their long association with another manual trade, barbering.[10] (So strong was this association that in parts of the Basque region, surgeons' houses traditionally had names that were variants on "Barberaenea," meaning "at the barber's."[11] In Paris alone, a separate guild of master surgeons, known as the Community of Saint-Côme (after their patron, Saint Cosmas, a physician and martyr of the third century), had existed since the fourteenth century; in the sixteenth century their calling won recognition as a "science among the liberal arts," and the "college" of Saint-Côme, as it was now known, was reckoned among the "dependents" (*suppôts*) of the University of Paris, though not actually a part of it.[12] Even in Paris, however, most practitioners belonged to the much larger guild of barber-surgeons, officially subordinated to the Faculty of Medicine; the faculty, which taught its own students in Latin, provided instruction in French for the barber-surgeons. This corporation grew far more rapidly than the college, and its members (who included such distinguished surgeons as Ambroise Paré) came to practice as wide a range of surgery as their rivals "of the long gown." In 1655, bowing to economic pressures, the smaller guild merged with the larger and joined it in subordination to the Faculty of Medicine. This union of short and long gowns brought Paris surgery into conformity with the nearly universal practice of seventeenth-century Europe, as well as the French provinces; a similar merger had taken place in London in 1540, and only Italy boasted a significant distinct body of academically trained surgeons, in addition to a much larger number of barber-surgeons.

Not until the eighteenth century did Paris surgery truly emerge as a liberal profession, independent of, and largely equal to, medicine. By the end of the seventeenth century, a distinct surgical occupation existed in the capital. An edict of 1691 separated the surgeons from the guild of the barber-wigmakers/bath attendants, whose growth had received its impetus from the vogue of elaborate wigs that began in the reign of Louis XIII, and whose rights were confirmed in a royal declaration of 1673; the surgeons' statutes of 1699 held that masters who performed only surgery, without any barbering, would be considered practitioners of a liberal art. In 1743 another declaration definitively separated surgery from barbering in Paris. Henceforth all candidates for the mastership in surgery would have to know Latin and possess a master of arts degree; barbering would remain entirely in the hands of the barber-wigmakers. The surgeons' academic aspirations won recognition as well, with the establishment, in 1724, of public courses in surgery outside the Faculty of Medicine; the creation, in 1731, of a surgical society (which received letters patent as the Royal Academy of Surgery in 1748); and the transformation, in 1750, of the courses at the "amphitheater of Saint-Côme" into an official College of Surgery, independent of the University of Paris. Under royal patronage, the college emerged as the most vital center of medical instruction in the kingdom, and the surgical discipline, with its emphasis on hospital training and pathological anatomy, made a major contribution to the subsequent development of Paris clinical medicine.[13]

The development of surgery in the provinces lagged behind the capital. A royal declaration of 1717 ordered the complete separation of the barber-surgeons from the barber-wigmakers; the two guilds, however, continued to share the barbering trade. Surgery gradually emerged as a distinct profession. The legislation of 1730 on provincial surgeons provided that those who limited themselves to surgery would be recognized as practitioners of a liberal art; and in 1756 the Edict of Compiègne imposed this status on the highest level of master surgeons: in theory they were now required to hold a master of arts degree and to renounce barbering. In practice, though, many surgeons lacked the M.A., and only Lyons, Bordeaux, and a few other major cities actually barred surgeons from working as barbers.[14] Elsewhere, barbering remained an important source of income for many surgeons, particularly during the period before their official reception into the community of master surgeons. Conversely, some barber-wigmakers dabbled in surgery, despite the prohibitions contained in the seventeenth-century guild statutes. Well into the nineteenth century, particularly in the southwest and the German-speaking regions of the northeast, barbers commonly practiced phlebotomy and minor surgery.[15] The medical elite complained repeatedly about their activities.[16]

On top of this distinction between old-style barber-surgeons and the members of the new liberal profession, the provincial guilds imposed a legal gradation of titles similar to the hierarchy established by the provincial medical faculties. The legislation of 1730 recognized three ranks: surgeons who could practice in a city that possessed a surgical community; those who could work in other cities and towns only; and finally those who were restricted to small towns and villages.[17] At one extreme, the *internes*, or *chirurgiens du grand chef-d'oeuvre* (literally, "surgeons of the major masterpiece" – a series of examinations) pursued a course of training comparable in rigor and cost to that of the physicians and wound up practicing the most exacting branches of their art, attempting serious operations as well as minor external procedures. At the other extreme, the *chirurgiens de petite expérience* received only the most rudimentary practical training; a single three-hour test (the *petite expérience*, or minor examination) gave them the right to "set up shop and hang out a sign," as their letters of reception characteristically put it. Often they were the only medical practitioners of any sort in their district. In addition to practicing medicine and performing minor surgery, they typically sold remedies (despite a decree of 1749 that prohibited surgeons from either prescribing or selling internal remedies); only a minority had been officially received by a guild of apothecaries. With rare exceptions, they possessed only a smattering of medical knowledge, and remained essentially village tradesmen and artisans.[18]

Any description of the surgeons, finally, has to take into account those practitioners who lacked a recognized place in the corporate structure. Surgeons of the army, navy, and merchant marine did not necessarily have the right to practice "civil" surgery, though in fact they often did so in garrison and port towns; many were younger practitioners preparing for later reception into the guilds.[19] In addition, some fully qualified practitioners had not bothered to seek official reception or could not afford it. Their ranks also included surgical students (an elastic term) and other half-trained practitioners, who worked in cities and towns (including Paris) as *chambrelans* (the general term for artisans who were not guild members) and throughout the countryside. As Toby Gelfand has argued, some practitioners whom the medical elite castigated as charlatans were in fact marginal surgeons.[20]

Experts

On the outskirts of official surgery worked the various surgical specialists, or "experts," as they were generally called. Specialization is a relatively recent phenomenon in modern medicine; in Paris, as late as 1845, all but about 12 percent of physicians were still general practitioners. It is common, however, among primitive peoples, and it flourished in the ancient world – in Egypt, for example, where medical practitioners devoted themselves to treating diseases of the eye, teeth, head, intestines, or "those which are invisible." This tradition continued in Western folk medicine, and it also survived on the fringes of the medical network of the Old Regime. These experts were not, however, specialists in the contemporary sense, practitioners who limit themselves to a single branch of medicine after completing the usual general training. They belonged, rather, to distinct occupations, with no extensive shared fund of theory; they were essentially artisans who applied highly developed mechanical skills to certain delicate operations. Before the eighteenth century, when the surgical profession began to coopt the various specialties, conventional wisdom held that procedures such as couching cataracts were best left to itinerant operators who did little else. The fourteenth-century physician Guy de Chauliac, for example, whose major text on surgery was translated from Latin into French in 1592, made this recommendation for ocular surgery; so, in the seventeenth century, did Lazare Rivière, professor of medicine at Montpellier, at least for cases in which "a cataract cannot be dissolved by any medicine."[21]

Though usually treated as a category sui generis, midwives constituted the largest group of surgical experts; like the others, they never had a guild of their own and were subject to the oversight of the surgical communities. The surgeons examined and licensed midwives. They shared responsibility for certification with the Church, which was supposed to attest to their good character. It was the midwife's duty to help ensure that the infant was baptized and that neither the afterbirth nor the cadavers of stillborn infants were used for witchcraft or illicit magical practices.

In principle, midwives were divided into the same three classes as provincial surgeons. Those in the highest rank might have received training at a level roughly comparable to that of a country surgeon, but they constituted a small minority of active practitioners. Through the celebrated efforts of the master midwife (*maîtresse-sage-femme*) Angélique-Marguerite Le Boursier Du Coudray, who traveled throughout most of the French provinces in the 1760's and 1770's, using a mannequin to demonstrate the various presentations of the fetus, a knowledge of obstetrics became more widely diffused. In practice, though, the fully qualified *sage-femme* remained a rarity, particularly outside the northern and northeastern parts of the kingdom. Women who wished to be delivered by a skilled practitioner increasingly turned (at least in northern France) to a male surgeon–accoucheur (obstetrician), and the vast majority of babies still came into the world with the help only of *matrones* devoid of formal training. Until the Napoleonic era, midwifery remained an essentially uncertified occupation.[22]

The term "expert" was more generally applied to a wide range of other practitioners, including dentists, "oculists" (ocular surgeons), herniotomists, lithotomists, bonesetters, and even corn surgeons. Many were itinerants, since they could not hope to find enough clients in a single town or expect patients to travel long distances to reach them. (For related reasons, the same individual sometimes combined two or more specialties: Pierre Guilleminot, for example, announced himself as a hernia surgeon and dentist at Troyes in 1797.)[23] Many such traveling operators were indistinguishable from the general run of empirics. But the surgical guild statutes of 1699 and 1730 did expressly provide for officially licensed experts, who would not join the regular corps of master surgeons but would be examined and approved by them. In Paris all the surgical specialists came under the nominal jurisdiction of the King's First Surgeon; a 1776 directory listed 6 oculists, 14 hernia surgeons, and 36 dentists in the capital. The king himself appointed royal experts; in 1787 the royal household had 5 bonesetters, 2 oculists, 2 dentists (one in reversion), 1 chiropodist, and 2 surgeons for stones trained in different techniques.[24] (One of the bonesetters, Dumont Valdajou, was a former cobbler from Le Val-d'Ajol in Lorraine, a village whose inhabitants were celebrated for their skill in treating fractures and sprains; this enterprising empiric had won the title not only of bonesetter to the royal army and to Monsieur, the king's brother, but also of "demonstrator in the city of Paris." He received an annual pension of 6,000 livres in return for treating indigent patients and maintaining six students to whom he taught his art.)[25] In the provinces, the local surgical guilds oversaw the experts' work. At Orléans, for example, truss maker/rupture surgeons were examined and allowed to practice on payment of a fee of 45 livres. At Bordeaux, special operators could treat cataracts, stones, and hernias, but only in the presence of two *agrégés* (regularly admitted members) of the medical *corps* and the lieutenant of the King's First Surgeon.[26] An exceptional situation existed at Lunéville in Lorraine; its special institute for lithotomy, established by Duke Leopold in 1715, continued to function after the province's permanent union to France in 1766.[27]

The medical authorities tried as best they could to distinguish authorized special practitioners from charlatans: they were not to advertise or put on public displays to attract crowds. In spite of these restrictions, the expert's practice could be quite lucrative: one operator is said to have treated eighty-two patients at Bordeaux in the space of three and a half months and to have earned more than 12,000 livres. Some practitioners also drew salaries from the local government; thus in 1770 the town of Grenoble paid a certain Dachino, a Neapolitan ocular surgeon, for operating on the poor.[28]

The most fully developed specialty was ocular surgery, whose status was recognized in 1765 with the creation of a chair at the College of Saint-Côme in Paris; licensed oculists were thereafter master surgeons.[29] Practice in this field was never completely regularized, however, especially in the provinces. Paul Delaunay has sketched its history for one district, the region around Le Mans, in the eighteenth century.[30] The only resident oculist was a certain Bizieux of Montdoubleau; the surgeon Levasseur of Le Mans also operated on cataracts. But a series of itinerant practitioners, some of them foreign, also visited the region; they ranged from established specialists to full-blown mountebanks. Louis Béranger, who had been certified at Saint-Côme, passed through in 1749 and 1751. The lieutenant general of police allowed one oculist/empiric a six-week stay in 1733, and another enjoyed three months of toleration in 1764. Some of these practitioners boasted of lofty connections in France and abroad – a practice widespread among, though not limited to, itinerant charlatans. The chevalier de Tadiny, active in Le Mans in 1754, called himself a count palatine and oculist of the duc d'Orléans, first prince of the blood. (Almost three decades later, Tadiny, who had now been settled in Nantes for eight years, wrote to the Société Royale de Médecine to criticize a visiting charlatan and to defend himself against charges of being an empiric; he still maintained that the duc d'Orléans had given him the right to treat everyone in his appanage, adding that he had operated in the presence of the comte de Vergennes, then minister of foreign affairs, when he had been France's ambassador to the Porte in Constantinople.)[31] In 1785 the surgeons of Le Mans wrote a certificate for the Councillor von Hilmer, "pensioned oculist of the court of Vienna in Austria, and consulting oculist of His Prussian Majesty." And a certain Gleize, when he visited in 1786, called himself the oculist of the comte d'Artois (the brother of Louis XVI) and the duc d'Orléans – a title he may have abandoned by the time of his next trip to Le Mans, which came in the Year IX of the French Republic (1800–1801). A more obvious quack was Mahé de Maisonneux, who styled himself "a physician who consults urines and a sur-geon-oculist." The physicians, surgeons, and apothecaries of Le Mans had him served with a writ in 1754.

Herniotomists had a more dubious reputation than oculists. Many em-ployed a technique involving castration (they closed the inguinal ring to provide a support for the herniated intestine, severing the spermatic cord in the process). According to local authorities and physicians, the operation was often unnecessary; some suggested, even into the nineteenth century, that such widespread sterilization might depopulate the country.[32] In 1776, the bishop of Saint-Papoul in Languedoc protested that operators had per-formed this procedure on some 500 children in his diocese, after removing the trusses that he had distributed to them.[33] Other *herniaires*, however, relied on trusses themselves, like a certain Le Brun, who in 1785 advertised in the local gazette of Le Mans, the *Affiches du Mans*, that he could "provide every appropriate means for [treating] ruptures in the two sexes."[34]

Of all the experts, though, bonesetters (who were called "*bailleuls*," "*re-noueurs*," "*rebouteurs*," and "*rhabilleurs*," among other terms) probably aroused the greatest unease among the medical elites. They were the most numerous, and their occupation crossed the blurred boundaries between official and popular medicine to an extent unusual even in the Old Regime. Bonesetters included, at one end of the spectrum, the licentiates of the surgical guilds and, at the other, folk practitioners with a healing "gift." (Although bonesetting was clearly a mechanical art, like the other specialties, in popular practice it was widely associated with the use of magic healing rituals.) Moreover, lack of formal qualifications did not necessarily preclude official authorization: at Bray-sur-Seine, for example, a shepherd was said to have been received as a *rebouteur* in 1767.[35]

Legally authorized bonesetters practiced in Paris under the provisions of a 1634 statute that subjected them to the lowest level of examination, *la petite expérience*.[36] Outside the royal household they had no special guild or official status; in the provinces, like the other experts, they came under the jurisdiction of the local surgeons' companies, which imposed their own requirements. At Orléans, for example, aspirants had to present certificates of experience, good character, and fidelity to the Roman Catholic religion; upon passing an examination on fractures and sprains, they paid 150 livres for the right to practice.[37] Many practitioners, though, simply enjoyed local toleration. Training was highly empirical, skills typically passing down from father to son. Several families became celebrated for their work, no-tably the Fleurot clan of Le Val-d'Ajol in the Vosges mountains.[38] According to an account from the late eighteenth century, male children were trained in osteology from an early age. At first they were allowed to play with isolated human bones to learn how to unite them; then they received a skeleton and mannequins to manipulate before being allowed to practice on live patients. At La Vallouise in Dauphiné, in the 1760's, a master bone-setter named Morand had a diploma stating that his ancestors had practiced for two centuries; another eighteenth-century Morand was said to have cured the king of Sardinia at the royal court in Turin. This family sustained the tradition into the twentieth century.[39]

In some towns of Old Regime France, bonesetting and related surgical procedures were performed as a customary sideline by another group of semihereditary skilled operators, the executioners. The public hangman enjoyed a sort of sinister charisma, and his medical functions included selling parts of the cadavers of his victims for use in healing (and doubtless in black magic as well). He also had a reputation as the local authority on human anatomy. His traditional duties included torturing suspects and dismembering the bodies of convicted criminals (the French word for executioner, *bourreau,* is sometimes said to derive from the verb *bourrer,* to maltreat); it was widely assumed that he could mend the same parts that he knew how to break.[40]

Some executioners set themselves up as full-fledged surgical operators. A few practiced illegally every branch of medicine, surgery, and pharmacy; one such practitioner at Nîmes, according to a physician's report of 1787, even succeeded in being relieved of his duties as hangman after some fifteen to twenty years of service.[41] At Le Mans, the executioner took the honorable title of *bourgeois de la ville et chirurgien restaurateur, "restaurateur"* being a more elegant synonym of *"rebouteur."*[42] And at Lille the executioner Pierre Forez treated fractures and sprains with great success, despite a challenge from local surgeons in 1768; he also earned a good income from the sale of hanged men's grease. In 1781 he went so far as to petition for an increase in his regular salary to reflect his surgical practice.[43] Despite the executioners' obvious encroachment on the surgeons' domain, the legal issue was never fully resolved in the Old Regime, and for much of the eighteenth century the courts tended to sustain the executioners' customary rights.[44]

The familiar types of surgical specialists were joined here and there by a variety of more exotic specialized practitioners whose work was recognized in local custom. The barony of Saint-Michel-en-l'Herm, for example, had (at least through the end of the seventeenth century) a "sworn bather," whose important duty it was to wash with sea water, in accordance with traditional belief, "all persons and all sorts of animals bitten by dogs, or other rabid or corrupted animals."[45] In the eighteenth century, bathkeepers (*baigneurs-étuvistes*) offered therapeutic baths (one thinks of Jean-Paul Marat in his tub), not as a sideline to surgery or barbering but as a separate occupation.

The work of both the experts and the master surgeons suffered encroachment from another order of artisans, the craftsmen who made and sold the apparatus used in surgery; though in principle they were not supposed to prescribe or apply it, some did, and their ventures into the surgical domain were widely tolerated. *Tabletiers*, or workers in ivory and inlaid ware, had the right to make false teeth. Since hernia trusses were usually covered with chamois, the right to produce them went to the pursemakers (appropriately called *boursiers* in French: *"bourse"* means purse, but *"bourses"* also means scrotum); they met with competition from blacksmiths, locksmiths, and cutlers.[46] In some cases, truss makers won recognition as a separate craft. Thus Jean Gautier, *bandagiste*, received an authorization from the mayor of Nantes in 1790 to make and sell trusses, though with the stipulation that he perform no surgical operations. He carried a certificate from the lieutenant of the King's First Surgeon at Orléans, where, according to his account, he had practiced for thirty-five years. When he met with opposition from the provost (*prévôt*, the surgeons' equivalent of the guild officers known in the other trades as *jurés*), he protested that his profession was a free calling, not subject to guild regulation.[47]

Despite this long tradition of pluralism, the status of experts was already in question by the end of the Old Regime. Difficult operations had passed into the hands of the surgical elite, who saw the old-style operators as little better than quacks. When the health committee of the Constituent Assembly carried out a national survey of surgery in 1790–1791, the great majority of surgical communities (all but 16 of 106 surviving replies) reported that they refused to receive experts. The reasons were at least partly economic. It is significant that eleven of the sixteen were among the larger communities. Presumably a resident expert could find a sufficient clientele only in a population center; and in the smaller communities, as some of the reports made clear, the regular surgeons believed that they could ill afford to give up a part of their practice to a specialist.[48]

Apothecaries

Just as the surgeons had long shared a guild with the barbers, the apothecary's trade had traditionally been associated with that of the spicers (*épiciers*). At the same time, like the surgeons, the apothecaries constituted one of the three medical *corps* and were legally subordinated to the physicians. The candidate for the mastership had to undergo an apprenticeship and submit a *chef-d'oeuvre* (as in other guilds); but he also had to pass an examination supervised by physicians. Like the goldsmiths and printers, the apothecaries were dropped from the purely mechanical trades in 1759 and hence escaped the provisions of the edict issued by Turgot as controller-general in February 1776, which abolished the trade guilds (*corporations de métiers*). In 1777, when the guilds were restored following the disgrace of Turgot, a special declaration established pharmacy as a liberal profession in the capital, separating the Paris apothecaries from the spicers and transforming their company into a College of Pharmacy.[49] In some of the larger provincial towns, too, pharmacy emerged as a distinct profession, complete with regular courses of instruction (though not actual colleges of pharmacy). The Academy of Dijon, for example, began in the 1770's to offer public courses on botany, chemistry, and materia medica; a local apothecary, Jacques Tartelin, the only apothecary member of the academy, served as demonstrator in botany from 1780 to 1793, and then again from 1798 until his death in 1822. After 1782 aspiring apothecaries were required to spend two years attending the courses in botany and chemistry.[50] Elsewhere, apothecaries normally combined pharmacy with the spice trade and the wholesale trade in drugs, la droguerie; only after the Revolution did these occupations definitively separate.

Professionally ambitious pharmacists clung jealously to distinctions and marks of rank – the use of Latin, for example, which set them apart from the simple grocer; when in 1789 the pharmacists of Angers drew up their cahier de doléances (list of grievances) for the meeting of the Estates-General, they asked that physicians be required to write their prescriptions in that language.[51] The terms for guild membership placed other obstacles in the way of the upwardly mobile; the statutes of one corporation, for example, stipulated that no child might be accepted as an apprentice "who comes from people who are of base origin, or in mechanical trades, or dishonored [notés d'infamie], and who is not at least a good grammarian."[52]

In theory, physicians were to prescribe and apothecaries to dispense. (Surgeons had the right both to prescribe and to sell remedies for external conditions and venereal disease. Where there was no apothecary, physicians were supposed to supply internal remedies, though in their absence surgeons might be allowed to do so. Where there was no physician, an apothecary might give advice and prescribe simple remedies, but only "in case of necessity.")[53] In actuality, nonphysician general practitioners were commonplace. In the seventeenth century apothecaries routinely worked as surgeons, especially in the smaller towns. By the eighteenth century, though, the surgeon-apothecaries outnumbered the apothecary-surgeons – in part because the guild structure was less well developed in pharmacy than in surgery, and where no community existed it was a "free" profession. Even in places with established apothecaries, surgeons sometimes doubled as pharmacists; at Mamers in Haut-Maine, for example, in the latter eighteenth century, the surgeon François Besnard du Buisson sold remedies at a droguerie-épicerie.[54] In small rural bourgs and villages, the surgeon largely displaced the apothecary. (The French experience here diverged from that of Britain, where apothecaries increasingly practiced medicine and surgery, all the while striving to affirm and raise the status of their original profession. After 1815 all general practitioners in England and Wales who wished to dispense were required to be licentiates of the Society of Apothecaries; the Royal College of Surgeons enjoyed no comparable monopoly.)[55] The total number of French apothecaries diminished; in many parts of the countryside they had all but disappeared by the end of the eighteenth century, leaving the distribution of remedies in the hands of hospital sisters, convent nurses, curés, and charitable persons, despite an article in the declaration on pharmacy of 1777 that restricted the religious foundations to dispensaries for internal use.[56] It is possible, as one historian of pharmacy has suggested, that their decline contributed to the widespread use of both proprietary and domestic remedies in the last decades of the Old Regime.[57]

Even at their acme, though, apothecaries never enjoyed a full monopoly in the Old Regime. As one of them complained in a doggerel quatrain,

> Est ainsy que chascun s'empresse
> A faire le pharmacien,
> Le marchand, le praticien,
> Et tous les fols y font la presse.[58]
>
> [Thus it is that everyone is eager
> To play the pharmacist,
> The tradesman, the practitioner,
> And all the fools flock round.]

In the guild towns themselves, other merchants sold remedies and the basic ingredients for making them, sometimes offering medical advice to their customers: druggists, herbalists, distillers, vinegar merchants, beverage vendors (*limonadiers*), confectioners, wax and tallow chandlers, and the rest.[59] Druggists, like the nonapothecary spicer-grocers (with whom they often combined, after the fashion of the barber-wigmakers), were entitled to sell certain remedies in bulk, though not in doses. Herbalists sold medicinal plants, as a few still do in France, although (according to the major eighteenth-century work on medical jurisprudence) "chemistry [having] so prevailed over Galenical [pharmacy], the herbalists are so forgotten that they are so to speak unregulated."[60] Various other members of the loose medical network encroached on pharmacy as well. Touraine, for example, boasted a dynasty of executioner-apothecaries. In Paris, the widow of the royal oculist Daviel sold a green water for weak and tired eyes, a white water for inflammation of the eyes, and a pommade for sores, pimples, and gum on the eyelids.[61] Virtually anyone might sell drugs as a sideline to some more regular trade, and outside the jurisdiction of the guilds they usually went unchallenged; part-time apothecaries included old-clothes dealers, bookbinders, and wigmakers, among many others. And the sale of secret remedies, although it theoretically required official approval of the remedy, was open to all.

Recasting the old corporate order

The tripartite division of the medical field was never fully realized in France, and by the last decade of the Old Regime it was visibly breaking down.

Not only did surgeons (and some physicians) sell remedies; the medical and surgical worlds also converged, well before their official union in the legislation of 1794 on medical education. Though it was rare for physicians to take a second qualification in surgery, a growing number learned surgical techniques. (One indication of their interest is the appearance, after mid-century, of lawsuits in which surgeons charged physicians with encroachment; in Artois, legislation adopted in 1757 expressly barred physicians from performing surgery.) Conversely, surgeons studied medicine and took second degrees as *docteurs forains*. Even the joint education of physicians and surgeons was adumbrated at Montpellier, where the medical faculty, after receiving a special bequest in 1737 from Pierre Chirac (an alumnus who had become the King's First Physician), offered a program leading to a doctorate in medicine and surgery. Following a slow start (only six graduates by 1760), Montpellier awarded more than 600 such doctorates between 1760 and 1794. In Grenoble, too, a "practical school of surgery" offered joint instruction, starting in 1771, to students who wished to combine the two fields.[62]

By the end of the Old Regime, many observers would no longer have divided official medical practitioners into the legally recognized *corps*. They thought instead in terms of two roughly defined orders. The higher comprised physicians (with the possible exception of those who held only degrees from the less reputable provincial universities), together with the first order of master surgeons; the lower included essentially the country surgeons. As Toby Gelfand has stressed, the latter might best be characterized as "ordinary practitioners." But this reorganization constituted only the first step toward unification. The relation of ordinary practitioners to the medical elite was not that of general practitioner to consultant, as it developed a century later in Britain. Even within surgery the two groups were so widely divergent in training and outlook that it may be preferable to treat them as separate occupations, rather than subcategories of a unified profession.[63]

The great penumbra: authorized empirics, charitable persons, and the clergy

Perhaps the strangest feature of the old medical network, to a twentieth-century observer, is that it extended so far into the murky regions beyond the three *corps* and their associated guilds. Either because of gaps in the legislation or because royal edicts were simply ignored at the local level, the regular medical occupations fell far short of establishing a complete de jure monopoly in their fields. In medicine, as in other domains, the Old Regime system of privilege (literally, private law: a right or immunity for an individual) continued to flourish.

Privilege in the medical domain took two basic forms. Certain regular practitioners – notably the royal physicians and surgeons, together with military surgeons – were entitled to practice outside the guild system by virtue of their appointments. Except in the lower ranks of the military surgeons, these practitioners were ordinarily fully qualified personnel – indeed, under the law, they had to be to receive a royal appointment.[64] But special "permissions" were also issued to empirics, despite a provision in the Edict of Marly that revoked all existing permissions (including those from the Crown) and barred local authorities from granting new ones. In theory, after Louis XV's regulations on surgery were registered in the sovereign courts (1752), such authorizations did not suffice to let the un-qualified perform surgical operations; this restriction, however, was widely disregarded.[65] For obvious reasons, the guilds themselves did not normally receive or issue warrants to empirics, though some practitioners described as "charlatans" (possibly half-trained surgeons) were said to have been admitted as country surgeons. At Rosières in Lorraine, "letters of limited toleration" were accorded to two nonreceived surgeons, one of them a former aide to a military surgeon.[66] The lieutenant of the community of Montmorillon in Poitou was accused of selling a mastership to the operator Edin, who was on the list of empirics proscribed by the Société Royale de Médecine, and at Montdidier in Picardy, which boasted three received bone-setters, the lieutenant was said to have received a "dangerous charlatan" in 1761; one respondent to the Comité de Salubrité's investigation of surgery in 1790–1791 complained that a trade in privileges existed in his district.[67] More typically, permissions and letters of toleration came from government officials, ranging from the Royal First Physician to provincial governors and commanders down to municipal magistrates and lieutenants of police; nobles exercising seigneurial justice also issued permissions.

Local authorizations sometimes took the form of regular appointments – an imitation, on a more modest scale, of the medical offices of the royal household. At Obensheim in Alsace, according to a 1779 report from a correspondent of the Société Royale de Médecine, not only was unautho-rized practice tolerated on noble lands "out of mercenary interest," but a noble lord had even named the executioner titular physician of his domain.[68] Municipalities sometimes made similar arrangements with empirics, usually for more specialized services; they enjoyed less independence, however, than a powerful seigneur, who could usually do as he pleased on his own estate. When in 1770 the council of Olette in Haut-Conflent proposed to pay a 24-livre annual subscription for the services of Jean Salvador of Thuir, called a *saludador* (a term usually applied to a mystic healer who used in-sufflation, or blowing on a wound, to treat rabies), the *viguier*, or regional administrator, rejected the request and the provincial intendant supported him, leaving the healer in a doubtful legal position.[69]

Among the tolerated and authorized empirics, one group deserves special mention. In many parts of France, practitioners of veterinary medicine customarily treated some human patients, especially victims of the bite of a rabid animal. The treatment of animals traditionally belonged to the farriers' guilds, but they met with competition from other occupational groups, notably the *affranchisseurs*, or gelders, who frequently practiced human medicine as well. In Poitou, the population was said to prefer to turn to veterinarians and *mégéyeurs* (a regional term for gelders, possibly related to *"mége,"* or healer) for the treatment of skin disorders.[70] In Maine, the *affranchisseur* of Saint-Cosme-de-Vair advertised in the *Almanach ou calendrier du Maine* for 1786 a "sovereign remedy for rabies." A more ambitious gelder asked the intendant at Tours in 1787 not only to allow him to practice medicine but also to compensate him for the assistance and remedies that he had given to the poor. The intendant instructed his subdelegate that it was necessary to belong to the local surgical community in order to practice, but that the petitioner's capitation tax might be reduced – a form of de facto recognition.[71] Something of this view of the veterinarian influenced the planning of the first regular schools of veterinary medicine in France; one was created at Lyons in 1762 and another at Alfort, outside Paris, in 1766, with support from Henri-Léonard-Jean-Baptiste Bertin (controller-general 1759–1763) and then from Turgot. Bertin hoped to see the veterinarians provide rudimentary human medical care in the countryside and advocated training them in midwifery and bonesetting; official veterinarians would in effect have become lower-level surgeons.[72]

Local authorities also granted merely temporary authorizations to passing itinerants. Some were traveling surgeons and special operators outside the control of the regular guilds.[73] More typically they were remedy vendors, often agents (or so they claimed) for a major distributor of proprietary remedies; perhaps the best known such entrepreneur, toward the end of the Old Regime, was Charles Dionis, a doctor-regent of the Paris medical faculty who had a warrant to sell one of the most famous concoctions of the old polypharmacy, orvietan.[74] A series of enactments, starting in 1728, held that such remedies had to be officially approved; vendors routinely cited approbations from the Crown or a medical corporation, among other possible sources. Not all such claims were true, but in fact the two men who held the post of First Physician in the middle decades of the century, François Chicoyneau, who succeeded Pierre Chirac in 1732, and Jean-Baptiste Sénac, the incumbent from 1752 to 1770, issued warrants quite liberally.[75] Local permission for actually distributing the remedies might be obtained from nobles, mayors, magistrates, and lieutenants of police, as well as from medical faculties and colleges.[76] The larger towns had a set procedure for according such approbations, which generally required the local physicians and apothecaries to inspect the vendors' wares. With the proper papers, approval was usually routine. Consider one case, which passed through the machinery of medical police at Angers in one day, 16 April 1776. An itinerant empiric submitted to the lieutenant of police a petition that began:

Annibal Rubini humbly entreats and informs you that he has obtained from sieur Dionis, doctor-regent of Paris, a warrant dated 2 September 1774, for a period of three years, which permits him to sell the antidote known as orvietan, in the form of butters, or powder, or liquid. The petitioner lived three months in the town of Le Mans, selling his drugs; according to the certificate which he has received from the mayor and municipal magistrates of that town . . . , he behaved there with all integrity.

Rubini asked permission to construct a theater in the marketplace and to stay at Angers for six months selling his orvietan. The lieutenant of police referred his petition to the royal procureur; he in turn transmitted it to the dean of the medical faculty, who verified Rubini's certificates and then examined and approved the drug itself. Rubini had only to appear before the mayor and municipal magistrates to obtain permission to erect a theater; the petition was sealed and approved at a cost of 35 sols.[77]

In theory such permissions restricted the beneficiary to the sale of a specifically approved remedy. It was common knowledge, however, that once a vendor had erected a stage in the marketplace, he hawked other medicines and frequently gave medical advice as well; customers, after all, came in search of a treatment for a particular ailment, rather than a preparation that had already been prescribed for them. Some remedy peddlers admitted that they were in fact more than traveling salesmen; Morel Delisle, for example, when he appeared in 1777 at Châtellerault in Poitou with a commission from Dionis, asked permission to sell *and administer* drugs in the forms of powder, syrup, balm, and liquid.[78] The medical corporations argued, justifiably, that such vendors were in fact being authorized to practice medicine.

The legal status of the authorized empiric nevertheless remained ambiguous; though he might fill his wallet with approbations and attestations, he could expect setbacks along his way. The oculist Hilmer, for example, who received local permission to work at Le Mans in 1785, had been prohibited from practicing at Bordeaux in 1780, despite two certificates from Nancy, one bearing the signatures (possibly forged?) of the lieutenant of the First Surgeon and other officials, and another from a professor at the Royal College of Surgery in Nancy. And in 1794 an oculist named Hilmer – presumably the same man – appeared on a list of charlatans at Troyes.[79] The line between regular and irregular was easily crossed.

In addition to authorized empirics, for whom medicine was a livelihood, the penumbra of the old medical network included a great variety of amateur practitioners for whom medicine was a public service sanctioned by tradition and even recognized in some cases by the local authorities. Often a *châtelain* or landed proprietor, like Montaigne in his rural domain, ministered to his dependents and neighbors.[80] In the eighteenth century, a noble living at Bussy-lès-Poix in Picardy, François-Joseph Leclerc, chevalier de Bussy (1681–1754), recorded in his journal how he had visited his tenant farmer, who was desperately ill and had just received the last rites. Bussy administered remedies and recommended that the patient be kept very warm.[81] Some chateaus maintained actual pharmacies, and many *châtelains* had specifics handed down in the family. Milon, lord of Le Breuil-Mangot in Poitou, had a miraculous tisane for victims of gout and rheumatism. Near Brioude in Auvergne, a seigneur who possessed a remedy against rabies took in patients, fed them, and treated them. According to local tradition, when he emigrated during the Revolution he passed on the secret to a family in the environs.[82] The more ambitious seigneurs' medical activities sometimes extended beyond the circle of their immediate dependents, as in the case of Perrochel, an eighteenth-century lord of the manor of Granchamp in Maine, who treated patients sent to him by the curés.[83] A noble or other major landowner could further extend his influence by employing servants to practice in his name. In 1782, during an outbreak of disease around Fougères in Brittany, the valet of the comte de Mué bled patients and gave remedies; they called him "the King's physician, sent from Paris for the epidemics."[84]

Every region also had its share of "charitable ladies" who cared for the sick poor. "Passing through certain cantons [of Auvergne, in the last years of the Old Regime]," one traveler noted, "I heard named with gratitude several respectable women, who, devoting themselves to the relief of the suffering poor, in their town or their country houses, worked hard at a few details of rustic medicine, treated wounds, distributed and administered certain ordinary remedies themselves, and won the gratitude not only of the peasants of their commune, but also of those in the neighborhood."[85]

The medical field in the eighteenth century also attracted well-intentioned laymen, drawn equally by Enlightenment notions of beneficence and by the growing prestige of amateur science, who saw themselves as inventors of novel therapies, with which they hoped to assuage the ills of suffering humanity. They bombarded the academies, parlements, intendants (and anyone else who they thought or hoped might listen) with suggestions for miraculous remedies and procedures, which they rarely hesitated to administer or apply themselves. Like the mercenary empirics, they urged that successful experience counted more than professional training. One amateur sent a remedy to the Estates of Brittany in 1774, after reading a published account of an epidemic disease marked by headache and fever:

Although I have [not even a] smattering of medicine and surgery, I am taking the liberty of sending you the remed[ies] I have made for headache and fever. Their effectiveness makes me bold enough to suggest it, although it may be that no one will believe in them, because neither one of them is expensive.[86]

These activities were widely tolerated, so long as the remedies were not noxious and were distributed gratis. As all the charlatans well knew, a little philanthropy went a long way toward legitimating a practitioner's work, though by the end of the Old Regime this argument was beginning to lose its force, at the same time that the academies began to close ranks against the intrusions of amateurs.[87]

Though the tradition of charitable medicine persisted until recent times, compensating during much of the nineteenth century for the inadequacies of social welfare legislation, the Old Regime system of public assistance much more clearly sanctioned the direct intervention of charitable persons in the medical sphere. During epidemics, they were often charged with distributing the boxes of "royal remedies" (*remèdes du roi*) that the provincial intendants received from Paris for emergency use in epidemics.[88] Some received compensation for their expenses or even quasi-official local appointments. When, for example, in 1742, the inhabitants of Tiercé in Anjou founded a school, they expected that "the schoolmistress will know how to treat the sick, and [how to practice] a little pharmacy to assist the poor. [This work will require] bleeding and medicines only . . . , the parishioners and other charitable persons furnishing her with what will be necessary to prepare these medications and make the balms."[89] Others benefitted from special approbations that allowed them to continue their work unmolested; under Louis XV, for example, the controller-general Bertin gave royal protection to a woman from Le Havre who treated the injuries of the poor with ointments and a cataplasm.[90]

Behind many of these activities lay the idea of a Christian vocation to minister to the sick poor, which the eighteenth-century notion of rational and secular *bienfaisance* (beneficence) coordinated by the government had not entirely displaced, particularly among the charitable ladies. Madame Fouquet (Marie de Maupeou, d. 1681, wife of a seventeenth-century controller-general and mother of the more famous superintendent of finance) remained the model; in the late seventeenth and eighteenth centuries, her handbook of charitable medicine became the most popular work of its kind.[91] The pious work of the charitable healer was a form of imitation of Christ and in some cases an exercise in self-mortification; as one of the manuals for charitable healers noted, the poor "smell bad," but the reader was to endure the stink for the love of God.[92] Numerous examples of devotional medical care can be found down to the Revolution and beyond, as in the parish of Saint-Barthélemy in Anjou, where a woman known locally as "*la dévote*" cared for the sick each Sunday.[93]

The religious orders and parish clergy performed a similar function on a much larger scale.[94] The "Grey Nuns" (Franciscan hospital sisters) were among those charged with distributing the *remèdes du roi* during epidemics. Most religious foundations had dispensaries, often the best local source of routine medical care in a district. A physician at Saint-Brieuc in Brittany noted in 1779 that it was

unnecessary to send a physician to Plévin, because among the Sisters of Charity in that parish, there are some women who are well educated and who are in the habit of caring for the sick daily, [and] even of prescribing remedies in ordinary cases. In difficult cases, we continue to give our advice, as in the past.["95]

Some local statutes also tolerated the surgical activities of the Brothers of Charity. Although the surgeons in 1724 won royal letters patent against the brothers of the Paris Charité hospital, and although the 1730 statutes on provincial surgery included ecclesiastics in their prohibition of unauthorized practice, a declaration of 1761 allowed the monks to practice surgery in their hospitals throughout the kingdom "in case of necessity."[96] (The Edict of Marly, however, specifically barred religious from practicing medicine.) One of the most celebrated of eighteenth-century lithotomists, Jean Baseilhac (1703–1781), known by his religious name as Frère Côme, belonged to the Paris monastery of the Feuillants. In some places the brothers went further – in Lorraine, for example, where the Edict of Marly (which antedated the duchy's union to France) did not apply. In 1750 Duke Stanislas Leszczyński signed a contract with the religious of Saint John of God to care for the victims of epidemics; following an outbreak of disease, a monk would be dispatched to the scene to provide bouillons and other assistance paid for out of a special fund established in 1748 for victims of epidemics, hail, and fire. The order also maintained a small hospital in Nancy, treated sick inmates of the local prison (using remedies paid for by the Bureau of Charity), and gave medical advice to the poor of Nancy.[97]

Even more pervasive than the monks, the secular parish priests occupied a central position in local public assistance; it was their responsibility to notify the intendant's subdelegate of epidemics, and they played a major role in distributing the *remèdes du roi*. In Burgundy, for example, in 1783, they accounted for 40 boxes out of 73; the contents of another 20 were distributed by private charitable persons, 9 by physicians, 1 by a surgeon, and 1 by a Sister of Charity.[98] Their work was very widely accepted, though the idea of actually training priest-doctors, as Johann Peter Frank proposed in Austria, seems not to have taken hold in France. (Some suggestions of this sort can, however, be found in the papers of the Société Royale de Médecine,[99] and one physician of the Nancy Medical Faculty half seriously recommended that the Brothers of Charity study medicine, since they already practiced it – though he clearly would have preferred to use available

funds to pay stipends to qualified physicians and surgeons, on the model
of the German *Physikus*, or public health physician.)[100]

Not all the medical activities of ecclesiastics and religious foundations
could be classified as strictly charitable, and the more mercenary they became, the less likely they were to continue to enjoy official toleration or
approbation; protracted lawsuits pitted medical against religious corporations. Hospitals sold remedies at a profit to outside customers, in theory
to raise money for the poor. Religious foundations advertised secret remedies, like the True Ointment of the Abbey of Le Bec in Normandy, "generally suitable for the cure of all sorts of wounds."[101] Members of the lower
clergy with modest livings, who sometimes resorted to farming to supplement their incomes, could turn to medicine as well; their numbers swelled
following the Revolution's anticlerical campaigns.[102] Rural surgeons and
sometimes even physicians protested that local ecclesiastics were robbing
them of their paying clientele; in 1786, for example, the physicians of Troyes
complained of the activities of the curé of nearby Montaulin, which extended
beyond his parish.[103] In 1790, according to the lieutenant of the King's First
Surgeon at Mende (Lozère), local practitioners included "curés, their assistants [*vicaires*], and often their domestics, who enrich themselves at the
expense of their patients."[104] Indeed, ecclesiastics could be found among
most categories of popular practitioners. The curé of a parish near Châtellerault in Poitou, who in 1777 was reported to distribute balms for the cure
of cancer, resembled many an empiric; so did a certain Desjardins, known
as Brother Alexis, a Capuchin at Nantes who had specialties against cancer
and venereal disease.[105] Others, who practiced magical healing or exorcism,
were locally regarded as a sort of *maige*, or folk healer. The First Estate,
then, so various in so many other ways, straddled the line between regular
and irregular medical practice.

This overview of the structure of the old medical network has suggested
both the great variety of regular practitioners and the difficulty of identifying
a precise criterion for distinguishing between official and unauthorized practitioners. In the eighteenth century, though, professionals – *les hommes de
l'art* – were clearly establishing their place as trained consultants at the center
of the network. The remainder of this chapter will focus on the emergent
profession and its position in the society of the Old Regime.

PROFESSIONAL INSTITUTIONS

The organization of the medical occupations in France followed two divergent lines of development. The first, as has been seen, was corporative:
local practitioners in the larger towns formed guilds and guild-like bodies
known collectively as *agrégations*. Although they had official statutes and

were subject to state supervision, they were essentially private institutions whose chief function was to further the interests of their members. The second, which might be called bureaucratic, derived from the state: the network of royal offices, together with the royal societies and academies, which (although they were technically privileged bodies like the professional corporations) performed certain functions for the government and reported directly to its ministers.[106]

In a handful of cases, the three principal medical occupations belonged to a single corporation. In Grenoble, the physicians, surgeons, and apothecaries formed a "medical *corps*" in 1614 and promulgated regulations "that must be followed by each one separately in his vocation, and by all unanimously, making up only one mystical body [like the Trinity]." The marquisat de Sévérac adopted a similar arrangement in 1694.[107] In general, though, the professions organized into three distinct bodies, whose respective rights, obligations, and boundaries were defined by statute. State institutions also respected these divisions, with the notable exception of the mixed commissions that examined secret remedies for the half century between 1728 and 1778, when the Société Royale de Médecine assumed this function (over the protests of the surgeons and apothecaries).[108]

Medicine

The medical profession at the end of the Old Regime was organized into some three dozen urban corporations: nineteen faculties of medicine (by most counts) and fifteen colleges of medicine. Despite what their names might suggest, the faculties and colleges were essentially *agrégations* whose most important function was usually to control professional privileges within their jurisdiction. The colleges offered only limited instruction and could not award degrees. As for the faculties, although they all had the power to confer higher degrees, fewer than half actively provided instruction on a regular basis: Paris, Montpellier, Toulouse, Besançon, Perpignan, Caen, Reims, Strasbourg, and Nancy. At some, instruction existed only in theory or was interrupted by periods of inactivity: Orange, Valence, Bourges, Poitiers, Nantes, Dôle. Not all doctor-regents of a faculty actually taught medicine. At Paris, and in the provinces at Angers, Bourges, Nantes, Poitiers, and Toulouse, the professors were drawn on a rotating basis from among the doctor-regents. At Montpellier and elsewhere, special professors were chosen through competitions – "*à la dispute*"; at Nancy, the professors, once named by the dukes of Lorraine, were selected through what was supposed to be an international search. But whatever the arrangements for providing instruction, the body of doctor-regents formed a single privileged and exclusive corporation.[109]

In a few cases, faculty and college coexisted in the same town – at Bordeaux, for example, where even professors of the medical faculty were required to be *agrégés* of the college in order to practice,[110] and at Nancy following the translation of the faculty from Pont-à-Mousson in 1768. The college of Nancy continued to promote free consultations with the poor, maintain order in the health field, and execute the laws against quacks – in addition to providing its own instruction in anatomy, botany, and chemistry (subjects frequently better represented at the colleges than at the faculties). Such arrangements sometimes confused even well-informed contemporaries. When Félix Vicq d'Azyr, permanent secretary of the Société Royale de Médecine, began to establish affiliations with provincial medical institutions, he erroneously assumed that his agreement with the College of Medicine of Nancy automatically included the faculty. The latter reminded him that the two bodies were separate; that it had existed almost two hundred years before the college; and that it had no intention of sharing its privileges.[111]

In principle a diploma from Paris or Montpellier (or Avignon, according to an edict of 1656) conferred the right to practice everywhere – *urbi et orbi* (in the town and in the world) and *hic et ubique terrarum* (here and everywhere on earth), in the words of the consecrated formulas. Where a corporation existed, however, it was normally necessary to become an *agrégé* in order to practice in the town and its suburbs; only physicians to the royal family were exempt from this rule. In the case of the faculties, *internes* who successfully completed the requirements for the doctorate were eligible, after paying some additional fees and observing certain formalities, to become doctor-regents. Graduates of other faculties had at least to pay a substantial fee and were often required to pass a new examination. The Edict of Marly established as a minimum a four-hour public examination (waived for practitioners who already had ten years' experience) and a fee of 150 livres; but it also empowered faculties and colleges that imposed higher standards to continue to do so. Nantes, for example, charged 2,000 livres and required five examinations over three to four years. Some faculties strongly resisted attempts by outsiders to gain admission, even when they met the legally prescribed conditions for *agrégation*. Moreover, in the case of Flanders, Artois, Hainaut, Tournésis, and Cambrésis, the edict specifically limited practice to graduates of the faculties of Douai, Paris, and Montpellier; at the same time, graduates of Douai were not to practice elsewhere.[112]

It would be a mistake to think of the corporations as forming a neat checkerboard covering the entire kingdom. True, some claimed to control medical practice throughout an entire province (though apart from the jurisdiction of Douai, the Edict of Marly required of physicians who wished to practice outside towns with an *agrégation* merely that they present their credentials and register with the authorities). Local physicians might chal-

lenge outsiders in court, as happened, for example, at the very end of the
Old Regime to three graduates of Nancy who wished to practice in relatively
small towns in Normandy, Burgundy, and the Nivernais.[113] But the question of corporate monopolies remained a controversial one, and in the
extensive litigation that it produced, at least some interlopers won their
cases, even in corporate seats. A nonregent with powerful protectors could
be hard to displace. In the 1770's, for example, Angers had a nonregent
physician protected by Monsieur, the king's brother, who resided there as
prince of the appanage of Anjou.[114] Some corporations, moreover, such as
the Faculty of Nancy, seem to have devoted more energy to promoting the
right of their graduates to practice throughout the kingdom than to defending their own privileges, and many accepted that their powers did not
extend beyond their urban seat. Such concessions, combined with the wide
dispersal of the urban corporations across the territory of the kingdom,
obviously left huge gaps; in Brittany, for example, only the Faculty of
Nantes and the College of Rennes strictly excluded outsiders.[115] It is difficult
to generalize about the situations in the different regions, but one point is
clear: nothing remotely resembling a national professional organization existed, or was even conceivable, in Old Regime medicine.

Royal institutions did not fill this lacuna, for the Crown's direct intervention in the field of medical practice remained quite limited. It is significant that the 1707 Edict of Marly, the only national legislation on medical
(as opposed to surgical and pharmaceutical) education and practice before
the Revolution, specifically affirmed the prior rights of the corporations.
The local *corps* had an ambiguous and sometimes tenuous relationship with
the Crown, which did not even technically administer all of them. True,
the king named the instructors at the majority of provincial faculties (they
were known as "royal professors"). The Crown maintained a special relationship with the faculty (or "university," as it styled itself) of medicine
at Montpellier, whose graduates, since the sixteenth century, had furnished
most of the King's First Physicians. Here the position of chancellor (an
official who, by the early seventeenth century, overshadowed the dean, the
senior active professor) became a royal appointment in 1664. But the Chancellor of France had to share jurisdiction over the faculties with the provincial
parlements, and some municipal oversight persisted: in Bordeaux, for example, questions involving the college of physicians – though not the faculty
– were referred to the jurats of the town.[116] No general mechanism existed
for coordinating the work of the corporations or even enforcing the standards imposed on all the faculties by the Edict of Marly.

A royal medical academy might have supplied the need for an institution
to oversee medicine throughout the kingdom, but corporate rivalries stood
in the way of any such project. Louis XIV's reign saw the creation of a
Chambre Royale de Médecine, inspired by Antoine d'Aquin, who was

named First Physician in 1667 and personally supervised the king's medical care from 1671 to 1693. Its only real purpose, however, was to allow graduates of provincial faculties (mainly Montpellier) to practice in the capital without being doctor-regents of the Paris faculty. The chamber, moreover, led a precarious existence and survived for only a little more than two decades; in the end, pressure from the faculty prevailed, and a royal order abolished it in 1694. In 1730, Pierre Chirac, the First Physician and a Montpellier graduate, again attempted to form a medical academy, whose members would be allowed to practice in Paris like the royal physicians; but this initiative collapsed with Chirac's death in 1732.[117] The Paris faculty, quite apart from the infringement on its local monopoly of medical practice, objected to the creation of an independent academy, for its doctor-regents saw themselves as the senior advisers to the Crown in matters medical. It was only in 1778, with the formal establishment of the Société Royale de Médecine, that France was endowed with a national medical body; and even then its charter restricted its principal activities to two domains, the study of epidemics and the regulation of secret remedies and mineral waters, leaving jurisdiction over professional issues in the hands of the corporations.[118]

Nor did the system of medical offices provide France with a significant medical bureaucracy. The First Physician licensed secret remedies and mineral waters during much of the eighteenth century, but he had no jurisdiction over the profession itself; Chirac as First Physician hoped to be elevated to the position of *chef de la médecine*, with powers to inspect and regulate the colleges and faculties, but this plan, like his project for a medical academy, ended in failure.[119] The provincial medical functionaries had similarly limited powers. The post of *conseiller-médecin-ordinaire-du-Roi-aux-rapports* (royal councillor and physician in ordinary for [expert] reports), created by an edict of 1692, was intended, in the words of a later commentator, "to correct and prevent all abuses which creep into the practice of medicine and surgery in the provinces."[120] Some royal physicians indeed entertained a grandiose notion of their position as "the only representative of the three *corps* of medicine, surgery, and pharmacy."[121] In practice, though, their function was soon reduced to that of forensic experts, with responsibility for conducting exhumations and testifying in legal cases. One important local exception to this pattern occurred in Roussillon, where the place of the *médecin du roi* was taken by a Spanish-style *protomédich* (from the Spanish *protomédico*, or royal physician, formerly named by the King of Spain), who enjoyed considerably greater powers. Significantly, though, this post was reserved after 1759 for the dean of the Medical Faculty of Perpignan.[122] French medicine lacked the sort of professional bureaucracy that could be found in many parts of Germany, Italy, and Switzerland.[123]

Surgery

As in medicine, surgical organization took the form of an uneven patchwork of local institutions; although the great majority were governed by the general statutes of 1730, Paris and the larger provincial towns had their own statutes, and each guild (*communauté*) had its own usages and traditions.[124] The nearly 400 surgical communities greatly outnumbered the medical corporations; whereas faculties and medical colleges existed only in major urban centers, the communities proliferated far more widely, subject only to the legal restriction that they be located in a town with a parlement or one of several other royal courts: a *chambre des comptes* (concerned with royal finances), *cour des aides* (tax court), *bailliage* or *sénéchaussée* (district courts that heard civil and criminal cases), or in an episcopal or archepiscopal seat. They varied enormously in the size of their jurisdiction and membership. The community of Seurre in Burgundy, for example, embraced the town and 9 neighboring villages, with a total of 5 surgeons; at the other extreme, the community of Moulins in the Bourbonnais encompassed 400 parishes or towns, with about 140 surgeons. Nearly half of the communities were in towns with populations under 4,000.[125] Some communities had so few masters that they barely constituted an organization. Where they existed, however, it was necessary to be admitted by them in order to practice legally in their jurisdiction (except for surgeons with Paris diplomas, who theoretically had the right to practice throughout the kingdom), and it was the duty of the community's provost, in the words of the statutes of Rennes, "[to] prosecute with care and justice empirics and all others who practice surgery without qualification."[126] Even in bourgs and villages without a community, it was still necessary, under the legislation of 1730, to be received as a master in order to practice.

Under the leadership of the King's First Surgeon, the communities came to form a centrally supervised network that brought surgery far closer than medicine to a national professional organization. Until the seventeenth century, the First Surgeon was simply a member of the king's household; it was the First Barber who headed the communities of barber-surgeons. In 1668, however, the First Surgeon purchased these rights, by order of the Royal Council; in legal terms, his position was now comparable to that of other royal officers (for bread and wine, for example) who oversaw the crafts and trades in France. In the eighteenth century, he further consolidated his authority over the profession; an edict of 1723 revived the old office of lieutenant of the First Surgeon in the provinces, replacing the post of sworn royal surgeon established, together with that of royal physician, in 1692. The masters of each community were to nominate three candidates for the lieutenancy, from among whom the First Surgeon would appoint one to serve for life.[127] The lieutenant would examine new members, help exclude the unqualified, prosecute unauthorized practitioners, and, in general, uphold the surgical statutes and regulations. In the words of one Breton community of surgeons, he was to be an "Argus," spying out impostors and repressing abuses in the surgical field.[128]

The authority of the First Surgeon and his lieutenants thus helped unite the surgical profession in the greater part of France. As could be expected in the Old Regime, however, certain outlying provinces and districts claimed exemption from his jurisdiction through traditional privilege: Artois, Roussillon, Alsace, Dombes, Lorraine and Bar, Franche-Comté, the Comtat Venaissin. In Roussillon, where, it will be recalled, the medical occupations were organized on the Spanish model, the surgeons of Perpignan answered only to the municipal consuls, and the surgeons outside the town precincts came under the jurisdiction of the provincial *protomédich*. When the edict of 1723 authorized the First Surgeon to name lieutenants, the surgeons and wigmakers vehemently opposed it; after the First Surgeon finally named a lieutenant in 1776 and asked him to examine candidates in the countryside, a great protest arose. In the end, a compromise allowed the *protomédich* to retain his functions, with the stipulation that he would have to conduct examinations in the lieutenant's presence.[129]

Perhaps the clearest symbol of the First Surgeon's influence was the Académie Royale de Chirurgie, which was his creature rather than the Paris community's. The masters of Saint-Côme had to content themselves with associate membership; the First Surgeon directly named the forty "counsellors," or active members.[130] Several decades later, fear of a comparable loss of status drove the Paris Medical Faculty to oppose the Société Royale de Médecine, which enjoyed government patronage and over which the First Physician nominally presided.[131]

Pharmacy

The apothecaries, finally, were the most loosely organized of the three *corps*. Their companies (later "colleges") were purely municipal corporations, though they sometimes included more than one town, and they left many apothecaries unorganized. In theory the First Physician had jurisdiction over districts that lacked a guild; in the 1660's, Antoine Vallot (First Physician from 1652 to 1671) had even hoped to group isolated apothecaries into a network of regional *jurandes* (guild masterships) organized by castellanies, provostries, and viscounties, but the project came to nothing.[132] Government supervision operated at the local level; in their capacity as tradesmen, the apothecaries were subject to the oversight of the municipal consuls until an edict of 1740 gave them their autonomy. Since the end of the seventeenth century, it is true, they had also come under the jurisdiction of the various lieutenants-general of police, who in theory represented the royal government. When the Crown in 1777 transformed the old apothecaries' company in the capital into a College of Pharmacy, the Paris lieutenant-general of police, the state councillor Jean-Charles-Pierre Lenoir, guided it with a firm hand; in a sense his influence extended beyond the capital, for the college had the right to receive provincial as well as Parisian masters, for towns that lacked a community of apothecaries or a college of medicine.[133] But this sort of administrative tutelage was a far cry from a national organization.

MEDICAL AND SURGICAL PRACTICE

It is sometimes said that, although official certification and some measure of professional organization set the medical men apart from their unauthorized rivals, as practitioners the two groups were largely comparable until well into the nineteenth century. The learned profession, according to this view, was distinguished only by its knowledge of the traditional Latin medical corpus and its proficiency in *disputationes*; it could not claim superior clinical competence, which its highly conservative training failed to provide. As for the lower-level practitioners, though they might through experience accumulate some practical skill, the bleeding, purging, and occasional minor surgical procedures that they performed were well within the capabilities of the average empiric. In any case, official medicine had only a few effective drugs in its armamentarium: cinchona for malaria, ipecac for dysentery, and perhaps one or two more. Otherwise, in the face of life-threatening disease, physician and empiric found themselves equally helpless.[134]

Because such a view may color our interpretation of professionalization, suggesting that the physicians' stance toward popular medicine derived solely from self-interest and class prejudice, the problem needs to be considered briefly here. (This is not, however, the place to take up the vexing question of the objective efficacy of therapeutics in the eighteenth and early nineteenth centuries: whether medicine, apart from public health measures, significantly influenced mortality – highly unlikely – or brought relief to substantial numbers of patients – almost certainly true, thanks to symptomatic remedies and the placebo effect.)[135] The history of French medical and surgical practice largely remains to be written, but enough work has been done to correct some of the stereotypes of pre-Pasteurian medicine. Among the medical elite, though not among all ordinary practitioners, training, technique, and a code of behavior did help define a professional community; the resemblance between some medical men and the empirics is less striking than the disparities between some medical men and others.

Training and competence

We have inherited from the luminaries of the Paris clinical school their disdain for the education provided at the old French faculties. Despite a section in the Edict of Marly intended to standardize and strengthen the medical curriculum, these institutions emphasized rote learning from classical texts and offered only limited instruction in a number of subjects, such as anatomy, that would now be considered fundamental. Clinical teaching had a small place in the curriculum; at Paris it was limited to, though not required of, *licenciés* preparing the doctorate. The unfriendly assessment of the old program by the physician, chemist, and statesman Antoine-François de Fourcroy (1755–1809) has often been cited: "the only foundations were introductory courses laden with sterile definitions. The physical and exact sciences, the only basis for solid instruction, were disregarded."[136] Some universities, moreover, were lax in awarding the title of *docteur forain*. A few were openly venal; the most notorious was the faculty of Orange, from which (according to one lieutenant of the First Surgeon) certain quacks, "on payment of the modest sum of 60 livres, are graduated in one day as physicians or surgeons."[137] Not surprisingly, the medical elite attacked the qualifications and methods of the average practitioner.[138] When François-Emmanuel Fodéré, the pioneer of French legal medicine, visited the Alpes-Maritimes in the early nineteenth century with a commission from the Minister of the Interior to conduct a statistical survey of the department, he found that most medical men relied almost exclusively on the old Hippocratic standbys of bleeding, purging, and strict diet, and that their methods were scarcely more sophisticated than those of the shepherds in the local mountains.[139]

Similar charges and worse were leveled against the deficient standards of training and reception in surgery. One correspondent suggested that the surgical corporations of the large towns would grant privileges to any applicant who paid the fee and presented certificates of apprenticeship.[140] In 1756, the Intendant of Brittany, Le Bret, complained of untrained practitioners received by surgeons who were themselves unfit to conduct an adequate examination; he could count only three or four surgeons at Rennes, one or two at Nantes, and a handful in the smaller towns who could rise above pure mechanical routine.[141] Criticisms of lower-level surgeons filled the responses that the lieutenants of the First Surgeon drew up for the 1790 survey of surgery; according to the lieutenant at Saint-Gaudens, for example, most surgeons in his district knew only how to shave and bleed.[142] Physicians told of patients killed by surgeons and apothecaries.[143] Each could recount a horror story, like the case of a surgeon near Sedan who in 1775 tried to remove a dead fetus in pieces and, having failed, attempted to perform a cesarean section with a razor, killing the mother.[144]

No wonder, then, that Jean-Gabriel Gallot, the physician from Poitou and future deputy to the Constituent Assembly, called the ineptitude of ignorant surgeons (and midwives) the greatest scourge of the countryside after charlatanism.[145]

The suggestion that most routinely licensed practitioners were in fact unqualified – and therefore threatened the lives of citizens and the interests of the state – was common enough to appear among the grievances in the *cahiers de doléances* of 1789. The College of Surgeons of Rouen, for example, denounced ignorant practitioners in its corporate *cahier*.[146] This is perhaps unsurprising, but similar complaints, evidently drawn up by laymen, appeared in the *cahiers* at the parish level: ignorant practitioners, who in a few months have learned to shave, bleed, and make up bad remedies, do more damage than "all the artillery of the most numerous army" (Cloyes, bailliage de Blois); they are nothing more than "patented assassins" (Courson, bailliage d'Auxerre).[147] A *cahier* from La Roë in the region of Angers singled out rural surgeons as a "destructive scourge" (a cliché of the medical reform literature), all the more pernicious because it afflicted those who did not have the means to summon "educated physicians." All told, 8 out of 177 surviving parish *cahiers* in the *sénéchausée* of Angers attacked the incompetence of country surgeons, and one (Vihiers) specifically asked for greater rigor in admissions.[148]

It is important to remember, though, the distinction between a highly trained elite of physicians and first-order surgeons and the less well-trained mass of practitioners. Serious medical students supplemented the admittedly limited faculty curriculum by taking courses elsewhere on such subjects as anatomy and materia medica (in Paris, at the Collège Royal, where Latin was the language of instruction, and at the Jardin du Roi, where lectures on botany, chemistry, and anatomy were given in French); by seeking out private instruction in fields like obstetrics; and by accompanying the attending physicians on their rounds at the hospitals and hospices. Many in fact received what by the standards of the day was a solid grounding in their subject. The regular graduates of the Paris College of Surgery were also well trained.[149] And even at the lowest level of the hierarchy, some country surgeons, although largely ignorant of medical theory, may have been less bound to mindless routine than the stereotyped portrait would suggest; one study of the records of a country surgeon who worked outside Angoulême, at the end of the eighteenth century and during the first decade of the nineteenth, shows that he used some hundred remedies and that he was willing to introduce new ones.[150] In the light of present medical knowledge, one could no doubt argue that the intervention of even the best-trained practitioner rarely benefitted the patient (beyond providing supportive care) if he used ineffective or potentially dangerous therapies such as bleeding and purging, and that in this respect the physician and the quack were interchangeable. But such an argument would be ahistorical and even unfair. The best medical practice, unlike that of empirics, was grounded in an excellent grasp of anatomy and an improving understanding of physiology and pharmacology; and it reflected the accumulated clinical experience of European medicine, disseminated not only in courses but also in the burgeoning medical periodical literature. The highly qualified physician was a far more skilled diagnostician than the empiric; and although bloodletting did enjoy a vogue in the early nineteenth century, particularly among the followers of François Broussais (1772–1838), the old armamentarium had been purged of much that was harmful or worthless, and the trained physician was far likelier than the empiric to use dangerous remedies judiciously.

The continued denunciations of *impéritie* (which remained a commonplace of discourse on medical practice well into the nineteenth century) essentially applied, then, to the lower-level ordinary practitioners; they reflect, not contempt for official medicine as a whole, but the accurate perception that France lacked a uniform standard of qualification. In the eyes of the professional elite, great numbers of their nominal colleagues were little better than empirics. These divisions are of great importance for the present study, for they long hindered the profession from forming a united front against unauthorized practitioners.

Professional conduct

Much the same observation applies to the charge that physicians and surgeons at times behaved liked charlatans or *maiges*. Some eighteenth-century physicians, including a few in high places, did exploit proprietary remedies, extolling their virtues in popular publications or even, in exceptional cases, hawking them in the public square. It was said that Charles Dionis, the doctor-regent of the Paris faculty who purchased from the Contugi family the royal privilege for distributing orvietan, had his own children get up on a stage to help peddle it. Another physician of the Paris faculty, Jean-Stanislas Mittié (1727–1795), promoted a putative vegetable remedy for venereal disease; when the Société Royale de Médecine dismissed his claims, he branded it a "company of physician-aristocrats" (this was in 1789) and blamed its decision on hatred for a rival *corps*. At Lille, an *agrégé* of the college of medicine distributed leaflets for a vendor selling the powders of the chevalier de Goderneaux. And in the Southwest, the holder of a medical doctorate from the University of Orange, named Coronat, traveled from place to place, announcing his arrival with trumpet blasts and boasting that with drugs of his own making he could cure all maladies; at Boulogne he promised to cure a madwoman in two years, using drugs costing 60 livres.[151] More typically, the regular practitioner who played the charlatan was a surgeon, sometimes a former irregular who had managed to win membership in a surgical community. At Dun-le-Roi in Berry a surgeon, the former secretary of the surgical community, was accused of peddling drugs in the public square to the sound of a trumpet. The surgeon Lescot, who had been admitted to practice in the market town of Saint-Georges-de-Ballon in Maine, was said to be an empiric who sold drugs from a stage.[152] Other practitioners used unorthodox methods. One respondent to the 1790 survey of surgery cited a physician and a surgeon who inspected urine and "administer[ed] remedies to the patient's rear end."[153] Urban physicians, caught up in the mesmerist craze of the 1780's, dabbled in animal magnetism.

Such cases were the exception, not the rule; but they could absorb a good deal of the energy of the corporations, whose statutes barred physicians and surgeons from consorting with charlatans and usually provided strict guidelines for professional conduct. In one *cause célèbre*, the Paris faculty struck from its rolls the physician Guilbert de Préval, who had given offense through excessive promotion of his *eau fondante anti-vénérienne* (resolvent antivenereal water) and other special remedies. In 1784, the Faculty of Medicine of Bordeaux excluded from its assemblies and barred its members from consulting with a Dr. Gibbon, who had persisted in experimenting with animal magnetism. (In a more notorious case, the Paris faculty suspended the physician Charles Deslon for two years for having consorted with Mesmer.)[154] The perceived charlatanish behavior of some colleagues, like the *impéritie* of others, militated against professional unity and complicated the campaign against unauthorized practice.

ACCESS TO A MEDICAL CAREER

The discussion so far has considered training essentially as an index of competency, but a system of education can also serve to restrict membership in a monopolistic occupation. Any account of professionalization must examine the ways in which the profession controls entry into the field and, from the aspiring practitioner's point of view, the obstacles that he must overcome in order to gain access. The effects of such barriers can be quite paradoxical. Educational requirements may raise standards within the profession, but high costs or arbitrary restrictions can swell the ranks of the empirics by driving into unauthorized practice potential candidates who might otherwise have received certification, thereby undermining the larger project of professionalization.

In order to become a physician in the Old Regime, it was usually necessary, first of all, to be a Roman Catholic. University degrees were refused to unconverted Jews (as well as to bastards and sons of executioners); at Nancy, a Jewish candidate denied admission in 1785 was not able to matriculate until after the Revolution. Strasbourg alone was allowed to grad-

uate Lutherans. Protestant physicians were legally denied the right to practice, and the medical corporations, like the guilds in general, excluded them
until the Edict of Toleration gave full civil rights to Protestants in 1787
(although in practice many were able to work unmolested).[155]

It was also necessary to be a male. In France, women were not admitted
to universities (as they were, in small numbers, in Italy), and they were
therefore excluded from the faculties of medicine. In the Middle Ages
women had legally practiced surgery, but in 1484 a decree of Charles VIII
barred them from the field, with the exception of surgeons' widows. In
1694, the ban was extended to widows (though they could maintain their
husband's "shop" by taking on a qualified *garçon chirurgien*, or surgeon's
assistant), and in 1755 the Parlement of Paris decreed that women could
not practice even the special branches of surgery, apart from midwifery.
Some women continued to work as surgeons in the eighteenth century,
though not as regularly admitted master surgeons; and since they could not
take a university arts degree, they were completely excluded from the liberal
profession that emerged in the latter part of the century.[156]

Beyond religion and gender, it is difficult to generalize about conditions
of access to the medical field. The old medical network characteristically
lacked uniform criteria for admission. (The costs of training, for example,
ranged from more than 7,000 livres for the Paris doctorate down to less
than 1 percent of that amount for the lowest level of the surgical mastership.)
It is therefore necessary to look more closely at the range of requirements
in medicine and surgery.

Medicine

Under the terms of the Edict of Marly, the aspiring physician had, first of
all, to study philosophy for two years and take the master of arts degree
(except at the Faculty of Nancy, to which the edict did not apply). Three
years of study were required for the baccalaureate degree in medicine; after
passing the necessary examinations, the candidate could proceed immediately, if he chose, to the examinations for the *licence* and the doctorate. The
edict, however, allowed the faculties to impose higher standards.[157] Paris
was the extreme case: four years for the baccalaureate (three for holders of
a Paris M.A.); then two years for the *licence*; then at least two more years
for the doctorate and two to attain the title of doctor-regent.[158]

In the provinces, the duration of studies was typically much shorter. As
a result, many candidates, after a few years in the capital, went on to a
lesser faculty to receive their degree. In 1785, for example, a certain Verdier
du Clos, after four years at Paris, proceeded to Nancy, where he received
the baccalaureate on the 18th of July, the *licence* on the 21st, and the doctorate
on the 26th.[159] Those pressed for time could find still shorter routes, notably

at the corrupt Faculty of Orange, which was so undiscriminating that it was said to have officially received one candidate with a warrant outstanding for his arrest. Here it was possible to get a doctorate in the space of a week, as did a former valet of the chancellor Maupeou, a certain Bignau, who had lost his job after his master's disgrace in 1774.[160] A few of the more venal faculties were said simply to sell diplomas for cash. If the physician then attempted to establish a practice in a town with a corporate monopoly, he normally had to pass new examinations and pay a fee for his *agrégation*, unless he was an *interne* of the local faculty. At Bordeaux, the college required two years of practice in the jurisdiction of the Parlement of Bordeaux and six examinations. At Nantes, where the faculty actively discouraged newcomers from joining, it was necessary to pass five examinations over a period of three to four years.[161]

Costs were predictably highest in Paris, where total expenditures for the regency could reach 8,000 to 10,000 livres in all. Charges in the provinces ranged from less than half that sum (4,000 livres for the *grand ordinaire* at Reims, 2,000–3,000 at some other faculties [Angers, for example]) to barely one-twentieth. The *externe* degree typically cost several hundred livres (about 425 for all expenses at Angers, for example), but as much as 2,000 livres at Montpellier.[162] Under the Paris faculty statutes of 1758, collection of the fees for the *licence* and the doctorate would be postponed for those who were "truly poor"; and in 1766 a few scholarships were made available, through a special competition, to pay for the expenses from the *licence* through the regency.[163] In most cases, though, the price differential drove candidates, even those who began their studies in Paris, to take a degree at a cheaper provincial university. The most attractive alternative was Montpellier, which was the second most prestigious faculty after Paris but cost considerably less. For the same reason, few provincial graduates sought *agrégation* in a major urban corporation outside the jurisdiction of the faculty where they took their degree. Some corporations deliberately set the admission fee prohibitively high–2,000 livres at Nantes, for example.[164]

Surgeons

The training of surgeons, as befitted what remained an essentially practical calling, depended heavily on an apprenticeship system; until 1772, all candidates in the provinces were required to sign a formal contract with a master. The apprenticeship might last a year or two; the candidate would then spend two or three years as a journeyman, working under a master surgeon in a town with a surgical community, in a frontier hospital, or in the army, navy, or merchant marine. A period of travel typically followed: for the more ambitious, a *tour de France*; for the future country surgeon, a tour merely of the district. After four years, the candidate for the highest level of the mastership might ask the King's First Surgeon to admit him to the *grand chef d'oeuvre*. Increasingly, though, candidates spent part of their time taking courses at schools of surgery or at the College of Surgery in Paris, which attracted growing numbers of students from the provinces until 1784, when its full three-year curriculum was made mandatory for all.[165] A few provincial schools already existed in the first half of the century (those at Rennes and Nantes, for example, dated from the 1730's), and in the 1750's, surgical teaching was established or expanded at Montpellier, Bordeaux, Toulon, Rouen, Orléans, and Toulouse. A royal declaration of 1772 required provincial surgeons to study at a surgical school for one year (the minimum was raised to two in 1784) and encouraged the establishment of schools in major provincial cities. By the end of the Old Regime, France had fourteen civil schools of surgery.[166] In one local study, an analysis of the qualifications of the received surgeons practicing in the diocese of Auch in Gascony at the end of the Old Regime has shown that half had some formal instruction and that nearly a third had attended the College of Surgery in Paris (though Gascony is probably the extreme case among the French provinces).[167]

Like the spread of formal schooling, the requirement for the master of arts degree reflected the transformation of surgery into a liberal profession. Already required by a few of the leading provincial communities, notably at Lyons and Bordeaux, the M.A. was imposed on Paris surgeons by the royal declaration of 1743 and on surgeons of the first order in major provincial towns by the Edict of Compiègne in 1756. In the provinces this rule was not strictly observed; at Rennes, for example, the community applied it only in 1776, and surgeons with the M.A. remained the exception. In Paris after midcentury, however, almost all master surgeons held the arts degree and defended a thesis in Latin.[168]

Under the terms of the surgical statutes of 1730, the cost of a mastership for a community town was set at 300 livres; approbation for a noncommunity town cost about a third as much, and the lowest qualification, the *petite expérience*, came to about 70 livres.[169] These were minima, however; the charges imposed by the larger communities, which had their own statutes, could run much higher. The community of Orléans, for example, asked 120 livres for the right to practice in a village or bourg with 100 or fewer households, and 150 livres for a larger one. The costs for the top grade in the more important community towns greatly exceeded 300 livres. In Rennes they came to 1,200–2,000 livres, plus 600–700 livres for the stages as apprentice and journeyman – more than the price of a medical degree from Caen or Angers and as much as a medical degree from Montpellier or Nantes. Paris cost even more – around 3,500 livres. (The requirement for the master's examination could be waived, however, for a *gagnant-*

maîtrise, or senior surgical hospital resident.) When the fees for the right to practice in a major community town were added to those for the degrees, the total could reach a sum comparable to the charges faced by the most ambitious physicians, attaining 8,000 livres in Bordeaux, for example, according to one calculation.[170] For the great majority of candidates, the reception fees constituted a formidable, and often insurmountable, barrier in the road to the mastership. Not surprisingly, many surgeons were admitted relatively late in life, if at all. In 1773, for example, when J.-B. Dagobert was received at Rennes and licensed to practice at Saint-Didier, he was thirty-eight years old and had been working as a surgeon for twenty years. The study of the diocese of Auch mentioned earlier shows that more than three-quarters of the received surgeons were over thirty at the time of the examination; the average age was thirty-nine.[171]

Midwives

Under the statutes of 1730, midwives in a town with a community of surgeons had to serve a two-year apprenticeship and take an examination administered by two surgeons. In a town without a community, one surgeon would conduct the examination; in small towns and villages the formalities were reduced to a bare minimum, and in any case no serious attempt was made to enforce the requirements until the middle of the century. For the vast majority of future midwives, the question of more formal training in the field simply did not arise; the only institution that provided it was the *office des accouchées* (lying-in ward) founded in 1630 at the Hôtel-Dieu in Paris. Toward the end of the Old Regime, the missionary work of Madame Du Coudray did much to make a higher level of instruction available in the provinces. She offered courses in some fifty cities and may have taught as many as 5,000 women; in addition, the surgeon-demonstrators she trained to carry on her work may have instructed another 10,000 women in the three decades from 1760 to 1790 (though most of them tended to settle in towns). But such courses, although government sponsored, were not a strict legal requirement, nor did they reach every part of France. Most midwives still lacked formal training, especially in rural areas. In 1786, for example, among the 51 registered midwives of the subdelegation of Le Vigan in Languedoc, where courses in obstetrics had not been established, only 7 had studied with surgeons in Montpellier or Nîmes.[172] The most serious impediment to formal reception remained the cost, which was of course highest in the towns with a surgical community. In Montpellier, the fees for the mastership totaled 37 livres – considerably less than the charges in surgery, but still a discouraging sum for a woman without means.[173]

SOCIAL AND ECONOMIC STATUS

We are of course accustomed to the notion that entering a medical career can be onerous and expensive, but we are also accustomed to thinking of the investment as a profitable one. The public perceives physicians as hand-somely paid and, almost without exception, upper middle class. Although some young physicians struggling to establish themselves in an over-crowded field or older ones coping with mounting premiums for malprac-tice insurance might take exception to this notion of uniform prosperity, physicians remain one of the most highly remunerated occupational groups. This was not always so. In the Old Regime and during much of the nine-teenth century, the range in social and economic status among medical men was so great that it spanned nearly all categories above the level of the lowliest artisan.

Physicians

The costs of degrees and of admission to the medical corporations limited recruitment into the medical elite to a small part of the comfortable bourgeoisie. The prejudices of the doctor-regents helped perpetuate this exclusivity. "It was an established usage...," wrote a member of an old Angevin family, "not to confer degrees on candidates known not to belong to honorable families in the bourgeoisie."[174] The curriculum's emphasis on Latin and a classical education also served to exclude candidates from the wrong background; in some places, too, the corporations explicitly required that an applicant never have practiced a manual trade.[175] The celebrated Swiss physician Samuel-Auguste-André-David Tissot succinctly stated the deeper rationale for a policy that ensured that medicine would not serve as a vehicle for social mobility: if the wrong kind of people were attracted, "then the Academies, the Universities would be filled with subjects who should plough the fields and ditch the vineyards."[176] Not surprisingly, then, the upper reaches of the profession were filled with men from established families. Guillaume-François Laennec (1748–1822), for example, uncle of the better known René (inventor of the stethoscope), was the son of a barrister at the Parlement of Rennes and a descendant of a family of royal notaries.[177]

Family tradition and explicit favors accorded by the corporations en-couraged the sons of medical men to follow in their father's footsteps. In some towns, a significant part of medical practice was in the hands of a virtual caste of medical dynasties. Of 31 doctor-regents received at Angers in the eighteenth century (1694–1785), 8 were sons of doctor-regents, 3 of master surgeons, 4 of master apothecaries, 4 of merchants (including 2 *juges-consuls*, or magistrates of the commercial tribunal), 2 of "bourgeois," and

1 of a holder of a seigneurial office.[178] A similar pattern appeared at a much more modest level in the countryside, where the *externe* was often the son of a country surgeon and a midwife.

The established physician in a provincial town ranked with the barristers among the bourgeois notables as a *"noble homme"* (man of noble standing); in the ordinances, physicians were styled *"gens de grand état et de grand salaire"* (people of high station and income). In some regions the title of doctor technically conferred nobility, as in Dauphiné and in the Comtat, where local custom made it hereditary, allowing children of physicians to enter the Order of Malta.[179] (In 1789, one correspondent of the Société Royale de Médecine went so far as to call for hereditary nobility for all physicians.)[180] Nobles could practice medicine without fear of *dérogeance* (fall from noble status), and the nobles' *cahiers de doléances* of 1789 specifically listed medicine as one of the callings that they wished to be able to pursue.[181] Not many in fact did – the law proved more attractive – but several became members of the Paris medical faculty. Other physicians started as commoners but acquired nobility. One option under the Old Regime, the purchase of ennobling venal offices, was too expensive for all but a handful of medical men (lawyers outnumbered doctors among purchasers twelve to one), but sixteen court physicians were ennobled in the eighteenth century through their positions in the royal household. Considerably more were ennobled for merit and service, in this case outperforming their rivals the lawyers.[182]

The privileged status of physicians made them exempt, like the nobles, from certain taxes and other impositions. Medical students were excused from the militia, and practitioners could normally escape the *taille* (the principal direct tax), *guet et garde* (a seigneurial imposition that theoretically replaced the old obligation to defend the lord's castle), *corvée* (labor owed to the seigneur or the state), *tutelle* and *curatelle* (public guardianship of minors), and *collecte* (the rotating position of tax assessor and collector) – the last, it is said, because "if a physician were a tax collector, his arrival, instead of consoling the patient, would frighten him and redouble his fever." At Angers, the physician of the Hôtel-Dieu was expressly exempted from the *tutelle*, *curatelle*, *guet et garde*, and quartering of soldiers.[183] These privileges saved money and inconvenience, but they were also status symbols. One practitioner in lower Poitou complained to the Société Royale de Médecine that he had been subjected to the indignity of billeting troops, which "degrades the nobility of the profession."[184]

As befitted their station as bourgeois notables and members of the intelligentsia, physicians occupied a prominent position in the provincial academies, which were to emerge in the latter eighteenth century as major centers for the diffusion of Enlightenment thought. About 1,000 medical men (predominantly physicians) belonged to the various academies, making up

28 percent of the regular members and 37 percent of the associate members; in five local societies, more than half of the membership came from medical backgrounds. Among academicians from bourgeois backgrounds (the academies also included significant numbers of nobles), 26 percent came from medicine (as compared with 23 percent from the clergy and 29 percent from the fields of justice and administration).[185]

The economic status of practitioners varied widely. Those at the top of the scale were wealthy – occasionally very wealthy – men. Jacques Daran amassed a fortune of more than a million livres, though he ultimately went bankrupt.[186] A few physicians accumulated enough resources to purchase major offices. La Chapelle-Hamart of Rennes was chief clerk of the *chambre des requêtes* of the Parlement of Brittany (this chamber primarily heard cases brought by parties who held royal letters of *committimus*, which gave them access to the court in the first instance). In 1781, the physician Dubois bought the office of royal councillor and secretary attached to the chancellery of Brittany: in the words of Jean Meyer, he was "in the world of the great capitalists."[187] At the other extreme, some practitioners had no fortune to speak of, even after long years of practice. When, for example, Dr. de la Croix of La Ferté-Bernard in Maine died of an epidemic disease in 1788, he left his widow destitute.[188]

In the larger towns, it was often possible for an established physician to live comfortably on the income from his practice. According to one study of 404 eighteenth-century Paris physicians, at least 219 appear to have lived off their fees alone. Some did quite well, though often with the help of other resources; Dr. Portal, for example, earned more than 40,000 livres annually. All told, 85 percent of Paris physicians at the end of the Old Regime enjoyed "bourgeois" incomes, if 5,000 livres per annum is taken as the cutoff point.[189] In Brittany, Robin de Kériaville, a physician at Josselin, had an income of 3,000 livres a year, and the earnings of La Boujardière, one of the most highly esteemed physicians at Rennes, attained 6,000 livres in 1788. Indeed, seven of the eight physicians at Rennes in 1789 paid more than 60 livres in capitation tax on incomes that derived in large part from their medical practice.[190]

Practice in smaller towns and rural areas was arduous and less lucrative; a physician working in the countryside, suggested one correspondent of the Société Royale de Médecine, might expect to earn 200 pistoles (2,000 livres, well above the average for many regions) and be worn out at 40.[191] Some towns found that they could attract physicians only if they offered pensions to supplement the inadequate fees a practitioner could expect to receive. The physician at Carhaix in Brittany, for example, collected a stipend of 400 livres. His less fortunate colleague at Le Croisic had only 200 livres and earned virtually no fees. Complaining of his insufficient earnings, he sought to eke out his income elsewhere – a practice that led the municipal officers to complain of his "lack of attention to the patients in the town, whom he has often abandoned in order to roam the countryside, where he has on more than one occasion passed entire weeks." The municipal physicians strained local resources, and starting in 1775, the intendant, Gaspard-Louis Caze de la Bove, systematically eliminated their salaries, arguing that "a physician, if he is worthy of confidence, must create for himself a respectable position without the help of this salary."[192] The unfortunate practitioners found themselves trapped in a vicious cycle of poverty and professional frustration.

Surgeons

The social and economic positions of eighteenth-century surgeons displayed even greater diversity than those of physicians, reflecting the disparity between the first order and the products of the *petite expérience*. So long as surgery was considered a manual trade, the master surgeons in most towns that had *jurandes*, or trade guilds, remained on a par with the master cobbler, and his best title in public documents was "*honorable homme*." The decree of 1756 added surgeons "living nobly" to the ranks of the bourgeois notables and allowed them to aspire to municipal honors. They were not to be included on the rolls of the arts and crafts or subjected to the tax on industry and certain other charges and duties.[193] The countryside, however, presented a very different picture. An occasional large proprietor who ministered to his neighbors and dependents might take his letters of mastership in surgery, but the typical practitioner remained on the level of the village artisan. He was, as one contemporary noted, "the son of a peasant or *laboureur* [a term usually applied to a peasant who owned some land and a team of draft animals], who, having learned to read only thanks to the efforts of the curé of his village . . . , goes off to a barber-surgeon of the environs to learn the elements of barbering with him."[194] The greater and lesser lights of surgery, though, had one thing in common; like medicine, the occupation was often a family tradition. In the diocese of Auch, for example, at least a third of the surgeons practicing at the end of the Old Regime were the sons of surgeons.[195]

Over the course of the eighteenth century, the first-order surgeons substantially improved their economic position. In Paris, perhaps three-quarters of the master surgeons of Saint-Côme enjoyed "bourgeois" incomes by the end of the Old Regime.[196] At Angers, a chart of the capitation taxes paid in 1715 would show the surgeons clustered near the bottom; in 1788 they were spread far more evenly, though their fortunes did not equal those of the doctor-regents.[197] A study of surgeons in nine Breton towns (not including Nantes) suggests that they did as well or better: those at the highest level of income were approximately on an equal footing with the physicians.[198] In general, though, the range was greater than for physicians, and the average income was lower. One study of surgeons in Paris and thirteen provincial cities speaks of three groups: a small number paying a capitation of a few livres; a majority paying 5–20; and a minority paying 30–60 or even 80 or 100. About half of the surgeons paid between 5 and 19 livres; about half of the physicians, between 10 and 29.[199]

The rural surgeon's chance of making an adequate living from his practice remained slim. One lieutenant of the King's First Surgeon noted in his response to the questionnaire of 1790: "it is now impossible for a surgeon in a small town or the countryside to support himself from his profession, unless he engages to a certain extent in trade." In the same year, a correspondent from Auch estimated that a country surgeon might earn in a year perhaps nine or ten bags of grain (rural practitioners were often paid in kind), compared with four or five bags for the average peasant.[200]

The medical occupations, then, were highly stratified, with the broadest division between urban and rural personnel, both physicians and surgeons. Practitioners ranged from established members of urban elites to village tradesmen for whom medicine was only a part-time activity. The persistence of such differences in wealth and status retarded professional unification; it also produced divergent attitudes on the question of illegal competition from empirics – typically a more urgent issue for the struggling rural practitioner than for his bourgeois colleague in a university town.

DENSITY AND DISTRIBUTION OF PERSONNEL

The discussion so far has examined the medical occupations chiefly from the practitioner's point of view, as a job or career. Medical practice obviously depends, though, on encounters between doctors and patients; to understand its social significance, we must also consider it from the client's point of view as a resource. To what extent could and did the population use the services of qualified personnel? The degree of contact with professionals, which varied over time and from place to place, essentially depended on three factors: accessibility (determined by the number of practitioners within easy traveling distance and the ratio of active practitioners to population); cost; and the population's attitudes toward official medicine and its representatives.

It is unfortunately impossible to say with any certainty just how many medical practitioners worked in eighteenth-century France. Physicians numbered at least 2,000–3,000; some estimates place the outside limit as high as 5,000 at the end of the Old Regime in a population of some 26 million.[201] Surgeons were far more numerous: perhaps as many as 40,000, counting all of the barber-surgeons, though other estimates would place the number considerably lower.[202] (In the regions for which good infor-

Table 1. *Regional densities of practitioners in 1786*

Généralité	Overall density (per 10,000 inhabitants)	Physicians (per 10,000 inhabitants)	Surgeons (per 10,000 inhabitants)
Amiens	7.38	0.56	6.82
Caen	5.53	1.71	3.82
Dijon	7.11	1.45	5.66
Rennes	2.21	0.45	1.76
Soissons	7.00	0.65	6.35
Tours	4.82	0.60	4.22

Source: Jean-Pierre Goubert, "The Extent of Medical Practice in France around 1780," *Journal of Social History* 10 (1976–77): 421. Used with permission.

mation has survived, the physician-to-surgeon ratio varied from 1:4 to 1:10.)[203] Even the most conservative estimates suggest that the density of practitioners was at least around 5 per 10,000 inhabitants and possibly 10 per 10,000 or higher, close to present-day levels.[204] (It is of course important to remember that the great majority of practitioners were lower-level surgeons. In Anjou, for example, the density was 7 per 10,000 in 1786, approaching that of the department of Maine-et-Loire in 1962 [8 per 10,000]; but 6 out of 7 practitioners were surgeons.)[205] Assuming that each practitioner had a clientele of about 500, it is theoretically possible that a quarter or more of the population saw an official practitioner – though this is only the crudest of guesses.[206] France, then, was among the more "medicalized" countries of Europe; the density in England and Wales during the same period works out to 5.7 per 10,000 on the basis of the available estimates of the number of practitioners (though these figures are probably too low).[207]

   Global densities are useful for cross-national comparisons, but a study that used them to analyze the availability of medical services would fall into the ecological fallacy. The density of practitioners in eighteenth-century France varied markedly from region to region. Statistics for six *généralités* (the districts administered by intendants) in northern France, drawn from a government survey of 1786, show regional densities ranging from 2.21 per 10,000 inhabitants for the *généralité* of Rennes to 7.38 for Amiens. (See Table 1.) The density for Rennes is so depressed that even the next-lowest-ranking *généralité* is still slightly closer to Amiens than to Rennes. (It should be noted, though, that two of the three regions with the most favorable overall densities had relatively low concentrations of physicians but exceptionally high densities of surgeons.) The estimated percentage of the population that might have seen an official practitioner would range from about 11 for the *généralité* of Rennes to about 37 for the *généralité* of Amiens.[208]

Table 2. *Disparities in urban/rural densities of practitioners, 1786*

Généralité	Urban			Rural		
	Global	Doctors	Surgeons	Global	Doctors	Surgeons
Amiens	7.99	2.63	5.36	7.19	0.04	7.15
Caen	11.45	5.15	6.30	3.95	0.79	3.16
Dijon	18.31	7.44	10.87	5.20	0.49	4.71
Rennes	7.70	2.97	4.73	1.27	0.02	1.25
Soissons	15.23	4.28	10.95	5.56	0.02	5.54
Tours	11.23	4.20	7.03	3.90	0.15	3.75

Note: Densities are expressed as number of practitioners per 10,000 inhabitants.
Source: Jean-Pierre Goubert, "The Extent of Medical Practice in France around 1780," *Journal of Social History* 10 (1976–77): 421. Used with permission.

Regional statistics still mask the even more pronounced contrast between town and country. Overall, the density of practitioners was three times higher in urban areas. Physicians, especially, were concentrated in towns: fully three-quarters of them lived there, as opposed to only one-quarter of the surgeons (though surgeons still made up 60 percent of urban practitioners). Even where town and country had roughly comparable overall densities, the rural areas had disproportionate concentrations of lower-level surgeons.[209] (See Table 2.) Moreover, the countryside was even more than usually disadvantaged in the least favored regions: in Brittany, the rural areas had a density of only 1.3 per 10,000.[210] A comparison with Anjou is revealing. The urban density in Brittany was half that of Anjou to begin with, but even so, cities had proportionally 148.5 times as many physicians and 3.8 times as many surgeons as the countryside; in Anjou, the ratio of the densities of urban and rural physicians was about 18:1.[211] A closer look at the Breton situation shows even more striking disparities within the province. Seventeen subdelegations, or about a third of the total, had no physicians at all. With one-seventh of the population, the towns had 99 percent of the physicians and 65 percent of the master surgeons, together with 90 percent of the authorized midwives.[212]

Even in the urban centers, finally, significant variations appear. The capital, not surprisingly, was exceptionally well supplied with medical men. It has been calculated that Paris in 1789 had 172 doctor-regents, 52 other physicians, 235 master surgeons, 113 privileged surgeons, 60 other surgeons, and 58 experts, for a total of 690.[213] Assuming a population of 600,000, the densities would be 11.5 per 10,000 for all practitioners and 3.7 per 10,000 for physicians. These results are comparable to those derived from a London list for 1783: 11.90 per 10,000 overall, and 2.29 per 10,000 for physicians.[214]

In the case of the provinces, it might be supposed that the largest cities had the highest concentrations of practitioners, but in fact an inverse correlation obtains: 10–35 per 10,000 inhabitants for towns with populations of 1,500–5,000; 7–15 per 10,000 for 5,000–10,000; and 5–10 per 10,000 for 20,000–80,000. On the eve of the Revolution, the small town of Saint-Rémy-de-Provence, with a population of only 4,500–4,700, had 10 medical practitioners, or a density of about 22 per 10,000.[215] (In England, similarly, some of the smaller provincial towns were traditionally better supplied per capita than London.)[216] Some of the lowest densities appeared in large manufacturing centers with a sizable laboring population that did not consult official practitioners. Some of the highest densities were realized in administrative centers of middling size that enjoyed a better average standard of living.[217]

The gap between all the urban densities and those in rural areas suggests that differences in levels of urbanization should help account for the broad regional variations discussed earlier. To some extent they do, but the correlation does not always hold; for example, Champagne and the Île-de-France, exclusive of Paris, had a low index of urbanization but a high concentration of surgeons.[218] Other factors played a role as well: economic prosperity; the presence of a thriving faculty like that of Montpellier; and even that great imponderable, popular receptivity to official medicine. Brittany, to take the extreme case, was deficient on every score. It was less urban and poorer than France as a whole. (Within the province, too, the pattern of medicalization clearly followed regional differences in wealth; the more favored areas, the littoral and the eastern extremity, were much better supplied than the hinterland.) Moreover, the faculty of Nantes was in such a sad state of decline that Breton students had to pursue their training at Caen, Angers, Nancy, or Reims. Medical men may also have perceived Brittany, where traditional beliefs were exceptionally tenacious, as an unattractive place to settle.[219] It is somewhat more difficult to explain the unusually high concentrations of practitioners in the Midi (10 per 10,000 and above), a singularity that survives to this day. This abundance of medical men in the South, which recalls the Italian pattern, may reflect the Mediterranean urban tradition and the proximity of the faculty at Montepellier. But surgeons were involved as well as physicians, and relatively small places as well as population centers. In the diocese of Toulouse, for example, though only 3 percent of communities had a physician, a quarter had surgeons; and only 5 percent of those that lacked surgeons (which had a mere 3.7 percent of the population) were more than a league (about 4 kilometers) from a surgeon. The overall density of practitioners was 13.6 per 10,000.[220]

More work needs to be done along these lines at the regional and local levels. The evidence now available makes clear, however, how difficult it is to generalize about what the French call the "index of medicalization."

The West was at an extreme disadvantage compared with the North, the East, and the Midi. In some of the less favored regions, large areas were almost entirely without authorized practitioners, though towns might be fairly well supplied. Nevertheless, if all surgeons, whatever their limitations, are counted as medical practitioners, it becomes clear that the picture of the provinces as a "medical desert" has been considerably overdrawn. It now appears that by the end of the Old Regime the majority of Frenchmen may have been in a position to contact an authorized practitioner. Whether they chose to do so is another question.

COSTS OF PROFESSIONAL SERVICES

Even where a regular practitioner was available, his charges placed his services beyond the reach of most peasants and workers, though the poorest and least urbanized regions had the lowest prevailing rates. Fees for a lower-level surgeon were half or a third of what a first-order practitioner might charge: 10–15 sous, as opposed to 1–3 livres (1 livre = 20 sous); in the subdelegations of Brittany that had the smallest towns, the fees never exceeded 10 sous. But that sum already equalled the daily wage of an agricultural worker or modest artisan and half that of a more prosperous urban artisan. The costs of travel, moreover, could vastly increase the charge for a consultation in the countryside, where many sick peasants could not even afford a nourishing soup. In 1778, for example, a surgeon of Loudéac in Brittany asked 2 livres to travel 3 kilometers; the visit itself cost only 12 sous. In the city, fees could range from 1 to 3 livres (3 to 6 in Paris) for a daytime visit, with the more prestigious practitioners in the larger towns charging up to 12 livres; the rate doubled at night. Although it was customary to use a sliding scale, the minimum was still at least 1 livre.[221] In some regions, it is true, physicians' fees were fixed by statute, but even then at levels that only patients who were fairly well off could afford. In 1734, the Parlement of Poitiers established a schedule of fees for the physicians of the town; a trip to the countryside would cost 10 livres a day. In 1748, the parlement imposed a scale of 6–12 livres for the same service.[222] This sort of price control could not have significantly expanded access to medical care.

The fee structure helped give medical practice its characteristic social contours. A regular practitioner would normally be summoned only in an emergency or when a patient had become gravely ill. (Occasionally, though, one hears of a form of contract practice that provided medical care for a fixed price: at Biarritz, for example, in the 1760's, 253 families paid 2 livres a year for the services of a surgeon, including visits, bleeding, and even amputations, though not childbirth.)[223] A patient was still less likely to send for a physician or surgeon if he lived any distance away. At Sartes in

Lorraine, which had no medical practitioners, the curé reported (c. 1780) that "the rich people send for them once or twice, never more; the poor, without any resources, are already too wretched without adding the costs of physicians."[224] And even in communities that had a practitioner, the regular clientele was socially circumscribed. The surviving daybooks of a Breton surgeon at Loudéac in the 1770's show a clientele made up of about one-third bourgeois (property owners and rentiers); one-third artisans and shopkeepers; and one-third well-off peasants. Even then, the incidence of bad debts reached 20 percent, presumably in part because of inability to pay (though it could be difficult to collect fees even from the rich).[225] In a cash-poor economy, moreover, rural practitioners were often obliged to accept payment in kind.

The problem of cost particularly affected the licensed midwife, who had to compete with the untrained but often more experienced *matrone* who could be found in nearly every village. The custom of having the infant's godfather pay the midwife may have made high charges still less acceptable to rural families. One case from among many in the late eighteenth century is that of Desforges Maillard, a master surgeon's wife who trained in Paris and passed her examination in Nantes, becoming a *maîtresse-sage-femme* in the parish of Pontchâteau. Her certificates were duly published, but she failed to win over a significant part of the local custom from her unqualified competitors. The peasants, who probably had more confidence in the *matrones* to begin with, considered her fee of 24 sous too high.[226]

In the peasant's view, money differed from the products of the organic realm in that it was not self-renewing. Nowhere is this attitude better expressed than in the old proverb "Plaie du corps peut se cicatriser avec le temps, plaie d'argent dure toujours" (A wound in the body will heal with time, [but] a financial injury lasts forever).[227] Nothing could be further from the current middle-class truism that good health alone is irreplaceable. Physicians' fees were perhaps the single most important obstacle to rural medicalization. Popular complaints about physicians repeatedly stressed their cupidity, and official reports on rural medicine almost invariably excoriated the peasants for their stinginess. At Guidel in Brittany, the *recteur* (priest) of this wealthy parish complained in 1779 that "the most well-to-do inhabitants let themselves die without help, through avarice, rather than have recourse to the physicians."[228] When the physician Moucet arrived with two surgeons at Plénée-Jugon in Brittany during an epidemic in 1758, the peasants refused to lend them horses, "saying that they were working their fields, and that [to help us] would be to take bread out of their mouths. They all say that they have no sick people, even though their houses are full of them."[229] There was much truth to the hackneyed observation of the chaplain in Diderot's *Supplément au voyage de Bougainville*: "The wretched peasant of our regions, who overworks his wife in order to spare his horse, allows his child to perish without succor and summons the physician for his ox."[230] Everything hinged on economic calculation. The draft animal might be irreplaceable; the wife and child were not. Moreover, the peasant's transactions with official medicine, like his relations with the market economy in general, were a source of confusion and distrust. Who had a legitimate claim on his limited reserve of cash? And what was a fair price – what money value could be placed on his health?

Not all patients, it is true, paid for medical services. A master would often pay for his servants, a seigneur for his dependents. Some practitioners received salaries from religious foundations: at Lille, for example, toward the end of the eighteenth century, one physician received 240 livres a year from the Abbey of Marquette.[231] Others were employed by the provincial estates or by municipalities, though this practice was far more limited than the system of the *Physikus* in Germany or the town physician in Italy. In the *élection* of Armagnac, for example, only 7 of more than 300 communities had a paid municipal physician.[232] In theory, too, private practitioners were supposed to care for indigent patients, making up for their losses by charging the rich more. This was the stated policy of the Faculty of Poitiers, for example, according to its deliberations of 1701; and the Edict of Marly required the dean and several physicians of the medical corporations to assemble with assistants once a week to give free medical consultations for the poor.[233] Some country practitioners did treat the poor gratis, if we are to believe the petitions they sent to the provincial intendants seeking compensation for their philanthropic services, but this work was never carried out on a regular basis. (Hence the various proposals that Enlightenment physicians put forward for creating and funding a network of district physicians; one scheme would have salaried a physician from an ecclesiastical prebend in every town possessing a cathedral or collegiate church.)[234] Nor did the hospital system, whose essential function was to serve the poor, offer an adequate alternative to individual initiative. Although it comprised several thousand institutions, only about a thousand provided medical services; only a few hundred (concentrated in the North) were primarily medical (*hôtels-Dieu*); and of these, only about a hundred had full staffs of residents and consultants.[235]

For the large part of the population that chose not to pay physicians' fees, exposure to the official personnel and their therapies might come only during an epidemic, when the intendants, following a practice well established by the middle of the eighteenth century, dispatched *médecins et chirurgiens des épidémies* to the scene, together with the boxes of royal remedies sent from Paris and kept in store for use in such emergencies. (The scheme for distributing remedies dated from the reign of Louis XIV. Begun in 1680 and then interrupted, the program owed its revival to the efforts of the Dutch physician Adrien Helvétius [c. 1661–1727], the promoter of ipecac and grandfather of the celebrated *philosophe*. At his death, responsibility for preparing the boxes passed to his son Jean-Claude-Adrien, and then in 1756 to a cousin, Jean de Diest. He in turn was succeeded in 1762 by Joseph-Marie-François de Lassone [1717–1788], the future First Physician and president of the Société Royale de Médecine; but by then the remedies were closely associated with the founding dynasty and were known, not surprisingly, as *les remèdes d'Helvétius*. Originally available to all the indigent sick, the medications were restricted after 1740 to the victims of epidemic disease in rural parishes.)[236] In this way, many peasants came into contact with official medicine for the first time, and physicians into contact with the peasantry. But their relationship was not yet that of consultant and client. Moreover, despite assurances that medical care would be free, many inhabitants of the countryside still feared that public assistance would have to be paid for, or that the result of the government's intervention would be to load them with new taxes.[237]

ATTITUDES TOWARD THE MEDICAL PROFESSION

In addition to accessibility and cost, a third factor influenced a patient's decision on whether or not to consult a physician or surgeon: the degree to which the practitioner could inspire respect and trust. We tend now to see early modern physicians through the distorting prism of Molière's satire, and it is easy to assume that the population, like Toinette in *The Imaginary Invalid*, saw them as pompous and ineffectual frauds; discovering what its views actually were is far more difficult. It is undoubtedly true that medical Pyrrhonism was a commonplace of educated discourse in the seventeenth and eighteenth centuries in France and abroad. "Physicians kill as many as they save," the English clergyman Robert Burton wrote in his *Anatomy of Melancholy* (1621), adding that "many that did ill under Physicians' hands have happily escaped when they have been given over by them, left to God and Nature and themselves." Many educated patients, like Thomas Hobbes, would "rather have the advice or take physic from an experienced old woman, that had been at many sick people's bedsides, than from the learnedst but unexperienced physician."[238] In the mid-eighteenth century, the article "Médecins" in the great *Encyclopédie* dilated on the harm done by physicians and concluded that "it would have been more advantageous if medicine had never existed in this world." A decade later, the baron de Montyon suggested that it was an open question "whether medicine destroys more men than it saves," at least outside the major cities.[239] The eighteenth century, however, also celebrated the physician as hero, an image that Peter Gay has described as central to the Enlightenment's "recovery of nerve."[240] The *philosophe* La Mettrie (a medical man himself, it is true) praised medicine in these terms in the dedication of his celebrated *Homme-machine*:

Everything yields to the great healing art. The physician is the only philosopher to whom his country owes anything.... The very sight of him calms the blood, restores peace to an agitated spirit, and revives sweet hope in the hearts of unfortunate mortals. He announces life and death as an astronomer predicts an eclipse.

And even the skeptical Voltaire, who held that "regimen is better than medicine..., [that] for a long time, ninety out of a hundred physicians were charlatans..., [and that] Molière was right to mock them," reminded his readers that "it is nonetheless true that a good physician can save our life."[241] But literary evidence can easily be cited on either side of the question.

What of the population at large? The evidence is fragmentary.[242] Some reports from the late eighteenth century suggest that patients with money to spend were increasingly willing to pay physicians and surgeons. In 1788, for example, the municipal officers of Moitron in Maine noted that "the patients who enjoy some degree of material comfort summon the surgeons of Fresnay and Beaumont" (the one a bit more, the other a bit less, than 10 kilometers away). In much of the countryside, however, physicians were never well accepted. The subdelegate at Morlaix complained in 1772 that "we have cantons where they want neither physician nor medicine."[243] As one doctor noted in 1750, the physician or surgeon was summoned only when old wives' remedies had failed.[244] When the *médecin des épidémies* arrived in the villages following an outbreak of disease, the peasants often refused to cooperate with him. During one such episode in the diocese of Quimper in 1741, the physician Bernetz estimated that only 10 patients in 100 were following his instructions. And during an outbreak of dysentery at Combourg in 1773, a quarter of the patients were said to have died "for lack of confidence in medicine."[245] Why did the people so frequently reject the physician? Contemporary writers on popular usages returned time and again to this question. If peasants called in the veterinarian but not the physician, a correspondent of the Société Royale de Médecine suggested in 1780, "they give as a reason that since God watches over man, he needs nothing; whereas animals are subordinated to men, who [therefore] must succor them." Another observer, who visited the Alpes-Maritimes in the early nineteenth century, remarked that physicians were rarely summoned outside Nice and three other towns. "Everywhere I was told that the days of man were numbered, and that there would be neither more nor less; moreover, in many places, people are unable to pay physicians."[246] Leaving aside the obvious question of cost, how helpful is the notion of peasant fatalism – exactly like "the conduct of Mussulmans in times of plague," according to one correspondent of the Société Royale[247] – which runs like a leitmotiv through all the rhetoric on rural medicine? Devastating epidemics that decimated entire villages could indeed lead to a state of listless resignation. Yet peasants were not resigned to every form of suffering and incapacity; indeed, popular medicine was usually interventionist, although it was better equipped to deal with routine ills than with serious infectious diseases and was less likely than modern technological medicine to attempt to prolong the life of an obviously moribund patient. But to the peasant's way of thinking, although the physician might know a thing or two, he was unfeeling, and his intervention was unlikely to benefit the patient. An old saying from Ambierle in the Lyonnais proclaimed that a dog's tongue is as good as a physician's hand. "The front of the miller's ass is worth more than the arse of a physician," ran another proverb. And of course, "God cures, and the physician collects."[248]

The physician was not merely ineffective; his procedures were at best an affront to modesty and at worst a threat to life. Female patients often rejected male surgeons as obstetricians and even as general practitioners; one Breton physician noted that "peasant women are prudish and never summon *messieurs les chirurgiens.*"[249] Men and women alike found enemas indecent. And certain therapies, notably bleeding and purging, were considered debilitating. Peasants expected to be purged and perhaps bled at certain times of the year; but in general, popular therapies filled patients up, whereas official medicine, as it was sometimes said, emptied them from above and below. One Breton *médecin des épidémies,* dispatched by the intendant during the major dysentery epidemic of 1779, reported that many patients refused to take the "king's remedies," instead "gorging themselves with wine and spirits, preferring, they said, to die with a glass in their hand than with an enema in their behind." Others cooperated for a few days and then refused the purgative that the doctor had ordered

because, according to their false way of seeing things, they were being purged naturally to a sufficient degree. Medical knowledge is beyond the grasp of peasants as coarse as ours. To tell them that alvine [intestinal] evacuations are to be evaluated, not by the frequency of stools, but rather by the quantity and quality of each one, is an enigma for them. I have never been able to persuade them of this truth, and when I have administered several purgatives to them, it was without their knowing.[250]

Above all, though, rural populations of the eighteenth and nineteenth centuries dreaded going to the hospital; peasants had heard that "they" killed people there by giving them nothing to eat (as Balzac reminds us in *Le Cousin Pons*) or dispatched incurable patients with "eleventh-hour bouillons."[251] If the patient died, his body might be subjected to the further indignity of an autopsy – a prospect greatly feared, an eighteenth-century observer wrote, by "a coarse people, who ordinarily have more respect for the dead than for the living."[252]

Another source of peasant resistance, as François Lebrun has suggested, was the progressive "desacralization" of medicine.[253] In some cases, it is true, the modern official practitioner may have assumed the sacerdotal or magical prestige associated with many forms of prescientific healing. One physician at the end of the nineteenth century found that his patients took chips from his carriage, benches, and waiting room to use as talismans;[254] another, in the middle of the century, boasted that he had won the reputation of a witch in part of the department of the Rhône because he had worked so many wonderful cures.[255] More typically, though, the physician lacked charisma. Popular practitioners said to possess the healing gift could lure patients away from the regular profession; often they actively discouraged clients from consulting physicians. These prohibitions were in keeping with a number of folk medical beliefs, well documented for the nineteenth century, that impinged on the peasants' relations with official medicine. Certain magical remedies, for example, were thought to lose their potency if the patient received medical treatment; the effect of a novena might be spoiled if the patient consulted a physician.[256]

Moreover, the rural practitioner, unlike the nineteenth-century country doctor mythified in Balzac's *Médecin de campagne*, was often not well loved by the people, who saw in the faculty graduate a haughty bourgeois. Unpopular practitioners occasionally met with violence. The diary-cum-commonplace book kept by a minor official of the Parlement of Grenoble in the 1760's records an incident in which a physician who had mocked a philanthropic rival (a surgeon) was stoned by the populace.[257] A report from Poitou pointed to a less dramatic, but telling, expression of local hostility: when the *taille* (the basic direct tax) was levied, rural physicians were arbitrarily overassessed, a practice the writer attributed to pressure from unqualified rivals.[258] In rural society, the city-trained physician was often an outsider, an interloper, less trusted than the local curé or empiric. The *médecins des épidémies* dispatched into the countryside and many of the surgeons who worked under their direction were doubly handicapped, for they had not even settled in the vicinity. "The surgeons appear here in vain," ran the report from a region of Brittany afflicted by the *"maladie de Brest"* (probably typhus) in 1758. The peasants "do not want to make use of them; they do not want to take any remedies other than what the *recteurs* distribute to them, and provided that they have wine with it they are content."[259] An account of a conflict between a surgeon and a urinoscopist in eighteenth-century Normandy notes that the surgeon may have been resented as an *"horsain,"* or outsider.[260] In his classic study of the counterrevolution in the Vendée, Charles Tilly emphasized the precarious role of the Revolution's constitutional curés as intruders in the village community.[261] Physicians often labored under the same disadvantage.

The physician, of course, was an outsider of a special kind, a figure of authority; he was a representative of the university, with its ancient links to the Church and its more recent links to the state. Peasants in eighteenth-century France sometimes felt threatened by doctors, particularly the *médecins des épidémies* and other physicians actually in the employ of the government. They might seem spies, agents of the fisc, the arm of an alien authority intruding into a traditional and in many ways non-French society. Voltaire caught something of this attitude in a whimsical part of an article on government, published in the *Questions sur l'Encyclopédie*, in which he satirized France's irrational institutions. The passage tells the tale of a traveler whose host had refused him a drink because the "leaseholders of the kingdom" had deputed physicians to visit the cellars of winegrowers and set aside just the amount of wine they needed for their health. At the end of the year they returned, and if the unfortunate proprietor had exceeded his ration, he had to pay the hated "*trop-bu*" (excess drinking tax); the recalcitrant were sent to Toulon to drink seawater.[262] Distrust of the medical profession may also express deeper assumptions of popular political culture; the same reaction against hierarchy and authority that produced medical Protestantism in seventeenth-century England gave rise to medical republicanism in late-eighteenth-century and nineteenth-century France: the view that medicine belonged, not to the doctors, but to the people.[263]

To recapitulate: the regular medical network of the Old Regime was highly diverse and only locally and imperfectly organized. It might in fact be better described as a congeries than a network. For the eighteenth century, it is obviously misleading to speak of "the" medical profession, though the phrase remains a convenient shorthand for the surgical craft and the liberal professions of medicine and surgery considered collectively. The network, moreover, was as much inclusive as exclusive; its boundaries remained unclear. Without a uniform monopoly and a clear line between regulars and irregulars, the concept of illegal practice loses much of its meaning.

The social and economic status of practitioners varied widely; many could not live from their practice alone, particularly among the lower-level surgeons. Even with other sources of income (such as barbering), they were insecure enough to fear as well as resent competition from unauthorized practitioners. Empirics devalued the investment they had made in their training and reception, on which they expected a reasonable return.

Recent research, finally, suggests that licensed personnel were well established in the provinces by the late eighteenth century, at least in many parts of the North, the East, and the Midi. The medicalization of the countryside increasingly brought physicians and surgeons into contact with rural populations. Only the bourgeoisie and the more prosperous peasants and artisans, however, consulted them on a regular basis. The interesting but hypothetical calculations of the proportion of the population that might have seen a regular practitioner, given the number of practitioners and the size of a typical practice, almost certainly err on the high side. It was partly that physicians and even master surgeons cost too much; partly that the peasantry was slow to overcome its distrust of official medicine. The countryside, then, was not entirely abandoned to quacks, *maiges*, and witches; they, the surgeons, and the occasional physician could be rivals. But the medical profession had yet to win a substantial popular clientele.

2

The medical profession in the early nineteenth century

The transformation of the old medical network began some hundred years before Pasteur and the new technical prowess attributed to medicine at the end of the nineteenth century. The medical revolution that occurred in France during the late eighteenth and early nineteenth centuries has become one of the most extensively studied topics in the history of medicine, thanks in part to the fascination of the larger political events with which it was associated and in part to the prestige of the French clinical school, which made Paris, for a time, the medical capital of the world. Much has been written on the mutations of French medical education, institutions, and thought;[1] and yet social historians have given comparatively little attention to the implications of these developments for the profession.[2] This chapter traces the evolution of the medical occupations and suggests how France began to move from the diffuse medical network of the Old Regime toward a tight network and a sharper distinction between authorized and unauthorized practice.

THE REVOLUTIONARY DECADE

The medical reform movement that reached its climax in the 1790's was already well under way in the last decades of the Old Regime. The convergence of medicine and surgery has already been discussed in Chapter 1. "Enlightened" medical men, as they liked to style themselves, also addressed a wide range of other problems in medical education, professional organization, and public health; the question that most preoccupied them was how to make adequate health care more widely available to the population, especially in the countryside.[3] But it was the revolutionary debates over public assistance and medical education that clearly proclaimed medical reform a task for the nation, and the Revolution's leveling of the old corporate structures that cleared the way for a radical reconstruction of the medical field.

Medical reform, 1789–1791

The inadequacies of French health care inescapably formed part of the revolutionary agenda. In 1789, the *cahiers de doléances* complained of the lack of qualified personnel in the countryside, and some expressed the hope that publicly salaried practitioners might be established there to provide free treatment for the poor.[4] The early years of the Revolution saw a flood of proposals for reforming the "medical constitution" of France at the same time as its political constitution; most remained unpublished and were duly deposited in the archives of the Société Royale de Médecine or of the revolutionary assemblies.[5]

Michel Foucault has described two utopian visions, inherited from the medical Enlightenment, that informed the early revolutionary debates. In one, a Rousseauist fantasy most forcefully articulated by the Paris physician and future member of the revolutionary National Convention François Lanthenas (c. 1740–1799), the regeneration of society would restore mankind's primitive good health and make medicine itself unnecessary. The other placed medicine at the center of the program for social reform and imagined a system of public assistance that would make medical care available to all.[6]

This latter conception inspired a series of detailed projects. In 1789, for example, the Paris physician Noël Retz (1758–1810), editor of the *Nouvelles ou Annales de l'art de guérir*, proposed a system of free health care to the Estates-General. The Toulouse physician and future regicide Jean-Marie Calès (1757–1834), in a memoir written for the Société Royale, called for a public physician in each arrondissement, and a memoir to the National Assembly's committee on poor relief by Michel-Augustin Thouret (1749–1810), one of the Society's founding members and brother of the more celebrated revolutionary leader Jacques-Guillaume, suggested appointing cantonal surgeons in the countryside; in a major report to the committee, its chairman, the duc de La Rochefoucauld-Liancourt, advocated a system of cantonal physicians as well as surgeons. To solve the problem of funding such a scheme, Sabarot de l'Avernière urged in 1789 that public doctors receive a living (*portion congrue*) like curés, financed by income from confiscated Church properties. (Since the state took over the Church's charitable role in maintaining hospitals and assisting the poor, the great wealth of the old ecclesiastical corporations seemed the obvious source of financial support for what promised to be a major public enterprise.) Such proposals also typically recommended that local public health agents take over some of the functions that the hospitals and hospices had served in the relief system of the Old Regime, helping instead to care for the poor at home; indeed, such plans were usually linked to a broad program of dehospitalization.[7]

The Société Royale de Médecine began its own formal deliberations on the creation of a new medical system, and on 20 August 1790 the National Assembly invited it to submit a new code for the medical field. The Society's views on medical practice were first summarized in a report by Jean-Gabriel Gallot, which he read at the Society's session of 31 August. But the major statement of the Society's position appeared in November, when Vicq d'Azyr presented in its name a "new plan for a medical constitution in France." In an oft-cited overview of French medicine, the plan decried widespread abuses and lamented the poor state of health care in the countryside. On the question of medical organization, it attacked the corporate and particularist institutions of the Old Regime; local and exclusive privileges were "repugnant to the French constitution." It went on to call for the fusion of medicine and surgery and for a system of state-salaried cantonal physicians.[8]

The new push for medical reform in the fall of 1790 coincided with the creation of a special committee within the Constituent Assembly charged with health matters – the Comité de Salubrité. Questions of public health had initially fallen within the jurisdiction of the committee on poor relief, the Comité de Mendicité, founded the previous February. Joseph-Ignace Guillotin, the only physician member of that committee, believing that the interests of medicine were underrepresented, on 12 September asked for and obtained the establishment of a separate committee on health whose members would include a higher proportion of medical professionals and which could give more specific attention to the problem of "regenerating" medicine in France.[9] The new body (which Guillotin chaired) included the seventeen physicians who were members of the Assembly, together with an equal number of laymen. Gallot was appointed secretary, a move that underscored the links between the committee and the Société Royale de Médecine; on 6 October he presented the report that he had previously given to the Society at the end of August.[10] The Comité de Salubrité represented a bow in the direction of professional, rather than social, solutions to the problems of public health. True, the Comité de Mendicité had endorsed the appointment of cantonal physicians. But in the spirit of Turgot and his collaborator, the economist and reformer Pierre-Samuel Dupont de Nemours, it had emphasized home care for the sick and nonmedical measures for relieving distress and indirectly improving health, such as providing employment for the poor. And far more than the Comité de Mendicité, Guillotin's committee was concerned with the practice of medicine itself, as opposed to general issues of health and health care.[11] Prominent physicians were invited to testify, and the committee soon became a clearinghouse for proposals on medical reform.[12]

The conclusions that the committee drew from its examination of French medicine pointed in the same direction as the reform projects of the Société Royale; its proposal for a decree on the teaching and practice of medicine, which Guillotin completed in August 1791, markedly resembled the Society's *New Plan*. (The committee would willingly have reported its project earlier, but a decree of 13 October 1790 had barred it from making recommendations for medical education until a general project for national education, the work of Talleyrand and the Comité de Constitution, had been presented; in the end it was never formally debated.) The proposal called for joining medicine and surgery; medical practitioners would be allowed to work anywhere in France. Agencies of "health and assistance" in each department would have jurisdiction over questions relating to public health. Cantonal physicians would provide free care for the poor in their homes; and in addition, each town with a population greater than 4,000 would have one or more doctors for the poor.[13]

At the end of the month, however, when the Constituent Assembly was dissolved, it had failed to provide a new dispensation for medical practice. The Comité de Salubrité had no direct successor in the Legislative Assembly, which met on 1 October. The Comité de Secours, which inherited responsibility for public assistance, did not try to keep alive Guillotin's ambitious and potentially very expensive project for medical assistance.

The assault on medical institutions, 1792–1794

The primary contribution of the Legislative Assembly and the Convention to medical reform was negative: without implementing the reforms debated by the Constituent Assembly, its successors hastened the dismantling of the institutional legacy of the Old Regime. The revolutionary principles of individualism and equality before the law led the legislators to oppose the privileged bodies, or corporations; in March 1791, the Constituent Assembly abolished the guilds and proclaimed professional freedom.[14] This measure in effect deregulated medical practice, and subsequent legislation specifically attacked the colleges and faculties and abolished the Société Royale de Médecine. The old hierarchy, the old corporate titles of doctor-regent, master surgeon, and even physician, were legally swept away; all practitioners would be brothers and equals as *officiers de santé* (health officers). For a decade, anyone could, in principle, set up as a medical practitioner after having paid the necessary *patente*, or tax on industry. At no other time in modern French (or European) history have the legal distinctions between professionals and irregulars been so blurred. Practitioners from the margins of the old regular network flourished in these conditions. (The bonesetter Dumont Valdajou, for example, received enthusiastic support from the Commune of Paris; following a report from L. Bailly, deputy from Seine-et-Marne, the National Convention ultimately voted in early 1794 to resume payment of his annual stipend, which had ceased in 1790.)[15] Empirics of all descriptions plied their trade almost without hindrance.

The anticorporate legislation of 1792 and 1793 also seriously disrupted medical education without entirely ending it. The Faculty of Caen enjoyed a special dispensation (although as Cabanis – the physician-philosopher turned legislator – later emphasized, this authorization applied to the professors as individuals, rather than to the corporation). Between the Year III (1794–1795) and the Year VI (1797–1798) of the French revolutionary calendar, Caen received thirty-nine doctors. Besançon also remained active; it had seventy students in the Year VI. Some other faculties functioned clandestinely, on a reduced scale, at least into the spring or summer of 1793; Montpellier conferred its last degree on 28 Nivôse Year III (3 April 1793). Some surgical instruction continued as well (at Rennes, for example, until March 1795). In Paris, though, only the school of surgery at the Hôtel-Dieu, under the direction of Pierre-Joseph Desault, maintained a program of instruction. And even where teaching continued, the regular reception of candidates lapsed until the Year VI (1797–1798); during the decade 1793–1802, the number of practitioners received was only a seventh of the total for the previous decade.[16] Pharmacy, however, fared considerably better; after a brief hiatus, the field was exempted from the antiguild legislation of 1791. The Paris college weathered the storms of the Revolution and re-emerged in the spring of 1796 as the École Gratuite de Pharmacie (decree of 3 Floréal IV/22 April 1796).[17]

The restoration of medical education

The renewal of medical reform that followed the revolutionary hiatus of 1792–1794 reflected different priorities from those embodied in the Enlightenment proposals of 1789–1791. Public assistance dropped into the background. The new program proposed to fill the gaps left by the collapse of Old Regime institutions, but without reviving these institutions themselves. The emphasis was, first of all, on medical education – in part because the French army was losing its health officers at an alarming rate and needed trained personnel to replace them. Of 2,700 *officiers de santé* in the army in 1793, almost 1,000 had been lost by the spring of 1794. Examinations for new officers revealed serious deficiencies in the qualifications of the available candidates and the need for effective educational institutions.[18]

In July 1794, the Committee of Public Safety called on the doctor and chemist Antoine-François de Fourcroy and the specialist in legal medicine François Chaussier to design a new system of medical training. Chaussier did most of the actual work. The project was debated five months later (27 November–4 December). In his presentation to the Convention, Fourcroy declaimed against the prevalence of ignorant doctors and charlatans; for five years, he told the legislators (with some exaggeration), the medical arts had had no masters and the sciences had declined. The project called for a central school of health in Paris, uniting medicine and surgery, with a program of clinical instruction that recalled the Société Royale's project of 1790. As a concession to local interests, the Convention added health schools at Montpellier and Strasbourg; the modified proposal passed and was slated to go into effect almost immediately, in January 1795. The three *écoles de santé* (which in October became part of a larger system of special training institutions and were renamed *écoles spéciales de santé*) provided the foundation for the national system of official medical instruction in nineteenth-century France. As expected, the capital dominated the provincial centers.[19]

Medical instruction did not in itself guarantee that qualified practitioners would be distinguished from the unqualified, though it was obviously a precondition. The military health services had a special interest in the certification of their *officiers de santé*, and in Fructidor Year IV (August 1796), the Directory called for a formal procedure for admitting health officers to practice (*mode de réception*). In 1798, the government authorized certificates of qualification for those who had passed three examinations at the *écoles spéciales de santé*, but this measure was still far from a general system of licensure.[20]

The Convention had intended the legislation on the *écoles de santé* only as a stopgap measure until a definitive law on education, licensure, and the regulation of medical practice could be adopted and put into effect. The legislators of the Directory period tried repeatedly to arrive at a permanent solution, but without success.[21] Their failure can be ascribed in part to political disruptions of the legislative process and in part to procedural difficulties and lack of consistent leadership: the various bills had a succession of different reporters. The greatest obstacle, however, was a striking lack of consensus on what form the new educational system and the reorganized profession should take. In general, provincial legislators resisted the complete unification of medicine and surgery.[22] Local attachments also led them to fight Parisian dominance and to argue over the number and distribution of the schools.[23] The 500 scholarship students at the three existing schools seemed insufficient; one proposal called for establishing "special schools" in ten cities and, in addition, a "secondary school of medicine" in each department.[24] The traditional medical centers struggled to reestablish instruction on the foundations of the old faculties and schools. In the meantime, some medical men and local administrators made temporary arrangements independent of the central government; Toulouse, for example, established an *école provisoire de santé*, and some *administrations centrales* in the departments arranged for candidates to be examined.[25]

Implicit in the argument over the form and scale of medical training was a profound disagreement over the structure of the new profession, which was to dominate the debate on medical legislation under the Consulate. If medicine and surgery were united (as Cabanis, Thouret, and Fourcroy had insisted), who was to replace the old lower-level surgeons, who had often been the only regular practitioners in the vicinity? For Cabanis, the answer was clear: it was better, he argued in 1798, for the countryside to have no practitioners than deadly ones. For others, though, a second order of practitioners remained indispensable. The deputy Louis Vitet, for example, a medical graduate of Montpellier and former mayor of Lyons, argued in the same year that it was unreasonable to try to banish to the countryside highly trained professionals who had spent large sums on their education.[26]

THE MEDICAL PROFESSION AND THE LAWS OF VENTÔSE AND GERMINAL

Continuing disagreements over the organization of the new profession delayed final action on medical reform for three years under the Consulate, although political conditions were now more propitious than under the Directory: the Constitution of the Year VIII, adopted the month after Bonaparte's coup d'état of November 1799, gave the government considerably more initiative and influence in the legislative process. Between 1800 and 1803, the councillors of state (including Fourcroy and the chemist Jean-Antoine Chaptal, a medical graduate of Montpellier who was named Minister of the Interior in 1800) examined five projects on medical education and practice. The discussion of education yielded the first result, a law of 11 Floréal Year X (1 May 1802) authorizing three new medical schools. Three unsuccessful projects would have provided for examinations and licensure. The last, in the Year X (1801–1802), distinguished two grades of physicians: doctors, who could practice anywhere, and health officers, who would be able to practice only in rural areas or in towns with fewer than 2,000 inhabitants; twenty "practical schools" would be established to train the second-order physicians. The project that finally won approval (introduced on 7 Pluviôse Year XI, or 27 January 1803) retained the basic two-tier model. Fourcroy and two other councillors spoke for the bill before the Corps Législatif on 7 Ventôse (26 February). On 16 and 17 Ventôse (8–9 March), Thouret and Michel Carret (a surgeon from Lyons) presented the bill to the Tribunat. The one real point of controversy remained the distinction between doctor and health officer. Carret defended the government's position, arguing that the inhabitants of the countryside had simpler mores and purer morals than city dwellers and therefore had less complex diseases, for which a more rudimentary training sufficed. The resolution carried unanimously, and the Tribunat designated Thouret, Carret, and Louis-Alexandre Jard-Panvillier (a physician from Niort) to report the result back to the Corps Législatif. Jard-Panvillier again defended the *officiat* (the health officer's credential): the lower order would be content in the rural districts, and the less expensive credential would have the added advantage of making a medical career accessible to young men from modest backgrounds. The result was a foregone conclusion, and the bill won final approval on 19 Ventôse (10 March) by a vote of 216 to 6.[27]

The law of Ventôse provided for the first time a uniform licensing system for all of French medicine. "Doctors of medicine" and "doctors of surgery" were to study for at least four years at a medical school and pass a set of examinations there that qualified them to practice throughout France. At least two of the examinations had to be in Latin. The *officiers de santé*, in contrast, were to receive a largely practical training reminiscent of the instruction given to country surgeons in the Old Regime. They might study for three years in a medical school if they wished, but two alternative routes were open to them: six years of service under a doctor or five in a hospital. The health officers would normally be examined not by a medical school but by a medical commission (*jury médical*) in each department, composed of two physicians named by the First Consul and a commissioner from one of the six medical schools. (In the departments with medical schools, the professors would form the jury.) Certain stipulations limited the scope of the health officer's practice: he could not work outside the department in which he had been received – a barrier to the ambulatory practice so common in the Old Regime – and he could not perform a major operation unless supervised by a physician. (Nothing in the legislation, however, limited the *officiers de santé* to the countryside, where in theory they would practice.) A separate title of the law provided for the examination and reception of midwives. With the exception of dentistry, the principal medical occupations of the Old Regime were included under the three rubrics of doctor, health officer, and midwife.

These provisions would apply to the next generation of medical men. The legislation also had to establish procedures for coopting existing practitioners into the new system. Physicians and surgeons received under the Old Regime and personnel in conquered territory annexed to France who had been licensed by foreign universities would continue to practice as in the past. Those who had set up their practice after the old corporations had been abolished had two options. If they had trained as physicians or first-order surgeons but the Revolution had prevented them from being officially admitted, they could sit for the examination for the doctorate; if they had been established for ten years as lower-level surgeons but had similarly been prevented from seeking formal reception, they could take the examination for the *officiat*. Both groups enjoyed a two-thirds reduction in the examination fee. (Students who had completed the program in the health schools of the Year III received a 50 percent discount, and practitioners who had served for two years as military or naval health officers first class would pay even less.) Alternatively, under article 23, anyone who had begun a practice after the suppression of the universities and had worked for at least three years could get a certificate from the subprefect of his district based on an attestation from the mayor of his commune and two local notables; this certificate would take the place of the health officer's diploma.

The doctor or health officer now enjoyed a special right to practice, not by virtue of membership in a faculty or college but as an individual whose competence had been certified by a medical bureaucracy. Apart from the restrictions placed on health officers, he could practice as he chose and where he chose; to this extent the revolutionary freedom of the practitioner was conserved. The various privileges of the Old Regime were not revived; the once blurred line between regular and irregular was now sharper; and in theory at least, the law of 1803 divided practitioners into legal and illegal, those within the state network and all the rest.

Pharmacy

The regulation of pharmacy followed in the month of Germinal, not long after the law on medicine. On the 10th (31 March 1803), Fourcroy presented his second project to the Corps Législatif. The bill called for six schools of pharmacy; the Paris College, a vestige of the old corporatism, would be abolished. The pharmaceutical profession would be divided, like medicine, into two tiers. The schools of pharmacy would examine candidates for the first order, who would obtain the right to practice anywhere in France. The medical juries, assisted by four pharmacists, would conduct examinations for the second order, whose members would be able to practice only in the department for which they had been received. (The juries would also examine herbalists.) The pharmaceutical monopoly was still not complete; although it was fenced off from the encroachments of spicers and other tradesmen, health officers were allowed to act as *propharmaciens* and furnish remedies in places where no pharmacist was available, though they could not actually set up shop. (Pharmacists, on the other hand, could not stand in for medical men.) Still, no one could acquire a *patente* as a pharmacist unless he had been duly received. The Corps Législatif, after hearing Fourcroy's reading, voted to transmit the bill to the Tribunat for discussion.[28]

In his report to the Tribunat (17 Germinal or 7 April), Carret defended several of the project's departures from tradition. If the College of Pharmacy were not abolished, it might become necessary to restore the medical colleges and other corporative institutions. Some critics, Carret acknowledged, might also object that widows would no longer be able to take over their late husbands' pharmaceutical practice. Here the male legislators' view of the other gender appeared explicitly (as it had not in the case of medicine): widows must be barred qua women, since pharmacy was "less a trade than a learned profession," which females could not expect to master. On the

19th of Germinal, the project on pharmacy was the question of the day; when no tribune asked to speak, it was put to a vote and approved unanimously. Three members returned the project to the Corps Législatif, where Carret defended it on the 21st (11 April); the bill passed by a vote of 202 to 4.[29]

Pharmacy finally emerged in the nineteenth century as a distinct profession, separate from surgery, on the one hand, and from the spicer's trade, on the other. The nineteenth century had no surgeon-apothecaries (though some pharmacists encroached illegally on the medical field). With the exception of the *propharmacien*, the laws of the Year XI insisted on the principle, lost to view during the Revolution, that the same person ought not to dispense what he had prescribed. Nor did apothecaries mix pharmacy with essentially unrelated forms of commerce; the *pharmacie-droguerie* existed during the nineteenth century, but not apothecary-spicers, although the law of Germinal did not explicitly separate the occupations.

The reorganization of the medical occupations in theory created an all-embracing national network in which every qualified practitioner could find his place, but it was still not a fully unified profession. Four legal groups could be identified: the physicians and first-order surgeons of the Old Regime; the old lower-level surgeons; the new doctors of medicine and surgery; and the *officiers de santé*. (Doctors of medicine and surgery followed the same basic program, though the former would take the last of their five examinations in *la clinique interne*, the latter in *la clinique externe*.) In 1803, practitioners received under the Old Regime still constituted more than half of the profession.[30] A more basic distinction, though, separated an upper order who could practice anywhere (new doctors and old physicians and first-order surgeons) from a lower order that could not (health officers and lower-order surgeons). Some of the old *licenciés* in medicine dropped into the lower order.

In establishing the *officiat*, it is true, the legislation of the Year XI did not exactly re-create the old distinction between physician and surgeon (though in the early part of the century, *officiers de santé* were commonly referred to as surgeons). Health officers were less-well-trained physicians, "*simples médecins*" as they came to be known – not members of a different profession. Indeed, the courts held that the *officier* could legally style himself a physician; only the title of doctor was beyond his reach.[31] Still, the continued existence of a lower grade, following the unification of medicine and surgery, bothered many physicians, and its long persistence (access was closed at the end of the century, but individual health officers remained active; there were still 200 in 1931)[32] preoccupied medical reformers as much as, or more than, the problem of illegal practice.[33]

Almost immediately after the law of Ventôse was adopted, the Ministry of the Interior began to receive pointed criticisms of its provisions.[34] Conservative practitioners objected to the blurring of distinctions recognized under the Old Regime.[35] They complained, too, of a lapse in standards. In 1808, P.-J. Marie de Saint-Ursin charged that since the "revolutionary disorganization," only surgeons practiced, to the detriment of the physicians and of public welfare.[36] Professional decline, it was said, not only lowered the quality of care that the official personnel provided but also constituted an implicit invitation to charlatanism.[37]

It soon became clear that for many members of the medical elite, the *officiat* represented an unacceptably dangerous compromise with empiricism and *impéritie*. Some objected to the title of health officer, in which they saw an illogical legacy of the Revolution that was unfortunately likely, with its suggestion of an official government function, to impress and mislead an ignorant clientele. (During the Restoration, one reformer proposed restricting the title to military personnel and calling civilians *bacheliers* if they had not received the *licence* or the doctorate. Another proposal suggested giving the title of "empirics" to a new, more modest second order – not because they resembled charlatans, but because they would have received a purely empirical training in domestic medicine and surgery.)[38] More generally, the critics castigated the health officers, like the country surgeons of the Old Regime, for their ignorance, their *impéritie*, and their presumption (one thinks of Charles Bovary in Flaubert's novel). Those who had taken advantage of article 23 of the Ventôse law and had obtained certificates in place of diplomas drew the most stinging attacks; in the countryside, it was said, farmers readily gave attestations to untrained empirics and medical students with a few months' training.[39] Overall, the health officers' level of training and even of general education seemed unacceptably low. In the early years of the Restoration, the medical society of the department of the Eure (to cite only one example) received a memoir from a physician who had collected a set of certificates, prescriptions, and letters of advice said to have been written by health officers, among other ignorant practitioners; they revealed an astonishing ignorance of anatomy, physiology, pathology, and the French language.[40]

Many commentators would have abolished the *officiat* altogether. In 1804, a letter to the Minister of the Interior (Chaptal) called for good apothecaries to take the place of health officers, especially those who practiced as *pro-pharmaciens*; the populace, dazzled by the health officer's title, took his drugs and were poisoned by them. (The writer himself was not well educated; his syntax was tortured and his hand practically illegible, and he begged the minister to read him "not for my rural style but for the truth.")[41] In the same year, the physician Royer of Nogent-sur-Seine, who had spent a large part of his long career promoting a program for a rural medical service, urged the government to replace the *officiers de santé* with a system of salaried and uniformed cantonal physicians, assisted by curés trained as physicians' aides – an innovation, he argued, that would destroy "ignorance and charlatanism."[42] In the following years, the chorus of protest mounted.[43]

Proposals for new legislation

Even under the Empire, the defects of the law of Ventôse prompted the government to consider possible reforms. A commission of the council of the Imperial University, headed by the naturalist Georges Cuvier, was appointed in 1812 to consider the problem of the *officiat*. Although its members contemplated the possibility of cutting off further receptions of health officers (as did the Council of State), their discussions soon focused on ways of improving training and making the examinations before the medical juries more rigorous. In November, a project was presented that called for creating "secondary schools of medicine" in the major hospitals, where all candidates would have to spend three years; several provisions of the project, however, drew sharp criticism from medical men with a vested interest in the existing system, and it failed to be adopted.[44]

The legislative achievements of the Consulate and the educational system of the Empire bore the marks of the Napoleonic settlement; order was reestablished in the medical field, but not the corporations and privileges of the Old Regime. With the restoration of the Bourbon monarchy, a number of influential ultraroyalists hoped not only to reform the profession, eliminating the *officiat*, but also to return to the old organization of medical education and practice, breaking up the Napoleonic university and once more separating medicine from surgery.[45] This program of medical restoration seems to have reflected the sentiments of at least a vocal conservative minority within the profession. One admiring monarchist (or opportunist), Dr. Édouard Lemaître, later wrote that "the restoration of French medicine, which dates from the days of the Bourbons' entry into France, and the elimination of abuses in medical practice... will be, with the Charter [of 1814], one of the greatest blessings that can inspire in Frenchmen true feelings of love, attachment, and gratitude toward the descendants of Henri IV." His colleague François Plantié, a graduate of the old Montpellier medical faculty, composed a treatise on medical anarchy in which he argued that all courses and theses should be in Latin.[46] Other physicians reiterated the complaint that fusing medicine and surgery had lowered standards in the profession, since no one could master all its branches.[47] The surgeons, for their part, chafed at the ascendancy of the Paris Faculty of Medicine; one group of practitioners in the capital urged the king to restore the old College of Surgery and the Royal Academy of Surgery.[48]

Following the Hundred Days and the Second Restoration, two prominent surgeons emerged as leaders of the revisionist campaign. Louis XVIII's First

Surgeon, Father Élisée (Marie-Vincent Talochon, 1753–1817), a Brother of Charity and former surgeon-in-chief and professor of surgery at the Charité hospital of Grenoble, pleaded for the independence of his profession. Another Ultra surgeon, Jean-Théodore Marquais, former principal surgeon of the Paris Charité, denounced the health officers and called for separate surgical teaching.[49] The two served on a royal commission on medicine and surgery formed in November 1815; Marquais, with the support of a narrow majority, wrote a report along the lines that he and the First Surgeon favored.[50] But so radical (and potentially unpopular) a move proved unacceptable to the government, and in the end the Council of State simply recommended raising standards of training for health officers (1820).

The proposal to separate medicine and surgery seems to have died with Father Élisée in 1817. During the remainder of the Restoration, the debates on medical reform revolved around the question of the *officiat*; a significant body of opinion still held that the rank should be eliminated and the medical juries abolished.[51]

After the succession of Charles X in 1824, two ministers presented further proposals for medical reform.[52] In 1825, the Minister of the Interior, Jacques-Joseph-Guillaume-François-Pierre Corbière, assisted by Cuvier, now chancellor of the University, drew up a bill that would have retained the *officiat* but required four years of study in "secondary schools of medicine." The medical juries would be abolished and the certification of new health officers entrusted to the schools. Although the deputies approved a modified version of this proposal, it encountered stiff opposition among the peers. The reporter of the commission that considered the bill in the upper house was the comte de Chanteloup – better remembered as Jean-Antoine Chaptal, the former Minister of the Interior under the Consulate, who had directed the initial implementation of the law of Ventôse. Chaptal was now dead set against the *officiat*, which he considered a failed experiment. He proposed instead that the secondary schools serve only to prepare students for the faculties. All candidates would complete a full course of training; those who lacked the two baccalaureates (in the arts and the sciences) required for the doctorate would become *licenciés*, who (unlike the health officers) would be able to practice anywhere in the kingdom. The legislative session ended shortly afterward. In the new session of 1826, Corbière presented his bill once more. Chaptal remained the reporter for the peers and now put forward an even more extreme counterproposal: the secondary schools would be entirely eliminated and three new faculties of medicine created. By a narrow majority, the chamber accepted his recommendation. Faced with a stalemate, Corbière dropped his project.[53]

In 1828, the vicomte de Martignac, Secretary of State for the Interior (and Prime Minister in all but name) proposed an even more drastic reorganization of the medical field. This time, however, the government deliberately involved the profession in the debate. In September, Martignac put a series of questions to the Académie Royale de Médecine (which had been founded in 1820); the academicians, however, were unable to agree on a response. In November, a ministerial circular asked the prefects and subprefects to make recommendations based on their familiarity with local conditions. As in 1789, provincial medical men sent proposals for reform to Paris, inundating the ministry and the Academy. In a more unusual step, Martignac allowed the Paris profession, which had begun meeting to discuss the question, to form an official commission; in December, more than 300 medical men, perhaps a third of the medical personnel in the capital, took part in electing its members. Provincial physicians formed their own commissions. In July 1829, the Paris body issued its recommendations: abolish the *officiat* and create two new faculties in the provinces.[54] The debate in the medical press rose to fever pitch, but the government had more pressing concerns. The Martignac ministry fell in the summer of 1829; the Polignac ministry plotted to contain the growing influence of the liberal opposition; and in July 1830 revolution erupted, toppling the Bourbon monarchy and burying the medical reform plans of 1828–1829 in the rubble.

Subsequent attempts at medical reform under the July Monarchy (notably in 1845–1848) and under the Second Empire bore little fruit; perhaps the most significant change came in 1854, with the abolition of the medical juries that had examined candidates for the *officiat*. It was the Third Republic that transformed medical education and, after protracted debates and several false starts, reorganized the medical profession in 1892. The new legislation closed access to the *officiat*, eliminated the title of doctor of surgery, and required certification for dentists.[55]

WHO WAS COOPTED INTO THE NEW SYSTEM?

The legislation of Ventôse represented an uneasy compromise between the aspirations of medical reformers and the needs of two major interest groups: the received personnel of the Old Regime and practitioners who had begun to work after the destruction of corporative regulation. If rigorously applied, it would have excluded from the new medical system the large number of practitioners who had worked on the fringes of the old regular network and the least well trained of the revolutionary health officers. But it was not so applied, and article 23, together with the other loopholes and defects in a hastily drafted piece of legislation, favored accommodating many less than fully qualified practitioners.

The new requirements were slated to go into effect on 1 Vendémiaire Year XII (24 September 1803). At the end of August, in a ministerial circular to the prefects, Chaptal addressed some of the ambiguities of the legislation.

He urged a narrow construction of article 23 in terms that suggested, among other things, the reformers' misogyny. The law, he directed, should not be interpreted to authorize things generally recognized as abuses, such as medical practice by "women, empirics, persons practicing another profession, or at public entertainments, [or] by men who are dishonored or reproved by public opinion." Practitioners received under the three-year rule needed the same evidence of having completed the appropriate studies as those regularly admitted as *officiers de santé*. Ideally, they should have trained with a physician or surgeon, or in a school; if questions remained about their qualifications, they could perhaps be placed under the supervision of a well-known physician or surgeon who could answer for their work. Military health officers of the second and third classes could easily get certificates from their superiors; in other cases, the medical juries could be of some help.[56]

In practice, the business of certifying and registering legal practitioners proved a slow and formidable task. The cases of lower-level practitioners had, in theory, to be individually reviewed to determine whether they would be admitted as *officiers de santé* or rejected as mere empirics. The results, however, were not as the drafters of the legislation, or Chaptal, had hoped. Some apparently qualified practitioners refused to be examined; at Gambsheim in the Bas-Rhin, for example, a former surgeon of the Army of the Rhine pleaded that he could not afford the examination fee.[57] In subsequent years, some new health officers, like the lower-level surgeons of the Old Regime, practiced for many months before actually taking their qualifying examination.[58] In addition, many persons "practicing another profession" (as Chaptal put it) continued to practice medicine as well without worrying very much about their legal status; the idea of coopting into medicine the ablest members of such occupations as barbering that were traditionally linked to medicine or surgery was slow to take hold. During the Empire, the cantonal physician at Soultz-sous-Forêts (Bas-Rhin), after denouncing a large number of incompetent barbers, singled out two "who, on the basis of their knowledge, would indeed be worthy of the title of *officier de santé*," but they were not officially licensed.[59]

At the same time, some patently unqualified practitioners were beyond the reach of the medical juries because they held certificates under article 23 or other credentials. Officials could not ordinarily refuse to register practitioners who possessed regular diplomas. (The exceptions involved egregious miscreants like Jean Picard, who had been received as a surgeon at Nantes in 1770 but was accused of immorality, drunkenness, and associating with a quack who attributed even the simplest illnesses to witchcraft; he was rejected primarily in order to hamper the activities of the empiric, whose prescriptions he had been signing.)[60] Disputes over these cases sometimes arose among the jury, the prefect, and other authorities. In 1808, for example, the medical jury of the Nièvre refused to admit a practitioner named Clément on the grounds that he was ignorant, despite a diploma issued in 1777 by a lieutenant of the King's First Surgeon. The Minister of the Interior, however, ruled that he must be allowed to practice.[61] One critic of the law of Ventôse cited the case of an empiric who had failed even to obtain a certificate from the subprefect under article 23 but had allegedly secured an order from the minister allowing him to be instated.[62]

The one point on which there seems to have been general agreement was that women should not be admitted. At Reuilly in the Indre, for example, Marie Daux hoped to practice as an *officier de santé*; she had been a Sister of Charity and then a "health officer" during the Revolution, and had practiced for seventeen years. She had secured the necessary attestation from the subprefect and local notables; the only question was whether a woman could practice medicine. The prefect refused his permission, and the Minister of the Interior declined to overrule him.[63] The legal grounds for excluding women from the medical field were in fact debatable; the Ventôse law did not address the issue, and even the Chaptal circular, which did, could be construed to mean simply that women could not benefit (as Marie Daux hoped to do) from article 23.[64] So long, however, as the medical schools continued to close their doors to women, they were effectively relegated to work as midwives or to illegal practice; the first Frenchwoman to become a doctor of medicine received her diploma in 1875.[65]

Trained practitioners heaped scorn on the certification system. Writing toward the end of the Empire, in a work on the influence of the Revolution on medicine, Dr. Sébastien Serrières recalled the triumph of quackery during the Revolution, when (he said) some physicians actually burned their diplomas and "ignorance replaced merit." Since then, medical education had improved, thanks especially to Fourcroy and Thouret, but the regulation of medical practice had not. The trouble, he suggested, began with the certification process itself: the examination of candidates was defective or nonexistent.[66] In the Seine-Inférieure, the health officer Poulain complained of abuses in the application of article 23; although the prefect had written a letter calling for greater stringency, this text was not regarded as law.[67] Medical juries met irregularly, and practitioners took advantage of the delays to secure "temporary" authorizations. In the Loiret, René-Georges Gastellier, physician-in-chief at the municipal hospital of Montargis and a member of the departmental jury, complained that the jury had not received a single *officier de santé* and that no juries functioned in the neighboring departments of the Cher and Loir-et-Cher.[68] Many similar cases could be cited. In the isolated and mountainous department of the Hautes-Alpes, for example, the medical jury held only three sessions before the system was abolished in 1854. Its last meeting took place in 1818; the occasional candidates who presented themselves in later years did not seem to justify convening the commission, and so they were directed to the administrative seats of other departments.[69]

In view of the gap between theory and practice, it is worth examining more closely how the certification system functioned, and in particular how it dealt with the fringe members of the old medical network – the experts, charitable persons, and privileged empirics. Would they be coopted or excluded?

Experts

The medical elite distrusted experts. Well into the nineteenth century, specialization in the treatment of a single disease or disorders of a single part of the body was considered a distinguishing mark of the charlatan, like the "celebrated physician-oculist" Dr. Guénon de la Chanterie, who advertised his services in Paris cafés and restaurants during the Restoration.[70] Ideally, anyone who treated or operated on patients should have undergone the normal general training – even the *mohel* who circumcised baby boys in the Jewish communities of Alsace.[71]

Some certified experts nonetheless survived from the Old Regime. During the Revolution, moreover, specialists had readily taken out patents as health officers; two executioner-bonesetters did so at Nîmes, for example, as did an executioner at Vannes.[72] In the nineteenth century, all types of traditional specialists and members of ancillary occupations continued to practice – bonesetters, dentists, ocular surgeons, lithotomists, herniotomists, truss makers, pedicures, masseurs, and the rest, joined by the growing tribe of "magnetizers" that had emerged from the mesmerist movement. (In the Bas-Rhin, for example, an official list of practitioners in 1812 included a bathkeeper as well as two dentists.)[73] Many such practitioners used anomalous titles unrecognized in current law, such as *botaniste expérimenté en médecine*, or *chirurgien-herniaire-mécanicien* (one of the latter actually objected to a provision of the law of Ventôse restricting the practice of "surgeons" – as he put it – to the department in which they had been received);[74] a fashionable "wigmaker-pedicure" named Arpon did a thriving business in secret remedies.[75] As in the past, itinerant oculists (some, but not all, regularly qualified) continued to couch cataracts, like Dr. L'Habitant, whose work in 1806 received the approval of the prefect of Ille-et-Vilaine.[76] Unqualified persons set themselves up as podiatrists, masseurs, or bathkeepers and then offered to treat medical conditions. In 1811, for example, a certain Royer began to work in the Loiret as a bathkeeper and in effect sought official recognition by offering to pay the professional tax on his new occupation as a therapist.[77]

Similarly, the trade in surgical appliances, despite efforts to regularize it and subject it to the oversight of the medical profession, persisted in the hands of small-time artisans eager to supplement the limited income from their recognized occupation. In 1820 the prefect of the Rhône, acting on a complaint from the "surgeon-truss makers" of Lyons, carried out an investigation of cutlers, buckle makers, and other unauthorized manufacturers of surgical trusses. His probe turned up 24 illicit practitioners of the trade, including 2 makers of *culottes*, a barber, 2 wigmakers, a wigmaker-dentist, an herbalist, 2 dentist-hernia operators, and an umbrella maker. (The licensed *bandagistes*, for their part, traded in more than trusses; toward the end of the Restoration, a prominent *bandagiste-herniaire* of Lyons sold not only such surgical articles as milk pumps, ear trumpets, condoms, and devices to discourage masturbation, but also suspenders, socks, gloves and other clothing accessories.)[78] None of this should surprise us; laws and institutions change more easily than long-established patterns of behavior.

What happened to all these people? Some were prosecuted. But others, particularly in the early years of the Ventôse regime, were tolerated or even received official recognition in their specialties through administrative fiat (since the law nowhere explicitly acknowledged their callings); some medical juries actually consented to examine experts solely in their special fields. Thus in the Doubs, a former executioner of Besançon was listed on the official rolls as a *chirurgien-bandagiste-herniaire*, despite the objections of the local physicians and surgeons.[79] A celebrated Breton bonesetter, Jean-Baptiste Guillard of Bécherel, was authorized to continue practicing while awaiting formal reception (although the prefect of Ille-et-Vilaine warned him that he could not give drugs without a physician's prescription).[80] In the Hautes-Alpes, another *rhabilleur* received the right to practice in 1807 (although it was later denied to his son).[81] A similar case was settled in the Loire the following year. Claude Péricard petitioned the emperor for authorization to practice, claiming that he and his father had worked as bonesetters for fifty years. To bolster his case, he submitted petitions from thirteen local mayors and deputy mayors; the mayor of his own commune, Lentigny, cited Péricard's services to the poor and the difficulty of traveling to consult a surgeon when none lived in the neighborhood. The minister ruled that Péricard should be inscribed on the list of *anciens rebouteurs* – that is, those who had been allowed to practice under the old dispensation – though the law in fact recognized only old-style master surgeons. If he had practiced before the Revolution, the minister suggested, he enjoyed a certain prescriptive right; the law was meant to destroy "abuses" due to revolutionary anarchy, not to hurt the old practitioners, even those authorized only by custom.[82] In the Loire-Inférieure, an Italian oculist named Rabiglia was similarly able to obtain authorizations from various mayors, subprefects, and prefects; he claimed to have been received as a surgeon in 1786. When the medical jury arrived, he moved on; finally, in 1837, when he was an old man, the jury (probably out of compassion) admitted him as a "consulting physician for eye diseases," but forbade him to operate.[83] And at Bondy, near Paris, an oculist claimed in 1848 to have been received eighteen years earlier as a specialized *officier de santé*, despite the medical corps's hostility to the "ophthalmological specialty."[84]

Despite this less than rigorist climate, no specialist could be sure of reception (or of toleration, if he decided to practice without official authorization). Some traditional experts bowed to the expectations of the times and secured regular credentials. In 1820, for example, the departmental executioner of the Yonne and his brother, a "student-executioner" in Seine-et-Marne, were said to be only one examination shy of qualifying as health officers.[85] At Sillans, in the province of Dauphiné, the Jollans family had for two centuries enjoyed a reputation as skilled bonesetters; in 1817 the celebrated hygienist François-Emmanuel Fodéré, who was professor of legal medicine at Strasbourg, met a member of this dynasty who had decided to enroll at the faculty.[86]

A still more curious case was reported at Bordeaux. In 1819, it was said, a minor had inherited the post of executioner from his father; his uncle Caron then stepped in and temporarily fulfilled his obligations both as executioner and as bonesetter. After a local physician denounced Caron, an investigation revealed that he held a medical degree.[87] This makes a nice story. The truth, which can be reconstructed from archival documents, is even more interesting. Caron (or rather Scaron, a native of Sardinia) was chief executioner of the Gironde until 1815; in August of that year he was replaced by his predecessor's brother and was apparently slated to take up the post of executioner at Versailles in 1816. The following year he received a health officer's diploma from the medical jury of the Seine. He claimed to have studied for six years under a doctor in the provinces and to have spent twenty years in practice; this latter statement, if true, would have made him eight to ten years old at the outset of his career. In 1818 he obtained a medical diploma from the Paris faculty through a ruse, apparently using the credentials of a J.-B. François Caron de Bretonnaux of the Somme, who had taken the five required examinations between 1808 and 1812 but had not presented a thesis.[88] Whatever the strength of (S)caron's bona fides, the story shows the importance attached to obtaining the new certification; under the Old Regime, he could have taken his case before the Parlement of Bordeaux and perhaps won a decree in his favor *as an executioner*.

In the second quarter of the century, several court decisions reaffirmed the intent of the Ventôse legislation: bonesetters, oculists, and other specialists were deemed to practice surgery, not some other profession. (The question remained sufficiently uncertain, though, to figure in the questionnaire that Martignac sent to the Academy of Medicine in 1828.)[89] Dentists remained the single notable exception, partly on the grounds that their work

consisted mainly of pulling teeth, which did not seem to require any particular address or to put life and limb in danger, and partly for more obscure
legal reasons. In an 1827 case, the Cour de Cassation (supreme court of
appeal), noting that Old Regime dentists had been received exclusively as
experts (rather than masters) under the 1768 surgical letters patent, ruled
that they did not practice the medical art "in its entirety" – an argument
that could equally well have applied to the other specialties.[90] Indeed, since
the profession required no diploma, the courts held that even a woman
might be allowed to practice it.[91] But by the same token, no formal certification could be issued to dentists; in 1837, a ministerial circular criticized
the practice by some juries of giving special examinations in dentistry.[92] It
should be added that since few popular dentists practiced that art alone,
they sometimes found themselves half within and half without the law, like
a certain Cartin, who in 1819 was allowed to practice as a dentist but not
to sell remedies and toothpaste as he had hoped.[93]

Charitable persons and the clergy

The Edict of Marly had specifically provided that unauthorized persons
who practiced medicine could be prosecuted even if they never accepted
payment. The law of Ventôse contained no such clause, but since it did not
explicitly exempt charitable practice from its provisions, the courts interpreted its silence to mean that even nonmercenary practice was illegal. As
in the past, though, the jurists were willing to make allowances for routine
first aid, and in particular for the work of "charitable persons, especially in
the countryside, where obtaining medical assistance is time-consuming and
difficult, who have given some initial advice to the patient, indicated some
remedies to use for the time being, or put the first dressing on an injury."[94]
Such practices were widespread; the physician Armand Trousseau, in a series
of lectures on empiricism delivered in 1862, suggested that there was "no
château, unless it has been purchased by commoners [!], which does not
conserve its traditions and its book of recipes."[95] Indeed, this custom continued in some places into the present century.[96] As in the Old Regime,
some amateur practitioners went much further; the writer George Sand,
for example, described in her memoirs how, out of devotion to the poor,
she became a "country doctor" and wore herself out in their service.[97] Some
had a reputation as specialists; thus the *châtelains* of an estate at Saint-Dolay
(Morbihan) treated ophthalmia.[98]

   Nevertheless, the seigneur or notable who doctored his peasants enjoyed
only toleration, not the quasi-official recognition he might have won in the
Old Regime. Many of the more active charitable practitioners were told
that however laudable their motives, they would be prosecuted if they did

not desist from treating patients. Like the surgical experts, a few took out regular diplomas as *officiers de santé* in order to practice legally.[99] The status of the clergy and religious who dabbled in the healing arts was more problematic, for successive governments chose to accord them a limited place in the health care system. The revolutionary Convention had alienated the old hospitals' endowments and hounded out many of the nursing sisters. The Directory, however, reestablished the hospitals under municipal jurisdiction; the Consulate then reconstituted the endowments and in December 1800 authorized the nursing orders to return (though some refused and preferred to work illegally outside the hospitals). A year later, an instruction of the Paris Medical School advised that it would be acceptable for them to use tisanes and other easily prepared remedies as part of their work for hospices and home relief agencies, though no more. (The law of Ventôse was not taken to abrogate this policy, which was more an attempt to define the limits of nursing care than an authorization to practice medicine.) In May 1805, a ministerial circular from Jean-Baptiste de Nompère de Champagny on public assistance during rural epidemics asked the prefects to encourage the Sisters of Charity to aid the sick poor. In September of that year, the Council of State confirmed a minor role in charitable medicine for priests as well; they were not, however, to charge fees, prescribe remedies, or practice medicine on a regular basis, even charitably. (Some, however, exceeded these bounds, among them émigré priests who had fled the persecutions of the Revolution and now returned to France, still faithful to the ways of the Old Regime.) The following year, the minister Emmanuel Crétet ruled that the sisters could use the internal hospital pharmacies to aid the poor without fear of prosecution under the law of Germinal.

The Bourbon Restoration heightened support for the medical activities of the Church, though even this regime never went so far as to recognize ecclesiastics as full-fledged physicians. In 1828, Martignac issued a circular that allowed the nursing orders to prepare and sell certain magistral remedies; despite an unfavorable court decision in 1830, this instruction was not annulled until 1840.[100] Religious dispensaries were to remain the primary source of illegal pharmaceutical practice in nineteenth-century France; in most places they outnumbered legal pharmacies.[101] Physicians bitterly criticized those priests and nuns who, as they saw it, interpreted the government's toleration of their role in public assistance as a license to practice medicine.[102]

Empirics

Under the Old Regime, some empirics had practiced by virtue of special privileges or authorizations; a few were received as surgeons or purchased medical diplomas from the University of Orange. The legislators of the

Year XI presumably intended to remedy this abuse by certifying only qualified practitioners. And yet, it was charged, many empirics had shown evidence of three years' practice and thereby obtained diplomas under article 23 of the Ventôse law.[103] At Château-Salins (Moselle), for example, the surgeon Vimont denounced a urinoscopist, Pilot, who worked at Sornéville. Vimont held a doctorate from Strasbourg and had served as a surgeon first class in the French army; Pilot had been admitted as an *officier de santé* by the subprefect of Château-Salins. Vimont could not understand how Pilot could have satisfied the requirements of the law, "as if an empiric could invoke any provision of a law whose essential goal is to purge society of all kinds of medicasters"; humanity would suffer if a certificate from a "bribed mayor" sufficed to justify the practice of medicine. In Ille-et-Vilaine, the subprefect of Fougères went so far as to suggest that the two notables asked to provide attestations under the terms of article 23 should be drawn from the ranks of the physicians and surgeons, because laymen were favorable to charlatanism – an impracticable suggestion, because the notables had to come from the commune where the candidate resided.[104]

It would be difficult to assess with any precision the credentials of candidates actually admitted as health officers. Some empirics with little or no formal training did petition for prefectoral certification or even appeared before medical juries. But for every success (like Pilot's), which inevitably attracted comment, there seem to have been several more obscure failures. At Troyes, for example, the empiric Raget petitioned unsuccessfully in 1804 to become an *officier de santé* for the Aube; he identified himself as a urinoscopist. In 1806, a certain Mas of Écouché appeared before the jury of the Orne, armed with certificates; but the jury, finding that the certificates were by "ignorant persons" and that Mas himself was unqualified, rejected him and asked the prefect to warn the mayor of Écouché about possible violations of the law.[105] Examples of comparable rigor can be found in the West, a stronghold of popular medicine. The jury at Vannes rejected the empiric Guillaume, who had worked at Questembert since before the Revolution and had been prosecuted for unauthorized practice. And at Rennes in 1806, the jury refused four out of eight candidates for the *officiat*, turning away a resident who claimed to have done good work with simples; it also forbade an herbalist to work on the grounds that in a small market town like his, the trade was conducive to charlatanism.[106]

Many of the disputes over licensed empirics actually involved ill-qualified or unscrupulous surgeons who had been received before the revolutionary hiatus or were authorized to practice under article 11 of the Ventôse law because they were former military health officers. The complaints recall the commonplace criticisms of marginal surgeons under the Old Regime. In 1806, the director of the Paris medical school denounced a "charlatan," Vital Gigun, who distributed handbills on the Pont-Neuf, the traditional gathering place of quacks and hucksters. Gigun had in fact studied at one of the old colleges of surgery and had spent nine years as an army surgeon; he had been admitted to practice, quite correctly, under article 11. In the Bas-Rhin, Jean Hildebrand of Biblisheim, who had been received as a surgeon under the Old Regime, was threatened during the Restoration with indictment for "charlatanism" [sic]; he had already been prosecuted, despite a certificate obtained in 1804 from the subprefect of Wissembourg. And in the Yonne, the subprefect of Joigny in 1811 sent the prefect a certificate of disability signed by an *officier de santé* called Laurent-Théophile Michel, who held a certificate by virtue of article 23 of the Ventôse law. Michel called himself a "corresponding member of the central committee of the City of Paris" and a "surgeon practicing major operations" (which health officers were forbidden to perform except under a doctor's supervision). This practitioner's conduct, in the subprefect's view, showed "the marks of charlatanism."[107]

We have the details of a confrontation between a dubious surgeon and a medical jury in the case of Chevrier, a practitioner of Neuvy-sur-Loire (Nièvre), who, not yet having met the requirements for certification as a health officer, presented himself to be examined in August 1805. According to the jury, he was asked about "putrid fever," the current name for what in most cases was probably typhus; although the questions were kept simple, Chevrier could not answer any of them, and his case was continued to the following session. When he returned, Chevrier balked at submitting to further questioning, maintaining that a man such as he ought not to be examined. After all, he enjoyed the confidence of the inhabitants of his canton. In the past, he had made trials of his skills that had perhaps cost the life of some of his patients, but now his knowledge was "consolidated." He defied the jury to prevent him from "completing his fortune" and offered to pay the fee for the health officer's diploma. He then presented his version of his case to the prefect in a rambling letter that betrayed his real lack of education. The jury, he complained, received "surgeons" only for the sake of fees. (There was perhaps some merit to this charge; each examiner pocketed 24 francs for every candidate admitted, 16 for those who passed two examinations, and 8 for those who passed only one.) In his own examination, he had merely failed to characterize a putrid fever, "an illness very useful to a physician who does not know what to say about a long illness"; the jury had sent him away until the next day and asked for 200 francs. He thought that under the law he was entitled to a diploma; he had been a surgeon for eleven years and had certificates to show it. If necessary, he concluded, he would obtain justice from the medical school at Paris. The prefect, who already had him under surveillance, took alarm at the prospect of one of his local malcontents traveling to the capital and warned the authorities there.[108]

No doubt many *officiers de santé*, especially among those who had been admitted under article 23, were guilty of *impéritie*, as were many pharmacists and midwives (like one, received by a medical jury, who was said to have asked whether a uterine hemorrhage could be stopped by making signs of the cross, tying a red ribbon around the patient, and giving her a piece of toasted bread in wine).[109] The evidence, however, does not support the charge that quacks benefitted in large numbers from article 23. For all its deficiencies, the new medical network was tighter than the old.

To make the network still tighter, both professionals and administrators seriously considered stripping already licensed but inept or unscrupulous practitioners of their titles. In 1807, the prefect of the Cher suspended a certain Pirot, called Pierrot, as a health officer after receiving a complaint from a physician who was a member of the medical jury; although Pierrot had a diploma, the doctor submitted that he was "grossly ignorant" and should be examined before being allowed to practice again.[110] Some medical juries attempted wholesale reassessments of *officiers de santé* practicing by virtue of certificates; they were usually well along in their careers, and some refused to submit to the indignity of an examination. In 1813, 21 of 42 candidates examined at Rennes were beneficiaries of article 23 whose credentials had been questioned; and at Vannes, the jury for the Morbihan barred four health officers from practicing.[111]

Such decisions were generally supported in Paris, although the government seems never to have issued a binding directive and did not itself always follow a consistent policy. In 1803, the prefect of the Belgian department of the Ourthe, acting on a complaint from a local physician, reported that some persons had received certificates as *officiers de santé* who did not deserve them. Chaptal replied that if the information against them was correct, the certificates should be annulled. Illiterates should not be allowed to practice medicine, however many years of experience they might have accumulated; the mayors and notables responsible for certifying established practitioners under article 23 should judge their character and capacity, and refuse certification to those who had never studied medicine. Nor, he added, should ecclesiastics be allowed to practice as health officers; before the Revolution they had been forbidden to practice medicine and surgery.[112]

In 1806, the Minister of Justice intervened in the case of Marin Fagot, whose name had appeared on a list of medical practitioners prepared for the arrondissement of Mamers (Sarthe) in 1803. Fagot called himself a health officer, but his claim was said to rest on a certificate from "another charlatan." The minister asked the *procureur-général* of the Sarthe to have his name struck from the rolls unless he conformed to the law. In the same year, the prefect of the Haut-Rhin, acting on orders from the Minister of the Interior, barred two health officers guilty of *impéritie* from practicing. And yet the minister (Champagny) refused to allow the prefect of the Doubs to deprive an ignorant practitioner of his title, since he had received the necessary attestations from two notables.[113]

In August 1809, Joseph Fouché, Napoleon's wily Minister of General Police (then acting Minister of the Interior), seized upon a technicality to invalidate the credentials of a large group of practitioners holding certificates under article 23; those who had waited longer than the three months prescribed by the law of Ventôse to register their certificates would now have to undergo an examination. But it was still not clear whether practitioners whose papers were in order could be challenged simply for *impéritie*. The following year, the prefect of the Loiret queried François Chaussier, professor at the Paris faculty and president of the medical jury, on the cases of two possibly incompetent health officers who held their titles by virtue of article 23; could they continue to practice without undergoing an examination? Chaussier suggested that they should be temporarily suspended until the examination, and that a decree should be issued to make the practice general. The matter was eventually referred to the Minister of the Interior, but his response is not indicated.[114]

We have fuller information on the case of Schmitt, a celebrated urinoscopist of the Eifel region of Germany (in territory annexed to Napoleonic France as the department of the Sarre). The 1804 list of official practitioners in the Sarre named him as an *officier de santé*. In the autumn of 1808, however, a physician of the neighboring department of Rhin-et-Moselle denounced him for violations of the Ventôse law. The prefect relayed the information to his colleague in the Sarre, noting that Schmitt apparently traveled around the entire region. A second complaint came a year later from Vetten, another physician of Rhin-et-Moselle, asking that a commission be formed to look into Schmitt's practice. The prefect again forwarded the report to the Sarre, requesting this time that Schmitt be removed from the list of authorized practitioners.[115]

The prefect of the Sarre referred the case to his own medical jury, whose members replied that they themselves, during the last examination of titles, had called Schmitt "the scourge of suffering humanity." Schmitt had recently submitted a new request for recognition, in which he claimed twenty years' experience; he included attestations from 2 notables, 10 mayors, and a subprefect. The jury observed that Schmitt was unfortunately within the letter of the law; indeed, its own response had virtually been dictated by its president, who showed a recent letter from the Minister of the Interior disapproving the rejection of several "charlatans" who had the prescribed certificates from two notables. Although Vetten's report seemed entirely justified, the jury felt powerless to act. Nevertheless, the prefect, arguing that Schmitt was ignorant and lacked adequate credentials, ordered his name struck from the list of health officers. A copy of his decree went to the Ministry of the Interior. Despite the jury's misgivings, the minister, the

comte de Montalivet, approved the decision in January 1810, observing that
the government had always intended to prevent the abuses that might result
from misapplication of article 23.[116]

In June, Schmitt's son protested the ruling. The prefect defended his
decision on the grounds that Schmitt was illiterate and that the only document supporting his title to practice was not an original but a copy, which
had apparently been obtained through fraud from the former government.
In short, the man was a charlatan. Neither his reputation in the countryside,
cited by his son, nor certificates in his favor were reasons to withdraw the
decision against him. Schmitt, however, persisted in his quest for recerti-
fication. By the summer of 1811, his representatives in Paris had obtained
and submitted to the minister 3 petitions, from as many cantons, signed
by 20 mayors, and 14 notarized certificates from 59 deputy mayors and
notables of other communes. It was all to no avail; the case remained closed,
and the elaborate documentation was returned.[117]

Appeals for authorization

The Schmitt case illustrates the persisting belief in a privilege system that
would bypass the normal licensing procedures, much as special authorizations had circumvented the corporate monopolies of the Old Regime.
Practitioners who failed to win approval in the ordinary way petitioned
their prefect or the Minister of the Interior, advancing arguments that they
hoped would legitimate their practice, even if they conspicuously failed to
meet the formal requirements laid down by the law of Ventôse. They spoke
of their well-attested skill; of their services to the poor or the state; or even
of their own need – a throwback to the latitudinarian attitudes of the Old
Regime, when the right to practice a little medicine or peddle a few remedies
had been widely accepted as a form of outdoor relief for the deserving poor.
Nineteenth-century jurisprudence rejected such claims; even royal warrants,
which were issued freely during the Restoration, were considered essentially
honorific and no excuse for illegal medical practice.[118] Still, many empirics,
charitable persons, and others beyond the pale of official medicine assumed,
especially in the early years of the Ventôse regime, that the government
could grant the right to practice medicine at its pleasure.

Some practitioners hoped to assume a regular title but wished to be
excused from courses or examinations, from the baccalaureate in letters
needed for the doctorate, or from the minimum age requirement.[119] In Paris
a certain Contrastin, who said he was a surgeon, asked to be examined
without taking the courses stipulated by the law. At Angers the director of
the botanical garden asked to be received as a doctor of surgery without
being examined; the minister reminded him that he would have to study
in the medical schools and pay the prescribed fees. A self-styled *officier de*

santé at Richelieu (now in Indre-et-Loire) asked permission to continue his work in medicine and pharmacy. He was sixty years old and had practiced as a pharmacist and botanist for fifteen years; this was his only resource, he said, for supporting his family. And at Chartres, an empiric named Rochefort boasted of forty years of miraculous cures and asked the Minister of the Interior to admit him as a health officer. That official refused, observing that medicine had to be distinguished from "the abuses of ignorance and charlatanism."[120]

Other suppliants asked in effect for special authorizations that would allow them to practice legally, but outside the regular system established by the law of Ventôse. Some of these petitions came from practitioners working in the penumbra of the old medical network, whose claims might well have been recognized in the eighteenth century but who now found access to the medical field closed off. Prominent among them were surgical experts who had been denied the title of health officer. Thus the Minister of the Interior received an appeal from an ocular surgeon and rejected it because he lacked general medical qualifications. The claims of the executioners of Loir-et-Cher and the Isère were similarly dismissed. The first, Ferey, protested that he used no surgical instruments but only reduced fractures and dislocations and used ointments to treat rheumatism and sores; executioners, he maintained, had always had the right to do so, as several decrees of the Parlement of Paris indicated. His Grenoble colleague, Jean-Baptiste Demorest, used balms to treat skin diseases. In both instances, the minister invoked the law of Ventôse as grounds for denying special authorization, although in the first case comte Portalis indicated that the executioner needed to be received before he could practice, whereas in the second, Crétet held that the executioner's status had always been regarded as incompatible with the profession of surgery.[121]

Another survivor of the old medical network, François-Antoine Maillet, an itinerant surgeon born in 1757, took great pains to distinguish himself from quacks who peddled nostrums from the stage; this sort of work was beneath him, he informed the prefect of the Yonne, although he did distribute circulars to announce his arrival in a new town. Like some other old operators and empirics whose practice had been engulfed by the new wave of health officers, Maillet saw himself as a victim of the Revolution. Some years later a fellow operator, named Guillot, was bold enough to draft his own authorization, which he submitted to the prefect of the Aube in 1828. This official-looking document, written in the prefect's name, identified Guillot as a native of Troyes living at Bérulle amd described him as an ocular surgeon who had operated on poor blind people; he had certificates from surgeons and mayors and from a physician of the Faculty of Medicine of Strasbourg. "Given that he has no other means of existence," the document would have allowed him to continue his practice, although it stipulated that he must be accompanied by a physician – an authentic-sounding touch, though far removed from anything allowed by the law. In a covering letter to the prefect, the empiric repeated that he had no other means of support and added, as a final claim to legitimacy, that the king had previously given him money. The prefect, who found it "strange" that Guillot should himself have written the text for his signature, refused his approbation.[122]

Still another pretender, in a new twist on an old theme, maintained steam baths at Nancy where he treated skin diseases with sulfur fumes and aromatics. The proprietor, an American named Hart, said that he had bought a privilege for Nancy from the inventor of the baths, a man with the suspiciously appropriate name of Galès (*gale* is the French word for scabies); he described himself as a former American naval surgeon and a member of the Society of Medical Instruction in Paris, and falsely advertised that he had been authorized by the prefect.[123]

Other petitions arrived from distraught empirics and remedy vendors who had long been accustomed to toleration or recognition. From Bétheny (Marne), the elderly practitioner Rousselet sent a crudely penned letter to the Minister of the Interior, asking to be excused from the formalities of the Ventôse law. He had studied plants, he said, until 1757, when he served in the French army; after leaving military service, he had studied urinoscopy. He could treat "scorbutic chancres," the bites of sick animals, and other disorders. Only two months before, ten persons had been bitten by dogs, and two had died; he had sent a memoir to explain his treatment and asked that a member of the medical jury come to his residence to evaluate his work. He knew now, he said, that his report had not been accepted because he lacked a diploma; but since he never left his home, he believed that this formality did not apply to him. Rousselet closed his petition by asking the minister to decide his case; but the latter dismissed the appeal with the curt notation, "requires no action."[124]

Self-proclaimed charitable practitioners and ecclesiastics among the petitioners are often hard to distinguish from the empirics. In an appeal to Napoleon, a Madame Le Plénier submitted that "surgery" for the poor was her only occupation after her fortune in revolutionary paper money had evaporated; she claimed to have practiced for forty years and to have received bouillon, wine, and remedies to distribute to her needy patients, as well as a small stipend for herself. The Minister of the Interior referred this case to the prefect of Maine-et-Loire, who in turn consulted the medical jury. The jury said no. At Les Molières, near Limours (Seine-et-Oise), the tenant farmer Béguin claimed that he provided free care to the poor when the professionals had abandoned them. He boasted of a good knowledge of simples, which he gave for chills, injuries, and ulcers, according to what his inspection of the patient's urine indicated. Two surgeons had criticized him, although the exercise of his talents involved no "trade or merchandise." He had certificates, but he was prepared, if necessary, to undergo an examination. The minister's reply invoked the legislation of Ventôse and Germinal and informed him that he was unconditionally obliged to submit to the examination.[125]

The problematic status of the clergy in the new medical network prompted petitions for special approval from ecclesiastics whose charitable medical activities had provoked opposition from local regular practitioners – sometimes, it is true, because they went well beyond routine first aid. At Oulchy-le-Château (Aisne), Charles-Marie Denis, who claimed to have treated the poor for eighteen years, had recently met with opposition from the profession. He asked for authorization to continue his work; if necessary, he would submit to an examination and pay the fees for the "free practice of medicine." In the Ardennes, not long after the Ventôse law went into effect, the priest Delvincourt inquired of the Minister of Justice whether he might continue to give advice and help. He had studied medicine at Reims and had been a curé since 1783. The Church, he argued, had approved a role in healing for its priests, and under the Old Regime the government used to give them boxes of remedies to distribute to the poor in the countryside. The minister answered, however, that he must submit to the regular examination.[126]

Some more ambitious ecclesiastics had well-developed specialties; they asked, in effect, for approval as experts. Pignot, a resident of the department of the Indre, hoped to be allowed to continue his treatment of sores. Despite the intervention of his brother, who described himself as a graduate of Montpellier and a member of the departmental medical jury, the minister refused his approbation, citing the Ventôse law – though he held open the possibility that Pignot's practice might be considered a "simple act of humanity" and left it to the prefect to decide whether or not to prosecute. In the Manche, a group of mayors submitted a petition on behalf of another priest, Hamec, citing his success in treating ruptures, deformities, and illnesses that the physicians (as the cliché went) had abandoned; according to them, he never accepted a fee. In support of their request, they pointed to an old decree of 1737 in the custom of Normandy, cited by the Minister of Cults in 1806; but the Minister of the Interior replied that Hamec must conform to the law of Ventôse.[127] In the diocese of Versailles, the curé of Étiolles, Father Bin, clearly saw himself as a physician manqué. "Family reasons," he wrote, had compelled him to become a churchman rather than a medical man, although he knew medicine "from nature." Now seventy years old, he had helped the poor for more than forty years, treating especially scrofula and epilepsy. His superior encouraged him, he said, and regular practitioners sometimes referred patients to him; yet he had recently been barred from practicing. The minister replied that he could not make an exception to the law of Ventôse; it was up to the prefect of Seine-et-Oise to judge whether distributing a few remedies in simple cases would be considered medical practice.[128] Very occasionally one hears of a priest or pastor who seemed to want to become a full-time practitioner of medicine. A certain Vaubaillon, of Landigou (Orne), announced to the Minister of the Interior in 1812 that he could cure several diseases (epilepsy, scrofula, hemorrhoids, fluxions of the blood, loss of blood . . .), although he had not studied medicine or anatomy. He added that he no longer "preached the gospel" and hoped to be more successful in the cure of bodies than of souls.[129]

Many of the various petitioners asked less for a legal title than for protection against harassment by regular practitioners or immunity from prosecution, much as they might have asked for protection from the corporations under the Old Regime. The curé Hugon complained about the "so-called *officiers de santé*" who had annoyed him, dismissing them as "ignorant or greedy." Sudan, a practitioner at Morteau (Doubs), saw himself in 1805 as the victim of the jealousy of his "colleagues." He claimed to have studied at Montpellier in 1778 and to have practiced at Morteau for twenty years. The place was in a mountain valley; only he had "distinguished" himself by performing cures there. His colleagues not only were threatening to deprive his family of "all resources," they also seemed to wish to force the inhabitants to do without the services of a medical practitioner, or else to entrust themselves to "a physician of two days trained and licensed during the storms of the Revolution." This was not the first time, he recalled, that he had been troubled by colleagues resentful of his success. A similar incident had occurred in 1786; on that occasion, however, he had received the support of the local aldermen, the special procureurs, and the principal inhabitants. In the Seine-Inférieure, the practitioner Valmory accused the subprefect of Dieppe of conspiring with local physicians and surgeons to prevent him from practicing. His skill was not in question, he said, but his opponents, narrow formalists all, invoked the law of 19 Ventôse. Thus he had come to Paris to escape the incessant importunities of the poor, who begged him for his services.[130]

The petitioners characteristically opposed the selfish interest of the profession to the larger interests of the communities whose needs they served; when possible, they supplied testimonials from satisfied patients and benevolent local officials to suggest that, whatever their legal status, they really did do good. The sort of popular support on which such practitioners could call appears in the case of Claude Dufay, a charitable "botanist" at Nemours, who had been arraigned before the *tribunal correctionnel* (the court that heard cases involving lesser criminal offenses) at Fontainebleau. Dufay wrote that he had special knowledge of the properties of plants and their saps and had helped the poor for more than twenty years; he claimed to enjoy the confidence of the inhabitants of twenty communes. A second petition, this one signed by some fifty residents of the region around Nemours, expressed regret that the surgeons and health officers had denounced Dufay. The petitioners insisted that he had a patent as a botanist for the years XI and XII (1802–1804) and had conformed to article 3 of the Ventôse law, which concerned practitioners received under the Old Regime. The formalities prescribed for physicians, surgeons, and health officers, they argued, did not apply to botanists. Why he had not produced his certificates they could not say, but they urged that he be allowed to continue his practice, while recognizing that it was difficult to reconcile "humanity" with the "particular interests of the physicians, *officiers de santé*, and surgeons."[131]

Even more impressive was the popular acclaim that surrounded Christophe Petitgand, a joiner of Maizières (between Lunéville and Sarrebourg in the department of the Meurthe), who had an extensive practice as a bonesetter and was convicted of illegal practice during the Restoration. In 1824, a petition signed by almost 200 inhabitants of Maizières asked the prefect to authorize him to practice as a charitable *rebouteur*. (According to the census published two years earlier, Maizières was a village of 293 households, comprising 1,139 souls; Petitgand appears to have won the confidence of a significant proportion of the adult inhabitants.) No surgeon lived nearby. The petitioners pleaded that a bonesetter was needed in the agricultural districts they inhabited, "where people handle carts, work around horses, and climb on high stacks of sheaves and hay, etc., [and where] accidents are common." The number of bonesetters, they said, had diminished since the Ventôse law, because of fear of prosecution for illegal medical practice. Petitgand was too good to lose; he even corrected the mistakes of official practitioners. The *rebouteur*'s cause received further endorsements from the mayors of ten surrounding communes, some nearly 9 or 10 kilometers distant, and from a lieutenant-general of the royal armies in the district.[132]

On the whole, the authorities ignored appeals that their counterparts a few decades earlier might have taken to justify the petitioners' claims. In the case of Petitgand, the prefect remained adamant, holding that the bonesetter would have to submit to an examination by the medical jury if he wished to practice; he asked the subprefect of Château-Salins to have the *gendarmerie* keep an eye on him. The very evidence that unqualified practitioners cited to legitimate their activities could be turned against them. So, for example, the traditional rhetoric might invoke a healer's great age for two reasons: as an index of experience and as evidence of special economic need, since he could not be expected to learn a new calling. But an administrator could reply, as a prefect did in the Schmitt case, that the empiric's advanced age was all the more reason to proscribe him, since it would have sapped his mental faculties. And in the end, as the prefect of the Meurthe pointed out in the case of Joseph-Isidore Grillet, who in 1827 asked to be excused at least temporarily from the examinations, the law of Ventôse made no provision for such exemptions; even if the prefect were to "authorize" him, the courts could still prosecute.[133]

Not that the medical bureaucracy remained completely insensitive to the plight of the neediest unqualified practitioners. In 1818, for example, an elderly German named Retler, who described himself as a "provincial herbalist," defended himself against accusations of illegal medical practice by saying that, infirm and unable to work, he could subsist only on the proceeds from the sale of a tisane and a purgative prepared according to recipes left to him by his wife. The Paris Health Council, in a report to the prefect of police, rejected Retler's plea but added that "an old foreigner, an octogenarian reduced to indigence, will arouse Your Excellency's compassion, and that, limiting [yourself] to depriving him of the dangerous trade that he practices, [you] will protect him in his misery."[134]

The authorities of the early nineteenth century, like the eighteenth-century "enlightened physicians," separated the domains of professional licensing, patronage, and public assistance, which, in their view, the traditional rhetoric on medical practice badly confused. The state might see that basic wants were satisfied, including those of both needy professionals and needy empirics, but the right to practice a profession involving the well-being of the public would depend on minimal competence, as attested by legal certification.

The persistence of toleration

This description of the tight medical network needs to be qualified, however. Even if under the new medical regime unqualified practitioners were refused formal privileges or authorizations, many enjoyed the equivalent of the Old Regime "tacit permission": they were allowed to work unmolested. One significant loophole was the lack of a rigorous definition of medical practice; not only dentists but also masseurs, podiatrists, orthopedists, and others who might sometimes treat medical or surgical problems could hide behind their primary (and unregulated) occupation. Moreover, the distribution of secret remedies, which the Société Royale de Médecine had ultimately hoped to ban, remained legal. A decree of 25 Prairial Year XIII (14 June 1805) allowed the sale of such remedies if they had been previously authorized or approved by a physician, continuing the Old Regime tradition of permitting, while attempting to regulate, this highly profitable trade; a new campaign in 1810 to reform the commerce in secret remedies by publishing all useful formulas and proscribing the rest proved a failure. In theory, an approbation for a proprietary remedy did not confer on the owner the right to practice medicine or pharmacy. Thus, in February 1810, Napoleon authorized the preparation, advertising, and sale of an "antipsoric essence," following trials at the Paris maternity hospital and the hospices of Lyons, Lille, and Saint-Denis, but it was to be made available only in pharmacies and on the prescription of a regular practitioner.[135] In practice, however, few proprietors of secret remedies could resist playing the physician.

Moreover, the administrative apparatus that Napoleon fashioned from the revolutionary bureaucracy did not operate efficiently at the local level. Mayors and even some officials further up the hierarchy connived at or encouraged the medical activities of persons not formally included in the newly defined medical profession. As has been seen, the central government itself moved in the same direction where the clergy were concerned. With the coming of the Restoration, the trend toward toleration gathered new momentum; the Bourbons had no great commitment to defending the prerogatives of a profession that had not, on the whole, rallied to their cause.

Municipal officials looked with a benign eye on the work of local practitioners whom they knew and trusted. In a report of 1812 on illegal practice, the mayor of Feurs (Loire) had only praise for the occasional practitioner Cartéron, one of the "best proprietors" of the commune of Jas. In 1818, the mayor of Seignelay in the Yonne hesitated to deprive the Polish woman who practiced medicine there of her means of existence, especially since she treated the poor gratis. The prefect, in a fulminating reply, pointed out that her practice was strictly forbidden by law and that the mayor should recognize free treatment of the poor as "one of the usual tricks that empirics and charlatans use to abuse the credulity of the people and seduce the authorities."[136] Near Bourbon-Vendée (as La Roche-sur-Yon was known under the Restoration), François Sibenaler, an itinerant dentist with a patent for what he called his "eau de Cologne," found a benevolent patron in the mayor of a local commune; although he urged him to obtain a diploma, the official nonetheless prolonged his stay. And at Auxerre, although the police commissioner purported to deal strictly with charlatans, he said that he allowed those with "diplomas from the faculties[!]" to sell Swiss vulneraries; a local physician had also approved a "maritime absinthe" for worms, which was being peddled at the municipal market (1821). The mayor justified this policy on the grounds that when the vendors' papers were in order, "we cannot be stricter than they are in Paris."[137]

Even more highly placed officials, though theoretically charged with enforcing the law of Ventôse, willingly tolerated illicit practice when the circumstances seemed to warrant it. A prefect might wink at the activities of an empiric where no licensed personnel were available.[138] In the Loire-

Inférieure, a certain Ordonneau of Bouguenais practiced as a "health officer," not only in his own commune but also at Nantes and Clisson, although
his name did not appear on the official roster; he had a room at Pont-
Rousseau where he worked every Saturday. The subprefect of Paimbœuf
hesitated to interfere on the grounds that if Ordonneau were educated, he
probably did some good; it was even possible that he might have some sort
of credentials.[139] Another empiric at Nantes, Olivier, a self-styled *officier de
santé* who used simples to treat epilepsy and other diseases, published a list
of his cures, prompting the prefect to ask the police commissioner for
information. The certificates that Olivier was able to produce greatly impressed the commissioner, and he found that the man was unlike other
empirics – despite his unfavorable reaction to "the very vulgar physique,
elocution, and manners of this *officier de santé.*"[140] Even flagrant empiricism
could find protection; two brothers circulated through the various departments, for example, winning approval for their treatment of tinea with a
special remedy consisting of cinders from their hearth; and in the most
notorious case involving a proprietary remedy, the Ministry of the Navy
approved Leroy's drastic preparation even after the Academy of Medicine
had denounced it.[141]

The medical profession repeatedly protested this laxity, but without effect. In 1818 an essay submitted for a competition sponsored by the medical
society of the Eure criticized rural mayors who authorized charlatans to sell
remedies from stages in the marketplace. Ten years later, Dr. Ulysse Trélat,
in his proposal for medical reform, denounced not only inadequately trained
licensed practitioners but also "a great many men practicing through toleration, thanks to local authorizations accorded by virtue of some sort of
right acquired over time, or an unfounded belief in [their powers of] inspiration."[142] To some observers, it seemed that little had changed.

The question of who was coopted into the new medical network has proved
complex. The legislators of the Year XI entertained a vision of the future
medical profession that was clear enough in itself; in practice, though, they
intended less to make a radical break with the past than to regularize, so
far as possible, the situation they had inherited from the Old Regime and
the Revolution. The results lend themselves to two different interpretations.
Like the proverbial optimist and pessimist who see the same container as
half full or half empty, historians may choose to emphasize either the survival of Old Regime categories – especially the role of the clergy in medical
assistance – or the attempts to create a network of practitioners that would
be governed by a single law and would eventually comprise only persons
who had met certain fixed standards imposed by the state. In the context
of the history of the Western professions, the latter view has more to
recommend it. For a major state to establish a uniform (if two-tiered)

national profession, with a coordinated national licensing system, was a novelty; long after Napoleon, Europeans continued to think of it as the French model.

PROFESSIONAL INSTITUTIONS

Under the Ventôse law, state-appointed examining bodies took over the licensing functions of the old corporations. Physicians, however, had no professional institutions of their own comparable to the prerevolutionary faculties, colleges, and communities. In 1810 Napoleon created for lawyers an Ordre des Avocats, in which membership was obligatory, while leaving the medical men unorganized. Some doctors urged a return to the old corporations (a move promoted in 1800–1801 by the Société de Médecine de Paris, whose president, Edme-Joachim Bourdois de la Mothe, had become friendly with Bonaparte as chief physician of the Army of the Alps);[143] new legislation, however, was not forthcoming. Any effort by practitioners to create their own occupational organizations would have conflicted with the Le Chapelier law of 1791, which prohibited members of the same occupation from organizing to promote their collective interests, and with a measure introduced in 1810 that barred all associations of more than twenty individuals formed without government approval. Nor was the Société Royale de Médecine immediately replaced after its destruction during the Revolution (although the Paris Faculty of Medicine attempted, with only limited success, to perform multiple functions, advising the government on epidemics, secret remedies, and other questions affecting public health, and making a few gestures toward stimulating and coordinating medical research). Physicians and legislators attempted, instead, to address in piece-meal fashion some of the tasks performed by the old institutions: promoting public health; encouraging medical science and disseminating new discoveries; aiding needy professionals and their dependents; and disciplining errant practitioners.

Public health

The development of "public hygiene" during the early Industrial Revolution is one of the great sagas of nineteenth-century French medical and social history.[144] But apart from a central sanitary commission that operated during the yellow fever epidemics of 1819 and 1821,[145] France had no real national institution in the field of public health until 1848, when the government established a national health advisory committee, together with a centrally organized network of local health councils that were to function through the Second Empire and into the Third Republic. The capital had a *conseil de salubrité* for Paris and the department of the Seine, founded by the prefect of police Louis-Nicolas-Pierre-Joseph Dubois in 1802; it served as the model for numerous local and departmental health councils in the provinces. But these were essentially advisory bodies that provided the various administrations with information and recommendations on medical questions.[146] Neither they nor the limited system of state-salaried epidemic physicians and (in a few departments) district physicians provided an organizational framework for the profession, as the Société Royale had done to some extent for the medical elite in the late 1770's and the 1780's.

Learned societies

Although the liberal individualism of the Revolution denied the medical profession corporate rights, the Directory Constitution of the Year III (1794–1795) did tolerate the formation of professional societies with a scientific purpose (article 3, title 10). Several quickly appeared in Paris, among them the Société de Santé (later Médecine) de Paris (1796), which included among its membership veterans of the Société Royale de Médecine and the Académie Royale de Chirurgie, and served after 1804 as an official consultative body of the city of Paris on questions of public health; and the Société Médicale d'Émulation (also 1796), which brought together an exceptionally talented group of young researchers and clinicians. Others emerged under Napoleon. The Société de l'École (later Faculté) de Médecine (1800), an official organization created by the Minister of the Interior, included mainly members of the Paris medical faculty; it inherited the archives of the old Société Royale de Médecine and pursued some of its interests in hygiene and medical topography. In 1804, a group of former doctor-regents of the Old Regime's Paris faculty, including Guillotin, attempted to organize an Académie de Médecine; the government obliged them to accept the more modest title of Société Académique.[147] Still other medical societies were formed in the provinces at the local or departmental level. The pharmacists, for their part, organized a Société de Pharmacie de Paris in the summer of 1803, shortly after adoption of the legislation of Germinal.[148] None of these organizations, however, came close to replacing the old Société Royale de Médecine.

It was not until 1820 that a medical academy finally emerged, following a campaign by baron Antoine Portal, First Physician to the king and president of the Cercle Médical. The Académie Royale de Médecine was a creation of the government, distinct from both the existing societies and the Paris faculty. Like the old Société Royale, it embraced surgery and pharmacy as well as medicine and was charged with promoting and coordinating medical science and work in the field of public health; it also inherited the task of examining secret remedies. But its role, which in a summary description sounds vast, was narrowly circumscribed. Like its predecessor, the Academy had to coexist with institutions whose licensing authority gave them the power to set standards for entry into the medical occupations; and contrary to what Portal had originally envisaged, it was not authorized to oversee medical practice and discipline members of the profession. Even more than the old Society, the Academy was ill equipped to function as a national professional organization; it served primarily as a scientific advisory body and a platform for reporting and discussing new developments in the field. Although it did sometimes debate the question of medical reform (as in 1828, at Martignac's direction), professional issues were not among its central concerns.[149]

Professional discipline

Unlike practitioners in the German states (which typically supervised medical activities quite closely),[150] the French physician, once he received his license, was free from regular oversight and subject only to legal responsibility for malpractice; the problem of professional discipline remained a perennial concern in the postrevolutionary era. The 1812 commission on medical reform headed by Cuvier and the surgeon Guillaume Dupuytren recommended appointing special councils (literally "chambers of discipline"), whose jurisdiction would include professional misconduct. Proposals for such bodies at the level of the department or arrondissement multiplied under Louis XVIII, and the two reform projects that the government sponsored under Charles X incorporated similar provisions: chambers of discipline in 1825 and less ominous-sounding "medical councils" in 1828. Corbière's proposal of 1825, as passed by the lower house, included an amendment by a physician-deputy of the Cher that called for the profession to elect the members of the chambers. None of these projects came to fruition, in part because they were linked to the highly controversial problem of reforming the *officiat*.[151]

Mutual aid

Among their other functions, the old guilds had worked to protect the material well-being of their members and to aid the neediest among them. Under the conditions of legal individualism and free enterprise promoted by the Revolution, only private persons and the state (or, after Thermidor, the various municipal agencies of public assistance) could, in principle, help out when a practitioner could not make a living, or labored under the handicaps of sickness or old age, or failed to provide for his widow. In medicine as in other domains, mutual aid societies did not prosper until the July Monarchy, which officially legalized them on a general basis in 1837, with the stipulation that they must have government approval. They took

their inspiration from the Association of Paris Physicians, which the practitioners of the capital established in 1833 under the patronage of the dean
of the medical faculty, Matthieu-Joseph-Bonaventure Orfila.[152]

Professional organizations remained weak, then, in the early nineteenth
century. Neither under Napoleon nor during the Bourbon Restoration did
the profession have any real hope of obtaining strong autonomous institutions. Indeed, during the Restoration, the government attacked even the
relative independence of the faculties, modifying the competitive examinations that the Empire had used to make appointments and at one point,
in 1822, temporarily closing the Paris faculty and dismissing its liberal
professors.[153] The physicians had their societies and then the Academy to
serve as forums for the expression of opinion; they also took advantage of
the great proliferation of medical periodicals that began in the 1820's.[154] But
they still lacked the institutions that might have contributed to making them
an influential pressure group – a handicap in their campaign for new reg-
ulatory legislation and against illegal practice. More effective French medical
organizations were a product of the second half of the century: the Association Générale de Prévoyance et de Secours Mutuel des Médecins de
France, founded in 1858 as a federation of mutual aid societies (by 1880
over half of French medical personnel were members of affiliated societies);
and medical unions (*syndicats*), devoted to promoting the profession's collective interests, which began to emerge in the 1880's and were formally
legalized by the new medical legislation of 1892. Even then, the relative
weakness of French professional organizations contrasts to the role of the
American Medical Association (founded in 1846) and state medical societies
in the United States or the British Medical Association (founded as the
Provincial Medical and Surgical Association in 1832 and renamed in 1856).[155]

ACCESS TO A MEDICAL CAREER

Together with the medical organizations of the Old Regime, the Revolution
swept away the traditional system of recruitment and the old restrictions
on entry into the profession. Protestants and Jews were no longer excluded.
The prejudice against female practitioners persisted longer; male doctors,
though perhaps willing to make a few exceptions for women of extraordinary talent and dedication, thought that in general the physical and moral
organization of their sex made them unsuited for the pursuit of scientific
studies, and that, as one of them put it, they were "destined to please through
natural grace and physical beauty."[156] In place of the requirements of the
Edict of Marly, the law of Ventôse instituted a new set of uniform and, in
principle, more stringent requirements – a minimum of four years of formal
study for the doctorate and, for the *officiat*, six years of training with a

doctor, five years in a hospital, or three in a school. As has been seen, the medical juries were often lax, particularly in the early years of the Ventôse regime; until 1836, they sometimes issued conditional authorizations, which allowed candidates to practice until they had fulfilled certain requirements. Some prefects, it will be recalled, also issued temporary authorizations to practitioners who had not yet been officially received.[157]

Over the first half of the century, however, the prevailing standards for the *officiat* rose, and an increasing proportion of candidates received a formal medical education (as opposed to serving an apprenticeship); at Rennes, for example, the percentage trained under individual doctors declined from 44 in 1819–1822 to 28 in 1839–1842.[158] Training was available at major hospitals and from "free societies of medical instruction" in some provincial towns. Under the Empire, the government gave the hospital schools of a dozen large provincial towns the status of "secondary schools of medicine," though they still did not have the right, like the faculties, to turn out health officers in three years. The sponsors of this project envisaged an extensive network of such schools, one for each academy of the Imperial University (there were twenty-seven within the old French borders).[159] Under the Restoration, an ordinance of 1820 placed the schools officially under the jurisdiction of the University, and subsequent legislation added several more.[160] Since credit from the schools could be transferred to the faculties, they somewhat enlarged access to the doctorate, though this procedure made for a long course of study.

The candidate for the doctorate had to know Latin (optional for the thesis but required for two of the five examinations); during the Empire he was expected to have completed the full secondary program at a lycée before entering the faculty, and starting in 1821 he was formally required to have a baccalaureate in letters. (A requirement for a second baccalaureate in science was added in 1823 and maintained for the next seven years, but it proved hard to enforce.) The demands of maintaining a son at a secondary school, especially with full room and board (which could cost more than ten times as much as tuition), significantly restricted entry into the higher order.[161]

The architects of the Ventôse settlement, although rejecting on principle cost-free entry into the medical profession, fixed the charges for the *officiat* at a level they hoped would not be prohibitive for candidates from modest backgrounds – 200 francs for the examination and 50 for the diploma. But these sums already exceeded the cost for the two lower levels of surgery in the Old Regime, and in any case they represented only a fraction of the total expenditure, which could amount to 4,000–5,000 francs for the years of training (plus possibly another 1,000–1,500 to pay for a substitute for military service). The legislation of 1803 fixed the fee for the doctorate at 1,000 francs – considerably less than the most expensive receptions in the

Old Regime, which had put legal practice in certain major towns beyond the reach of all but a small elite. Estimates of other expenditures (which might include fees for private instruction) varied widely. Cuvier calculated in 1826 that a student might have to spend 1,200 francs a year (for a minimum of four years). The average cost may have reached 12,000 francs by the 1830's.[162] The nineteenth-century reforms, then, appear to have compressed somewhat the extraordinary range of the Old Regime occupations, making recruitment slightly less socially selective at the upper end and perhaps slightly more so at the lower end.

For all concerned, entry into this not very remunerative field required a significant commitment of time and resources; medicine as a career seems to have attracted some young men who could barely afford it. Doctors came from the middle classes – the liberal professions and the ranks of the less wealthy property owners; only later in the century did sons of notables appear in significant numbers. The *officiat* did offer opportunities to candidates from modest rural backgrounds, but completing the requirements was often a struggle; one hears, as in the Old Regime, of financial difficulties and delayed receptions.[163] A few such young men, it is true, went as far as the doctorate and occasionally achieved real success. The celebrated Paris surgeon Alfred Velpeau (1795–1867) was the son of a village farrier in the department of Indre-et-Loire; as a teenager he taught himself a little medicine and practiced illegally until a nearly fatal outcome led him to reconsider and undertake formal medical studies at Tours.[164] But this was an exceptional case.

SOCIAL AND ECONOMIC STATUS

That the restructured medical profession of the early nineteenth century should have been nearly as stratified as its Old Regime counterpart should not surprise us. Many practitioners were in fact survivors of the Old Regime network – still more than 18 percent of medical personnel in the West at the beginning of the July Monarchy. Moreover, the new profession, with its distinction between doctors and health officers, had inequality built into it.

The lower order, old and new, constituted the majority of the new profession – more than three-quarters of practitioners in the West in 1803 and still more than 40 percent at midcentury.[165] At the bottom of the scale, the humblest *officiers de santé* lived on the same social plane as the peasants whose way of life they shared. One physician in a non-French-speaking region of Alsace scoffed at a local health officer, a native of Soultz who had been apprenticed to a barber in Switzerland and knew no Latin, French, or (according to the physician) medicine or surgery: "he joins in the funeral processions of his victims and eats the meal at the home of the deceased, in accordance with the despicable custom of this region."[166]

At the top of the scale, a few doctors numbered among the great notabilities of the Empire. Napoleon, who favored scientists and scholars, appointed doctors to government positions (Jean-François Barailon, for example, who had distinguished himself in the legislative debates on medical reform under the Directory, became an imperial procureur), and he ennobled almost fifty physicians, surgeons, and pharmacists.[167] A less exalted but still highly privileged group managed to combine several public appointments with a lucrative private practice. The tendency of a small professional elite to accumulate a disproportionate number of honors and offices irritated their more modest colleagues; the latter also suspected them of lacking enthusiasm for the crusade against illegal practice, which, as one commentator put it, did not hurt practitioners with a rich clientele but "crushes the modest and honest medical democracy." The same writer attacked as an elitist scheme a newly formed "sanitary association," a prepaid health care plan organized by medical luminaries that would have allowed subscribers to obtain comprehensive coverage for 22 francs per annum; the professional aristocracy, he suggested, not content to monopolize public appointments and the most remunerative work in the capital, was now invading the realm of ordinary practice.[168]

On the whole, however, even the doctors did not figure prominently in the ranks of the *grande bourgeoisie*. Among Napoleonic notables, as defined by membership in the electoral colleges (which depended to a large extent on wealth), lawyers greatly outnumbered physicians. A study of local notables in the West shows that the proportion of physicians who appeared on the electoral lists ranged from about half of the profession in the Mayenne to about a tenth in the Côtes-du-Nord; a roster of notable persons that the prefects prepared in 1810 confirms this impression for France as a whole. If physicians distinguished themselves, they did so through service rather than wealth, and mainly in modest local offices.[169] Jacques Léonard has aptly characterized the physician of early-nineteenth-century France as a "deminotable."[170]

Large fortunes, then, were rare among medical men, and those that existed typically came through inheritance, marriage, or a shrewd investment (such as the purchase in the 1790's of property that the Revolution had confiscated from the Church or from émigrés). In the West, Léonard estimates that the average wealth of physicians may have been around 20,000 francs in 1815, though with striking disparities between the first and second orders – a ratio, on the average, of about 5:1.[171] Another study suggests that in the Ardèche many physicians could have been characterized as poor. In the Rhône, thanks to the economic influence of Lyons, they were more

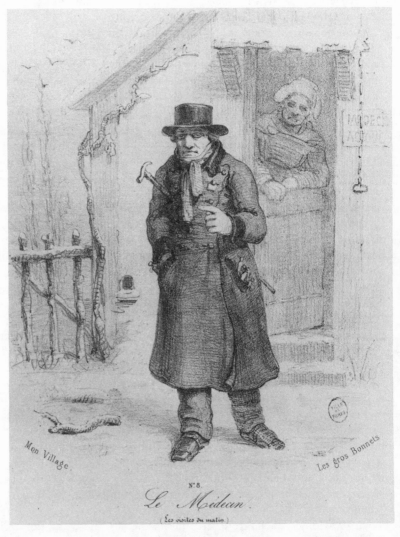

The physician: morning visits. The country doctor as village "bigwig."
(Courtesy of the Cabinet des Estampes, Musée Carnavalet. Photograph
by Jean-Loup Charmet.)

prosperous, tending to come from moderately well-off rural families and
to enjoy modest middle-class status.[172] Only in the 1840's, though, did
substantial numbers of physicians begin to reach the upper-middle range
of wealth.

A physician with limited independent resources could scarcely expect to thrive on his professional income.[173] Around the time of the First Empire, a modest *officier de santé* might earn 600–800 francs a year from his practice, half the income of a curé first class (although this figure does not include payment in kind). A good doctor might earn 4,000 francs or even as much as 7,000 in the better regions, but 2,000 was more typical. (Paris, as always, was an extreme case. At the end of the Restoration, the 200 most prominent physicians earned an average of 10,000 francs per annum, though it should be added that their joint income exceeded that of all the other 1,100 physicians in the capital combined.) Many rural practitioners, especially *officiers de santé*, depended on the sale of remedies as *propharmaciens*, which might account for half of their revenues.[174] Practitioners sought to supplement their regular income by exploiting their land holdings or, when possible, by accumulating official positions. On the whole, such posts were not handsomely paid, however, except for appointments as prison physicians. Government policy discouraged allowing *médecins des épidémies* much more than their expenses; a study of the Hautes-Alpes suggests that after 1818 an official vaccinator might receive between 75 and 125 francs a year.[175] At midcentury a practitioner in the Morbihan could still complain that "we would be in a precarious state if we had to live only from the practice of medicine."[176]

Over the course of the *monarchie censitaire* (1814–1848), the more prosperous members of the profession improved their position while the more vulnerable ones sank deeper into poverty. In the first half of the century, the number of physicians in difficulty trebled; the period after 1820 saw the growth of a new group of medical men entirely dependent on their practice for a livelihood and therefore less secure than those with independent means. As would be expected, health officers in economic trouble outnumbered the doctors (by about 2:1 in the West during the period 1814–1851, although they constituted only a third of medical personnel).[177] Some were obliged to accept public assistance. The less fortunate practitioners were particularly sensitive to fluctuations in the economy; they suffered from the crisis that followed the Napoleonic Wars, just as they later profited from the good years of the 1850's and 1860's. Yet they saw themselves primarily as victims of excessive competition in an overcrowded profession. Conditions reached their worst in the difficult decade of the 1840's, but they were perceived as bad throughout the early years of the Ventôse regime. A health officer at Elne (Pyrénées-Orientales) complained in 1811, for example, of the excess of *officiers* in the department. How could a father put his son through medical training knowing that he would later be poor and insecure?[178] A minority in the profession suggested that the number of practitioners in any place be fixed by law, as for the notaries.[179]

Lacking such protection, physicians tried as best they could to adapt to a free market, sometimes resorting to the entrepreneurial stratagems that the French collectively labelled *l'industrialisme*. Aspiring practitioners, it was said, might seek to make an impression by rushing about town, supposedly on an urgent summons from aristocratic clients, or by making patients wait "when one is in one's study, with slippers on one's feet, engaged in chewing one's nails or trimming one's quill."[180] They advertised; split fees and accepted kickbacks; contributed potboilers to the medical literature; exploited secret remedies; and fronted for empirics.[181]

The medical man who promoted proprietary remedies or special cures was so commonplace a figure as to be almost unremarkable. It was a surgeon, Jean Pelgas, who promoted the enormously successful Leroy purgative and vomi-purgative; according to his publicity, all diseases stemmed from a unique cause in the blood, which infallibly yielded to his remedy.[182] A physician in the Vaucluse promoted the powders of Irroé, which he said had been in his family for sixty years.[183] P. Le Pelletier, who described himself as a former surgeon and accoucheur, had a biscuit concocted to disguise the taste of purgatives; he angrily denounced the apothecaries who criticized him for keeping the recipe a secret.[184] Under the Restoration, a physician named Gout, who had won a doctorate from Montpellier despite what the Academy's commission on secret remedies described as an astonishing ignorance of the French language, proposed to treat goiters in the inhabitants of the foothills of the Pyrenees; but this project would clearly have served as a cover for ambulatory medical practice and the sale of remedies, one of which, an "English purgative," was so powerful that, according to the commission, a few drops could kill a man.[185] Other medical men dabbled in Mesmerism and the occult. At Nantes in the 1820's, one physician sold magnetized water from the river Loire, at 3 francs for the small bottle and 6 for the large.[186] (No doubt cabalism, animal magnetism, and somnambulism genuinely fascinated some physicians of the Romantic era; many, however, were driven by economic need.)

Other physicians practiced empiricism at second hand, collaborating with or protecting the unqualified. At Chantenay in the Loire-Inférieure, for example, an obscure health officer signed blank prescriptions for a urinoscopist and shared his earnings. In the early 1830's, a physician and a pharmacist of Paris were said to cover the medical activities of a shoemaker, who paid them 10 francs a day for their services.[187] Sometimes, too, a physician's family worked as empirics, like the Mazureau women, daughters of a physician from Martinique who had come to Nantes at around the time of the Revolution.[188]

To be sure, the more flagrant behavior involved only a minority of the profession, principally in the major urban centers; but there was more than a grain of truth in the caricatures that Honoré Daumier drew during the July Monarchy of the grasping Robert Macaire as a medical man, or the Dr. Saint-Ernest of Louis Reybaud's *Jérôme Paturot* (1842), who turned to quackery so as not to die poor.[189] Throughout the century, professional misconduct remained as lively a topic of debate as illegal medical practice; the projects for establishing *chambres de discipline* were meant to deal with both. Indeed, the two problems were closely connected in the minds of insecure professionals, who felt as much threatened by unfair competitive practices as by empiricism. Some of the medical elite (who professedly cared more about honor than about lucre) proposed applying an ounce of prevention; they would have restricted medical careers to young men from safely comfortable backgrounds by raising tuition, imposing an excise tax on practice, or simply requiring candidates to possess a certain sum of capital that would serve to guarantee their future conduct.[190] None of these projects was actually adopted; they would almost certainly have exacerbated the problem of illegal practice, whatever their influence on the dignity of the profession.

ACCESS TO A PRACTITIONER

As in the previous chapter, the profession needs to be considered from the patient's, as well as the practitioner's, point of view.

Density and distribution of personnel

How accessible, first of all, were the services of a licensed practitioner? This question is not easily answered (see Appendix A). Contemporary estimates of the number of practitioners in France in the last years of the Restoration ranged from 24,000 to 72,000. These figures are almost certainly too high if only fully qualified, registered personnel are counted. Léonard suggests a total of 21,000 in 1844, which was about the peak for the country as a whole in the nineteenth century; the profession then shrank, for the slow growth in the number of doctors did not suffice to compensate for the rapid decline of the *officiat*. Léonard's figure would mean a density of roughly 6 practitioners per 10,000 inhabitants – slightly higher than comparably conservative estimates for the Old Regime, which implied densities of from 4 to 5 per 10,000. This level was within the range of optimal densities suggested by nineteenth-century medical reformers, though still well below recent levels (about 11.5 per 10,000 in France in 1965).[191] If a "doctor glut" existed in France during the July Monarchy, it was not because the country had more physicians than were required to meet the perceived needs of the population; it was simply that not enough people could afford to pay for them.[192]

Just as for the Old Regime, it is important, when considering the global statistics for the early nineteenth century, to distinguish the various categories of practitioners. The lower order naturally predominated. The department of the Deux-Sèvres, according to its prefect, had about 20 physicians at the time of the passage of the Ventôse legislation, but four or five times as many surgeons.[193] In 1821, Fodéré counted 44 physicians but 80 "surgeons" in the Alpes-Maritimes.[194] The situation in the nineteenth century was more complex, however, than in the eighteenth; the ratios were in constant flux, especially since entire categories – Old Regime practitioners and those admitted by certificate through the grandfather clause – were not renewed. Léonard's study of the West shows that in 1803, 55 percent of practitioners had been licensed under the Old Regime; by 1816, that figure had dropped to 31 percent. Lower-level surgeons made up 40 percent of medical personnel in 1803 but 21 percent in 1816; *officiers de santé* by certificate, 40 percent in 1803 but 24 percent in 1816 and less than 10 percent in 1830. The overall ratio between the first and second orders changed more slowly, because although the number of doctors grew, so did the number of health officers received by juries, at least until 1841 in the West; the total number of health officers began to decline only in 1826. Physicians of the first order comprised 20 percent of practitioners in 1803 and 34 percent in 1816. At the beginning of the July Monarchy, *officiers* still made up 42 percent of medical personnel, whereas doctors constituted 40 percent.[195]

Densities continued to vary widely from region to region (see Appendix A). As in the eighteenth century, the Midi had unusually high concentrations of practitioners; the West, unusually low ones. Even within the West, great disparities are apparent. In 1814 the Côtes-du-Nord had only 107 doctors, surgeons, and health officers – a density of roughly 2 per 10,000. The Finistère and Morbihan were in about the same situation (though later in the century the density of the latter descended as low as 1.2 per 10,000). But the Loire-Inférieure had a density approaching 5 per 10,000, and in Ille-et-Vilaine the concentration was around 6 per 10,000. The contrasts at the arrondissement level are even more striking: densities ranged from about 8 per 10,000 for the arrondissement of Saint-Malo (Ille-et-Vilaine) to 1.1 per 10,000 for Châteaulin (Finistère).[196] An 1827 manuscript on folk medical usages around Saint-Malo noted that such practices could not be blamed on a lack of regular personnel, since "there is probably no market town in the environs of the city that does not have one or two *officiers de santé*; and in the little town of Dol, whose population consists of 3,800 persons, including the rural section of Cotentin, there are four physicians, two master surgeons, three *officiers de santé*, and a few marine surgeons [for an overall density approaching 30 per 10,000!]."[197]

The ratio of first- to second-order practitioners also varied greatly, though it correlates rather poorly with the overall densities. Some contrasting cases will illustrate the problem. In the 1840's, the old province of Gascony (departments of the Landes and Gers) had a high overall density (10 per

10,000) and a high percentage of health officers (66.7), whereas the Seine, including Paris, had a very high density (15.5) and a low percentage of *officiers* (12.2). The Lyonnais region (the Rhône, including Lyons, and the Loire) had a modest density (4.5) and a low percentage of health officers (16.1); the Artois/Picardy region (Pas-de-Calais and Somme) had a roughly comparable density (5.3) but a high percentage of second-order practitioners (73.7).[198]

In most regions, the absolute number and density of practitioners both increased during the first half of the century, though at varying rates. In the Rhône, for example, during the period 1805–1825, the population and the number of medical men rose roughly pari passu; then for the next twenty years the profession expanded more rapidly, so that the density, which had once been about 2.5 per 10,000, increased to around 5 per 10,000. In the West, the profession reached its highest overall density in 1841 and then, as a result of population growth and some slippage in the number of personnel, dropped to a lower level in 1851 than in 1803. In the Ardèche, however, the peak in both absolute and relative terms was attained in the early 1800's, a level not reached again until the twentieth century.[199] It should be noted, too, that some regions had significantly lower densities in the early nineteenth century than at the end of the Old Regime. A study of the arrondissements of Gap and Embrun in the Hautes-Alpes, for example, shows an increase in the density of doctors from 0.56 to 1.1 per 10,000 between 1789 and 1831, but a decline in the density of all practitioners from 4.2 to 2.7 per 10,000.[200]

How are these differences to be explained? Prosperity and urbanization alone do not account for all the variation; indeed, Léonard suggests that the correlation with literacy is somewhat closer. Nor is the ratio of health officers to doctors simply a function of wealth, as one might expect. Some poor departments had many more doctors, proportionally, than some wealthier departments where sons of the bourgeoisie tended to enter other professions.[201]

It is obviously difficult to generalize, then, about the accessibility of licensed practitioners. The situation in the early nineteenth century is roughly comparable to that of the last decade of the Old Regime, except that the masses of lower-level surgeons were replaced by increasingly better-trained health officers, who were in turn supplanted (though not entirely replaced) by doctors. Physicians remained concentrated in towns (Lyons, for example, with one-third of the population of the Rhône, had three-fourths of the physicians), but they had not yet deserted the countryside in droves, as happened in the late nineteenth century.[202] We should also bear in mind that they were willing to travel 7, 8, or 9 kilometers to see patients, and occasionally as much as twice that distance. The study of the Hautes-Alpes just mentioned shows that in 1823, only 14 percent of the communes in the two arrondissements, with 12 percent of the population (according to the census of 1820), lived more than 10 kilometers from a medical practitioner's residence or from a place regularly visited by a physician.[203] Only a small fraction of the population was more than a few hours' walk from a physician, and it should be remembered that the practitioner himself normally had a horse. And yet the massive medicalization of the population had not yet arrived; though he might have been geographically accessible, the typical practitioner saw, on the average, fewer than ten patients a day, and often only two or three.[204]

Costs of professional services

Cost remained the principal reason for low utilization of professional medical services; before the advent later in the nineteenth and early in the twentieth century of major third-party systems of payment (mutual aid societies, private and state insurance schemes, social security), regular medical care was simply beyond the means of most Frenchmen, as of most Europeans. Medical economics had not changed much since the Old Regime. Fees remained stable; one long-lived Breton practitioner, for example, who worked at Loudéac as a surgeon in the 1770's and as a physician at Lamballe during the Restoration, hardly raised his charges above what they had been at the beginning of the reign of Louis XVI.[205] In a town a visit would cost under 1 franc, or even less than 50 centimes, especially for a health officer. (Doctors, on the average, charged two to three times as much as health officers.) In major cities higher rates prevailed: 1–3 francs (6–10 in Paris). Fees were doubled or trebled at night; and, as in the past, the charge for travel (at least 1.50 and often 3–5 francs per league, and double at night) could quickly exceed the cost of the visit itself. Even 50 centimes was about the daily wage of an agricultural worker and perhaps half that of an urban artisan.[206] Calling a physician to the countryside might cost two to three weeks' wages, not even counting the price of the remedies he prescribed. Over the first half of the century, moreover, the cost of living rose; the period when medical personnel were most numerous unfortunately coincided with the hard times of the 1840's.

Methods for distributing private medical care more widely had changed little since the Old Regime. Physicians still adjusted their fees somewhat, typically on a sliding scale of 1–3 (though sometimes as much as 1–10). A minority of families signed annual contracts with practitioners at a fixed cost, which entailed a not insignificant outlay but at least afforded protection against the medical costs of a major illness. One health officer in the Hautes-Alpes had an agreement with the town of Ribiers, from 1818 until at least 1862, under which, for an annual stipend of 300 francs, he made his services available to the middling classes of the commune for 50 centimes a visit and to the bourgeoisie for 1 franc.[207] In another case, from 1845, a year's subscription cost a fifth of a hectoliter of wheat.[208]

Few Frenchmen who lacked the benefit of such an arrangement could find the cash to pay the prevailing fees. As the last example indicates, many rural patients paid physicians in kind. Nevertheless, practitioners could expect to write off perhaps a fifth of their fees, and sometimes more, as bad debts. In the area of Redon (Ille-et-Vilaine), a health officer was forced to leave in 1830 after two years' practice, claiming that he had not been able to get any money from the inhabitants.[209] As would be expected, the price of medical services resulted in a clientele whose social composition resembled that of its Old Regime counterpart: comfortably off landowners (and their servants), merchants, the professional classes, and the more prosperous artisans.

Those who could not afford to consult a physician complained, not unnaturally, about excessive costs, which they often attributed to the physicians' cupidity. In 1812, for example, the mayor of Feurs in the Loire blamed the lack of peasant patients on the exorbitant fees that the profession demanded. These assertions are not easy to judge; in the absence of fixed fee scales (which became widespread only later in the century), charges varied very widely, and it was difficult to say what a fair rate was. It is of course possible to find examples of gouging. During the Napoleonic vaccination campaign, to cite just one, a resident of the Nivernais denounced three "leeches" (*sangsues* – there is no automatic pun in French) who had extracted 3–6 francs from the poor for this very simple procedure, and a gold *louis* (worth 20 francs) or more from the well-off – a sliding scale, it is true, but starting from too high a base.[210] But even the normal charges could seem excessive to impecunious patients, who found it easier to understand paying for remedies than for an intangible like professional advice.

Public assistance

After the failure of the Revolution's grand vision of a state welfare program, medical assistance was reorganized essentially along the lines of the Old Regime system.[211] The major institutions were municipal: physicians or health officers were attached to the welfare centers (*bureaux de bienfaisance*) or appointed as doctors for the town's poor.[212] Some were quite active; at the end of the Restoration, the municipal health officer at Vannes (who could be summoned by mayors of nearby villages) received payments for his services amounting to more than 3,000 francs per annum.[213] Private charity supported some additional dispensaries and home visits; the most prominent example was the Société Philanthropique de Paris, whose consultants included some of the leading lights of French medicine.[214] The countryside, however, was far less well provided for. As in the Old Regime,

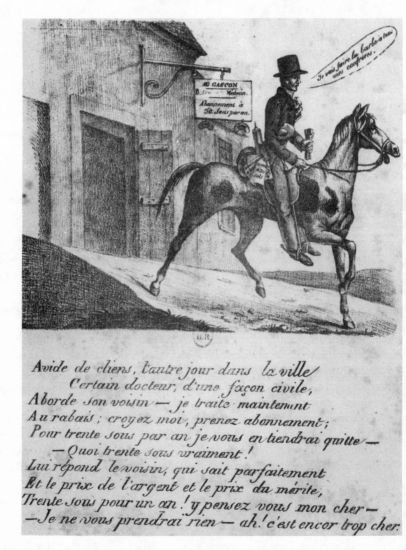

Avide de chiens, l'autre jour dans la ville
  Certain docteur, d'une façon civile,
Aborde son voisin — je traite maintenant
Au rabais; croyez moi, prenez abonnement;
Pour trente sous par an je vous en tiendrai quitte —
  — Quoi trente sous vraiment!
Lui répond le voisin, qui sait parfaitement
Et le prix de l'argent et le prix du mérite,
Trente Sous pour un an! y pensez vous mon cher —
— Je ne vous prendrai rien — ah! c'est encor trop cher.

The physician in search of subscribers. Lithograph by Deletain. "The other day, in town, a certain doctor, eager for clients, civilly approaches his neighbor: 'I now treat at a discount; believe me, take a subscription; I'll let you have it for 30 sous a year.' 'What, 30 sous, really!' replies the neighbor, who knows perfectly well the value of money and of merit. '30 sous a year! You mean it, my dear fellow?' 'I won't take anything from you.' 'Oh, it's still too expensive.' " On the shop sign: "At the Gascon's place [Gascony was a traditional source of barber-surgeons]; subscriptions for 30 sous a year." The doctor, with his subscription forms and an old-fashioned syringe in his saddle bag: "I'm going to shave all my colleagues" (i.e., I'm going to be one up on them – an idiomatic meaning of *faire la barbe*). (Courtesy of the Cabinet des Estampes, Bibliothèque Nationale.)

médecins des épidémies were dispatched during major outbreaks of disease. A ministerial circular of 1805 called for the prefects to organize them on a more systematic basis than in the eighteenth century: there would be one in each arrondissement; they would be paid according to the work they did, rather than given a fixed annual salary; and where Sisters of Charity lived, they were to administer the remedies prescribed by the physicians.[215] In the Year XIII (1804–1805) the central pharmacy of the hospitals of Paris began to supply boxes of remedies on the model of the old *remèdes d'Helvétius*.[216] But no regular system of routine medical assistance existed, apart from the ubiquitous sisters. Hence the urgent tone of Dr. Royer's proposals for rural dispensaries (one version called for 3,500), which in his old age he continued to press upon the ministries of the Consulate and Empire. The Paris medical school advised against his scheme on the grounds that it would cost too much and would compromise professional standards by involving curés as *desservants en médecine* (*desservant*, a priest who serves a parish church).[217]

The early nineteenth century saw one significant, if limited, innovation in rural medical assistance. The German-style district physician, the *médecin cantonal*, who had figured in so many medical reform schemes of the late Enlightenment and Revolution, was introduced in a few departments of eastern France. The institution had its roots in Alsace. Even before the Revolution, the towns of Strasbourg, Haguenau, and Bischwiller had employed communal physicians; the office vanished during the Revolution but reappeared in more systematic form in 1810, together with a health council – thanks to an aggressive prefect, Adrien de Lezay-Marnésia, who had been transferred that year from Koblenz to Strasbourg. His salaried cantonal physicians were charged with, among other things, caring for poor patients and regulating wet nurses, as well as preparing reports on forensic medicine, like the old *médecins jurés*. The neighboring department of the Haut-Rhin adopted the system in 1825. It later spread somewhat farther, to the Vosges, Haute-Saône, Moselle, and Saône-et-Loire (1838–1843), and then to the Meurthe and the Loiret (1849–1850).[218]

Proposals at the national level, however, collapsed before the strictures of physicians who saw in salaried practitioners a threat to medicine as a liberal profession; they recoiled from the idea of a network of medical functionaries who would be dependent on the state, as many German physicians were. The critics drew additional support from economic liberals who feared that increasing support for health care would have the unintended effect of encouraging pauperism. Medical assistance in France expanded only gradually in the latter two-thirds of the nineteenth century. The July Monarchy saw the emergence and growth of mutual aid societies, which the Second Empire then encouraged and subsidized. Under the Empire and in the early years of the Third Republic, the government promoted programs of public medical assistance, organized (and largely funded) at the department level, but with mixed results. Even the law of 15 July 1893, which guaranteed assistance for indigent patients and made it the obligation of the communes, departments, and central state, failed to impose a uniform national system of social medicine.[219]

ATTITUDES TOWARD THE MEDICAL PROFESSION

Apart from the problem of cost, distrust of the profession and its methods continued to impede contact between official medicine and a large part of the population. Whatever gains the profession may have made in winning confidence during the Enlightenment, it appears to have reached a plateau on which it remained for the better part of a century; significant change came only during the Third Republic. The reports of the *médecins des épidémies* in the early nineteenth century are filled with virtually the same complaints about popular resistance that their predecessors had written in the reign of Louis XV.[220] The drastic depletive methods applied by the disciples of François Broussais alarmed the rural populace; at the height of the vogue in the use of leeches, one physician complained that he and his colleagues never succeeded in applying more than thirty of the bloodsuckers to their peasant patients.[221] As in the past, many women with gynecological complaints (which appear to have been widespread) refused to submit to an examination at the hands of a male physician.[222]

Nor were the sources of popular distrust confined to the physicians' therapeutic methods. University-trained doctors belonged to a culture that remained alien to much of the population. Only in some twenty of the ninety-odd departments did the inhabitants regularly use French, and as late as the Second Empire about a quarter of the population still did not speak it; when urban *médecins des épidémies* were dispatched to the mountains of the Ariège during the cholera epidemic of 1854, they needed interpreters.[223] Physicians also belonged to a different social class; the bourgeois practitioner who sought a popular clientele met with suspicion in the best of times, and it is not surprising that during the panics associated with the cholera epidemic of 1832, not only the rich but also doctors and medical students were accused of poisoning the poor; a few were beaten up by mobs. Physicians might also incur local enmity as agents of the state; a health officer at Montivilliers in the Seine-Inférieure complained, for example, that after he had served for several years examining conscripts, "I have been insulted by the families, who at present are taking their revenge."[224] Resident practitioners who wished to be accepted had to adapt, learning if necessary to speak the local patois and deferring to the more innocuous popular medical beliefs, such as the tradition of being bled on Saint Valentine's day or the feast of Saint Matthias (14 May), or purged on the feasts of Saint Paschal (17 May) or Saint Leodegar of Autun (2 October).[225]

It was possible, then, to accommodate to local expectations; but many physicians naturally chafed at the refusal of a large part of the population to accept professional authority – all the more galling at a time when some elements both in the profession and among influential laymen (notably the Saint-Simonians) shared a greatly expanded conception of that authority and of the social and political role of medicine.[226] Thus Dr. Ulysse Trélat declared in 1828:

The influence of physicians ... must extend to the movement and progress of society. They have, indeed, a higher mission than that of concerning themselves only with the preservation of individual life: it is to modify and improve collective life; ... it is their physiology, their public hygiene (which remains to be created) ... that must preside over the perfecting of mores and legislation.[227]

Dr. Édouard Lemaître put forward a concrete proposal: every medical doctor should automatically become a member of the municipal council of his town or commune.[228] Many other such examples could be cited. One can only speculate on the effect so grand a vision of the profession may have had on doctor–patient relations, but it is clear that conflicting views of the professional role remained a source of irritation on both sides.

The first two chapters of this study have provided no more than an overview of a vast and complex subject; its basic contours, however, should by now be clear. A few major points deserve to be underscored. Although many ambiguities remained, France began to move in the early nineteenth century from a diffuse toward a tight medical network. The profession, first of all, was reorganized: medicine was officially united to surgery, starting with the educational reforms of 1794; under the Ventôse regime, the nineteenth-century profession began either to coopt the various specialties or to relegate them to the domain of illegal practice (with the signal exception of dentistry, which remained essentially unregulated until the new legislation on medical practice of 1892). The profession, it is true, retained upper and lower tiers. For the first time, however, the state effectively imposed national standards for training, and it made considerably more sense than before to speak of the "medical profession." The legislation of Ventôse also encouraged a second, related development: the spheres of regular and irregular practice, though their boundaries were not yet perfectly clear, took on sharper outlines than in the past. Despite the latitude allowed the clergy and the individual concessions made to some formally unqualified persons who had established practices before 1803, it had become considerably harder for empirics and all the marginal practitioners of the Old Regime to win official recognition. Both of these developments obviously facilitated the campaign against illegal practice; it was more evident who the offenders were, and the regulars dissipated less energy in battles over intraprofessional encroachment.

It is also important to recognize what did not change or changed only very gradually. The density of practitioners in the early nineteenth century was not very different from that of the Old Regime; the total number grew slowly, peaking in most places in the 1840's. Nor did the percentage of the population that consulted physicians rise dramatically; no greatly expanded market for medical service developed until much later in the century, if then. The social and economic status of physicians remained similarly un-improved until later in the century. The strong sense of professional over-crowding, coupled with the loss of the corporation as an instrument of professional defense, made many practitioners in the early nineteenth century feel acutely insecure and directly threatened by illegal practice.

Because of the disparities between institutional and social change, the French medical profession of about 1830 did not closely resemble either the contemporary profession or its traditional antecedents, as described in ac-counts of the rise of professionalism.[229] On the one hand, it still lacked broadly accepted authority (one thinks, for example, of its conflicts with mayors favorably inclined toward empirics), and its average social and economic status was not high. On the other hand, it was no longer an elite learned calling far removed from a mass of consultants without formal training and barely distinguishable from empirics.

The development of the French medical profession in the late eighteenth and early nineteenth centuries carries implications for theories of profes-sionalization. The formation of a tight regular network began in an essen-tially preindustrial society without a mass market for professional services; it cannot be explained by profound social and economic transformations. The role of cognitive developments is more problematic. The functionalist explanation of medicine's professional success emphasizes its scientific pres-tige and perceived utility, dating from the discoveries of Louis Pasteur and Robert Koch in the field of microbiology.[230] The changes described here preceded by two generations Pasteur's major discoveries of the third quarter of the century; but they coincided with the age of pathological anatomy and the "birth of the clinic," and an era of extraordinary prestige for French science in general. To what extent can developments within the discipline help explain the fortunes of the medical profession? Surely they cannot be ignored; it is difficult to make sense of the fusion of medicine and surgery (to take the most important concrete example) without referring to the influence of the surgical tradition of anatomy and hospital training and perhaps even the positive efficacy of certain surgical procedures, such as lithotomy. And yet it is also difficult to explain why surgery developed and exercised the influence that it did without referring (as Toby Gelfand has done) to the institutions, supported by royal patronage, in which it flourished.

To understand why the French professions developed as they did, when they did, it is essential to look at the nexus between the state and scientific and medical institutions. It was the revolutionary state that abolished the old corporations and joined medical and surgical training; and it was the Napoleonic state that reestablished the profession on new foundations. To a far larger extent than in Britain or America, the profession in France, somewhat like its German counterpart, was shaped from above.

This is not to say that reforms were imposed arbitrarily, without consultation. The relationship between professionals and the state, as Charles Gillispie has suggested in a survey of science and polity at the end of Old Regime, was a partnership that gave large scope to application by the professionals of their special expertise, even in setting policy.[231] In medicine, the professional elite would have had a large say in the reforms proposed in 1789–1790, had any of them actually been enacted, and it greatly influenced the legislation of 1794 and 1803. It is no coincidence, obviously, that all the physicians in the Constituent Assembly sat on the special Comité de Salubrité, making up half of its membership, or that the reporters of bills on medical education and practice were physicians. But it is nonetheless important to see how institutional change followed political trends over which the profession had no direct control. The profession clearly did not will the legislative failures of the early Revolution, the "medical Terror," or the impasses of the Directory.

Nor did the compromise of 1803 simply reflect a professional vision. The legislation of Ventôse and Germinal constituted an integral part of the post-revolutionary Napoleonic settlement, just as much as the contemporaneous civil code (Code Napoléon), whose various articles were voted between 1801 and 1803; the later law codes; or the creation of the University. The guiding spirit is much the same throughout. The French would enjoy fewer liberties than under the Revolution but equal civil rights, with no return to privileges, corporations, or the economic relations that the revolutionaries called "feudalism." The only *corps* would be those organized by the state; rights and duties would be the same from one region to another; economic activity would be free, except insofar as the state used its police powers to regulate it in the name of the general good. Rights in property (including its intangible forms, such as an inventor's discovery, an author's text, or a professional's access to authorized practice) would be respected. The transition in the medical field from the localism and corporatism of the Old Regime to liberal individualism tempered by a strong state followed the political course of the nation; the history of the profession was in many ways French history writ small.

PART II

Popular medicine

3

Irregulars: itinerants

Many commentators of the eighteenth and nineteenth centuries thought that unauthorized medical practice had no history, that it was the timeless result of the encounter between gullible or desperate patients and the swindlers who cynically exploited their weakness. Strictly speaking, they were wrong; it is possible, for example, to trace the spread of popular mesmerism after the 1780's or the prolonged decline, in the nineteenth century, of the large troupes of traveling mountebanks that crisscrossed the French provinces. But the changes came very slowly; a typical empiric of 1830 is barely distinguishable from his counterpart of 1770, and many popular beliefs and practices of nineteenth-century rural France can be documented for the sixteenth century and even earlier, as far back as classical antiquity.[1] This chapter and the two that follow are therefore intended primarily to suggest a *typology* of unauthorized practitioners who worked in France at the end of the eighteenth and the beginning of the nineteenth centuries.

The most familiar taxonomy of unauthorized practitioners divides them roughly into "quacks" and "folk healers," catchall terms that usually imply some of the following assumptions:

Quacks are mercenary and insincere; they often travel; they advertise their wares; they have at least a smattering of book learning; and in their methods they sometimes ape the professions.

Folk healers are sincere and rarely accept payment; they operate within their village; they do not advertise; they are a product of indigenous popular culture.

The defects of these stereotypes will become apparent in the pages that follow, but it is difficult, if not impossible, to find adequate categories to replace them; certainly no simple dichotomy can adequately describe the range of practitioners.

Indeed, any such attempt at classification is so fraught with methodological difficulties that it is worth saying something about them explicitly at the outset. It is not necessary to be a radical nominalist to recognize that social categories do not form a neat Linnaean array of genera and species. The would-be natural historian of unauthorized practitioners encounters at least three major problems. The practitioners, first of all, are too various to be divided into clear-cut groups with generic labels, such as "quack" or "folk healer," that would accurately predict the significant traits of each individual. Some village healers, for example, expected to be paid. The second point is related to the first: since we are classifying not organisms but behaviors, it is important to recognize that an individual might engage in a variety of activities that seem to belong to very different categories, and that these activities might change over time. Thus a woman who worked as an herbalist in nineteenth-century Lyons had a reputation as a "witch" (an extraordinarily elastic term); sold not only herbs for tisanes but also hernia trusses and orthopedic appliances; and possibly worked as a *faiseuse d'ange* (abortionist; literally, angel-maker) on the side.[2] Finally, in this fundamentally synchronic exercise, a diachronic note intrudes: however constant the various types of popular behavior, their context – and therefore their social significance – changes. For the sixty-year period that is at the center of this study, this consideration is not always crucial, but for the longer term it almost invariably is. A *toucheur* who healed with saliva in 1700 is not the same as one who used an indistinguishable technique in 1900; the range of alternatives is different. Joseph Levenson, the eminent historian of China, reflecting on this problem of the persistence of tradition amid change, invoked the Taoist principle that an idea must be understood not only by what it is but also by what it is not, and suggested that "an audience which appreciates that Mozart is not Wagner will never hear the eighteenth-century *Don Giovanni*."[3]

If one tries to do justice to the full variety of possible behaviors, the number of categories multiplies unacceptably, until the result begins to look like the irrational taxonomy of Jorge Luis Borges's fantastic Chinese encyclopedia, which Michel Foucault took as the inspiration for *Les Mots et les choses*.[4] If, on the other hand, one chooses to focus systematically on a few key traits, the result inevitably is to some extent arbitrary, depending on the problem that one wishes to emphasize: a practitioner's relation to the market, the profession, or the authorities; the nature of his or her relationship with patients; the type of medicine practiced. Moreover, labels such as "urban" and "rural," "empirical" and "magical," "mercenary" and "charitable" represent as bipolarities what is in fact a complex gamut of possible behaviors; the significance of any descriptive term may be only relative. Thus a prosecutor in the Bas-Rhin cleared up a confusion between two empirics with similar nicknames by distinguishing between "our Dr. Hans," who he thought practiced a harmless domestic medicine, and Dr. Johann, who was a "true quack and dangerous empiric."[5] And yet Dr. Hans himself was a full-time practitioner of medicine, very different from the type of the benevolent Alsatian *Hausvater* (paterfamilias) who might have occasionally used a few home remedies. Ideally, then, we would not put individuals into boxes at all; rather, we would map them by locating them along a series of descriptive axes in a multidimensional space, in which their position would shift as their behavior changed.

The trouble with wielding Ockham's razor in this fashion is that it makes it all but impossible to use general terms of any sort. The object here is not to provide an exhaustive description of the entire population, but rather to find a way of talking about both similarities and variety in behavior. As a practical matter, it has been necessary to fall back on a number of rough, historically derived, constructed types which are neither perfectly exhaustive nor mutually exclusive. (These are not Weberian ideal types, defined in their "purest" form for the purpose of theoretical analysis; they are intended as approximate groupings of actual individuals.)[6] The various irregulars are broadly divided into itinerant and sedentary practitioners; each of these groups included a wide range of operators, remedy sellers, urine scanners, mystical healers, and many who combined some or all of these roles. (A separate chapter is devoted to *maiges* – a general term for local popular healers – and witches.)

This general distinction between itinerant and sedentary practitioners primarily reflects the bias of the authorities, on whose testimony so much of this study depends; travelers without a fixed abode (*sans domicile fixe*, in the hallowed formula of the French administration) were always of special concern to the police. Medical personnel also distinguished between outsiders and residents, usually contrasting the visiting charlatan to the local *maige*. One of the responses to the Comité de Salubrité's questionnaire of 1790–1791 observed, for example, that "charlatans rarely pass through our cantons, [where] the people are beginning to recognize the knavish tricks of these people, and there is every reason to hope that we will not see any more in the future. This is not true of *les gens à secrets* [healers; literally, people with secrets], especially those who deceive credulous people by passing as sorcerers."[7] The itinerants, by definition, were not established members of the community; they had no permanent relationship with their patients and could not rely on local prestige to maintain a practice. By the same token, though, they did not need to worry about the long-term consequences of their ministrations.

The most conspicuous figure among the itinerants was the classic charlatan, who set up a stage in fairs and public markets and, after drawing a crowd with popular entertainments, hawked his drugs, offered medical advice, and sometimes performed surgical operations. Many surgical experts also traveled, as was stressed in the first chapter, because their skills (such as couching cataracts) could not be fully employed in any one place. Even in the nineteenth century, the line between regulars and irregulars

among the traveling specialists is particularly hard to draw. Some were
licensed doctors, like the oculist (ocular surgeon) Forlenze, who received a
number of official appointments (among them the post of oculist to the
lycées of Nancy, in 1806). He also traveled through the provinces, visiting
Lyons, for example, in 1814 and 1819; and in 1818 his complaint about
inept rivals who followed in his wake triggered a more general investigation
of illegal practice by the *directeur de la police générale*.[8] Others, like the oculist
Rabiglia, had more dubious credentials and dabbled in various forms of
empirical medicine;[9] some crossed over into frankly criminal activities, like
Gosset, an ambulatory oculist from Bourges, who was found guilty of
"frauds" in Angers and wound up in the house of detention at Tours in
1796.[10]

Itinerants also included peddlers, who sold medicines, among other wares;
often they offered medical advice as well, making them occasional practitioners of a sort. Even a traveling journeyman might have a few remedies
to offer, like Jacques-Louis Ménétra, an eighteenth-century glazier who left
an boastful autobiography. Ménétra had a remedy for venereal disease; while
on the road, he acquired another against fever, which he supposedly used
with such success to treat an innkeeper's daughter that he attracted patients
to the inn, where he was allowed to stay for several days without charge.[11]
Others came from the ranks of a variety of wanderers, usually economic
marginals who made a meager living from the sale of medicines, among
other things. In the department of the Eure, for example, in the early
nineteenth century, a woman sutler who traveled about the countryside
following the regiment practiced medicine in the small market towns along
the way.[12] Still other itinerants saw themselves as having a religious mission
or vocation to heal. And a few were plainly mentally ill, by both eighteenth-
century standards and our own; whether by choice or necessity, they lived
on the road until the authorities intervened.

THE OLD-STYLE MOUNTEBANK AND OTHER CHARLATANS

The medical charlatan of early modern Europe was an immediately recognizable type. According to Jean de Gorris, who in the early seventeenth
century published a treatise on the subject (largely borrowed from an Italian
source), the typical quack got up on a bench (hence "mountebank"), told
lies, mocked the simplicity of the people, and sold boluses (large pills).[13]
More than a century later, the *Dictionnaire de Trévoux* offered a similar
definition of "charlatan" (and "charlatanne" in the feminine):

Empiric, false physician, who gets up on a stage in the public square, to sell theriac
[an elaborate antivenin and panacea] or other drugs and who gathers the people by
magical tricks and clowning, to sell his drugs more easily.[14]

Similar language appears in the many denunciations of individual practitioners written by local medical personnel and officials. The empiric Audey, for example, reported at Seurre-sur-Saône in the Côte-d'Or in 1790, "gets up on a stage in the town square and begins by amusing the public. Then he sells pills and salves, and he takes the liberty of going to treat patients in the town and perform operations."[15] The quack was also a familiar literary figure. Scarron's *Roman comique* (1651–57), for example, included a supposed Venetian nobleman (actually a native of Caen in Normandy), Signor Ferdinando Ferdinandi, whose retinue consisted of his wife, an old Moorish servant, a monkey, and two valets. And in a passage of the *Mémoires d'outre-tombe*, Chateaubriand evoked the image of an old-fashioned quack who had been passing through Combourg and stopped at his bedside: "a green coat laced with gold, a broad scrubby wig, large cuffs of dirty muslin, imitation diamonds on his fingers, breeches of worn black satin, silk stockings of a bluish white, and shoes with enormous buckles." This was the uniform of the classic mountebank, who traveled from town to town, selling nostrums and offering consultations to the public.[16]

One final comment on usage: although "charlatan" (like the English "quack") has come to mean anyone who makes false or exaggerated claims to knowledge or ability, the term originally denoted an unqualified practitioner of medicine and, more specifically, an itinerant mountebank. One etymology derived the word from the Latin *"circulator,"* stroller or peddler (but also mountebank); another traced it to the Italian *"ciarlare,"* to chatter (much like the English "quack"). Each version emphasized a characteristic trait of the old mountebank: he was ambulatory and loquacious. As a matter of convenience, "charlatan" has been retained here to refer to this class of itinerants, although in general this study uses the more neutral word "empiric" to designate unqualified practitioners. In eighteenth-century France, it should be added, *"charlatan,"* though distinctly pejorative, was not quite so loaded an expression as it is today; it was used interchangeably with *"empirique"* (and occasionally even *"maige"*) as a generic term for a self-styled physician. Some empirics were even said to apply the term to themselves, though of course they usually adopted such titles as operator, surgeon, physician, or botanist. One source (admittedly unfriendly) relates that Denis Laffecteur, the former clerk who promoted and gave his name to an enormously successful antisyphilitic vegetable "rob," encountered his old employer one day and, when asked what he did for a living, naively replied, "Monsieur, je suis charlatan."[17]

Many charlatans in early modern France were primarily glorified drug peddlers, sellers of remedies like orvietan, the complex electuary said to have been brought to France by an Italian operator from Orvieto.[18] The Italian Desiderio Descombes, for example, arrived in Poitiers in 1624 announcing an orvietan "to preserve from contagious diseases and guard

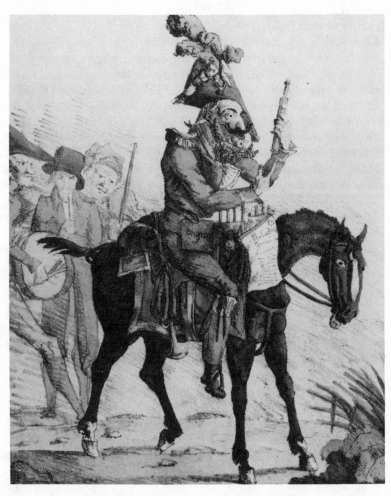

The orvietan vendor (1817). The quack carries a syringe. A bag of ointments hangs from his waist and a trumpet behind his saddle. The flyer
announces the diseases cured by his remedy. (Courtesy of the Cabinet des
Estampes, Musée Carnavalet. Photograph by Jean-Loup Charmet.)

against all kinds of venoms and bites of vipers, wolves, rabid dogs, and
even poison, with a view to relieving the [sufferings of] the people."[19] In
the seventeenth century, a Paris family of Italian descent, the Contugis,
acquired a royal privilege, later renewed for each successive generation, to
prepare and sell their orvietan; in the early eighteenth century one descendant, Florent-Jean-Louis, went so far as to challenge the right of the Paris
apothecaries to sell the drug. In 1741, Charles Dionis, of the Paris medical

faculty, acquired the privilege; with his death in 1776, the business appears to have passed into the hands of one of his associates, the spicer Julien-Edme-Marie Regnard, who received royal letters affirming his own privilege in 1778. The Contugis and their successors were not alone. The Toscano family, for example, had a privilege for the sale of an antidote reaching back to 1685; in 1771, Algaron Toscano, who was to be one of the most active empirics of the last years of the Old Regime, received a confirmation of this privilege. But Dionis and Regnard operated on an exceptionally wide scale, sending salesmen throughout the provinces.[20]

Few such agents confined themselves to selling the licensed remedy. When, for example, Salomon Cuchet (also know as Cuchet-Salomon) arrived in Dijon in 1769, he promised to sell only the orvietan of Dionis. But he then proclaimed himself a physician, chemist, botanist, and former military surgeon; and he distributed handbills informing the public that he examined eyes, inspected urine, and used stomachic remedies, orvietal quintessence, vegetable purgative, sympathetic powder and water, and philosophical balm. Similarly, the empiric Tadiny carried a commission from Regnard, and Vander, who had a contract to sell Belloste's pills (one of the few proprietary remedies authorized by the Société Royale de Médecine), was denounced at Mortagne-au-Perche for setting up a stage from which he hawked various other drugs and for consulting with patients and writing prescriptions (this enterprising practitioner even made house calls).[21]

The itinerant empirics typically announced their arrival in advance and sought to secure official approval from the police authorities in the place where they wished to distribute their remedies. They attempted to legitimate their activities in the eyes of the public and the police by invoking testimonials, official certificates, and titles (often foreign ones). The well-prepared charlatan could always present letters of approbation, some spurious but others authentic. When the practitioner Fedeau arrived at Vermenton in the Auxerrois in 1773, for example, he sent his agent to the local royal judge with a petition in which Fedeau styled himself a "privileged royal operator" and claimed that, in letters patent of 1741, he had obtained permission from the Crown to distribute his salve and orvietan throughout the kingdom.[22]

Charlatans' flyers

The petitions that the charlatans submitted to the local authorities are models of sobriety compared with the handbills that they used to advertise their activities to the public. The petitions usually concentrated on the empirics' right to sell one or two remedies; but the practice of most itinerants was in fact much wider, and their flyers and newspaper advertisements seemingly promised anything and everything. This promotional literature deserves to be examined in detail, for here the empirics speak directly to us, without the mediation of the medical profession or the police. It constitutes a rich source of information on the authors' practice. More than that, it reveals the way in which the itinerants appealed to a popular public; although the advertisements themselves assumed a literate audience, they closely resembled the harangues that the charlatan delivered to the crowd assembled before his stage.

The handbills survive in large numbers. The four that appear here in translation are from the period 1786–1801.

1. [Brittany, 1786]. The veritable Grassy, Italian, residing at Moissac, in Quercy, near Montauban. He successfully distributes the true Swiss vulnerary, approved by the medical art, [and] composed of medicinal plants which fortify the stomach and facilitate digestion. He has traveled in several European courts, where he has dedicated himself to seeking and experimenting with simples, by means of which he treats many illnesses regarded as incurable, which he cures radically. . . . He cures different disorders of the eye, without applying anything, by means of a reflection from liquids that are held in the hand. He also cures epilepsy and does not require payment until a year after the cure, provided that the patient has not lost his senses. He also cures scrofula, tinea, and all sorts of dartres [a vague generic term for various skin diseases]. He has a special secret for the feet, which is infallible. *Nolite confidere verbis, sed factis* (do not believe words, but experience). The aforesaid sieur Grassy does not know how to speak French well, but his experience will speak for him. At Nantes he cured a large number of persons afflicted with cancers, wens, and scrofula [*humeurs froides*]. His most powerful remedy is his philosophical oil, a miraculous composition, whose effects are incredible. It even causes goiters to melt away. Patients who cannot travel to him will send their urine. His knowledge of it will win him the confidence of the public.[23]

2. [Gosset; arrived at Troyes in 1791, calling himself a botanist]. He cures all eye disorders in general, [and] cures cataract in a short time by applying a new invention. He performs the operation by extraction. . . . He treats and cures hernia in both sexes. He cures scrofula, anal fistula, and ulcers on the legs. He works on ruptures, fractures, dislocations, and makes every [case of] malignant ringworm go away, without causing the hair to fall out, or doing violence to the brain. He cures epilepsy, known as *le mal caduc*. He cures jaundice. He makes the menses appear when the reproductive organs [*la nature*] are barren. He is familiar with and cures all venereal deseases, as well as undeveloped cases of dropsy. He cures prolapse of the uterus, whether caused by effort or by childbirth. He causes all sorts of malignant fevers to go away in less than six days, using a remedy that is very easy to take. He cures internal and external hemorrhoids. He cures purpura, fluxions of blood, hepatic fluxions, or diarrhea, even if it has lasted for ten years. He has a remedy for those who void urine involuntarily. He cures deafness, provided that it is not congenital, and in the space of three minutes. He cures disorders of the heart, of the stomach, weakness, colics, ulcers of the kidney, womb, and lung, [and] cures hectic fever. He has a remedy to provoke menstruation, calm griping pains, and staunch accidental losses of blood, cure cases of gout, rheumatism, vertigo, hypochondriacal vapors, apoplectic syncopes (serous or sanguine), spitting of blood, colics. He also cures erysipelas.[24]

3. [Normandy, 179?]. Citizen Morand, native of Mémain in Limousin. . . , ocular surgeon approved by the First Physician of Paris and by several colleges of medicine and surgery, announces to the public that he has arrived in this place for a stay of some time; he has given particular attention, moreover, to finding new remedies to cure several disorders that are regarded as incurable, which have resisted the usual remedies, such as stone, retention of urine, scurvy, dropsy, effusion of milk, bile in the blood, all kinds of dartre, powdery and inflamed, [and] all other disorders of the skin.

He cures ringworm radically, without using a skullcap, without irritation, without pain, and with the advantage of restoring the hair at the end of two months; he has given special attention to perfecting this remedy, which he is bold enough to assure to be infallible. . . .

He will continue to sell his elixir and an oil distilled from plants, whose effects have been recognized for eight years in Normandy, and especially at Caen.

This oil is a sovereign remedy for sciatic gout and the pains of rheumatism; it is a great resolvent for all sorts of glandules and tumors, and similarly for disorders of the nerves; it cures scrofula, cold humors, ulcers, and sores on the legs, and also causes children to pass worms; it also cures every type of burn and the bite of mad dogs and other venomous animals.

This elixir is admirable; a large number of persons have used it and been cured of tertian and quartan fever; [it] torrefies and cleans the stomach, removes from it all the fatty and sticky humors, and cures indigestion and purifies the blood, cures flatulent colics, provokes women's menses; it is a preservative against contagious diseases, and a perfect counterpoison. This elixir has produced great effects in cases of epilepsy and vapors.

He cures hernias in small children in very little time. He also makes trusses, for children as well as for adults, without iron or wood; they are of a small volume, which does not hinder [the patients] in any way.

He has an unguent prepared without sulfur or mercury, of a very agreeable odor, which cures scabies in three days. He also operates on cataracts by extraction, with knowledge and dexterity, using a single newly invented instrument, without hemorrhage or pain; this operation lasts only three minutes in order to restore vision. He performs all operations and cures all disorders which relate to this part [of the body]. He has also a sovereign Water that cures spots and inflammation of the eyes. . . .

He cures secret [venereal] diseases, without obliging the patient to stay in his room [as during a course of treatment with mercury].

He consults urine and gives the best directions for obtaining a cure. He can be found every day at his place of residence.

The cures that he has performed in hospitals and everywhere else have won him the most authentic certificates.

The aforementioned citizen Morand also radically cures persons who might be afflicted with epilepsy, by means of an operation which is little known in the art of surgery.

[There follows a list of the persons said to have been cured by Morand during the first month of his stay in Caen.][25]

4. [Bas-Rhin, 1801. Original in German]. Citizen Albertina Dränkler, living at Bischheim-am-Saum, near Strasbourg, informs her fellow citizens that she has recently arrived on the outskirts of the aforementioned community, where she will stay a little while. Everyone knows that medicine is the result and the true union of the three kingdoms, viz. the animal, mineral, and vegetable kingdoms. Through full knowledge of these different kingdoms and by means of their assistance, in the most eminent cities of France as well as in foreign countries, the aforesaid Citizen Dränkler has cured many dangerous illnesses which had been considered incurable; and she can prove this through the testimony of credible witnesses.

I advise my fellow citizens that from my tender childhood on, I have devoted myself to the study of the healing art; a serious and incessant industry has enabled me to heal the pain of stones, fractures, and other maladies. Nothing is greater, dearer, and more precious for mankind than the art of healing, especially when the result answers the confidence of the patient. This art should be practiced only with understanding, wisdom, and prudence, and not through ignorant temerity, as happens daily with the quacks and visionaries [*Schwärmer*], who deceive and abuse the credulity of the people. If the citizen needs to seek help from medicine or surgery, he should choose an experienced and learned person and place his trust in God alone, who watches over all of us without mystery and without miracles and dispenses blessings. The earth yields herbs and various other means [of healing]; one must therefore make use of them, but only with prudence and with the assistance of men who have especially devoted themselves to knowing illnesses and the means of curing them. I offer my talents to the public, as one who has been approved by the medical and surgical faculties, which give my views their due, as [those of] an operator fully experienced in medicine, just as much in the French Republic as in Holland, England, Switzerland, Germany and other states, where I maintain authentic witnesses, whom I am in a position to produce. Here is a closer description of my knowledge:

(1) I heal all diseases of the eyes; thus a person who has lost his sight for twelve to fifteen years because of grey cataract or leucoma I relieve in a few minutes, so that they see, provided the eyeball is intact. (2) I heal all defects of the body with a convenient truss, wearing which one can easily perform anything; what is more, I heal the same things in a short time with medicines. (3) Using subtle instruments, I remove painful stones from the bladder; I cure grit and gravel in the loins with medicines. (4) I operate on hideous cleft palates, harelips, congenital moles, and other repulsive excrescences. (5) I cure gnawing cancers, on the breast as well as on the mouth or nose, with instruments or drugs. (6) I also cure all old, open wounds on the feet or arms, with beneficial remedies. (7) Chronic tuberculosis, bleeding, consumption, dropsy, even if the patient is swollen up like a balloon. (8) Epilepsy, spleen disease, which often makes patients insane and robs them of their senses. (9) Ringing in the ears, and especially all persons who have lost their hearing for several years. I cure most of them before they even leave my apartment. (10) Women who have lost their menses, or never had them, and are infected with the whites. (11) Women who are troubled by a rupture of the womb and other accidents, or who were neglected in a difficult birth by ignorant midwives. (12) I cure victims

of scabies or mange, even if the skull should be eaten away. (13) I cure all venereal diseases in the greatest secrecy, without using the salivation [mercury] cure. (14) Apoplexy, rheumatism, and other diseases of the limbs. (15) In the space of twelve hours I expel tapeworm painlessly. If someone does not know what his disease is, let him merely put his morning urine in a clean vessel and send it to my residence; I shall then say where the illness comes from and whether or not it can be treated. I may flatter myself with being experienced at scanning urine, so I do not give any medicine without first having seen the urine.

At her place she also sells Turkish balm, already famous for so long, which has been declared good by the medical college in Paris; the excellent qualities of this balm are indeed admirable; it is composed exclusively of oily gum and soothing, beneficial herbs; externally it heals all old wounds and sores; it expels stone and gravel in the loins; it cures consumption and spitting of blood; it purifies the entire blood system; it is also good for chest diseases and asthma; it strengthens the stomach and restores lost appetite; it preserves all internal parts against any kind of decay; allays pain in the stomach and womb; starts the menses going again; also cures venereal diseases; removes all tumors; it is good for hot and cold fever; it strengthens the temperament of men and women; in most of these cases it brings relief within fourteen hours. This balm is also good for catarrhs and external diseases; it is generally very highly esteemed.

It is possible to speak with me at any time.

Citizen Dränkler reminds you that she does not go out to work; she explains, therefore, that all those who make house calls in her name are abject tramps, who should not be believed.

She is living in Bischheim-am-Saum near Strasbourg, in number 216; if you come out from Strasbourg and go through the central square, it is the last house on the right; and if you come from La Wantzenau, it is the first house on the left.[26]

The typical flyer has a basic tripartite construction. The opening announces the empiric's stay and offers some form of credentials; the main body of the text describes his operations and remedies; and the closing (not included here) usually offers a list of successful cures or testimonials from satisfied patients.

The empiric, first of all, attempted to establish his authority to speak on medicine by invoking some commonly recognized source of legitimacy: official medicine, royal favor, or, best of all, some combination, such as a supposed approbation from the First Physician (text 3). However much the irregulars boasted that they had cured diseases that baffled the doctors, or accused the physicians and surgeons of professional jealousy, they almost invariably sought to borrow the prestige of medicine and medical institutions. Often they took a title such as physician, surgeon, or (after the Revolution) *officier de santé*, without necessarily claiming to possess an actual degree. Salomon Cuchet said that he had spent twenty years as a surgeon-major, until he received a head wound that cost him his sight and would have killed him, if it were not for his remedies. Some simply identified themselves as relatives of qualified practitioners or scientists. The empiric Fleury, one of the most active irregulars at the end of the Old Regime, announced himself as the son of a former surgeon-major; Scipion, who peddled a *Faltranck balsamique des Alpes et de Suisse* (Swiss and Alpine balsamic remedy for injuries; [*Falltrank*: literally, "fall-drink," drink given to persons who have suffered a serious fall]), called himself the son of a celebrated Swiss botanist.[27]

In addition to associating himself with official medicine, the empiric nearly always claimed some sort of government approbation – partly, of course, in hopes of staving off prosecution, but also as a way of enhancing his standing in the eyes of the populace. The empiric Desmarest, who appeared in the Meurthe in the Year VIII, announced himself as a public functionary; some self-proclaimed health officers wore official-looking uniforms to go with the role. A few practitioners boasted of appointments as physicians to royalty and the great. (The oculist Hilmer said that he was a councillor of the King of Prussia, had been appointed oculist of the Republic of Geneva, and was salaried by the Queen.) More often they simply claimed a privilege or warrant that allowed them to carry on their work unmolested. These putative authorizations sometimes contained a comminatory clause threatening with a heavy fine anyone who dared to interfere with the empiric's exercise of his rights. A few boldly asserted the privilege of *committimus*, which in the Old Regime allowed a party in a legal dispute to bring the case directly before a high judicial authority (usually at great inconvenience to his opponent); Salomon Cuchet and the "botanist" Philippe [Ramay] warned that their cases would automatically be heard by the Hôtel du Roi, whose jurisdiction included litigation involving officers of the court and royal household. In Brittany, the empiric Demarest went so far as to claim that a decree of the parlement empowered him to arrest all "operators, charlatans and false empirics" working without warrants, imprison them, and fine them 1,000 livres.[28]

Just as important, though, the empiric claimed extensive experience: he had traveled widely, seen foreign places, performed experiments, and in general developed great familiarity with the ills that afflict mankind (texts 1, 4). Fleury said that he had traveled in Spain, Italy, France, and Germany. Philippe had made long voyages in foreign countries and accumulated twenty-five years of experience. Some empirics posed as foreigners, and actual foreigners sometimes tried to make themselves seem even more exotic than they really were; thus a certain Franki announced himself in eighteenth-century Lyons as a Turkish operator, although he was actually of Italian origin.[29] Strange garb and speech served, of course, to stimulate the curiosity of the crowd; they also betokened rare skills or knowledge brought from distant lands. For the empiric, practical knowledge counted more than book learning, results more than theory. Text 1 contrasts words (including, pre-

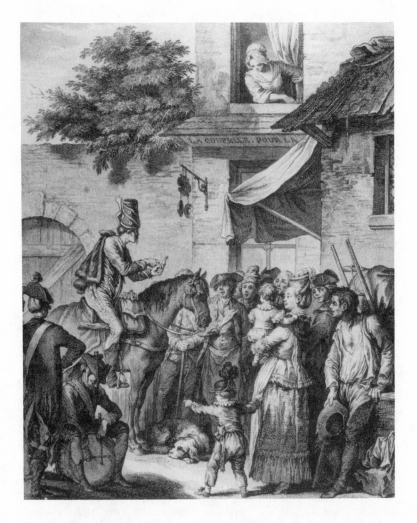

The German charlatan harangues the crowd in the public square. Drawing by Bertaux, 1776; engraving by Helman, 1777. Note the drummers in the left foreground. (Courtesy of the Cabinet des Estampes, Musée Carnavalet. Photograph by Jean-Loup Charmet.)

sumably, the eloquence of physicians) to experience; the Italian Grassy, we are told, barely knows French, but his experience (and the results that it produces) will speak for him. Philippe begged his readers "not to pay attention to his style, because, always having lived in the mountains, he devoted himself more to learning about simples, with which he composes his remedies, than to trying to impress people with the beauty of his discourse."

The charlatan then described the various services he had to offer: he sold medicinal plants (1, 3, 4) and drugs; made trusses (3, 4); and performed operations. The precise composition of the remedies was almost never revealed, for they were trade secrets; but they were usually said to be prepared from plants – from "simples," as Fleury's flyer put it, "which the Supreme Being has placed on the earth for the preservation of men and even animals." Philippe said that he had distilled a liqueur from plants gathered from around the world (America, Canada, Chile, Peru, and China) and from Switzerland and other parts of Europe. Occasionally an empiric offered more occult-sounding therapies: text 1 speaks of a cure for eye disorders that uses the reflection from liquids held in the hand, suggesting some sort of sympathetic magic. The typical flyer also offered instructions for use, like a modern-day package insert. Fleury's antidotal gold pills were to be taken in the evening, before retiring, rather than in the morning on an empty stomach, as with many other purgatives. Cuchet's sympathetic powder was to be snuffed up. His cordial and stomachic water could be given to children; the dose was graduated according to age, one drop for each year. Almost invariably, the empiric offered to make diagnoses and give medical advice; though he might do some business in tonics and preservatives, his main source of income was the patient in search of a cure for some disease or disorder. Most charlatans made the commonplace claim of diagnosing from an inspection of the patient's urine (1, 3, 4), an ancient practice that had the practical advantage of facilitating consultation at a distance, since a messenger could convey the urine of a bedridden patient to the practitioner, who would then prescribe and sell the necessary remedies.[30]

The critical part of the flyer was, naturally, the list of diseases that the charlatan offered to treat; he boasted that he could cure the incurable (1, 3, 4), perform the "miraculous" and the "incredible" (1). The treatment of many of the disorders mentioned in the prospectuses had fallen by default into the hands of the empirics, because these conditions required risky procedures, defied therapy, or were considered shameful. The empirics operated on hernias (2, 3) and eye disorders (1, 2, 3, 4) and had remedies for intractable skin diseases and epilepsy (1, 2, 3, 4). They also had compounds for venereal disease and emmenagogues to start the flow of the menses; one obvious use of the latter would have been to procure abortions, although they were not explicitly advertised for that purpose.[31] Nor was this all. The authors of all four texts – and the great majority of itinerant empirics – were panacean practitioners. Although one adopted the specialist title of ocular surgeon and another the title of botanist, they used surgery and medication to treat a variety of conditions. Moreover, many of their remedies, like Morand's elixir and oil, were themselves panaceas.

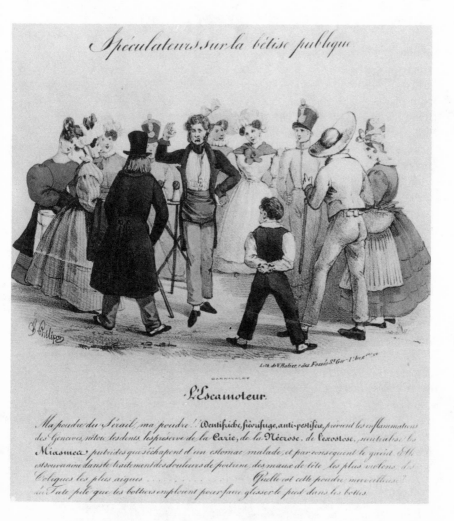

Speculators on human stupidity: the conjuror [or sneak thief]. By Charles Philipon; lithograph by V. Ratier. "My powder of the seraglio, my powder!! Dentifrice, febrifuge, antipestilential, prevents inflammation of the gums, cleans the teeth, preserves them from caries, from necrosis, from exostosis [a bony growth arising from the surface of a bone], neutralizes the putrid miasmas that escape from a sick stomach and therefore cures it. It is sovereign in the treatment of chest pains, the most violent headaches, the most acute colics. . . . What is this wonderful powder? Talcum powder that bootmakers use to make the foot slip into the boots." (Courtesy of the Cabinet des Estampes, Musée Carnavalet. Photograph by Jean-Loup Charmet.)

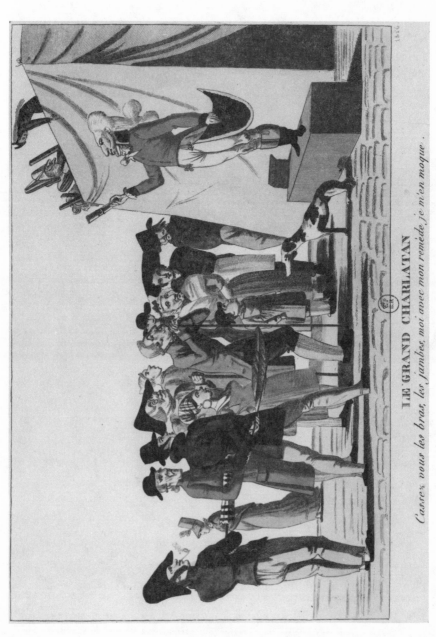

LE GRAND CHARLATAN

Cassez vous les bras, les jambes, moi avec mon remède, je m'en moque.

The "great charlatan" harangues the crowd (1816). "Break your arms, your legs – with my remedy I make light of it." (Courtesy of the Cabinet des Estampes, Bibliothèque Nationale.)

How, then, did the empiric cure? Unlike many *maiges*, he had no special personal gift to cure a specific disease. But unlike the trained physician, he was not a truly universal healer, applying basic principles to the treatment of any and all diseases. He diversified his activities through the accumulation of empirical secrets, which, unlike the the healing gift, anyone could acquire. The very rhetoric of the texts proceeds through enumeration and repetition – a recapitulation, as it were, of the charlatan's own career of empiricism.

The charlatan supported his boasts with lists of cures performed (1, 3); in some cases he offered to let the client defer payment until the cure was assured (1). Morand provided detailed information on the cases of patients he claimed to have treated successfully, such as a certain Vitard at Caen:

All the surgeons who treated him could not recognize his disease. Citizen Morand went to see him and found a considerable abscess in his body, which he removed in twenty-four hours; he suffered besides from dropsy and from an inflammation of wind such that for two weeks he could not even go to stool, being reduced to the sad situation of remaining recumbent night and day in an armchair. Citizen Morand having lavished his care and talent on him, he was perfectly cured in the space of six days, to the point where he walks very well and even saw citizen Morand back to his lodgings. . . .

The basic elements of the testimonial are here: the failure of regular medicine and the images of the patient before and after treatment, made vivid here by the descriptions of prostration and then the trip back to the empiric's apartment.

No information appears to have survived on how the flyers were composed or who actually wrote them (in some cases, they were surely the product of a hired pen). But they constituted a recognizable genre whose rhetoric is almost as revealing as the specific claims that they make. Although charlatans did not speak the language of doctors, their texts were filled with their own version of scientific discourse, liberally sprinkled with technical terms and seasoned here and there with a dash of Latin.[32] The underlying medical assumptions were basically humoralist. Cuchet, for example, promised that his cordial water would make the defective humors come out through the sweat, urine, and feces. There was nothing specifically demotic about these concepts. Charlatans rarely dabbled in witchcraft, or offered to raise "fallen stomachs," or indicated which saints to invoke for relief of suffering. Nor did they necessarily speak patois (which in any case the more active itinerants could hardly be expected to learn for each new locale), though they did have German flyers for Alsace (Dränkler) and Dutch ones for Flanders (Scipion). The charlatan did not pretend to be of the people; he dressed up, not down, and he spoke down to his audience or over their heads.

The empirics' rhetoric, however, struck the educated elites as defective, not only in its use of medical concepts but also in its composition and grammar. The texts are hopelessly disorganized; the succession of baroque boasts reminds us of the comically exaggerated lists of Rabelais, who in some places deliberately pastiched the pitches of the mountebanks of his day. The empirics use bad French. The third author, for example, is guilty of defective syntax: he cures cataracts, he says, "sans épanchement de sang, ni rendre la partie douleureuse" (without effusion of blood, or making the [affected] part painful – though in English, which has a gerund form, the effect is less jarring). The second is guilty of redundancy; his text mentions colics and amenorrhea in two separate lists. For contemporary observers, solecisms were a distinguishing mark of quackery; in the case of Salomon Cuchet, the authorities at Dijon remarked that "the language alone of this foreigner indicates the crassest ignorance and the most extravagant and most dangerous quackery."[33] It is worth recalling the importance that the "classical age," as Foucault calls it, attached to the parallel between social order and regularity in language; quackish discourse was subversive almost in itself.

This discussion has focused on the main characteristics of empirics' flyers in circulation in the late eighteenth and early nineteenth centuries. Further research should shed more light on the rhetorical variety of the texts and the ways in which they may have evolved over time. One unusual concrete example illustrates the process of borrowing, adaptation, and refinement that helped keep this essentially conservative genre alive for several centuries. Albertina Dränkler (text 4) was either the widow or daughter of a Johann Georg Drenckler, who settled at Bischheim-am-Saum in the last years of the Old Regime. (Her prospectus nowhere mentions this fact, although he must surely have been remembered in Bischheim in 1801; most empirics would have boasted of the connection. Possibly she wished to dissociate herself from his style or methods.) Drenckler had said that he was a native of Bavaria, and was not only an oculist, lithotomist, and herniotomist, but also a sworn mine inspector. Albertina clearly modeled her handbill on his; both the similarities and the differences are interesting. Albertina promised to cure the same diseases as Johann Georg; her list of fifteen boasts is almost identical to his. She also culled from his introduction the reference to the three kingdoms of nature (though she gave them their German names, where he used Latin) and a number of other rhetorical touches: having studied medicine from childhood on; the importance of meeting the patient's expectations; the temerity of quacks (though Johann Georg had a longer list of offenders, including practitioners of black magic); and the importance of trusting in God. But the overall impression is quite different. Johann Georg wrote a much less limpid German. He hinted at knowledge of alchemical secrets: miners had studied the mineral kingdom not only on the earth but beneath it; they had wrested its products from the hidden depths and worked on them in their laboratories. And where Albertina, perhaps because she was working in the French Republic, only briefly alluded to God, her predecessor dilated on the religious significance of the healing act, citing illustrations from Scripture to show that God has placed remedies on the earth. Sickness comes from sin; the healer is a weak instrument in the hands of God. Curiously, Albertina's great panacea, the Turkish balm, was unknown to Johann Georg, who promoted vegetable pills, a worm powder, a plaster for wounds, and a "mountain essence" for the eyes. The significance of the change in remedies is unclear, but the shift in rhetoric is unmistakable: Albertina had, in her way, accommodated to the Enlightenment.[34]

In the last decades of the Old Regime, as the number of journals in provincial towns increased, charlatans began to place advertisements there to announce their arrival (starting in 1772, for example, in the *Affiches du Poitou*).[35] With sufficient publicity, the empiric did not need to appear physically in the marketplace at all; his advertisements could draw a clientele to his rooms, at an inn, at the lodgings of a local resident, or some other fixed place. Flyers often included (like no. 4 here) detailed instructions for arriving at the empiric's residence. Although some physicians hoped that a better-educated public would learn to avoid the snares of empiricism, growing literacy helped as much as it hindered their activities.

The charlatans at work

The classic mountebank traveled through the provinces in a carriage that could double as a platform for haranguing the crowds. (One charlatan who appeared at Dax in 1787 was so fond of clambering up on his vehicle that he was commonly known as "Cabriolet.")[36] The more successful practitioners brought with them a large entourage of assistants and performers; a certain Saqui, for example, who sold a panacea in Eure-et-Loir in 1797, had a retinue of sixteen persons.[37] The assistants were sometimes dispatched into the countryside, while the bulk of the troupe worked a market town. Such a town could serve as a base for several weeks or even months. The line here between itinerant and sedentary practitioners easily becomes blurred; whereas some charlatans hawked their wares in the marketplace on a Sunday or market day and then vanished, others established, for a while, a sort of regular practice. In 1788, a troupe of charlatans "armed and dressed in military fashion," who had announced themselves as army surgeons, practiced medicine for over a month at Béthisy in the Île-de-France; their only competition came from an elderly surgeon whose independent income relieved him of any financial incentive to practice medicine.[38]

The mountebank used criers and entertainers to draw crowds at fairs,

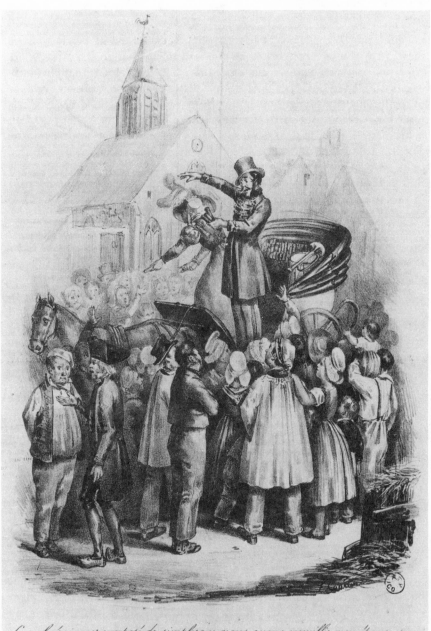

Ce vulnéraire est composé de simples que nous avons recueillis mon épouse et moi sur de hautes montagnes situées dix lieues plus loin que le soleil levant.

The boastful itinerant on his cabriolet with drum and trumpet. "This vulnerary is composed of simples that my wife and I have gathered on high mountains situated 10 leagues farther than the rising sun." (Photograph courtesy of the Musée National des Arts et Traditions Populaires; © Musées Nationaux.)

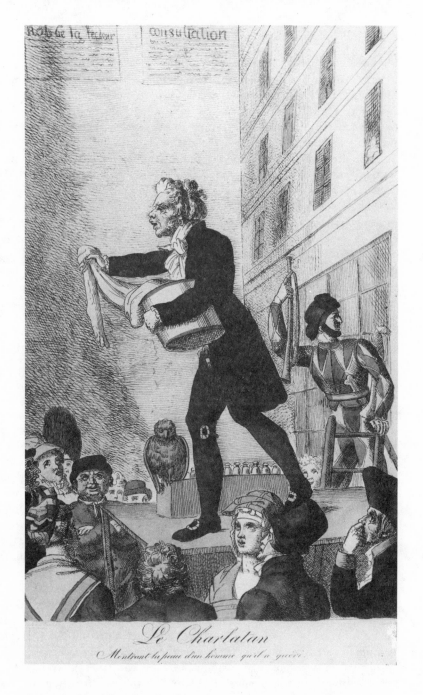

Le Charlatan

Montrant la peau d'un homme qu'il a guéri

"The charlatan showing the skin of a man he has cured." The signs advertise his consultations and a rob, or syrup. (Courtesy of the Cabinet des Estampes, Musée Carnavalet. Photograph by Jean-Loup Charmet.)

markets, and public squares; typically they traveled with skilled *baladins* (Merry Andrews or "zanies," as they were known in English).[39] The performers at the medicine show later doubled as clerks and agents, Paillasse and Pierrot serving as secretaries, Scaramouche distributing drugs, Sganarelle collecting payment (according to a report on a nine-member troupe working at Château-Thierry at the end of the autumn of 1780).[40] Various other devices might catch the eye of passersby. At Dreux in 1791, an empiric with a "brilliant equipage" had his four carriage horses prance in circles.[41] Some charlatans displayed trophies of their wonderful cures, such as tapeworms they had extracted from patients, together with other curiosities or precious objects; one empiric exhibited a 5-foot silver tube for curing deafness, as well as a monstrous artificial fetus (whose "mother" supposedly owed her safe delivery to the empiric's elixir), some large silver spoons, goblets, and a basin. The quack himself was usually magnificently dressed – in this last case, in a splendid coat gallooned with gold and decorated with a Maltese cross.[42]

Once the charlatan had drawn his audience, he began to hawk his wares, relying on a special patter and well-established repertory of high-pressure sales techniques familiar to carnival pitchmen and door-to-door salesmen everywhere. The harangue resembled the language of the flyers, but it usually sought to project what educated observers often described as an "air of mystery" – hence the term *baragouin* so often applied to it.[43] A correspondent of the Société Royal de Médicine at Le Blanc-en-Berry noted with disdain the oratorical exertions of one Paul Meda de Triulsi: "since he is Italian, he is absolved from using reason."[44] Demonstrations on volunteer patients (often confederates) and other stunts served to impress the audience with the empiric's prowess and the potency of his remedies. Empirics often operated in full view of the audience; surgery became another form of popular entertainment, rather like an execution. The physician Gallot described how d'Angleberme, in his carriage, removed a growth near a patient's eye; at Gerbéviller a troupe of empirics staged a public operation for what they called a "sarcocele" (fleshy tumor of the testicle), excluding from the audience only the local *officier de santé*, on the grounds that their method was a secret.[45]

To dramatize the wonderful virtues of their remedies, the empirics drew on all the usual tricks of the trade. A charlatan peddling an alexipharmic (antivenin) might line his stomach with oil before swallowing a dose of (genuine) corrosive poison. Or he might delegate this task to his toady (toadeater, an assistant who swallows noxious substances). Certain devices could simulate the appearance of a poison victim by distorting the face or making the pulse seem to disappear. If the charlatan were promoting a salve for burns, he might plunge an assistant's hand into a vase of mercury, which passed for a vessel full of boiling lead. A long empirical tradition, moreover,

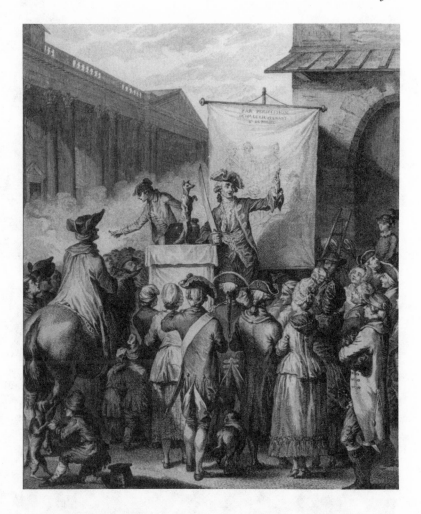

The French charlatan. Drawing by Bertaux, 1776; engraving by Helman, 1777. The inscription on the banner reads: "by permission of the lieutenant-general of police." The animal on display might be a fox – a symbol of deceit (cf. Ben Jonson's *Volpone*). (Courtesy of the Cabinet des Estampes, Musée Carnavalet. Photograph by Jean-Loup Charmet.)

had taught beggars, reluctant conscripts, and charlatans how to imitate the external signs of disease, which the empiric's remedies easily "cured."[46] Other stunts impressed the audience with the charlatan's special powers. In one case, two empirics inserted a long speaking tube into the ear of a patient whose urine was being inspected and whispered their diagnosis through it. They may have intended this procedure to ensure confidentiality for clients

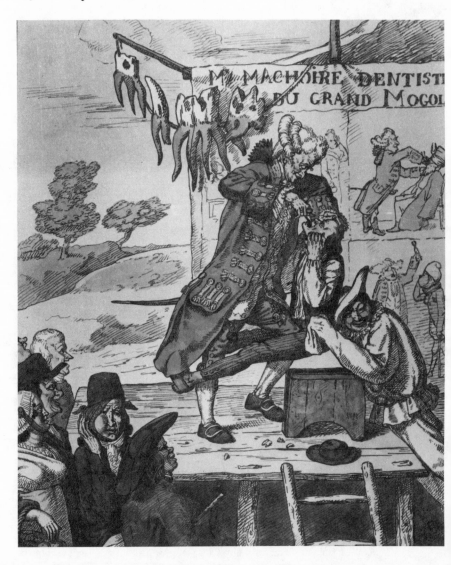

"Without Effort" (1818). The dentist on the public stage. The sign behind the giant molars reads: "Monsieur Mâchoire [jaw], dentist of the great mogul." (Courtesy of the Cabinet des Estampes, Bibliothèque Nationale.)

who might be suffering from venereal disease, but it also astonished and impressed the crowd; unable to understand how anyone could make himself understood over such a distance without being overheard, they attributed the phenomenon to magic.[47]

As a final touch, the empiric might distribute one remedy gratis, or offer it to the poor, or invite the local clergy to designate a number of deserving paupers for free treatment. At Clermont in the Île-de-France, one group of empirics even gave bread to the public; at Avallon, now in the Yonne, a "Venetian" intent on promoting his reputation as a philanthropist distributed bread, meat, and rice.[48]

The empiric then invited the public to buy his remedies or to submit to an examination (usually free), perhaps voiding a specimen of urine for immediate inspection. The charlatan's diagnostic techniques were sometimes less conventional than his printed prospectus might suggest; in face-to-face encounters with illiterate patients, he pandered to what he took to be their prejudices. At Mauperthuis-en-Brie in 1788, one empiric inspected water with a golden écu in it. He had a woman spit in the water and then revealed her complaint: she had a four-footed beast in her stomach. (That an actual living animal might inhabit the body was a widespread popular belief, linked to the long prevalent notion that cancer was a gnawing beast that had to be "fed.") His remedy, he said, would make her eject it through the mouth. Here she protested. What if she were to choke? Not to worry, he replied; he would make her pass it by the nether route.[49]

As their handbills suggested, the charlatans supplied a perceived need by treating intractable or shameful conditions. An inguinal hernia, for example, which most surgeons would have preferred to manage with trusses and bandages, they radically "cured" (if the patient survived) with a crude version of what would otherwise have been a very delicate operation, in the tradition of the Old Regime herniotomists described in Chapter 1: they simply sewed up the inguinal ring to serve as a base for the herniated sac of the intestine, severing the spermatic cord in the process. (The profession perceived such operators essentially as castraters; "I do not know," mused a correspondent of the Société Royale in Comminges, writing to inform the society of one such case, "why this man was working for the Cathedral of Saint-Bertrand, which has never prided itself on good music.")[50] As for remedies, although the empirics had some for patients stricken by epidemic disease (in 1832, for example, they commonly distributed specifics against cholera),[51] their preferred targets were victims of chronic illness, which official medicine either saw as unresponsive to therapy or else attributed to climatic influences or errors in regimen – problems whose solution could not come out of a medicine bottle. The charlatans were radical interventionists; the mainstays of their armamentarium included drastics such as calomel purges and other mercury-based drugs. (So closely was the quack associated with mercury, particularly as a treatment for syphilis, that one popular etymology for "quack[salver]" derives the word from "quicksilver.") Many of these preparations were intensely irritating and potentially lethal. One purgative was said to make patients pass clots of blood.[52] The Academy of Medicine's commission on secret remedies said in 1828 of another, which an itinerant practitioner proposed to distribute in the regions at the foot of the Pyrenees, that a few drops could kill a man.[53] And in Brittany at the end of the Old Regime, a German charlatan named Michel was blamed for numerous deaths directly or indirectly attributed to his mercurial remedies. One victim was said to have succumbed after six weeks of repeated purges; another died of a throat inflammation, having caught cold (the physicians charged) as a result of "spending every night on the pot, owing to the purges which this man gave."[54] (Like some other empirics of the 1780's, Michel dabbled in animal magnetism, but his obeisance to medical fashion did not prevent him from relying mainly on the old stock in trade.)[55] Many such cases could be cited; heart-rending stories were told of patients, including children, who died in terrible agony after taking an empiric's remedy.[56] In general, however, the public welcomed medicines that acted violently. When the purgative bolus distributed by a troupe of empirics at Clermont produced as many as thirty stools, the peasants found this "admirable," according to a correspondent of the Société Royale.[57] Although they may in many cases have disagreed with the profession on the need for depletive remedies, they shared the basic notion that corrupted matter sometimes had to be evacuated from the body. And as Charles Rosenberg has argued, the drastic remedies were in a sense conspicuously efficacious; calomel really did purge, undeniably and dramatically.[58]

When he was not on the stage, the empiric was busy behind the scenes, searching for patients confined at home and drumming up support among local residents. An innkeeper or another local contact might supply the names and addresses of sick persons and invalids. The oculist Hilmer was said to have won a particularly friendly reception among local artisans, when he visited France as a very young man, because they recognized him as a fellow Free Mason.[59] So far as possible, the empiric also sought to discredit his opposition, which might include rival charlatans as well as local professionals. At Dax in 1787, the "most magnificent" of four charlatans produced a patent as an "inspector of operators" and called on the other three to recognize his authority and show him their papers; in another similar case, also at Dax, one of the others, presumably a confederate, actually complied.[60] Empiricism was not for the indolent or fainthearted.

The political economy of charlatanism

To appreciate the social significance of charlatanism, it must be seen not simply as an illicit form of medical practice but also as a special type of economic activity. Whether or not they believed in their remedies, the itinerant empirics sought to make money. Unlike most local practitioners, they rarely accepted payment in kind, though they were adept at extracting drink and victuals from their dupes. (An informant in the Aube at the end of the revolutionary decade suggested that an empiric might require thirty bottles of white wine to prepare a topical remedy. One practitioner told his patients that in order to cure them he needed spirit of butter and essence of eel, and asked them to provide the raw ingredients.)[61] The charlatans' drugs were expensive, and when they charged for consultations, their fees were typically higher than those of a regular practitioner; at Carency in Normandy at the end of the Old Regime, for example, the empirics Le Fort and Darnet charged 24 sous for an oral consultation and 3 livres for a written one.[62] The most successful entrepreneurs accumulated fortunes in the tens of thousands of livres, if not more. Fleury's operations expanded to the point where he licensed other empirics as his agents, at least one of whom actually used his name.[63] But the business could be a rough and competitive one: apart from confrontations with the profession and the authorities, empirics had to be wary of rivals who tried to run them out of town, or impersonated them, or counterfeited their proprietary remedies; all were vying for a limited and not very elastic market, and since the charlatan was by definition outside the guild system, he could hardly hope to benefit from its protection. The ambitious charlatan was a prototype of the entrepreneur, taking great risks in hopes of earning a high return and using intense promotion to stimulate demand for his product; it was highly appropriate that he sould be known as an *industriel* (*chevalier d'industrie*, or swindler, but also industrialist). In this respect he resembled Robert Darnton's unauthorized booksellers, the "protocapitalists" of the eighteenth-century book trade, who peddled Enlightenment literature and pornography at significant legal and financial risk, while their licensed colleagues were using the privilege system to earn a safe return on religious books, official publications, and the like.[64]

Hard as it is to determine the size and distribution of the profession, it is obviously harder still to map the activities of the charlatans. They could be found in every region of France, perhaps slightly more commonly in the south than in the north. The geographic range of individuals varied enormously. At one extreme, the grand adventurers followed a circuit of European capitals, stopping for long periods there and in major provincial towns. Cagliostro, for example, who was among other things a medical empiric, entered France at Strasbourg in September 1780. In May of the following year, a correspondent of the Société Royale de Médecine denounced the medical activities of a certain "Caillostro"; a similar report followed in July from Oberbronn, 40 kilometers to the north. Between then and June 1786, when the Count fled to London following the scandal of the Queen's necklace, he stayed at Paris, Bordeaux (where he was denounced by yet another correspondent of the Société Royale), and Lyons, among other places.[65] At the other extreme, some itinerants simply traveled into the countryside from a single urban base, like a former porter of the Paris School of Medicine who, in the early nineteenth century, made weekly trips in the environs of the capital.[66]

Between the two extremes can be found a great variety of travel patterns. Some itinerants traversed the kingdom. D'Angleberme was reported in Bas-Poitou in March 1779, at Nantes in December 1780, and at Albi in 1781.[67] Algaron appeared at Saint-Malo in 1779, at Nantes in 1780, at Saint-Quentin in the 1780's, at Le Mans in 1790 – and reportedly even farther afield. The Société Royale found that he was denounced "everywhere."[68] The versatile Salomon Cuchet, who appeared at Dijon in 1769 (already claiming to be eighty years old), surfaced at Nantes in 1781 and at Dun-le-Roi in Berry in the summer of 1783.[69] Many circuits, though, apparently took in only a few contiguous provinces, if that. Edin was reported at Guingamp in Brittany, Le Blanc in Berry, and Gien-sur-Loire in the Orléanais.[70] Fleury appeared at Saulieu in Burgundy in 1780, at Auxerre in 1781, at Château-Thierry in the Île-de-France in 1785, and at Saint-Malo in Brittany in 1791.[71] Ramay appeared at Nogent in Champagne in 1779, at Vendôme in the Orléanais in 1786, and at Vierzon in Berry in 1786.[72]

Other practitioners worked a province or two for a few years and then moved on. Grassy, reported in the Île-de-France near Champagne in 1784, was said to have stayed in the region for eight years at three different residences (although in 1781 he – or someone using a similar name – was denounced at Dax, in Gascony). In 1785 and 1786, he made his way through Brittany, stopping not only at Nantes and Rennes but also at Guingamp, Quintin, Morlaix, and Josselin, among other places.[73] Some of these routes crossed national borders: Germans passed into Alsace and beyond, and Gascons ventured into Spain. Indeed, many of the most prominent practitioners in France were foreigners: Swiss, Germans, Italians, a few Englishmen.[74]

The key stopping places included major cities and towns. Charlatans did not simply fill the gaps where no physicians or surgeons were available; they went where the money was.[75] The city of Lyons, for example, at the intersection of major trade routes, long attracted large numbers of showmen, jugglers, operators, and charlatans, many of them Italian, although a vigorous campaign by the corporations may have reduced their number by the beginning of the Revolution.[76] In the town of Soultz (in Alsace near the German border) charlatans received police permission to erect their stages about twenty times a year.[77] But charlatanism was not exclusively a phenomenon of the major population centers. Contemporary observers believed (as one correspondent of the Société Royale put it) that the "capital continually inundates the provinces with this wretched breed," and that from the provincial towns they passed on to the countryside when pressure from municipal authorities and corporations became too great.[78] There is some truth to this explanation; in rural areas the empiric was free from most police controls and from harassment by medical and surgical corporations. But if he went into the countryside, to fairs and markets in small bourgs and even to villages, it was because money could be had there. The reports to the Société Royale suggest that the countryside represented an increasingly important market for the charlatan, who brought the popular medicine of the preindustrial city to a rural clientele. Societies without urban centers have no mountebanks; industrial societies that have been successfully medicalized have very few. The classic charlatan thrives at the urban/rural frontier: he is in the countryside but not of it. (The history of popular medicine in the American West points to a similar conclusion.)[79]

Charlatans circulated in that large space where the market economy overlapped what remained of the peasant closed economy, extracting money from the countryside and spending most of it in nearby towns – for which they sometimes received praise from the local authorities, who pointed out that a successful empiric meant trade for the druggists and other merchants.[80] The economic role of the provincial charlatan in some ways recalls that of the bandit. Like the bandit, the mountebank extracted money and valuables from his victims (the image of the quack as bandit recurs repeatedly in eighteenth-century rhetoric, and some itinerants literally mixed robbery with illegal medical practice and other forms of deviant ecomomic behavior). And then, like the bandit, he went to town and spent his gains to support himself and his band of dependents. "A successful brigand chief," Eric Hobsbawm writes, "is at least as closely in touch with the market and the wider economic universe as a small landowner or prosperous farmer. Indeed, in economically backward regions his trade may draw him close to that of others who travel, buy and sell."[81] So, too, with many a *chevalier d'industrie*.

If charlatanism is to be understood as an economic activity, it must be considered as an occupation and even as a career. How did people become charlatans? And how did they fare? The evidence is fragmentary; this problem did not greatly interest the authorities, and the contemporary literature on quackery has more to say about the charlatan's moral failings than about his social and economic background. But the question is worth pursuing. We are so used to seeing the charlatan through the eyes of the medical historian, as one possible source of medical advice for the population or as the embodiment of medical folly, that we sometimes forget that for the empiric his work was, after all, a job.

It was possible to become a charlatan in one of three ways: by starting from scratch, by being born into a family of charlatans, or by joining an existing troupe. Setting out on one's own was not a highly attractive option to a young man dissatisfied, say, with his work as a journeyman in a small market town. It was necessary to begin modestly; the equipage of a full-fledged mountebank, starting with a well-appointed carriage and horses to draw it, would have been beyond his means. Women faced even more discouraging prospects; they rarely emerged as successful charlatans and troupe leaders. One does hear of solitary female itinerants, like Catherine Barjon, from Lagery in the Marne, who turned up selling remedies at Blesmes in the Aisne in the spring of 1818. It was common, moreover, for a male charlatan's wife or woman companion to participate in the work of his troupe; some simple husband-wife teams were also reported, like the Vacherons, who were active around Châlons-sur-Marne in 1780.[82] The Madame Fleuri reported leading a troupe in the same year was probably associated with Fleury's business, whether or not she was actually his wife.[83] Widows or daughters (like Albertina Dränkler) sometimes inherited a family calling. But classic charlatanism remained a male-dominated occupation.

Charlatans' children were among the prime beneficiaries of the informal apprenticeship system that prepared a young person to be an independent operator and remedy vendor and, ultimately, a troupe leader. Philippe Ramay's son, for example, followed quite literally in his father's footsteps.[84] Some of the most prominent empirics of the Old Regime, such as Algaron Toscan, were members of well-established dynasties.

It was possible, finally, for an outsider to attach himself to an existing troupe or to join an itinerant solo practitioner as a sort of assistant-apprentice. Philippe Ramay was a chairmaker and former soldier from Dôle who had served as the *garçon* of an operator named Cherchin. Another itinerant of the early Restoration began as a village bootblack (*décrotteur*) who hoped to improve his lot by leaving in the company of a passing band of charlatans.[85] As circumstances later changed, the empiric adjusted. In the Yonne, a young practitioner who had worked in 1818 as the associate of a major charlatan named Léger, returned on his own in 1821, claiming to be his son-in-law; when the mayor of Toucy refused to authorize him to peddle remedies and extract teeth in the public square, he joined another troupe – but this time a troupe of acrobats, for whom he worked as a musician.[86]

For many charlatans, indeed, itinerant empiricism (sometimes interspersed with periods of more sedentary practice) was only one stage in a checkered career; they belonged to a breed of economic floaters or drifters, who never secured a definite niche, even as empirics. Consider two careers from the period of the Revolution and Empire.

Michel Girault

Known as Frère Ange, he was born in 1777 at Pontailler-sur-Saône, in Burgundy. According to his own account, his father was a *commissaire des poudres* (an official of the royal gunpowder company that Turgot established in 1775 under the direction of the chemist Lavoisier); in fact his father was an artisan, a *maître poudrier*, not a *commissaire*. The son professed to have studied surgery "from early childhood on," saying that he left home in 1790 and traveled in Holland, Switzerland, and Germany. After returning to France in the Year VIII (1799–1800), he spent several years in Holland and then passed several more in a Trappist monastery. His travels then took him to Strasbourg (where he received a passport in July 1807) and on to Lyons and Geneva. Finally he began to practice medicine at Chaux-des-Crotenay in the Jura, where he lodged with the curé. Girault may have fabricated much of his account in an attempt to promote and justify himself, but it is clear that he led an itinerant life as an adolescent and young adult during the Revolution. His means of support, apart from medical practice, are uncertain.

The medical career of Frère Ange unfolds in his police file of 1808. Girault now called himself the son of the Baron de Vaudré, owner of a property at Morveaux (Morval?). Since Girault himself was suffering from some sort of disease, the curé of Chaux took him to the hospital at Arbois (Jura), where he continued to work what were described as "miraculous cures." His patients (who were said to have come to him from the Doubs, the Côte-d'Or, and even farther away) were lodged and fed at the hospital. The miraculous healer was said to refuse payment, since he received funds from his family and from investments in Holland. Girault's triumph ended, like a popular farce, in an unmasking. The authorities found that his father was still living at Vonges, near Pontailler-sur-Saône, contrary to what the empiric had reported, and that he was a simple artisan; worse, they confirmed that Frère Ange's income came from patients, rather than from independent sources. Within two days of the revelations, he fled Arbois, in search of another livelihood and another identity.[87]

François Royer (the would-be bathkeeper mentioned in Chapter 2)
Nicknamed "Va-de-bon-coeur" (loosely, Good Fellow), he was one of six or seven children of a farmer in the Sarthe. He may have acquired some rudiments of medicine from an uncle who was a charitable practitioner; he probably also worked for the Brothers of Charity for a few years before the Revolution. During the Revolution, if we are to believe the rather naive report of the subprefect of Gien, Royer traveled with General Kellermann, the hero of the battle of Valmy, to Turkey, where he began to treat wounds and ulcers. He continued his practice after returning to France, although "quarrels with *officiers de santé*" forced him to change his place of residence frequently. Eventually he learned weaving and settled in the communes of Les Bordes and Ouzouer-sur-Loire (Loiret), where he nevertheless continued to treat patients. Royer was convicted of illegal

medical practice and sent to jail; a second conviction resulted in another sentence that could not be enforced, the empiric having gone underground. His recidivism was not surprising; as the subprefect observed, Royer had "no means of support other than those he obtains from the credulity of the inhabitants of the countryside who are afflicted with a few sores."[88]

Clearly, it is dangerous to generalize about the rewards of charlatanism as an occupation. Some charlatans – a rough guess would place the number at no more than several hundred – carved out successful careers during the reign of Louis XVI. Others, though, knew only fleeting triumphs and seem for the most part to have dragged out a pathetic existence. One comes away from some of their dossiers with the sense that their grandiosity was as much an effort to bolster self-esteem as a scheme to delude and defraud the public, and that their itineracy was less an expression of entrepreneurial ambition than an indication of repeated local failure.

Traditional charlatanism: persistence and decline

Classic charlatanism probably reached its acme in the seventeenth and early eighteenth centuries; in the last decades of the Old Regime it may well have been on the decline. In 1748, a Dr. Ganiaire at Beaune remarked on the diminution of *le grand charlatanisme*.[89] By 1789, according to some accounts, old-fashioned mountebanks were rarely seen in the larger towns; a correspondent of the Société Royale de Médecine at Aubagne, near Marseilles, noted in that year that "bedizened charlatans mounted on their equipages no longer appear in Marseilles," although he added that they were "inundating the villages and small towns in the environs."[90] The Comité de Salubrité survey of 1790–1791 unfortunately does not provide usable statistics, but some respondents commented on the dwindling number of itinerants. "During the last few years, traveling empirics and charlatans have begun to disappear" (Boiscommun, Loiret). "Charlatans rarely pass through our cantons; the people are getting to know these fellows' dirty tricks, and there is every reason to believe that we shall not see any more in the future" (Hyères, Var). Other reports say simply that the district has no charlatans, or that empirics are not tolerated and rarely pass through.[91] Such observations multiplied in the early nineteenth century. The itinerants seemed to be yielding to competition from fixed retail outlets (both pharmacies and local distributors of proprietary remedies) and then to the mail-order trade. The Swiss physician Gallot wrote in 1829:

The charlatans of today differ from those of times past. They are no longer seen in costumes trimmed with lace, a sword at their side, up on a stage and haranguing the astounded multitude, drawn by the piercing sound of the trumpet. I do not know whether eloquence has diminished among them, or rather whether they have not wisely calculated that by means of the divine art invented in Mainz in 1440 by the immortal Guttenberg, and with the help of a hundred thousand messengers who unceasingly convey thought between wrappers into every corner of Europe, they could, without going to so much trouble to travel about, send the advertisement of their precious discoveries from one end of the continent to the other in the twinkling of an eye. What is certain is that now they earn a million more easily and more quickly without moving from their den, than they formerly accumulated ten pistoles by moving their pompous, cheap finery from place to place and exhausting all the resources of the oratorical art on their traveling theaters.[92]

The old-style charlatan yielded less to modern medicine than to modern communications and marketing.[93]

But despite this long-term trend, the itinerants remained highly visible figures in the rural landscape.[94] Appendix B lists some representative cases of itinerant empiricism from the first half of the nineteenth century. About half of the cases involve traditional mountebanks, with their stage, drum, and trumpets, outlandish costumes, clowns, and tumblers. Others are locals who traveled a bit among the villages of their region. Three Alsatian cases – the Traber brothers, Propheter, and Volk – show that an itinerant could establish a regular regional practice. The Trabers apparently journeyed up and down both banks of the Rhine over a period of at least eight years. The other two, known as Dr. Hans and Dr. Johann, won so loyal a following in the Bas-Rhin that they effectively served part of the population as physicians, in keeping with their nicknames. These last cases warrant closer examination, for they suggest the extent to which an empiric might compete directly with local professionals.

In February of 1811, the cantonal physician of Sarre-Union denounced to the prefect a "quack and famous ignoramus who is called Dr. Johann":

I have been told that he is from around Bischwiller, arrondissement of Strasbourg, travels about the region, wreaks terrible havoc, and swindles money from the credulous and superstitious inhabitants of the countryside. The people, who are gladly drawn to miracles and extraordinary things, chase after him in a mob in order to consult him. He gives prescriptions transcribed from an old German medical book, which he has others write down.[95]

He required the assistance of others because (according to the mayor of Bergzabern in the annexed department of Mont-Tonnerre, where Dr. Johann had his main practice) he could neither read nor write.[96] The empiric's background was obscure. The prosecutor at Wissembourg reported that he came from Switzerland originally and was already "getting on in years."[97] Other accounts said that he came from Bischwiller or was a native of Bergzabern (so the subprefect of Wissembourg reported, although he added that he had "long since lost his rights as a citizen and his domicile").[98] The cantonal physician at Wissembourg called him a baker.[99] Propheter had traveled widely in the department, practicing medicine in the cantons of

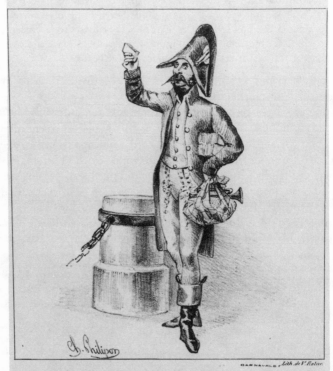

Surgery without a Surgeon: a quack peddles his self-help book. Drawing by Charles Philipon; lithograph by V. Ratier; from the *Petites affiches parisiennes*. "A work destined to destroy charlatanism by teaching a simple and easy way to cut off one's own arms, legs, etc. . . . The publisher, who has no other goal than to be useful to humanity, provides with a copy of this work an ear-pick and a bodkin."

Sarre-Union and Wissembourg, as well as around the arrondissement of Strasbourg, and had previously been arrested several times at Deux-Ponts (Zweibrücken), just over the border in Mont-Tonnerre. So well established was Dr. Johann's reputation that the local apothecaries filled the prescriptions he wrote for his patients.[100] His practice in the Bas-Rhin continued for at least two more years, for he appeared again in a census of illegal practitioners in 1813.[101]

The police record of Dr. Hans suggests that his career was both longer and more varied than Dr. Johann's. Jean Volk probably came from Freiburg in the Grand Duchy of Baden; originally a shoemaker, he sometimes went by the second sobriquet of "Schumacher Hans."[102] The first mention of Dr. Hans comes in a report of January 1811 by Hoffmann, a physician at Wissembourg, on an epidemic in the communes of Ober- and Niederbetschdorf. Volk was a "foreigner . . . who, after being driven from his own country, came to seek refuge in ours, where he wanders with no fixed abode and works hard at making dupes."[103] In 1812 Lion, cantonal physician of Soultz-sous-Forêts, provided further details on Volk's activities. "To give his business a certain mysterious air, he has the patients' urine brought to him, or uses several words that makes no sense." His remedies were "certainly deadly poisons for the majority of patients," but they "produced nevertheless a momentary good effect on patients who still had any strength." Lion added that Volk sometimes sent patients to pharmacists, who split their fees with him.[104]

Volk's activities ranged so widely that he appeared in the reports of several different cantonal physicians in 1813. In the canton of Brumath, Dr. Hans had been "very much in vogue a year ago in and around [Gambsheim]," where he "kept hidden during the day and traveled at night to see his patients, in communes that were sometimes very far away."[105] Buchholtz, cantonal physician at Wissembourg, also denounced Volk, noting that he had already mentioned him in his regular report to the prefect in January 1811.[106] And at Woerth, the cantonal physician complained that the "vagabond who calls himself Doctor Hanz . . . wreaks great havoc in my canton."[107] Volk became a notorious recidivist, probably the best-known illegal practitioner in the Bas-Rhin.

Volk and Propheter were perhaps exceptional; but some forms of itinerant practice flourished at least into the 1880's, and may even have expanded for a while after midcentury, thanks to the development of the road system. Even after the turn of the century, itinerant empirics lingered on. In the early 1900's, for example, the Italian Madame Chiarini traveled conspicuously around France on horseback, sometimes accompanied by one or more tooth pullers; she had snakes in alcohol and sold "purifying" plants, laxatives, and vermifuges, as well as a *baume de la guerre* (war balm) for aches and bruises. Other cases could be cited, some of them from as late as midcentury.[108] On the eve of World War I, "ambulatory physicians" remained prevalent enough for one deputy from Meurthe-et-Moselle to propose taxing their activities.[109] Like many groups long perceived as being on the decline, the itinerants proved a remarkably persistent lot.

VARIETIES OF ITINERANCY: PEDDLERS, MARGINALS, AND INSPIRED HEALERS

The discussion so far has concentrated on itinerants who practiced medicine as a full-time occupation, and particularly on the classic mountebank. But the sphere of the charlatan merged into a much larger world of wanderers, who lived by peddling, begging, and crime, with which they sometimes mixed a little medicine and remedy vending.

Peddlers

Even among the empirics, many itinerants were primarily ambulatory pharmacists. The Italian Saqui actually used this title (*pharmacien ambulant*) when he asked permission to sell his "universal panacea" in Eure-et-Loir in 1797.[110] Traveling operators, too, often derived a good part of their income from the sale of drugs. In the early years of the Restoration, for example, the dentist Cartin of the Haute-Loire peddled a dentifrice in the countryside; another dentist, François Sibenaler, working in the Charente-Inférieure, sold eau de Cologne (to be taken internally as a remedy).[111] In addition, the more modest and more numerous *porteballes* (packmen) simply bought discarded or spoiled drugs and resold them at fairs and in the countryside.[112]

Some itinerants were still less specialized, offering a wide variety of wares and services. The dentist Hoffmann, according to his advertisement in the *Affiches du Mans* (1776), extracted, transplanted, and preserved teeth and sold an infallible balsamic elixir that was guaranteed to calm neuralgia within three minutes; but he also sold a secret for "learning in three days how to paint all sorts of pictures, without it being necessary to know how to draw." The chiropodist Bonnesse not only removed corns, cured toothache in one minute, and whitened teeth in four (in addition to making and installing dentures), but also sold a secret for eliminating bedbugs – a mixed bag of empirical tricks.[113] Conversely, the familiar *colporteur* (peddler) might carry a few medicinal products along with other supplies. In 1747, for example, the Le Noir brothers, Piedmontese traveling through Maine, obtained permission to sell steel buckles and ibex's blood. The latter, like many of the peddlers' wares, was a regional specialty. The Swiss peasants, it was said, nourished ibexes on aromatic plants, bled them, and dried the blood in an oven or in the sun after separating the serum.[114] In general, the authorities of the Old Regime allowed peddlers to hawk simples in the provinces,

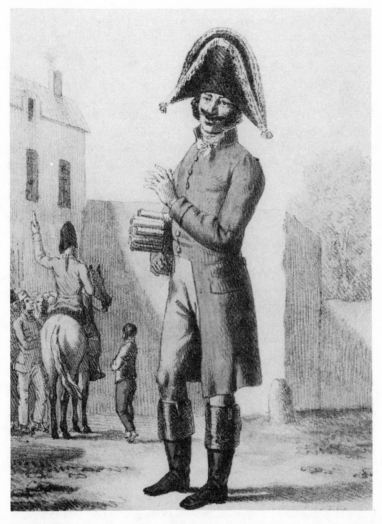

Vendor of Swiss vulnerary, in the classic charlatan's costume. (Courtesy of the Cabinet des Estampes, Musée Carnavalet. Photograph by Jean-Loup Charmet.)

although not officinal remedies (standard compounds stocked by pharmacists) or other compositions. Since they generally sold these products directly to patients or potential patients, their activities spilled over into medical practice.

The sale of drugs by itinerant peddlers continued through the nineteenth century, often tolerated at the local level. At Auxerre, for example, according to a report of 1821, traveling merchants "licensed" by a medical faculty could sell Swiss vulneraries, eau de Cologne, and sometimes even stones for use as a remedy against toothache; according to a widespread popular belief, a nail, stone or other small object might be imbued with the property of drawing off the pain from the afflicted tooth. (Three years earlier, though, the authorities had taken action against a vendor named René Léger, who sold an aromatic oil, eau de Cologne, and a dry grass in the guise of "Swiss tea" in the public square at Vermenton.)[115] Swiss tea or "Swiss pectoral tea" (that is, an herbal infusion for chest complaints) was a specialty of Tirolese and other foreigners, according to an 1834 report in the Bas-Rhin; one of them also sold vials of a reddish liquid containing sulfuric acid, apparently using the herbals as a come-on.[116] A similar trade was also associated with the great seasonal cycles of migration in provincial France, when villagers left isolated mountainous and rural regions for months at a time to make a living on the road. Dauphiné was especially renowned for exporting medicinal plants to other regions of France and to Spain; each village had its herbal specialty. During the winter expatriation of men, many became *colporteurs*; the plant sellers of the Oisans region (where late in the century one of every three heads of household worked as a peddler) were familiar sights in the nineteenth-century countryside.[117] Some emerged as full-fledged empirics. A local historian has left an unusually full, if unsympathetic, portrait of the plant-sellers of Oisans:

They needed innocuous remedies, the makings of cataplasms and vesicatories, aloes, antimony, cade oil, phenic acid, purgatives and vermifuge syrup, with the inevitable arnica and a little fuchsine added in order to have attractive colorings. To all this pharmacopoeia . . . , it was necessary to add a quantity of cabalistic signs and above all a flood of words; they scarcely operated unless somewhat drunk, "so as to give themselves courage and loosen the tongue." Never surgery or bonesetting; at most a few may have practiced the pulling of rotten teeth. They often traveled in pairs and tried not to return too soon to communes where they had swindled people. Sometimes, to inspire confidence, they provided themselves with sham diplomas on which the impression of a 100-sou piece imitated the official seal. On arriving in a village, in order to be sure not to make a mistake, they discreetly gathered information on the patients and their illnesses. There was a convenient method for revealing the illness or getting around difficult cases – the magic bottle. A flagon containing both water and ether, separated by the difference in density, allowed [the operator] to pour at will a drop of one or the other liquid on the back of the patient's hand, using a simple motion of the wrist. The slow evaporation of the water signified that he needed a remedy, the rapid evaporation of the ether that he was cured. . . . The more enterprising offered cheap protection against pregnancy, or even the risks of military conscription. There were also veterinarians and disenchanters of stables. An accomplice took care of hobbling the horses and cattle of a village with inconspicuous thorns, and the traveler from Oisans triumphantly cured them in the evening. It cost 40 francs.[118]

Unlike the theater of the old mountebank, though, these activities were confined to the countryside.

Almost as familiar as the Oisans peddlers were the *colporteurs de saint Hubert*, popularly called "Saint Huberts," who helped attract pilgrims to the monastery in the Ardennes that was consecrated to the saint, the patron of hunters, and, in the popular imagination, a source of protection against dangerous wild animals and their bites. They sold the prayer of Saint Hubert, a printed summary of his miracles, talismans to protect against the serpent, wolf, and mad dog, and trinkets such as rings (for girls) and hunting horns (for boys).[119]

The Saint Huberts illustrate a more general point: in popular culture, the peddler was more than an economic middleman. He could serve, for example, as a religious intermediary. One mid-nineteenth-century broadsheet offered this bonus to prospective customers:

Anyone who buys 10 sous of merchandise from the peddler will earn a half-mass at the chapel.
Someone who buys 20 sous' worth will earn a complete mass, whose benefits will last, not one day only, but, on the contrary, all eternity.[120]

Moreover, peddlers were sometimes seen as a source of good or bad luck and were widely believed to possess magical powers, some of which could affect human health. Thus in this century, a peddler who came annually to Boullay-les-Troux (Essonne) was believed to be capable of paralyzing a man by laying a hand on his shoulder.[121] But the hand that crippled might also heal.

Marginals

If charlatanism and peddling were regular trades for some, for others ambulatory medicine was but one stage or facet of a checkered career, which sometimes led them through the world of shady acquaintances, police spies, and revolutionary politics that Richard Cobb and Robert Darnton have described.[122] We have the testimony of a Paris spy that a certain Saule, who in 1793 was an *inspecteur des tribunes* (a police official charged with maintaining order in the public galleries of the National Convention), was formerly a tapestry maker, then a peddler, and then "a charlatan with boxes selling for four sous, filled with the grease of a hanged man for curing pain in the loins."[123] A typical wanderer of the early nineteenth century, Jean-François-Michel Boulogne, worked in the Var and the Bouches-du-Rhône, sometimes as a surgeon, sometimes as a music teacher. He called himself a native of "Sicillano in Tuscany" and in one place styled himself a Sicilian officer (although when he taught music he adopted the name Hippolyte Dupuy). He had in fact been born in Arles, but he used his father's Italian birth certificate with a false date. In 1817, Boulogne was charged with practicing surgery at Cotignac in the Var, including an operation for anal fistula; the *juge d'instruction* informed the court that in one commune he was suspected "of having spoken against the government," which he took to indicate that he might be "an emissary of ill will" – not a surprising charge in the case of so disreputable a character.[124]

Other itinerants were still more miserable economic marginals, mere vagabonds, as the police saw them, who derived a small income from the sale of medicines and other goods and sometimes from begging and theft. Étienne Lhôpital, called Dumas, was a semivagabond who set dislocated bones in the countryside around Lyons in the middle of the eighteenth century.[125] In 1787 the "dentist-conjuror" Charles Piogé and his wife, Fran-çoise Bartolle, were arrested at Faye-l'Abbesse in Poitou, where they were selling orvietan; the couple was accused of committing a theft at an inn. Among their belongings the authorities found "wooden figures or mari-onette characters, with packets of powders of various colors and pills. Plus a large panel to serve as a signboard." Theirs was not a highly profitable business; the woman had collected only 15 sous in the town that morning.[126] In the early nineteenth century, "vagabond empiric" became a standard notation in the police records, applied, for example, to a certain Louise-Magdelaine Jacquette, who had been in prison in Nantes, had been separated from her husband for several years, and in 1815 was found without papers in La Merlatière (Vendée).[127]

Such wanderings were in some case seasonal or occasional, like the mi-grations of the plant peddlers of Dauphiné. In the winter, according to a report from the Landes to the Comité de Salubrité (1791), shepherds came down from the mountains to sell remedies and secrets and apply plasters.[128] In Dauphiné, a few years earlier, a band of former shepherds from Montbrun (a contemporary source refers to them as *"maiges,"* an elastic term) de-scended on Barret-le-Bas, claiming to have been sent by the intendant; they were said to have collected 60 livres from a neighboring village in a quarter of an hour.[129]

A fuller picture of a vagabond and occasional empiric, this time from the early nineteenth century, can be reconstructed from a dossier in the archives of the Loire-Atlantique. Pierre-Jean Renou (or Renaud), a native of Vitré in Ille-et-Vilaine, was variously described in the police reports as a black-smith and a locksmith; they gave his age in 1820 as thirty-seven. In August 1819 he had been arrested at Nantes and charged with practicing surgery without a license. Renou, who had represented himself as a physician, claimed to be divinely inspired. Released from prison in July 1820, he turned up once more at his former place of residence, again practicing "inspired medicine."

Like many such deviants, Renou was a frequent recidivist. In 1812, he had been sentenced to two years' imprisonment for vagrancy and illegal medical practice in Beaupréau. According to the mayor of Saint-Macaire, a town in Maine-et-Loire where Renou had stayed, he had also been in prison in Angers. A year after his arrival in Saint-Macaire, he left for Angers and was arrested for robbery along the way. After serving a prison sentence, he returned and worked as a locksmith, taking his trade to neighboring Saint-André, where he committed another theft.[130] Renou belonged to a category of offenders whose behavior defied classification in terms of contemporary legal and social thought. Was he a simple *mauvais sujet*, a criminal, or a madman?[131]

The knights of Saint Hubert

The inspired itinerant sometimes traveled by religious vocation (or so he said), and his journey then assumed the character of a pilgrimage. The most prominent exemplars were the pilgrims who traveled to the monastery of Saint Hubert in the Ardennes to be preserved from rabies and to receive the power to cure and preserve others.[132] One remarkable example from 1808 has been briefly described in an article by Roger Vaultier, but the case is interesting enough to warrant a full presentation here, for it strikingly illustrates the ways in which the marginal itinerant could be both victim and victimizer.[133]

Marie-Joseph Hué was arrested near Boulogne-sur-Mer in March 1808; she called herself a *grande chevalière* in the order of Saint Hubert and claimed that after fasting and doing penance at the abbey of Saint Hubert, she had received from dom Bernard, formerly a monk at the abbey, the gift of curing rabies and conferring protection against the disease for ninety-seven years. At the time of her arrest, Hué was carrying certificates from local mayors permitting her to stay in their communes. The *magistrat de sûreté* at Boulogne, however, took her for a fraud; it was notorious, he wrote, that at Saint-Hubert there were "swindlers" who created "so-called knights," who then crisscrossed the countryside of France.

At her police interrogation, Hué stated that she was sixty-eight years old and a native of La Gorgue in the Nord; she had no profession, and the consecrated police formula *"sans domicile fixe"* marked her as a vagrant. Until the difficult Year III (1794–1795), she had lived *en puissance de mari* (under a husband's authority) – a phrase that says more than any commentary could about the perceived connection between the marriage bond and social order. Her husband, a mason named Louis-Joseph Legue, a native of Hersin-Coupigny near Arras, had wanted a divorce, newly permitted under revolutionary legislation; she, however, had not. In the end he left her and, according to her account, married two other women, probably bigamously, who were still alive near Saint-Omer.

At some point in the Year III, probably during the terrible winter of 1794–1795, when wolves left the forests and roamed through villages in northern France, Hué was bitten (or so she said) by a rabid wolf. Her reaction was to mortify herself. She followed the popularly prescribed ritual for the victim of the bite of a rabid animal, spending forty-three days at the chapel of Saint Hubert, subsisting on water and unleavened bread. She even eschewed two other foods normally allowed the penitents, hard-boiled eggs and fish with scales.[134] At the end of her ordeal, famished and delirious, she had a vision in a cave of the saint with his popular attributes, two dogs and a trumpet (hunting horn); it was the saint himself, according to one version of her story, who gave her the power to cure rabies and to preserve people for ninety-seven years from the bite of rabid animals.

It was then that she began what the police called her "wandering life." To prevent rabies, she said, she used prayers and what she called the "star" of Saint Hubert, a kind of coat hook with a figure in enamel, which she said dom Bernard had given her. The document uses the word "*étoile*"; the usual legend depicts the saint with a stole (*étole*), and a fragment of what was purported to be this miraculous vestment was sometimes implanted in the forehead as a preservative against rabies. Hué called the screw of the coat hook the "key" of Saint Hubert; the Saint Hubert's key, sometimes heated red hot, had a place in the healing ritual for rabies.

Hué's travels took her through at least five departments in France and what is now Belgium (Nord, Pas-de-Calais, Somme, Aisne, Lys); Map 1 shows her itinerary over a period of about four years before her arrest, from 26 Frimaire Year XII (18 December 1803) to 7 October 1807, according to the certificates from local mayors she was carrying at the time of her arrest. At her interrogation she insisted that she had never been arrested before. She wandered, she said, because she had taken a penitential vow and would not sleep in a bed until her death. Why she had imposed such a severe regimen on herself she could not say.

The incident that led to Hué's arrest took place at La Poterie near Boulogne. According to her account, she heard mass in Boulogne and then traveled south as far as a village between Hesdin and Montreuil, whose name she could not recall. There she tried to pass the night at two places where she had been taken in before, but they had no space for her; in the end she slept under a hedge near the church of Saint-Léonard, perhaps 5 kilometers from Boulogne. She apparently then proceeded north, past Boulogne to the commune of Wimille, where she arrived at the farm of the Hautefeuille family in the village of La Poterie. The husband, she said, gave her a tartine, and she stayed until Tuesday (evidently meaning two nights), sleeping on straw, though invited to sleep in a bed. The family, she suggested, may have kept her this long out of a desire to be preserved from rabies for ninety-seven years; in any case she had touched all the members of the household with the "star."

Angélique Leclercq, wife of Hautefeuille, a laborer at La Poterie, testified that the stonecutter who worked for her had admitted Hué to the house while she was at the market. When she returned, she found the woman sitting near the fire, crying. Hué said that she was from Cassel, 20 to 30 leagues away, and that she could only accept assistance in the stretch from Boulogne to Wacquinghen (a town between Wimille and Marquise; see Map 1). She showed a paper whose contents she said she did not know, because she could not read; since the Hautefeuille woman could not read either, they had to await the return of her worker to decipher the text for them. The paper recommended the "knight of the great Saint Hubert"; on the back, according to the police report, was written "Marie Joseph Hué, farmwife at La Gorgue [*à la gorge fermière*], and thirty horned beasts and fourteen horses" – presumably a reference to her supposed property holdings. The paper was unsigned, but the woman argued that coming from the hand of God, it could not very well have a signature. She asked for clothing and promised as recompense 30 measures of land out of the 166 that she owned, saying that this was as true as that she had the holy star in her pocket.

Her clothes, she said, were blessed, and she could not return to her own country unless she stopped at a distance of 6 leagues, had a service said for her, and buried her own clothing. She would then go to her own place, where she would have to spend six weeks without being able to give orders to servants or children or ask for anything to eat, unless it was brought voluntarily; she was also obliged to sleep on marble. If she fulfilled all of these conditions, she would then be able to "enjoy all her faculties." These self-imposed hardships were clearly intended as an imitation of the lives of the saints; she had merited the title of *chevalière*, she said, by enduring the same setbacks as Saint Hubert.

The Hautefeuille woman prepared a package following Hué's instructions, including three skirts (of ratteen, linen, and wool), a blouse, a round bonnet, five handkerchiefs, a pair of new stockings, a pair of new shoes, an apron, a gold cross with a *maintenon* (small crucifix), a pair of gloves, a pair of purses, and a snuffbox. Hué did not exactly request all these things (although the Hautefeuille woman did ask her whether she wanted the gold cross, and she replied yes), but she directed her hostess "to dress the *chevalière* of Saint Hubert." She asked, moreover, for 15 francs in a handkerchief for the divine service and an unspecified amount for her expenses on the road. The Hautefeuille woman gave her 18 écus in 6-franc pieces; her worker gave 9 francs and two pieces of 20 sous. Thus provisioned, Hué left the farm at seven on Tuesday morning.

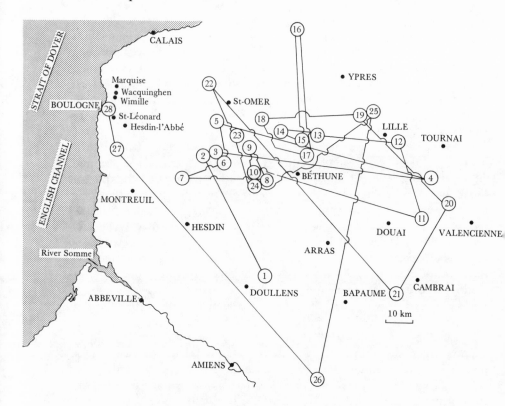

Map 1. Hué's itinerary, 1803–08. Wanderings of a *chevalière de saint Hubert*, reconstructed from a list of mayors' certificates found in her possession at the time of her arrest. [Dates of certificates do not always correspond exactly to Hué's arrival; connecting lines are schematic and do not represent her actual path between different points.] Numbers correspond to key below. (*Source*: Archives Nationales F⁸ 157.)

Place and date of issuance of certificates: (**1**) Saulty (Pas-de-Calais); 26 Frimaire XII/18 December 1803. (**2**) Wandonne (Pas-de-Calais); 9 Pluviôse XII/30 January 1804. (**3**) Dennebroeucq (Pas-de-Calais); 9 Pluviôse XII/ 30 January 1804. (**4**) Aix (Nord); 15 Pluviôse XII/5 February 1804. (**5**) Pilhem (Pas-de-Calais); 15 Pluviôse XII/5 February 1804. (**6**) Beaumetzlès-Aire (Pas-de-Calais); 24 Pluviôse XII/14 February 1804. (**7**) Créquy (Pas-de-Calais); 30 Pluviôse XII/20 February 1804. (**8**) Camblain-Châtelain (Pas-de-Calais); 12 Ventôse XII/3 March 1804. (**9**) Liettres (Pas-de-Calais); 18 Ventôse XII/9 March 1804. (**10**) Amettes (Pas-de-Calais); 19 Ventôse XII/10 March 1804. (**11**)Vred (now in Nord); 12 Floréal XII/2 May 1804. (**12**) Ronchin (Nord); 27 Prairial XII/16 June 1804. (**13**) La Gorgue (Nord); Hué's birthplace. 29 Messidor XII/18 July 1804. (**14**) Saint-Floris (Pas-de-Calais); 9 Fructidor XII/27 August 1804. (**15**) Lestrem (Pas-de-Calais); 27 Fructidor XII/14 September 1804. (**16**) Wulveringhem (Lys); 29 Fructidor

The *chevalière* came to grief by stopping too soon after La Poterie on the way to Marquise; at a cabaret in Wimille she consumed a large lunch with brandy, although according to her announced program she was not supposed to stop en route. Hautefeuille's worker caught up with her, learned about the meal, and had her arrested at Marquise. The police found in her possession the effects given her by the Hautefeuille woman, together with her own meager belongings, which included only the miraculous coat hook, a tin snuffbox, and two knives.

That Hué practiced a minor sort of confidence game is probable, but it is possible that this pathetic woman, abandoned by her husband and destitute at the age of nearly seventy, may have half believed the tale she spun in her quest for alms. She was typical, in any case, of the displaced persons who had to live by their wits, and who sometimes turned to medicine, empirical, mystical, or religious, as one source of a precarious livelihood. It took youth and a certain amount of daring to join the predatory *bande d'Orgères*, which Richard Cobb has so vividly portrayed.[135] Popular medicine was easier and safer.

The tradition of the knights of Saint Hubert persisted into the nineteenth century; a few itinerants (some of whom appeared sincerely convinced of their divine vocation) made a modest living by offering to protect farm animals against rabies. The *Gazette des tribunaux* of 1827–1828, for example, reported the trials of self-styled *chevaliers* at Reims and at Arcis-sur-Aube: Joachim-Agathe Voilmy, twenty-five years old, and a certain Nicolas, also twenty-five.[136] Voilmy appeared in January 1828, at Trois-Puits near Reims, at the house of a landowner named Menu. The head of the household was absent; his wife, a serving woman, and a third woman received Voilmy. The *chevalier* pulled out a medal and applied it to the three women, muttering prayers and making signs of the cross. He next asked for holy water and palm fronds that had been blessed on Palm Sunday and inquired about the number of animals in the house. Taking some bread, he knelt, surrounded by the three women, and recited prayers from a book. He sprinkled the water on the bread and recommended giving a piece of it to the animals

Caption of Map 1 (*cont.*)
XII/16 September 1804. **(17)** Locon (Pas-de-Calais); 30 Fructidor XII/17 September 1804. **(18)** Blaringhem (now in Nord); 27 Vendémiaire XIII/19 October 1804. **(19)** Frelinghien (Nord); 10 Brumaire XIII/1 November 1804. **(20)** Hasnon (Nord); 11 Frimaire XIII/2 December 1804. **(21)** Graincourt (Pas-de-Calais); 8 Nivôse XIII/29 December 1804. **(22)** Éperlecques (Pas-de-Calais); 15 Germinal XIII/5 April 1805. **(23)** Mametz (Pas-de-Calais); 30 Germinal XIII/20 April 1805. **(24)** Floringhem (Pas-de-Calais); 8 Floréal XIII/28 April 1805. **(25)** Deûlémont (Nord); 14 Messidor XIII/3 July 1805. **(26)** Vauvillers (Somme); 5 February 1807. **(27)** Widehem (Pas-de-Calais); 7 October 1807. **(28)** Boulogne (Pas-de-Calais); Hué arrested, March 1808.

over a period of nine days. He then asked payment for a novena. At first he required 50 sous, but he accepted 10 and even returned 6, saying, "these 10 sous will do you no good." Voilmy had also been seen at neighboring Montbré and Cormontreuil.

Nicolas, according to the reporter for the *Gazette*, was a native of the Meuse who chose to practice in Champagne because "no one is a prophet in his own country"; he had spent sixteen months in the prisons of Reims and Châlons. Nicolas told the familiar story of having been bitten by a rabid wolf and making the pilgrimage to Saint-Hubert, where he received the vocation of protecting against rabies by applying the "key" of Saint Hubert; his practice, however, seems to have been confined to animals. He said that he had taken the title of knight of Saint Hubert because village mayors had conferred it on him. Nicolas was an epileptic; some mayors may in fact have tolerated his veterinary practice out of compassion. In addition to applying the key, he asked a fee of 10 sous for a forty-day novena. The police found in his possession and confiscated seven rosaries, five necklaces, twelve rings of St. Hubert, twenty-eight pictures, a hartshorn, a Saint Hubert's trumpet, a key of Saint Hubert, and two hafts. Even in prison Nicolas persisted in his belief in Saint Hubert and the power of his key.

Other itinerants included self-styled witches, magicians, conjurors, and a general assortment of confidence men, whose worst offense in the eyes of the police was usually their vagrancy.[137] The old fear of vagabonds – some of whom were in fact bandits – lingered on; hence the continuing obsession with certificates, passports, and anything that might regularize the existence of a man or woman who lacked a fixed residence and *état*.

Itinerant empiricism should be seen both as a type of medical practice and as a significant form of economic activity. The major charlatans and *colporteurs* had an established place in the regional economies of France in the eighteenth and nineteenth centuries. Through further research it may be possible to establish with greater precision their itineraries and their connections to the various markets. Jean-Jacques Darmon has plotted the standard routes of book peddlers in the nineteenth century, and it is possible that a similar map can be drawn for empirics.[138]

For the individual, physical mobility as an empiric, charlatan's assistant, or remedy vendor promised a limited form of upward economic mobility; this was equally true for the bootblack who joined a charlatan's troupe, for the artisan turned ambulatory botanist-physician, and for the peasants of the Oisans who sold local herbs and sometimes turned charlatan. But not all were equally successful. Perhaps the most important conclusion to be drawn from this chapter concerns the great inequality that prevailed among the itinerants, who ranged from literate, hugely ambitious entrepreneurs to illiterate, often quite desperate marginals, like the epileptic or the elderly divorced woman who earned a living as knights of Saint Hubert. For many of the latter, occasional medical practice was simply one among several expedients in the "economy of makeshifts" (to borrow Olwen Hufton's phrase)[139] that sustained the poor of preindustrial France. To some extent, the field rewarded ability and punished lack of it; although it dressed itself in the trappings of the Old Regime privilege system, empiricism existed in a free market economy of the most unforgiving sort. Some practitioners were adept at seducing the crowd and even public officials. Others seem to have been effective only at preying on the most defenseless peasants; one suspects in certain cases that they deliberately selected isolated farms and waited until the better-educated husband was out of the house before knocking on the door. But if empiricism was to some extent the *carrière ouverte aux talents* (career open to talents) proclaimed by the Revolution, it was also a product of economic circumstances. Vagabond empirics appear to have multiplied during the hard times of the revolutionary era and the post-Napoleonic economic crisis; charlatanism on a grand scale appears to have been sustained by the economic expansion of the latter eighteenth century. The two phenomena should perhaps be distinguished; the question deserves further exploration.

4

Irregulars: sedentary empirics

"Besides the wanderers who follow in each other's footsteps daily," the physician René-Georges Gastellier wrote to the Société Royale de Médecine in 1782, "we have [empirics] right here at home [*dans nos propres foyers*]."[1] What is the significance of this distinction? As police officials saw it, the resident empiric was an easier object of surveillance than the vagabond, whose movements around the countryside could be difficult to trace. As some physicians saw it, his constant presence made him a greater threat to public health.[2] For the historian of medical practice, the distinction is worth making because the resident practitioner necessarily belonged to the community in which he or she found a clientele. The itinerants, with some exceptions like Dr. Hans, rarely succeeded in establishing a regular following in the regions where they worked; some, indeed, took care not to visit the same place twice with the same bag of tricks. The sedentary empirics, if they were to practice for any length of time, needed a permanent pool of patients. Their economic position, too, differed from that of the passing vendors. They occupied a more stable place in the local medical market, and some acquired sufficient notoriety to support themselves as full-time rivals to the profession. More often their medical practice was only occasional, but they could treat medicine an an avocation or sideline only because they had some other regular role in the local economy: many were artisans, shepherds, or farm laborers.

Like all of the taxonomic labels used in this study, "sedentary empiric" requires a caveat. No hard and fast distinction is possible, first of all, between ambulatory and sedentary practitioners. Some of the empirics discussed in the last chapter had a fixed residence but traveled in the surrounding countryside or left for several months during the winter migrations. Some changed from one way of life to the other. A practitioner who had been established in one place for a number of years might take to the road when he had saturated the local market with his remedies, lost public confidence, or had to bow to pressure from the profession and the authorities. Or an

itinerant might tire of the wandering life, like one former clown in a charlatan's troupe who settled down as an empiric at Boësse in the Loiret at the
beginning of the nineteenth century.[3] Nor is it possible to differentiate
sharply between empirics and "folk healers," if by folk healer is meant a
practitioner who draws on the concepts and methods of popular medicine.
One example will illustrate the possible ambiguities. A midwife in the
department of the Meurthe was said to practice medicine and surgery; during
an epidemic of a rash-producing fever (which the physicians took to be
either smallpox or scarlet fever), she bled and puked her patients. But she
also had recourse to an old "folk" remedy widely used for treating fevers
(notably meningitis): she took a live pigeon, cut it in half, and placed the
still palpitating bird on the patient's stomach.[4] This one practice does not
make the midwife a *maige*, but it is very different from the purges and secret
remedies characteristic of the empiric's armamentarium. It is worth emphasizing once more that a natural history of unauthorized practice might
better be conceived as an ethology, a study of ranges of behavior, than a
taxonomy, a classification of specimens.

But human history is ultimately concerned with individuals, and this
chapter is about people: a very diverse group of men and women who
conformed more or less closely to the ideal type of the sedentary empiric.
They lived in one place, rather than on the road, and, although they lacked
professional qualifications, supported themselves at least in part through
the sale of remedies, medical consultations, or both.

REMEDY VENDORS

Just as some itinerants were primarily traveling apothecaries, so some sedentary empirics were essentially vendors of pharmaceutical specialties. As
always, the line between pharmacy and medical practice is hard to draw;
although not all vendors made diagnoses, nearly all offered a form of medical
advice by prescribing their remedy for various disorders. They sold not
drug substances but cures for disease.

Even more than in the case of the itinerants, the enterprises of the sedentary vendors varied enormously in scale. The most successful – often
men with medical or surgical credentials – were prominent merchants,
sometimes supplying apothecaries as well as their own salesmen and retail
outlets; they are more akin to the great patent medicine manufacturers of
the late nineteenth and early twentieth centuries than to the local empiric.[5]
When the business of the physician-cum-empiric Jean-Pierre-Gaspard Ailhaud, baron de Castelet, failed in 1786, he left 180,000 livres in credit and
630,000 doses of his grandfather's celebrated purgative powders, which
brought 756,000 livres.[6] Among the most widely distributed specialties were
remedies for venereal disease, particularly those that were promoted (dis-

honestly in some instances) as containing no mercury. The *rob Laffecteur*, perhaps the most celebrated proprietary remedy at the end of the Old Regime, was an antisyphilitic;[7] so was the rob of Jean Giraudeau (1802–1861), a physician who published various popular medical handbooks mainly to stimulate interest in his products.[8] The most ambitious promoters aimed for a truly national market. The former military surgeon Mettemberg, for example, arranged for trials of his remedy for scabies in hospitals at Paris, Saint-Denis, Lille, and Lyons and received Napoleon's authorization to advertise and sell his remedy throughout the French Empire; in 1810 he proposed to the prefect of the Loire (and presumably to his colleagues in other departments as well) that he be allowed to establish outlets for his remedy in the chief town (*chef-lieu*, or administrative seat) of each arrondissement.[9] The "American elixir" of Courcelle was sold in seventy-eight towns. The *poudres d'Ailhaud* reached an international market; in France itself, the baron established an extensive network of local offices that served up purges and medical advice.[10] But success of this sort did not come easily and (as Ailhaud's bankruptcy suggests) could be hard to maintain. Although the actual ingredients of the remedy might cost almost nothing, this was not true of the packaging, and it was necessary to invest heavily in distribution and, above all, in promotion – as Balzac's César Birotteau learns when he tries to sell his *double pâte des sultanes* and *huile céphalique* on a major scale. In addition to newspaper advertising, vendors churned out publicity in formats ranging from handbills similar to those used by itinerant charlatans to elaborate prospectuses and books.[11] Such an enterprise could lead to financial disaster, as César finds to his sorrow. And even success had its costs. The owners of the most widely recognized products often found themselves undercut by producers of counterfeits and imitations; to counteract this trend, a group of patent holders established a central depot in Paris and published a prospectus in 1789 – a hopeless undertaking.[12]

Not surprisingly, remedy owners leaped at opportunities to defeat or circumvent competition in the free market, accepting legal monopolies (though these were hard to enforce) or, better yet, selling their formula outright to the Crown or some local governmental body. The most celebrated case in the Old Regime was the English physician Talbor, who secured a monopoly on cinchona and made a large fortune from it.[13] French monarchs also paid great sums for more dubious remedies. Louis XV bought a preparation based on male fern for 13,000 livres from the widow of its developer, a surgeon. The Estates of Provence gave 24,000 livres in 1764 for a secret against anthrax, which turned out to be a mixture of vitriol and egg yolk.[14] Old traditions died hard. In 1810 an enterprising empiric from the Niort region asked for a government subsidy and the assistance of three chemists to prepare his special elixir, which he said would restore

Napoleon (then in his early forties and visibly past his prime) to what he had been at the age of twenty-five.[15]

At the other end of the scale, owners of secret remedies who attempted to exploit them only locally found that they could derive a limited but fairly reliable income from a small investment – the charges for a few handbills or newspaper announcements. In the countryside, still more modest proprietors of "secrets" relied on word of mouth. In between could be found a whole gamut of local empirics, from rising entrepreneurs who employed assistants and salesmen to self-styled "physicians" for whom medical practice was essentially a pretext for marketing expensive special remedies.

The best markets for this sort of enterprise were, of course, urban. Hopeful provincials (and foreigners) gravitated to the French capital, like the Corsican Stefanopoli, who came to Paris in the 1770's, not long after France acquired his native island, to sell his "Lemithochorton" and coraline (a submarine plant).[16] A tanner from the Perche region who moved to Paris in the early 1780's to sell his eyewash – an ophthalmological panacea whose ingredients included dog dung, cuttlebone, alum, and green vitriol (iron sulfate) – soon found his apartment crowded with clients, although according to a disgusted correspondent of the Société Royale de Médecine, he had distributed his remedy in his native Verneuil for years "without anyone at all going into raptures over it."[17] One self-proclaimed "Swiss physician," a former painter named Deveyl, sold a "water of health" to credulous Parisians at 3 livres the pint bottle, available from his agents and depots in the various city neighborhoods. According to an anonymous denunciation received by the Société Royale de Médecine, Deveyl's remedy was simply Seine river water, "which he has clarified by letting it sit in butter pots on the bottom of which he has previously put a little pulverised antimony and a little oxydized tin." Another self-styled physician, who called himself Dor, lived on the rue Saint-Thomas-du-Louvre, across from the stables of the duc de Chartres, where he distributed a water, a "universal medicine," for 24 livres the bottle. (Although illiterate, he had an authentic-seeming master's diploma from Montpellier, which he may have stolen or obtained through fraud; the empiric, whose real name was Dol, was a former joiner and clockmaker from Aix.)[18]

But the sale of medical "secrets" and other remedies flourished in the provinces as well, even in sleepy villages, where it formed an integral part of popular medical practice. An 1833 work on popular errors claimed (with only some exaggeration) that each village had its "miracle worker who possesses a sovereign and infallible remedy against [rabies]."[19] Some such remedies were quite widely distributed and might enjoy reputations that reached back for generations. At Le May-sur-Èvre, near Cholet in Anjou, a certain Tharreau distributed, over a radius of 50 leagues (well over 100 miles), a syrup against dropsy, a violent purgative that sold for the substantial sum of 24 livres a pint.[20] In the early nineteenth century, at Neulise (Loire), a major property owner named Tixier drew patients from as far as 30 to 40 leagues away who were willing to pay 1–6 francs for his treatment against rabies. Tixier's remedy (which was said to be equally effective against the bites of snakes and other venomous animals) had reportedly been handed down from father to son for two hundred years; it was said that a knight of Malta had first transmitted the secret to an ancestor, and that under Louis XV one of Tixier's forbears had been called in to treat the abbé Terray, who served as controller-general of finance from 1769 to 1774. Tixier would not divulge his formula, except to say that it consisted of an infusion of plants in wine, and he insisted that he would pass it on to his successors in secrecy, as it had been transmitted to him. (One informant suggested that Tixier used a more mystical procedure, asking patients to drink water from a glass with an animal's tooth in it and then kneel while he read the Bible, prayed, and made signs of the cross. Tixier, however, denied using anything but his secret remedy.)[21]

Tixier's success probably owed something to his position as a local notable; he was not only rich, but mayor of his commune. Other examples could be cited, expecially after 1789, of remedy owners who were local officials. Antoine Esslinger, miller and revolutionary mayor of Châtenois in the Bas-Rhin, actually boasted to the departmental administration of the "miraculous cures" wrought by his sympathetic powder.[22] Ecclesiastics, too, could capitalize on their status in the community to administer or distribute special remedies, a practice that went well beyond the traditional role played by the clergy in charitable assistance. Toward the end of the Restoration, for example, an abbé in rural Eure-et-Loir kept in his cellar two barrels of infusions of native herbs, which he sometimes took to Dreux. In the Orléanais, the prior of Amilly sold water from a special well.[23] Clerics were joined by another marginal member of the traditional medical network, the executioner, who frequently practiced a little pharmacy. Executioners were the unique source of such prestigious remedies as hanged men's fat and the rope used in executions;[24] some also sold less exotic medicines such as tisanes or mixtures of simples.[25]

As was seen in Chapter 1, all sorts of tradesmen might sell remedies, often as a casual sideline. In 1770, the stock of a jeweler-hardware dealer at Dijon included a variety of remedies and cosmetics: water of pearls for the complexion; pectoral tablets; Scotch plasters for corns on the feet; sticking plasters for burns and cuts; a preparation for bleaching the teeth; a "ribbon of health" to purify the air of apartments; Greenough's volatile essence; eau de Cologne; Stoughton's elixir; Greenough's pectoral tablets; vulnerary tea; Greenough's stomachic tablets; English mustard; elixir of Ganus.[26] At Levier in the Doubs, another hardware dealer who was blamed in 1812 for the death of "a poor person" sold some *articles d'épicerie et de droguerie* and was accustomed to give wine, syrups, and sugar gratis to the indigent.[27] At Le Mans, a bookbinder, Gastineau, sold the balsamic pectoral syrup of the ladies of the Royal Abbey of Chaillot at 3 livres the bottle, and the French sticking plaster of *sieur* Vollant, which replaced English plaster; Le Monnier, a dealer in old clothes, sold Swiss vulnerary saffron.[28] And at Morlaàs-en-Béarn, near Pau, a local practitioner accused Jewish merchants of selling "bad drugs" on credit to the peasants, for which they paid through the nose at the next harvest.[29]

On a more modest scale, some occasional practitioners of medicine and practitioners of certain minor trades related to medicine earned a few sous from the sale of remedies. A Mademoiselle Blanc, tried for illegal medical practice at the end of the Restoration, applied leeches, attended women in childbirth, and also sold a benzoin liqueur.[30] Snake hunters (*chasseurs de vipère*) used their quarry to prepare ingredients used in popular pharmacy: viper brandy, dried snake vertebrae, and viper grease. (This trade survived in the Grenoble region until very recent times.)[31] Another pharmaceutical compound, known in the learned pharmacopeias as *album graecum* and more popularly as *merde de chien*, was prepared from the excrement of a dog fed on bones. Charitable persons sometimes concocted the remedy and distributed it gratis, but many suppliers offered it for sale; an inferior grade was produced from dog droppings provided by poor women who had collected them from public ways, as others collected horse and cattle manure.[32]

Finally, some artisans and small tradesmen simply sold a few empirical remedies on the side to eke out the meager income from their regular occupation. Some of these trades were traditionally associated with popular medicine; blacksmiths and farriers, for example, had a prominent place. In other cases the connection seems to have been purely fortuitous. The Lieutenant of the King's First Surgeon at Vouvant-en-Châtaigneraie in Poitou reported in 1790 that village match sellers peddled leftover remedies from shops.[33] A man who made a living primarily by selling crosses and little religious books asked the Société Royale de Médecine to approve his other source of income – the sale of a root recommended as a remedy for toothache and headache. In the early nineteenth century, Jacques-Félix Gelain, a former old-clothes dealer at Les Andelys (Eure), sold an *eau de commère*, a "spiritous, vulnerary, and cosmetic water." A folklore study of Languedoc cites a more recent case, that of Pierre Crespin, who repaired umbrellas and sold drugs until his death in 1909.[34] Clearly, the remedy trade could supplement a wide variety of regular callings. Appendix C lists some remedy vendors, reported between 1773 and 1830, whose occupation is known. The data are too scattered for statistical analysis to be meaningful, but they do suggest the range of possible backgrounds.

Though a few individuals made fortunes from the remedy trade, most of course did not, and a significant proportion – just how many cannot be determined with any certainty – came from the ranks of the poor and near-poor and relied on their excursions into pharmacy as a significant economic makeshift. Economic need recurs as a leitmotiv in the petitions for official approval sent to the Société Royale de Médecine and the later agencies that had jurisdiction over secret remedies. One author describes himself as "not rich" and another as "poor"; a third confesses that he needs the income from his remedies to live.[35] The sale of remedies also supported a handful of eccentrics and marginals who, by choice or necessity, lacked any other trade. A nineteenth-century hermit in the Morvan region lived in a grotto and supported himself by selling infusions of plants in white wine.[36] The Lancelotte widow who sold remedies for rheumatism and cancer in the Loire-Inférieure in the early nineteenth century was a former mental patient; an unsympathetic mayor of Nantes called her a "madwoman" and noted that she had been treated in a sanitarium.[37] (More generally, widows occupied a prominent place among the occasional vendors of secret remedies.)

It is very difficult to gauge how widespread these activities were or how many individuals participated in them. It is possible to get some very rough sense, in a few areas, of the number of resident empirics who saw patients regularly, but almost anyone could prepare remedies from a few local herbs and sell them close to home. A map of the trade would probably resemble a map of the French population.

VARIETIES OF EMPIRICISM

The remainder of this chapter is devoted to empirics in the more usual sense of the term: unqualified persons who frankly practiced medicine. The most famous quacks of early modern Europe have already found a place in a kind of rogues' gallery of medical history: Nicolas de Blégny and Valentine Greatrakes in the seventeenth century; John Taylor, Joshua Ward, James Graham, and Mesmer in the eighteenth, among others.[38] The discussion here will focus instead on the small fry, especially in the provinces. But the literature on the celebrities of unorthodox medicine illustrates a point that is of considerable importance for the history of charlatanism more generally: the lack of sharply defined boundaries between regular and irregular practice. Some "quacks" had a form of authentic professional credentials. Mesmer was a medical doctor; *le grand* Thomas, toothpuller and empiric on the Pont-Neuf, had been a surgeon of the Gardes-Françaises and a surgeon's assistant at the Hôtel-Dieu.[39] Conversely, some unqualified empirics eventually won privileges that legitimated their practice. Blégny, for example, was eventually admitted to the College of Saint-Côme.[40] In the century that separated Mesmer from Blégny, the possibilities for nonphysicians to secure official recognition by an alternative route diminished. In France, as has been seen, the law of Ventôse further accelerated this process. And yet, a gray area remained between licit and illicit practice.

Marginal regulars and impostors

The first two chapters have explored the sometimes perplexing problem of identifying the regular practitioner; the problem of defining the empiric is, of course, its mirror image. Many contemporary observers lumped together completely unqualified practitioners, practitioners with legal but dubious qualifications (such as a medical degree from the University of Orange), and the borderline surgeons who might have received some training in their field but had not been officially licensed (like the fifteen surgical operators known to be practicing in the subdelegation of Péronne north of Paris in the last years of the Old Regime).[41] Ambiguous cases included "empirics" who had spent time as military surgeons; Jean Lanoë, a practitioner in eighteenth-century Anjou, was known as "le Major," a contraction of *médecin* (or *chirurgien*) *major*, medical or surgical officer.[42] Veterans of the revolutionary and Napoleonic conflicts subsequently swelled the ranks of these practitioners. In the early nineteenth century, many *officiers de santé* who should have been admitted by a medical jury continued to practice without having passed their examination. One list of illegal practitioners in the Nièvre names eight such unlicensed *officiers* – almost surely a mere fraction of the total.[43]

More clearly in the camp of the empirics were those practitioners who, without any claim to formal training or regular professional experience, usurped official titles and, in some cases, stole or forged legal credentials. By doing so they set themselves apart from many of their colleagues, who, although they may have coveted official recognition, distinguished themselves from the medical profession in their methods, manner, and even their titles, and claimed to be able to cure diseases that had baffled the doctors. Cases of outright fraud may have been more common in the eighteenth century, when credentials (particularly from foreign institutions) were harder to verify. One young impostor, who went under the name of the chevalier de Raigondeau de Chastenac and claimed to be a *gentilhomme d'honneur* of the comte d'Artois, cut the ground from under his own feet in 1786 by claiming to have received a doctorate from Montpellier in 1767; since he was only twenty-nine years old, he would have completed his studies at the precocious age of nine or ten. He also boasted of having served for five years as a lieutenant in a regiment of dragoons and for six years as a physician in the hospitals of the Îles de Bourbon et de France (Réunion and Mauritius).[44] More problematic was the case of the American Hart, who attempted to practice medicine at Nancy in the early years of the

Restoration: he claimed to have lost his medical diploma in a shipwreck, although he did possess an authentic-looking document certifying that he had served as ship's surgeon aboard an American privateer.[45]

The widespread usurpation of the title *officier de santé* in the early nineteenth century suggests the degree to which this official-sounding credential had won popular acceptance (and probably also the freedom with which it had been conferred during the revolutionary era). Napoleonic officials had to deal with a strange assortment of self-appointed health officers inherited from the turbulent 1790's, most of whom believed quite sincerely in their right to practice medicine. At Mamers in the Sarthe, an illiterate former weaver named Marin Fagot announced himself as an *"officier de santé* at Saint-Cosme,"* a smaller commune some 10 kilometers distant. His only attempt at official legitimation struck the authorities as bizarre: a certificate from an apothecary ("another charlatan") at Bonnétable dated 10 Thermidor XI (29 July 1803), which testified that Fagot had taken drugs from the writer for eleven years without himself suffering any ill effects.[46] Another empiric, Jean-Pierre-Noël-Gervaise Suzov, signing himself *officier de santé*, naively appealed to the Ministry of the Interior in 1803, asking for authorization to continue to practice medicine and sell remedies at Richelieu (now in Indre-et-Loire), where he had been active for fifteen years, especially in the countryside. His knowledge of botany and pharmacy, he claimed, allowed him to cure refractory diseases; not having studied surgery, however, he performed no other manual operation than pulling teeth, a procedure that the (genuine) local health officer disdained to perform. In support of his case, he fell back on the usual sort of ad hominem pleading: healing was the only resource available to him, at the age of sixty, for supporting his family. He also submitted a voluminous set of testimonials and a list of the various diseases he had cured, which showed him to be a sort of specialist in dermatology: cancer, cancerous warts, carbuncle, leprous scurf, leprous scabies, scrofula (*humeurs froides*), hemorrhage, discharge of milk, diffused bile, ankylosis, leprosy and tinea of different kinds, and abscesses.[47]

Operators

The surgical specialties formed another terrain where regular merged rapidly into irregular practice; for every received expert in the Old Regime, there were probably several operating outside the law, and empirics continued to work in the various fields long after the end of special receptions. Some empirics were accused of meddling in every branch of surgery, but many, perhaps most, concentrated on a single condition or procedure. At the end of the eighteenth century, for example, the town of Dourdan in the Île-de-France possessed scrofula surgeons.[48] Half a century later, around Allaire and Rieux (Morbihan), an "ocular healer" used a horsehair to operate on pterygium (a thickening of part of the conjunctiva).[49] The operation for hernia by castration was a commoner specialty. Two instances among many, reported in 1796 and 1807: a day laborer in the commune of Étré-pagny (Eure), named Bétréau, who treated young children, and a woman in the Ardennes who boasted of having operated on 4,000 patients.[50]

Some of these operators acquired a certain mechanical proficiency, but the bolder among them applied caustics and wielded the knife as recklessly as their medical colleagues employed drastic purgatives. Each provincial physician knew at least one horror story. These tales are almost always impossible to confirm or disconfirm individually, but like the mutilation of mothers and fetuses by bungling *matrones*, the sorts of tragedies they describe undoubtedly did occur; this form of practice was not an innocuous domestic medicine. At Clisson in Brittany, the physician Duboueix cited one surgical intervention by a certain Lahaye, known as Chambaudière, a former low-ranking officer in the merchant marine who had turned to medical practice, beginning with relatively innocent salves and waters and then trying his hand at operations. He dispatched one patient suffering from an abscess, which he misdiagnosed as a double hernia, by plunging an old pair of rusty scissors into the scrotum.[51]

Of all the specialties, far and away the most important was bonesetting, a calling that cut across all the spheres of medical practice, from the fringes of the old regular network to folk medicine.[52] The bonesetter was most commonly known as a *"rebouteur"* or *"renoueur,"* from *renouer*, to join together. Other terms included *"adoubeur,"* *"radoubeur,"* *"remetteur,"* *"rha-billeur,"* and even *"ossier."*[53] The regional variants recorded by folklorists point to the bonesetter's established place in local popular culture: in Berry, *"rebouteux"* but also *"arbouteux,"* *"remigeaux,"* and *"ermieux"*; in Languedoc and the Pyrenees, *"adoubaire"* or *"adouaire"*; in Burgundy, *"rebriauleur"* and *"rangueunieur"*; in Morvan, *"regôgnou,"* *"gôgneux,"* or *"gougneur,"* from *gougner*, to rub, or possibly *gôner*, to dress; ; in parts of northern France, *"poucheux"* or *"paucheux,"* because of the importance of the thumb (*pouce*) in rites used by mystical *rebouteurs*. Some of the terms in patois have a broader sense than "bonesetter"; *"rhabilloux"* could take on the sense of tinker or itinerant cobbler; *"regôgnou,"* *"remanceau,"* and *"raimangeou"* could apply to physician, veterinarian, and sorcerer.[54]

Bonesetting was in many places a hereditary calling; the popular *rebouteur* of the nineteenth century was often descended from a recognized or tolerated bonesetter of the Old Regime. At Sivry in the Ardennes lived one of the many families that had handed down the craft from father to son; the member active at the end of the Restoration enjoyed a practice extending throughout the arrondissement of Vouziers.[55] Another such dynasty could be found at Lentigny in the Loire, where in 1808 Claude Péricard affirmed

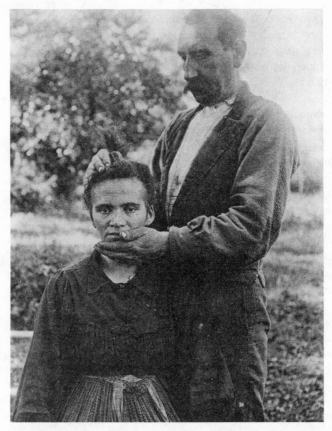

A Breton *rebouteur*: popular medicine captured by photography. (Courtesy of the Musée National des Arts et Traditions Populaires; © Musées Nationaux.)

in a petition to the emperor that he and his ancestors had practiced for fifty-eight years.[56] The most celebrated tradition was sustained at Le Val-d'Ajol in Lorraine, where the legacy seems to have been claimed not just by one principal clan but by the population at large. One enterprising inhabitant, a former cobbler named Dumont, moved to Paris when he was in his fifties, established a flourishing practice, and (as was seen in Chapter 2) won special recognition from the Crown and the revolutionary legislatures.[57]

Few *rebouteurs* devoted themselves exclusively to their surgical practice. Many came from rural occupations that traditionally involved a little veterinary medicine; they were farriers, for example, or gelders or shepherds.[58] At Jas in the Loire, a certain Cartéron, an established *rhabilleur*, treated domestic animals and was also accused of giving "remedies from the horse stables" to men (1812).[59] (This pattern continued into the present century; of the eight *rebouteurs* active between 1924 and 1955 at Noyant-Méon, in the Baugé region of Maine-et-Loire, six were gelders and one was a far-rier.)[60] Bonesetting also appeared in association with other occupations, usually manual crafts. In Perche and Maine, for example, *rebouteurs* were usually weavers.[61] In 1726, Bellet, a master roofer at Paris, was prohibited from practicing as a *chirurgien-bailleul*; he probably drew a good part of his clientele from among fellow members of his trade, for whom broken bones were an accepted occupational hazard.[62]

Bonesetters were among the most widely distributed of major empirics. Map 2 shows the location (by commune) of the principal *rhabilleurs* around Ancenis (Loire-Inférieure) in 1827. Such a map is somewhat misleading, for it does not show the range and penetration of an empiric's practice. Like many small-time tradespeople, rural *rebouteurs* went to towns on fair and market days. We learn from the Comité de Salubrité's questionnaire, for example, that a bonesetter named Charry, from the district of Pamiers in the Ariège, used to come to Carcassonne the first Saturday of each month.[63] Since a supply of suitable patients was not always available, the more active practitioners dabbled in medicine and pharmacy; at Guémené-Penfao in Brittany, for example, Denis Bernard administered drugs in addition to treating fractures and sprains.[64] The most successful won wide notoriety, like a celebrated *rebouteuse* of Châtillon, who attracted patients from the environs of Paris in the mid-nineteenth century.[65] In the eighteenth-century Auvergne, a bonesetter named Heyrauld traveled on horseback to patients and even gave them room and board in his home; he made so much money that an envious local peasant asked that his *taille* be increased.[66] Activity on this scale could make the empiric a serious rival to the local profession. In one late-nineteenth-century case in the Deux-Sèvres, an *officier de santé* re-solved the problem by paying his brother, who was a *rebouteur* at Frontenay, not to practice in the town of Niort.[67]

Of all the popular practitioners, talented bonesetters normally won the greatest respect from the educated elites and even the professionals, who were sometimes said to send members of their family to be treated by them. (The medical men recognized that the best among the *rebouteurs* had highly developed special skills and that they knew how to prepare a patient for a painful procedure; the famed bonesetters of the Vosges successfully used wine as a muscle relaxant to facilitate the reduction of a dislocated mem-ber.)[68] Local populations considered them indispensable for dealing with the injuries that regularly befell agricultural laborers. But bonesetters were commonly accused of treating as fractures mere bruises or sprains that would have healed nicely if left alone, and their interventions could be destructive. Some treatments for bruises and muscle strains, like Dumont Valdajou's cataplasm of candle tallow and urine, seem innocuous enough, but violent

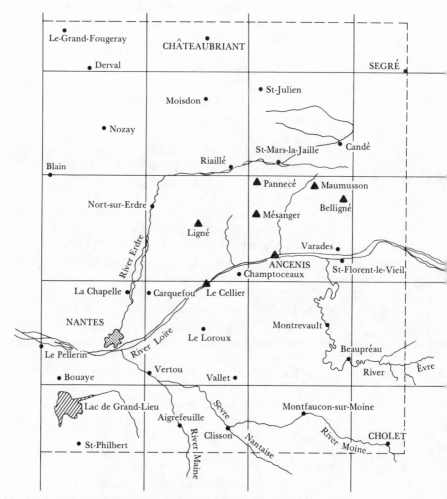

Map 2. *Rebouteurs* around Ancenis (Loire-Inférieure), 1827. A triangle indicates a commune in which a known *rebouteur* practices. Each side of the
squares in the grid corresponds to 20 kilometers. [*Source*: Archives Départementales, Loire-Atlantique, 1 M 1358, no. 321A.]

manipulations of the injured part could disable a patient, and incorrect
setting of a fracture might leave him crippled for life. Some ignorant bonesetters (who, according to one informant, said that broken bones were made
of glass) wrapped sprained, dislocated, and broken members in cardboard
coated with mastic or soaked in a decoction of tripe.[69] One peasant accident
victim at Nérac was told that he should walk upstairs to "accommodate"

his injured leg.[70] At Mantes in 1769, a *renoueuse* simply wrapped a bandage around a patient's arm after a cart wheel had passed over it and severed the humerus. A surgeon summoned a week later found that the arm was now "hinged," with a three-inch separation between the two sections of the bone; the hand still worked, but it had to be guided by the other.[71]

Medical practitioners

Some empirics had a medical rather than surgical specialty, usually based on possession of a secret remedy. In early-nineteenth-century Nantes, for example, a woman named Lecadre built her practice around a supposedly nonmercurial remedy for venereal disease, which she advertised in the sort of announcement used by itinerant charlatans:

La Dame Lecadre, having acquired the highest reputation in the treatment of venereal disease, would think that she failed humanity if she did not inform the inhabitants of this commune of her successes in medicine. She possesses a vegetable liquor that destroys all venereal diseases, quickly and with no possibility of relapse, however intractable they may be, even if they have the most stubborn symptoms. This remedy, in which mercury is not included in any form, is suited to all ages and temperaments, requires no regimen other than sobriety, and does not prevent [the patient] from attending to his business. It can be taken in every time and place, even when traveling by sea or by land. It is such a gentle specific that nurses and pregnant women can make use of it, without its affecting the most sensitive organs or viscera. The modest price of the remedy of *la dame* Lecadre cannot prevent even the poorest persons from receiving treatment; she has no other goal than relieving suffering humanity. The greatest secrecy can be assured. She also treats the whites [and] cures scabies, ringworm, and deafness, provided that it is not congenital. She can be found at any time. Her residence is in the Bisson house . . . in the allée du Boulanger, on the first floor, opposite the staircase, at Nantes.[72]

Other empirics specialized in equally stubborn or frightening disorders. In the village of La Débaudière, near Vallet in Brittany, a peasant named Oger won a reputation in the late eighteenth century for healing cancer (although he was willing to take on all other diseases as well).[73] Dr. Nicolas, the Société Royale's energetic correspondent at Grenoble, cited an old woman whom he had known in the little town where he had lived before coming to the provincial capital, who treated scabies with a supposed specific.[74] Under the Empire, a glazier of Avranches (Manche) had a reputation for treating rabies; and during the Restoration, a certain Du Mont-Plainchant, at Decize (Nièvre), sold a bracelet to restore the fertility of women who could not conceive, predicted the sex of the unborn child of those who could, and even promised the nulligravida a technique for making her first baby a boy or girl, as she chose.[75]

The most active empirics, however, were generalists, serving the local population as parallel physicians. They typically bled, purged, and applied topical remedies, like their official counterparts; many also relied on herbal remedies drawn from local flora.[76] They were often accused of supplying abortifacients to pregnant women (as were the popular *matrones*, or unqualified midwives).[77] A large part of their technique probably differed little from that of the modest village surgeon or *officier de santé*. Occasionally, however, one hears of less conventional procedures in stories that physicians seem to have related both as entertainments and as cautionary tales. In the region of Sainte-Reine in Burgundy, near the end of the Old Regime, a young man with an "inflammation" in his abdomen consulted a priest who enjoyed a reputation as a healer; this empiric, judging that the patient had a fire consuming his entrails, and that it was necessary to cool it, applied a bellows to his rectum, with lethal effect. Or so a local surgeon informed the Société Royale de Médecine.[78] Other empirics drew on a popular tradition reaching back to Pliny. One practitioner in the Eure, for example, during the early years of the Restoration, advised a patient who had suffered a fall that his liver was engorged; he was to follow a regimen that excluded calorific foods and contact with women (heating) but encouraged consumption of cress salads (cooling). The specific complaint, though, was to be treated with a powder obtained by grilling two moles alive between two plates that had never touched grease.[79] (This recommendation was preserved in a written letter of advice; many empirics were literate and aped the medical profession by writing out prescriptions and consultations.)[80]

Though the therapeutic methods of the empirics varied widely, many shared a diagnostic technique: they "inspected" or "scanned" the patient's urine. The flask of urine, in which the medieval physician had hoped to see, smell, or even taste characteristic signs of the patient's disease, became the symbol of the empiric in early modern Europe.[81] (Inspecting the urine remained, of course, a common procedure in eighteenth-century medicine, but physicians would have denied that it could replace the patient interview and physical examination.) At the end of the Old Regime, every region in France had its network of urinoscopists – in French, *jugeurs d'eau* or *uromantes* – and the tradition was still very much alive half a century later.[82] The full-fledged *uromante* was as much a diviner as a physician; in the patient's urine he or she was supposed to be able to read not only the nature of the complaint but also the age and gender of the patient, the patient's marital state, the circumstances of the accident that might have caused an injury, and so on. (The author of a history of urinalysis carefully distinguishes between "urinoscopy," or simple inspection of the urine to detect such indications of disease as an odd color or sediment, and "uromancy," or divining from the urine; in common usage the distinction was less clear.)[83] One empiric of Champagne, toward the end of the Old Regime, introduced a further refinement: she boiled the client's urine and then told him the details of his illness. The procedure of divining from the urine satisfied a basic expectation shared by many patients. The skilled physician would not *take* a patient's history; he would *tell* it to him.[84] The most successful urinoscopists invariably had confederates who gathered information on potential clients, which the magus could then triumphantly produce during a consultation.

Uromantes of one sort or another could be found at almost every level of the traditional medical network. Even licensed professionals sometimes dabbled in the more occult forms of urinoscopy to attract or hold a popular clientele. In 1830, for example, the mayor of Nantes learned that a moonlighting pharmacist not only sold composite drugs to the inhabitants of the countryside but also practiced as a *jugeur d'eau*.[85] (Occasionally, too, a licensed practitioner collaborated with an *uromante*, like the *officier de santé* Gosseaume at Chantenay in the Loire-Inférieure, who signed blank prescription forms for his colleague and shared the earnings.)[86] Urinoscopists flourished, too, on the margins between regular and irregular practice. A late-eighteenth-century empiric at Sougé in Maine, for example, had letters patent to practice surgery but worked mainly as an *uromante*, the faithful heir of the doctrine of his father-in-law, a *maître* Beausé, who had practiced for more than forty years.[87] Another practitioner at the limits of the old network, a certain Blanc, worked as an *officier de santé* (he said) from 1766 until he wound up in court at Bar-sur-Aube, not long after the Ventôse legislation went into effect. Although he had studied botany during the Revolution, he had received no surgical or medical training; nonetheless he consulted urines, used cream of tartar, and prescribed other drugs.[88] Some apparently philanthropic practitioners, including ecclesiastics, also used urinoscopy;[89] they seem to have believed in it as a medical tool. One such charitable urinoscopist, a tenant farmer named Béguin at Les Molières, near Limours (Seine-et-Oise), wrote to the Minister of the Interior in the Year XIII in an effort to secure official approval for his work. He was not a diviner in the larger sense; he had merely studied simples and learned uromancy, he said, and treated chills as well as the wounds and ulcers of the local military personnel.[90]

The ease with which a patient's urine could be carried to the *uromante*, thereby eliminating the need for either a house call or an office visit, favored the growth of local practices, which might reach a day's journey by foot, or more, into the countryside. At a village in Champagne called Allemant, for example, lived a woman urinoscopist who was said to be consulted for 10 leagues around; she employed "urine agents" to help ferret out information on clients (her prowess at divination earned her the reputation of a witch) and prospered by selling two medicines, both drastic purgatives, for substantial sums: 4 livres for one, 7 livres, 10 sous (though sometimes as much as 9 livres and a few sous) for the other. Her daughter carried on the practice in the 1770's and 1780's.[91] Another *uromante* of the 1780's, an illiterate peasant, reportedly drew patients from as far as 12 to 15 leagues away; after he was jailed for unauthorized medical practice, his loyal clientele continued to bring their urine to him in his prison cell.[92] Still other urinoscopists extended their practice by traveling, like an *uromante* denounced at Gomené in Brittany for having visited that town and seven other parishes;[93] and, as has been seen, urinoscopy formed part of the standard repertory of itinerant charlatans.

The most successful urine scanners made substantial fortunes;[94] during the Napoleonic era one of them, in the annexed department of the Sarre, was described by local authorities as the richest man in the region.[95] This last case merits a fuller description, for it shows how a skilled empiric, even if he were an illiterate peasant or artisan, could win popular and possibly official recognition as a physician.

Jean Schmitt (or Schmitz) was a cobbler and the son of a cobbler in the Eifel region of Germany. It was his father-in-law, for whom he had worked as a ploughman, who passed on to him the art of divining from urine. After the older man's death in 1767, Schmitt, in the words of one official, abandoned the plough for the more lucrative calling of the physician. He was still in practice at the beginning of the nineteenth century, in the town of Stattfeld; his son, the town's parish priest, served as his secretary, since Schmitt could neither read nor write. Messengers brought him flasks filled with patients' urine; he himself never left home. Normally the clients would also come to see him; two confederates posed as patients in his waiting room to gossip with them and extract the information that Schmitt would later divine from the urine. After discarding the contents of the flasks, he refilled them (a standard practice) with his usual remedies – jalap, sulfate of potassium, Armenian bole, and anise seed, according to one account.

Schmitt's practice was not confined to routine ills. During an epidemic he treated patients from two cantons, and one physician blamed him for the high mortality occasioned by a fever at Waldkönigen in 1802–1803 (a calamity that seems to have discomfited Schmitt as well, since it prevented his patients from taking the complete course of drug treatments). The frustrated physicians found, however, that Schmitt enjoyed both popular and official recognition, at least at the local level. The inhabitants of the Eifel venerated him as a prophet; and at the same time, despite his illiteracy, he appeared on the list of authorized *officiers de santé* for the department of the Sarre. His name was eventually expunged from the roster (as described in Chapter 2). But it must have taken a shrewd entrepreneur to achieve such a social and economic promotion from his station as the illiterate son of a cobbler. Schmitt first turned to medical practice as an economic necessity after the death of his father-in-law, who, although he may not have left him tangible property, ensured his livelihood by teaching him urinoscopy;

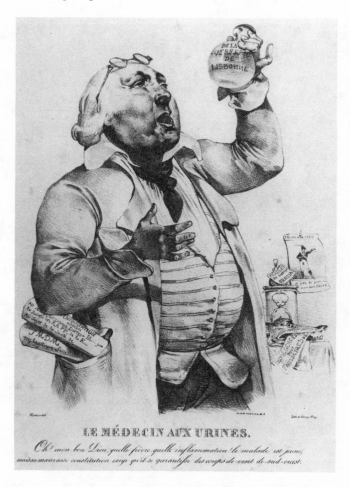

The urine doctor. By Wattier; lithograph by George Frey. "Oh, good Lord, what a fever, what inflammation! The patient is young, but his bad constitution requires that he protect himself from gusts of wind from the southwest." On the flask: "from the glassworks of Lisbon." In the pocket: "Consultation addressed to the most serene Dr. M... by the Society of the Reverend Fathers of F... about the health of...." On the table: crocodile holding in its mouth "indulgences for forgers [or perverters of the truth]"; fetus in a jar; "Pills of Doctor FRNCIA." (Courtesy of the Cabinet des Estampes, Musée Carnavalet. Photograph by Jean-Loup Charmet.)

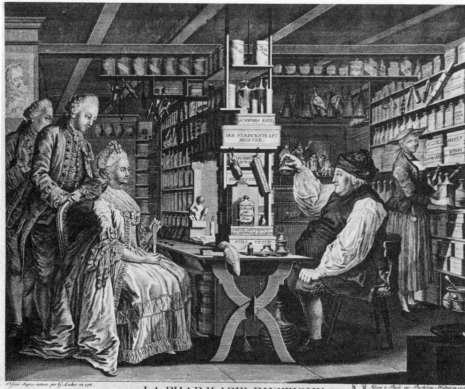

LA PHARMACIE RUSTIQUE,
*ou Représentation exacte de l'intérieur de la Chambre, ou Michel Schuppach connu sous
le nom du Médecin de la Montagne, tient ses Consultations.*

*Cet homme devenant s'est acquis une celebrité qui fait époque dans l'histoire de l'esprit humain. Il naquit l'an 1707 à Bigle village du Canton de Berne, et ne fut d'abord
qu'un simple Chirurgien de village. Mais une sagacité peu concevable à découvrir les maladies par l'inspection des urines, et nombre de cures surprenantes ont attiré chés lui
depuis quelques années de presque toutes les parties de l'Europe, une foule incroyable de Malades, la plûpart distingués par la naissance ou par la fortune.
C'est surtout à son genie et à sa longue experience qu'il doit ses rares lumieres, n'etant jamais sorti des environs de Langnau lieu de sa residence actuelle.
Sa bienfaisance envers les pauvres, la franchise de son caractere et l'originalité de son esprit, ajoutent encore un merite de ce rustique Hippocrate.*

"The Rustic Pharmacy: or exact depiction of the interior of the room where
Michel Schuppach, known as the Physician of the Mountain, holds his
consultations." Drawn from life by G. Locher, 1774; engraving by Bar-
thelemi Hübner, Basel, 1775. "This astonishing man has acquired a celebrity which marks an epoch in the history of the human mind. He was born
in the year 1707, at Bigle, village of the Canton of Bern, and at first was
only a simple village surgeon. But an almost inconceivable sagacity at
discovering diseases through the inspection of urine and numerous surprising cures have for several years attracted to his place an incredible
throng of patients from almost every part of Europe, most of them distinguished by their birth or fortune. He owes his rare understanding above
all to his genius and his long experience, never having left the environs of
Langnau, the site of his current residence. His beneficence to the poor, the
openness of his character, and the originality of his mind, add still more
to the merit of this rustic Hippocrates." The shelves are lined with remedies

in the end, his success was such that he could have renounced the trade and lived on his accumulated fortune.[96]

Occult healers

When urinalysis became urine casting, it took on the aura of an arcane science; a knowledge of the secret arts served to elevate the empiric's popular prestige above that of the practitioner who could claim only ordinary experience, however long, of disease and remedies. A similar role was played by those occult theories of medicine that held that a special power inhered in the healer's body, or that he or she made use of invisible forces or emanations to diagnose and cure disease. Stories of magical powers surrounded many of the most revered popular healers. Cécile Mazureau, the "black virgin" of Rezé (Loire-Atlantique), was said, for example, to have used her special gifts to reattach a joiner's severed fingers; in a moment of distraction, the story went, she placed them with the nails on the bottom, but she then noticed her error and turned them around to the correct position.[97] Other empirics explicitly claimed powers based on the same occult and mystical belief systems that won such extraordinary currency among the intelligentsia of the Romantic era.[98] The heyday of popular occult medicine came in the first half of the nineteenth century, as the Mesmerist fad trickled down to popular medical culture and local *somnambules* and *dormeuses* proliferated.[99] By the century's end, one student of popular medicine noted that these clairvoyants lacked prestige and were mainly used to find lost objects.[100]

High-culture medical magnetism (which still survives in various avatars) had emerged by the middle decades of the nineteenth century as a fairly well-defined movement, with its own journals (such as the *Revue magnétique*) and a characteristic doctrine, rather different from Mesmer's own system of tubs and electrical fluids. The central feature was a trance state, which one of Mesmer's disciples, the marquis de Puységur, had found he could induce through his personal "magnetism" (or hypnotic suggestion, as we would now say). In their magnetic sleep, the "somnambulists" seemed to

Caption to "The Rustic Pharmacy"(*cont.*)
and boxes (containing special compounds or perhaps urine specimens?), some bearing the names of such luminaries as the king of Prussia, Louis XIV of France, and Pasquale di Paoli, the Corsican patriot; funnels and other equipment hang from hooks. In the center, a motto: "The strongest is master." (Photograph courtesy of the Musée National des Arts et Traditions Populaires, © Musées Nationaux; from the collection of the Conseil National de l'Ordre des Pharmaciens.)

display extraordinary powers that allowed them (among other things) to diagnose disease and prescribe the necessary remedies; indeed, they were commonly called "physicians."[101] In the popular form of magnetic healing, the key figure was generally not the mesmerist (though it was recognized that he could, for example, induce insensibility in a part of the body), but the somnambulist or *dormeur* (*Schläfer* in Alsace). The *dormeur* was thought to possess extraordinary receptivity to things beyond the ordinary senses, including the spirit world. By exploiting this state, the gifted somnambulist-healer was supposed to be able to diagnose disease and even "x-ray" the body (as we would say) to determine whether an operation might be necessary.[102] A report from the Bas-Rhin suggested how in cases of colic, for example, a somnambulist might "see" yellow water circulating through the mesentery (though the practitioner might also diagnose from an article of the patient's clothing).[103] The same gift might be used to locate lost or stolen objects.

Some such practitioners worked in association with medical doctors;[104] though the methods of diagnosis were highly unorthodox, the prescriptions generally drew on the standard armamentarium of medicine and surgery. More typically, the popular somnambulist worked in tandem with a specialized "magnetizer," whose principal function was to induce the trance and record his partner's recommendations, though he might sometimes make magnetic passes over a tumor or a sprained hand or foot. Most magnetizers were men and most somnambulists women. (The folklorist Marc Leproux mentions one male somnambulist, a farmer who worked as a healer in the middle of the nineteenth century at Sonnac in the Charente-Inférieure; and the informant in the Bas-Rhin suggested that somnambulists of "both sexes" worked in Alsace.) The vocation often passed from father to son, or – more often – mother to daughter, through a sort of apprenticeship.[105]

One such pair included the wife of a hemp grower, Barbe Richert, and a notary named Jean-Pierre Küchel, or Kiechel, who appeared before a justice of the peace at Strasbourg in the Year VII. Küchel induced Richert's trances; when she emerged from them and prescribed remedies, he recorded them for her, since she did not know how to write. The patients then had the prescriptions filled at local pharmacies; the couple gave medical advice only. Küchel's own magnetic practice was not limited to hypnotism; he reappeared in 1808 as a solo mesmerist healer, or, in his own terms, as the discoverer of a "new infallible means to cure most of the external disorders of the body promptly and radically, whatever may have produced them, without the help of medication, by a light laying on of the hand, or by a simple touch."[106]

The line between occult healing and other magical practices is not easy to draw, and in the nineteenth century the police tended to lump them together as deviant behavior. In the Aube, for example, the archival dossier on the regulation of medical practice contains the records of an investigation of a local sorcerer named Houssant, who practiced cartomancy and helped young men avoid conscription; a police raid in 1813 turned up magic books, a book of obscene engravings, a magic lantern, and a microscope.[107] Angélique Martin, a native of Saint-Étienne, practiced medicine but also visited houses as a fortune teller.[108] Similarly, a woman in the faubourg Du Breuil at Le Puy (Haute-Loire) practiced medicine and urine casting in addition to cartomancy, and was said to procure abortions as well.[109]

As in other areas of popular practice, successful individuals could work full-time. A white witch in nineteenth-century Angers, "Père" Proust, began as a weaver, then worked as a *rebouteur*, and finally became a noted healer and diviner, using tarot cards to predict the future; he was described as a big spender.[110] More common, though, were the occasional practitioners, some of them established members of other occupations, some social marginals. Consider the case of Marie Prélat, a widow from Raon-l'Étape (Vosges), accused in 1802 of practicing cartomancy and magical medicine for money. Prélat described herself as a *"petite marchande foraine"* (small-time peddler), who told fortunes with cards merely for amusement. When she was called to see a sick farmer at Raves, she did so only to be obliging, she said, and accepted no fee. The prosecution maintained, however, that she called herself an inspired person and used magical practices. In treating one patient, she was said to have lit a candle; traced a cross on a plate covered with salt; and arranged for a cat to be killed without spilling its blood, after which its head, paws, and tail were cut off and buried separately, and its belly was opened without skinning it. On another occasion, she was said to have pretended to see corpses, upside-down chapels, and bell towers in a glass of water. It is likely that she did all these things, and for money. A widow with an inadequate income from peddling, she was typical of the occasional mercenary healers of the eighteenth and nineteenth centuries.[111]

There was no limit to the occult services that the small-time practitioner could provide – communing with the dead, providing advice on troublesome "secret" worries, and much more.[112] An operator-dentist in the Deux-Sèvres was a (probably insincere) sorcerer who sold a panaceac oil and gave advice to conscripts who wished to avoid military service.[113] An even wider range of services was offered in the early eighteenth century by a Marie-Madeleine du Colombier, widow of a man named Gaillard, who was arrested in 1709 by *lettre de cachet* and accused of transmuting metals, making gold, telling fortunes, giving secrets for love and gambling, and even using mysterious means to remove freckles. She boasted that she was able to cure everything, provided the liver and lungs were not rotted, and professed to have secrets for winning love and producing the philosopher's stone, although she denied using sorcery. The Gaillard widow was typical of the displaced persons who turned to healing, although more successful than most. When her husband died and left her without resources, she learned medicine, she said, with "all there was in the way of great minds and foreign physicians." In fact she was almost illiterate, but she insisted that she did not need to know how to read in order to understand simples and "secrets." And in one sense she was right; she had managed to earn between 7,000 and 8,000 livres.[114]

A case of alchemy combined with medical practice was prosecuted as late as 1830 (and no doubt further exploration would turn up still later examples). Laurent Debrou, the son of a former shoemaker of Tours and by his own account a *prêtre de la petite église* (a priest who did not accept the Concordat of 1801), claimed to possess not only marvelous healing secrets but also mystical means to find treasures and make gold and silver. The exhibits at his trial included alchemists' instruments. The authorities, facing either a clever fraud or a madman, leaned toward the latter conclusion. Debrou spoke with "verbose facility" but ignored the rules of language and grammar; although this combination of fluency and disorder was always considered a hallmark of charlatanish discourse, it could betoken mania as well.[115]

Religious and inspired healers

Even more than belief in the occult, religion was a pervasive presence in popular medical culture. Patients invoked saints for the relief of specific illnesses; *bonnes femmes* might say a few prayers for their neighbor's recovery; in Brittany, empirics themselves participated in *pardons*, the great processional pilgrimages to local shrines.[116] Many *maiges*, as will be seen in the next chapter, could be called religious healers; they relied in part on prayers, saw themselves as instruments of divine power, and required that their patients be baptized Christians. In addition, some popular medical practitioners, whom one would hesitate to classify as folk healers, claimed that their curative powers or their healing mission came from God. They might differ in a number of ways from the typical *maige*. Most were in some sense outsiders, not familiar members of a village community; some were religious visionaries, almost prophets; a few had extensive practices comparable to those of the most successful empirics. In most cases their powers did not derive, as those of the *maige* typically did, from a personal gift transmitted from generation to generation; some, indeed, were simply swindlers who exploited popular credulity.

These sorts of empirics were not so numerous or well-organized as faith healers in Protestant countries, and no indigenous movements comparable to Swedenborgian spiritualism or Christian Science emerged in France, though the sects won some converts there, and the practice of healing through prayer and the laying on of hands existed in the Protestant communities of the Midi and Alsace-Lorraine.[117] But their appeal could be enormous and frightening to the authorities, attracting, as it did, the faithful, the sick, and the merely curious in a way that adumbrated in miniature the extraordinary popular success of Lourdes in the latter nineteenth century. When in 1828, for example, a woman announced herself at Nantes as having the power to cure any illness through prayer, a great crowd gathered, and armed force was needed (according to the prefect) to prevent disorder.[118] François Oudot, the "saint of Varennes," created a sensation in 1759–1760, healing with holy water and five Ave Marias, until the royal lieutenant-general in Burgundy had him removed to a hospital at Dijon, where he died two years later.[119] Perhaps the most celebrated religious healer of eighteenth-century France, a former shepherd named Pierre Richard, received 500 to 600 patients a day at the height of his vogue.

The case of Richard illustrates particularly well the social ambiguities of religious healing. Known as "the saint of Savières," he was born in 1716 in the village of that name on the Seine in the province of Champagne, whose inhabitants had a reputation for curing sick animals. The local shepherds also practiced some human medicine. Richard probably did so himself for many years, but he in no way stood out from his fellow shepherds until he reached his early fifties. Around 1767 he began working cures with holy water; his reputation grew after he was found one morning in a locked church, to which he said an angel had admitted him. It was reported that he never asked directly for a fee, but grateful patients regularly made payments, which were accepted for Richard by the woman with whom he had begun living after his initial successes. Having a concubine seems not to have dimmed the saint's glory; but when in 1770 he went so far as to marry her, this rash display of worldliness shook the confidence of his clientele, and his practice rapidly declined. He died in 1787, never having reestablished his earlier reputation.

Richard's motives in all of this cannot be determined with any certainty. In his first police interrogation, he called himself a simple day laborer (*manouvrier*) who had fallen from the higher status of *laboureur* (who usually owned at least a plough and a team of draft animals). This story might suggest that it was a reversal of his economic fortunes that drove him to practice medicine. In his second interrogation, however, he stressed that his family enjoyed a healing gift, which he had received from a brother who was a tailor at Savières and was too busy to use it. Perhaps the *don* was passed on as an economic resource to the needier brother. In any case, Richard spoke freely of his medical practice. He did not deal with fevers or other "internal conditions," as he defined them, or with fractures or hernias, but only with rheumatism, sciatica, and other "catarrhal and nervous disorders," cancers, ulcers, epilepsy, and disorders of vision. Blind people had recovered their sight, provided they had not lost the pupil of the eye; some deaf people had recovered their hearing, but they cost him "a good deal of trouble, since it is difficult to have them learn by heart the prayers they have to say." He added that his remedies would not work on those handicapped since birth, but only on those who had become blind, deaf, mute, rheumatic, or epileptic through "accidents." Why, he was asked, did he continue to see patients? Because they continually tormented him, he replied; they came from everywhere, even from Normandy, 50 leagues beyond Paris. Who exactly these patients were he could not say. He contented himself with praying for them, without asking their names. But he knew that if they were cured, it was because they had faith; his remedies were useless otherwise.[120]

Similar cases can be found in the nineteenth century. Under the Restoration, for example, one religious healer, a woman named Milfort, who boasted of a gift to cure through prayers, enjoyed a vogue almost as great as Richard's, attracting patients to Charleville (Marne) from as far as 90 kilometers away (see Map 3). Her income came in part from the sale of a booklet containing printed formulas and invocations.[121]

Some religious healers ascribed their curative powers to the special favor of a saint or even claimed descent from a saint (such as Hubert) who had married before renouncing the flesh and taking orders. Several noble families in the Old Regime were believed to be of his "race" (lineage) and took the title of Knights of Saint Hubert. Georges Hubert, gentleman of the king's household, received letters patent as a knight of that order in 1649 and three years later won permission from the archbishop of Paris to claim the saint as a direct ancestor.[122] Other more modest *chevaliers de saint Hubert* "touched" for rabies, like the itinerants described in Chapter 3. Nicolas Clément, who wore a sort of shoulder strap (*bandoulière*) in lieu of the usual saint's stole, treated four persons bitten by a probably rabid dog near Lagny, at the edge of the Brie district, in 1780.[123] In the early nineteenth century, a *"grand chevalier de saint Hubert,"* a certain Falot or Fallot of the Marne, offered therapy in the form of regimen and prayers to victims of dogbite. He also applied a hot iron to the heads of dogs and farm animals to preserve them from rabies. Falot may have been literate; he was said to use medical books. The *chevalier* accepted whatever payment was offered. In one recorded case, four persons from the environs of Vitry-le-François paid him 20 sous apiece.[124]

The sincerity of these practitioners is usually difficult to gauge. A few religious healers, though, were clearly outright frauds, such as the practitioner to whom an *officier de santé* in the Hautes-Alpes referred only as the "ex-saint" from Peyrolles-en-Provence. This man, after playing deaf and dumb and offering his "catholico-magico-medical" prescriptions to the local populace, confessed his imposture to the authorities – which did not prevent

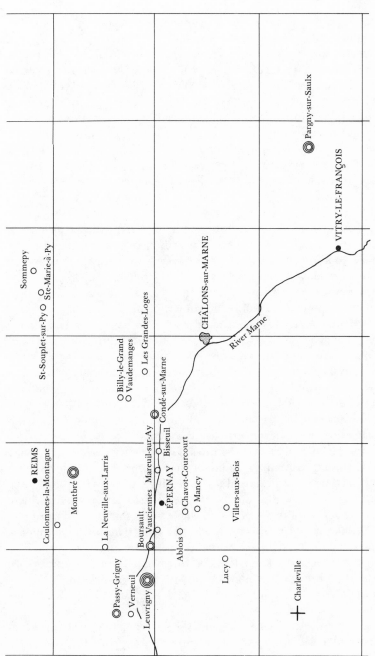

Map 3. Milfort case, 1822: Origins of patients traveling to Charleville. Each circle represents a passport issued to a patient traveling to consult Milfort at Charleville (in the lower-left-hand corner of the map, marked with a cross). Each side of the squares in the grid represents 20 kilometers. [*Source:* Archives Départementales, Marne, 33 × 8.]

him from continuing to treat rickets, congenital deafness, and other "incurable" ailments in the canton of Ribiers.[125]

Other cases of inspired healing challenge the would-be labeler. A seventy-three-year-old woman named Boucher, who believed that she had received a healing mission from on high, told a court in 1828, "I work for honor, [since] money is nothing to me"; she had dressed as a man for four years and had already been prosecuted twelve times.[126] Healers of this kind were not simply economic marginals, but outsiders in a larger sense. Their medical practice may have been not merely a financial link, but their only tie to society. Healing was an accepted career for eccentrics, one of the ways in which deviant behavior could be made socially acceptable – up to a point – in preindustrial Europe.

Whatever these healers' motives, it is important to remember that medical practice was for them, as for other empirics, a source of income, and sometimes a very good one. Two cases from the early years of the Restoration suggest how a medical practitioner could successfully exploit religious belief. The first empiric is closer to a confidence artist, the second seemingly more sincere; both could be called social marginals.

When we first hear of Magdeleine Aunievan, she is a wandering mendicant. The widow of the stonecutter Tassy, from Collobrières in the Var, she arrived in 1816 with her two children in the town of Saint-Maximin (about 40 kilometers away in the same department), in rags, covered with lice, and begging for bread. Soon, though, she had won the confidence of another widow, Colombe Menut, whose husband, a farmer, had left her some property; in the view of the local authorities, Menut was "a little deranged," and her inheritance must have seemed to Aunievan a fruit ripe for picking. The two widows and their children began living together; according to Menut's daughter, her mother and Aunievan even slept together. The guest promised to "cure" her hostess with prayers and to reconcile her with God; though her disease was not specified, Menut was clearly in poor health (or at least believed that she was). Three times each day, Aunievan put a crucifix in Menut's hands and lit three candles, saying that she could make Jesus Christ descend three times into the bedroom; she also directed Menut to have three masses said. (One cynical observer predicted that she would soon be working miracles like those of the saint of Peyrolles.) A surgeon who had been attending Menut was dismissed.

Aunievan's parasitism began on a small scale. She advised Menut to eat good soups; each day four pounds of mutton went into the pot. Soon Aunievan and her children were consuming "good meals," followed by coffee. She obtained high-quality clothing of India cloth and velvet for her children and took for herself a flannel corset, shirts, rings, and two crosses. Then, in a maneuver that finally landed the case in court, she defrauded the other widow of 800 francs, the proceeds from the sale of wine and some "capital" (property). Aunievan enjoyed playing the role of seer, and when Menut's son sold the property at her instigation and wanted to place the funds with a third party, she warned that the man would die a sudden death and the money would be lost. She even predicted the son's own death.

Like most confidence artists of this kind, Aunievan insisted that she had no material interest in treating her patient, having means of her own. According to one story, her brother, an officer of the Legion of Honor, was to arrive from Paris with an inheritance; according to another, she would take Colombe Menut and her children to live with her "in a beautiful house" on an estate that she owned at Collobrières.[127]

Aunievan's exploits at Saint-Maximin were not her only venture into empiricism or her last brush with the law. Subsequent police records contain another file on a "Magdeleine Tassy," accused of illegal practice of midwifery. It was also alleged that she and her husband beat up a horse trader in a quarrel over water in a canal running through their lands.[128]

Compared with Aunievan, Joseph-Xavier Tissot was a major medical entrepreneur. Tissot, or Father Hilarion as he was known in religious life (he was a brother of Saint John of God), appeared at Piolenc in the Vaucluse at the end of 1815 and established himself as a "physician," prescribing a few remedies such as arnica and recommending prayer. A certain Rodier, for example, who had a tumor on his knee, was told to pray to God, say novenas to the saints, give alms, and hear masses, and was promised a cure in ten to twenty days; Tissot also gave him a little bottle containing a remedy.

Tissot was fond of boasting that he had been sent by God to support religion and the king (this was reported in May 1816, when Tissot identified with most ultra of the ultraroyalists) and was widely known as *le bienheureux* (the blessed one). Local opinion, however, was divided. Some said that he worked miracles, others that he was a "clever rogue," and still others that he was a madman just released from Charenton. The subprefect at Orange leaned toward the last interpretation, noting that members of Tissot's family suffered from mental illness – "additional presumptive evidence against him." One point is clear: Tissot knew how to make effective use of publicity stunts, such as having a man arrive in a suburb, coming from Piolenc, with two crutches on his shoulders, proclaiming that Tissot had cured him of a "gouty rheumatism," which for two years had prevented him from walking.

Tissot's activities expanded further in 1817 as his conception of his religious mission grew more grandiose. Although in his petitions to the local authorities he modestly stressed the experience he said he had acquired in a Trappist novitiate, in his popular harangues he spoke of having performed miracles and announced that he had been sent by God to rekindle faith, that he had a mission to regenerate the Church, and that he would wind up being persecuted like Jesus Christ. By this time he was surrounded by adherents – "accomplices" in the eyes of the authorities – who claimed to be blind, lame, and paralyzed because of demons. Patients flocked to the barn where he lived.

Tissot's ultimate mission, as it turned out, was medical: God had directed him to establish a *mission de charité*, or almshouse, where penitents would be healed through true prayer. He promoted his scheme in a printed announcement, according to which the almshouse was to specialize in the treatment of nervous disorders – alienation, vapors, epilepsy. This plan greatly discomfited the authorities; Tissot's staff, the subprefect complained to the prefect, were to be directed in curing insanity "by a man who is greatly in need of treatment for this disorder himself." But the enterprise prospered. Patients paid 3 francs for a consultation, although the poor might receive free care on Saturdays if they could show a recommendation from their curé. Tissot even succeeded in recruiting two licensed practitioners, a surgeon and a Montpellier physician, who provided a legal front for his operations.[129]

Like Tissot, other inspired healers built a deeply loyal local following. One visionary empiric, a farmer at Coligny (8 kilometers south of Vertus in the Marne), who won popular favor in part because he accepted payment only reluctantly, was elected to the municipal council by a part of the population hostile to the mayor.[130] This kind of local solidarity, from which sedentary empirics of all types benefitted, was to prove a major obstacle to the repression of illegal medical practice in rural France.

THE POPULATION OF EMPIRICS: NUMBERS, DENSITY, DISTRIBUTION

Ideally, having sketched a typology of empirics, an analysis of irregular practice would say something about the number and distribution of the various types. Unfortunately there is no reliable way of ascertaining the actual number of unauthorized practitioners. Where unqualified practice is legal, as in Germany after 1871, it has been possible to establish official registers (though even these rosters probably omit many obscure or occasional practitioners).[131] In France of the Old Regime and early nineteenth century, however, empiricism remained a largely clandestine activity; and even if it had been fully legal and above board, censuses of unauthorized practitioners in this protostatistical age would have been at least as undependable as those of the profession, which leave much to be desired. In any case, no systematic attempt was made to count empirics until the mid-nineteenth century, when the Association Générale des Médecins de France polled its member societies, with spotty results.[132]

In the Old Regime, the closest thing to a census of empirics was a register maintained by the Paris police; when it was turned over to the Société Royale de Médecine in 1778, incomplete and badly in need of updating, it contained 1,746 names accumulated over seventeen years. The inspector in charge, Patté, estimated that about half of the practitioners and remedy vendors had moved or died or were no longer active, but that about an equal number of new practitioners were not known to the police or had not been registered.[133] If the overall number is roughly accurate, it would mean that empirics outnumbered the various authorized practitioners by about three to one.

No comparable figures exist for the provinces, although some well-informed observers did make guesses; Nicolas, for example, the Société Royale's faithful correspondent at Grenoble, estimated in the late 1770's that there might be about forty "operators" in Dauphiné – adding however, that nearly every village had some sort of *guérisseur*.[134] Some fragmentary evidence on specific empirics can be gleaned, though, from a variety of sources: multiple denunciations written by individual physicians or medical societies; the Comité de Salubrité's investigation of 1790–1791; and, in the nineteenth century, the reports of medical juries, health councils, and, in the few departments where they existed, the cantonal physicians. This information rarely provided meaningful absolute numbers, but it suggests the proportions or distribution of the various practitioners in a given region, at least as physicians or government officials perceived it.

Multiple denunciations are the least satisfactory source; their authors normally included only the most conspicuous practitioners encroaching on the work of the profession, although occasionally an informant, apparently driven as much by scientific zeal as by annoyance, attempted to compile an exhaustive enumeration. One general pattern emerges. Urban lists comprised mainly major empirics and tradesmen who impinged on the medical and pharmaceutical domains; these practitioners, unlike some of their rural counterparts, did not simply fill gaps where physicians or apothecaries were unavailable. Rural lists embraced a more varied group of small-time practitioners, including priests and nuns. They rarely included, however, the more obscure healers of the sort that modern folklore studies would lead us to expect in large numbers; either they remained invisible or their activities were deemed too trivial to count.

Consider first two urban reports, one prepared by the Faculty of Nantes in 1781, the other by a Parisian *officier de santé* in 1825. The faculty was able to identify four major practitioners (not counting the itinerant Salomon Cuchet, then residing at Nantes): the oculist Tadiny, who offended the physicians by selling phials of eyewash; an empiric named Romain; a "chemist-herbalist" named Duvrignau; and a joiner named Mercier, who practiced medicine and inspected urine. The Paris list actually included two of the author's fellow *officiers de santé*: one who was said to have usurped the title of physician, and another who kept a pharmacy (where he sold groceries and knickknacks as well as drugs) and peddled his wares. The latter's wife also practiced medicine and sold remedies. In addition, a stonecutter practiced surgery and sold remedies, and a herbalist kept a pharmacy and saw patients.[135]

A more rural range appears in a list for the canton of Orpierre in the Hautes-Alpes, submitted to the prefect in 1800 by an *officier de santé*. The author complained of passing charlatans, but he also provided a list of *maiges* (his term) and a parallel list, by commune, of the eleven *officiers de santé* practicing in his canton. The empirics included three *rhabilleurs* and six others, among them a priest and a former curé who had become a mayor: all told, nine irregulars, two fewer than the number of licensed practitioners.[136] A similar but more detailed list was compiled three years later by a physician at Saint-Vith, in the annexed Belgian department of the Ourthe, shortly after passage of the new legislation on medical practice. His report covered the cantons of Reuland and Bütgenbach, as well as Saint-Vith. These were his findings (summarized or paraphrased here, as in subsequent lists, except as indicated by quotation marks):

> Roth, at Reuland, is an illiterate who has been a shoemaker and a soldier. Most recently he was a customs employee; discharged, he became a "physician."
> Linden, at Born, can read and write a little. A joiner, he abandoned that calling to become a hunter. "Too clumsy to kill animals, he began to kill people."
> Hecking, at Amblève, can perhaps read and write a little; he settled there a few years ago, after traveling around the region. Three or four years ago he killed a girl afflicted with rabies by opening her veins and suffocating her.
> Ducombe, at Rocherath, is an old man with a reputation as an *uromante*, although he has been blind for two years.
> Hubert Boehmer, at Wirtzfeldt, has been deaf since childhood; he learned only the craft of shoemaking, which he still practices, together with medicine.
> Théodore Gierzen, a priest (*vicaire* at Hunnigen), is an "exorcist who finds supernatural causes where a few routine remedies have been ineffective."
> Feydet, *vicaire* at Wirtzfeldt, is an "*accouchant*" and physician.
> Alexandre Lamberty, a young priest at Wirztfeldt, practices medicine.

Marginals and occasional practitioners figure prominently here; three ecclesiastics carry on the traditional healing role of the clergy.[137]

The Comité de Salubrité's survey of surgery, although suggestive, provides almost no usable information on numbers of empirics. One of the fourteen items on the questionnaire read: "Are charlatans, empirics, and *gens à secrets* (healers; literally, people with secrets) very widespread in your arrondissement? What degree of toleration is accorded them?" Since the respondents were not asked to provide statistics, it is not surprising that very few did. The report from Luxeuil (Haute-Saône) indicated that every village had three or four persons who practiced medicine. The response from Saint-Sever (Landes) estimated that the arrondissement included about fifty *well-known* charlatans, counting surgeons not officially received; this was about the same as the number of surgeons received in the previous two decades (since 1770).[138] The great majority of replies, however, simply offered an impression: in most cases, empirics were seen as common or very common; other reports described them as rare or even unknown in the arrondissement.[139] The first group of responses outnumbered the second by more than two to one. In a suggestive article, Toby Gelfand has argued that the "high-density" responses tended to come from larger towns, the "low-density" responses from smaller and more isolated ones.[140] Empirics, like professionals, clustered near the most promising markets. It should be remembered, though, that the responses do not make it possible to distinguish systematically between itinerant and sedentary practitioners, and that they generally counted only the most conspicuous empirics.[141] Minor sedentary empiricism may have been a more rural phenomenon than this analysis would suggest. A few regional patterns also appear: more high-density responses in the South, and above all in the Southwest, thanks no doubt to that region's large numbers of partly-qualified surgeons, notably in Gascony.[142]

The survey yields somewhat more information on the types of practitioners whom the lieutenants of the First Surgeon saw fit to denounce: mainly surgeons not received by the local *communauté*, religious, and *rebouteurs*. Laon mentioned another category of special operator – dentists, who, according to the report, represented a new kind of charlatanism. Nuits cited a woman oculist. Poitiers complained about its executioner. Many of the bitterest complaints concerned unqualified surgeons, who in some cases had been received by the previous lieutenant.[143] Occasional practitioners and marginals appear with far less frequency in the reports. Lyons-la-Forêt (Eure) complained of two persons "without resources" in the parish of La Feuillie; and Arras mentioned a few who had no other livelihood than the sale of remedies – though it is not clear whether these were economic marginals or successful entrepreneurs.[144]

For the early nineteenth century, reports from medical juries or local health councils, which often summarize information received from individual physicians, are generally the best guides to local empirical practice, though none claims to be exhaustive. In 1805, for example, the medical jury at Strasbourg sent to the local tribunal a list of nine persons who "as a matter of common knowledge" practiced medicine in the city without authorization. Two of the names in the list will be familiar: Küchel, the hypnotist, accused of practicing medicine and distributing an elixir; and the Richert woman, "known by the name of *la Dormeuse* or Barbe *la Dormeuse.*" The others included an abbé; a weaver who treated external conditions and consumption; a *graissier* (grocer dealing in grease) who treated cancers; a shoemaker who practiced medicine "without being on any list"; and a self-styled *officier de santé* who had signed a spurious certificate. Among those whose occupations were identified were two "clerks" – the abbé and a notary (Küchel); two artisans; a peasant; and a small tradesman. One was the wife of a hemp grower (or dealer). Medicine appears here chiefly as a secondary activity, sometimes linked to the principal occupation: the shoemaker made use of his manual dexterity, and the *graissier* no doubt applied lard to the cancers.[145] A later report from the health council at Nantes (1827), summarizing information supplied by several Breton physicians, included a similar range of practitioners: no major empirics, but a woman who sold purgatives and emetics; another woman, who used a razor to make incisions on patients' palates (a traditional treatment for a vaguely defined condition known as *les hunes*); and seven *rebouteurs* in the arrondissement of Ancenis (see Map 2). One informant denounced the curé of Touvois (Loire-Inférieure) and a certain Guibert, from the commune of Beaufou (Vendée), who practiced urinoscopy.[146]

The Bas-Rhin survey

More complete information than this was compiled in one notable case – the closest thing to a real census of illegal practitioners carried out in France during the early nineteenth century. In 1813, the prefect of the Bas-Rhin ordered the cantonal physicians of the department to conduct a survey of unauthorized practice in their jurisdictions, including all types of practitioners.[147] The responses cover, first of all, a familiar range of traditional empirics, among them itinerant peddlers and charlatans (including Drs. Hans and Johann); barbers; and the executioner at Memmelshoffen (Henri Heid, known as Master Henner) who dabbled in surgery.

Itinerants (other than Drs. Hans and Johann)
    Justin Breit, a "vagabond" no less dangerous than Dr. Hans, in the view of the cantonal physician at Soultz-sous-Forêts, usually lives with a farmer at Birlenbach. Breit, also known as Justul, is a native of Wissembourg. He has no known trade apart from empiricism.
    A gardener of Strasbourg, living just outside the town, "makes frequent circuits in the communes of the [neighboring] canton of Oberhausbergen, to undertake the treatment of the most serious diseases," as does a fruit seller living within the town walls.
    In the arrondissement of Saverne, two persons coming from outside the region "enter the communes furtively and practice medicine and surgery." The cantonal physician at Soultz-sous-Forêts (arrondissement of Wissembourg) denounces "Tirolese" and other vagabonds, peddlers of "very strong drugs."[148]

Barbers

The cantonal physician at Benfeld (arrondissement of Sélestat) reports two barbers at Huttenheim. Dürr, sixty years old, practices medicine and surgery "with extreme audacity." The inhabitants of the commune "have a blind confidence in this individual despite the fact that he is under the influence of wine from the morning on, and that he dispatches a good many victims each year." The other barber, Wolff, about fifty years old, also practices surgery, but since the inhabitants have no confidence in him, "he is in no way dangerous to society."

At Stotzheim, in the same canton, two barbers are mentioned. Brenner, who practices medicine and surgery, "would be very enterprising if he enjoyed the confidence of the inhabitants"; Hess, "extremely mild, in no way enterprising," limits himself to bleeding and applying vesicatories ordered by a physician or surgeon of the region.

The cantonal physician at Soultz-sous-Forêts cites four barbers, of whom the most offensive is François-Adam Birckbüchler ("Fraentzel") of Rittershoffen, who "practices medicine with unbelievable audacity." (But two other barbers practicing medicine actually deserve the title of *officier de santé*.)[149]

The prominence of barbers reflects the persistence in Alsace, as in Germany, of the old association between barbering and surgery.

Midwives and unauthorized *matrones* had an important place in the reports. Two of them, apparently authorized *sages-femmes*, were accused of practicing medicine and surgery: a sixty-five-year-old woman in the arrondissement of Strasbourg, who worked in two cantons, and another in the same arrondissement, canton of Geispolsheim. Among the women accused of practicing midwifery without a license were the *accoucheuses* of five communes in the canton of Woerth (arrondissement of Wissembourg) and three in the canton of Soultz-sous-Forêts, in the same arrondissement. In the arrondissement of Saverne, sixteen accusations out of twenty-seven were directed against unauthorized midwives; they included two anonymous "old women," one of whom, from the commune of Adamswiller, enjoyed the protection of the mayor, who refused to divulge her name.[150] In general, the physicians complained of the dubious competence of the local midwives, and according to some reports nearly all the *accoucheuses* practiced medicine and surgery, bleeding patients, administering remedies, and dosing small children with opiates.[151]

In addition to the midwives, a small number of women empirics (about a fifth of the women on the list) practiced only other branches of medicine and surgery. In all, almost half the practitioners on the 1813 list were women.

Women practitioners (other than midwives)

At Marckolsheim (arrondissement of Sélestat), a Catherine Lehmann, daughter of a barber and wife of a country policeman (*garde-champêtre*), performs surgical operations and sells drugs. According to the cantonal physician, "although bleedings are rarely indicated in our region, this woman would not hesitate to bleed an entire commune for six sols."

In the canton of Brumath (arrondissement of Strasbourg), the wife of a dealer in rope and twine makes ointments and plasters and dabbles in surgery. "In spite of her lack of skill," the cantonal physician complains, "she knows how to win men's confidence."

Two women appear in the reports for the arrondissement of Saverne: at Hambach, a married woman practices medicine and surgery, and at Burbach, the mother of the Protestant pastor is an "oculist" (ocular surgeon). (If the midwives are included, two-thirds of the empirics on the list for Saverne are women.)

In the arrondissement of Wissembourg, the cantonal physician at Kandel reports a Marianne-Françoise Reinhard, a resident of Rheinzabern, who says that she has once been a nun. She sells remedies and visits patients in several communes of the canton.[152]

Except for the former nun, all the women are identified by association with a male; she was once "married" to Christ, but has now broken free.

For the remaining empirics, the reports usually indicated some primary occupation other than healing. The few exceptions may have been full-time medical practitioners. A certain Lettenberg, living at Hausen in Baden, practiced medicine without authorization at Schoenau (canton of Marck-olsheim, Sélestat) "with extreme audacity." In the town of Brumath (arrondissement of Strasbourg), a "harmful quack" named Diebold practiced medicine and surgery. Also cited were three surgeons whose names were not on the official rolls, among them a surgical student and the grandson of a surgeon. In the canton of Soultz-sous-Forêts, a former schoolmaster's clerk, Mathieu Treibel, had practiced medicine "without the least knowledge of the subject" for eight years since quitting his previous employment, according to the cantonal physician. He was commonly known as "Provisor," the German word for a pharmacist's aide, perhaps a reminiscence of an earlier calling, perhaps simply a tribute to his skill in dispensing.[153]

Among the part-time practitioners, one was identified only as the mayor of the commune of Dürrenbach (canton of Woerth, Wissembourg). Others included three "clerks" – a schoolmaster at Eywiller and two clergymen. At Brumath, arrondissement of Strasbourg, the cantonal physician cited a certain Stolz, a former priest living at Mertzwiller, canton of Niederbronn (in the arrondissement of Wissembourg, more than 15 kilometers from Brumath). Stolz had been denounced by the cantonal physicians of Brumath, Niederbronn, and Haguenau during an epidemic that had raged at Bernolsheim the previous year. The physician at Haguenau even made a collection of Stolz's recipes "in order to reveal this man's charlatanism." And in the arrondissement of Saverne, a Protestant minister who had taken courses in medicine at the University of Heidelberg practiced illegally.[154]

A larger number of popular practitioners covered in the 1813 survey were artisans or tradespeople, although in a few cases they achieved such success in their medical practice that they abandoned the earlier occupation altogether. The sobriquets by which they were sometimes known typically referred to this calling.

Occasional practitioners, with occupation

Gasser, a shoemaker at Baldenheim, canton of Marckolsheim (arrondissement of Sélestat), sells amulettes to cure rheumatism.

At Ehnwihr, in the township of Muttersholtz (canton of Marckolsheim), a weaver named Éberlé "undertakes to cure every kind of disease, sometimes using mystical and sympathetic remedies, sometimes chemical drugs, depending on the status of the people who consult him."

The cantonal physician at Geispolsheim (arrondissement of Strasbourg) reports a Jean-Michel Fritsch, nicknamed "Pfiffenschneider" (*Pfeifenschneider*, or carver of smoking pipes), who "practices exorcism and other superstitious exercises and also abuses in various ways the confidence with which the lower class favors him."

In the town of Woerth (Wissembourg), a cartwright named Scheuk practices medicine; the cantonal physician adds that he is "adept in the magical arts and sorcery."

In the commune of Hoffen (canton of Soltz-sous-Forêts), a former weaver, Jacques Vern, practices medicine. His sobriquet, "Weber Jockel," recalls his previous occupation.

In addition, the list of empirics in the arrondissement of Sélestat includes the name of a wet cooper at Rosheim.[155]

The regular métier did not necessarily dictate the decision to practice medicine or the choice of therapeutic methods; indeed, the 1813 cases do not even suggest a transfer of empirical skills. The part-time empirics had recourse to the sale of remedies or occasional medical practice as a source of extra income that required no additional training and almost no initial investment.

Folk healers remained less visible than these empirics and went almost unnoticed in the 1813 survey. It is significant that among the practitioners whose occupation is known appears one "gardener," but no farmer or peasant. Indeed, most of the practitioners were based in towns or resided there permanently. In the canton of Brumath, for example, three of the six resident empirics cited by the cantonal physician practiced in the town of Brumath itself; and in the arrondissement of Sélestat, it appears that none of the reported empirics had a rural practice.[156] The most visible empirics, then, were urban, though they sometimes sought a wide market in the countryside. The Bas-Rhin survey falls midway between the urban and rural ranges of practice seen earlier – perhaps because the cantonal physicians who provided the reports were based in towns but were required by their official function to provide services in the rural districts as well.

Table 3. *Unauthorized medical practitioners in the Bas-Rhin, 1813*

Occupation	No.	Type of practice	No.
"Midwife"[a]	26	Medicine and general empiricism	29
Barber	8	Surgery[c]	24
Artisan	9	Midwifery[d]	24
Other	10	Sale of remedies	7
No second occupation,		Magic/sorcery	5
or unknown	18		
Total	71[b]		—[e]

[a]Includes 2 midwives practicing medicine illegally and 24 *matrones* practicing midwifery illegally.
[b]Of the 71 empirics listed, 32 were women and 39 were men.
[c]Includes 2 surgeons not on the official lists.
[d]Unauthorized midwifery only.
[e]The same empiric has in some cases been counted in more than one category; the total therefore exceeds 71.
Source: Compiled from reports of cantonal physicians in Archives Départementales du Bas-Rhin 5 M 22.

In view of the types of practitioners on which the survey of 1813 was likely to touch, it is not surprising that their methods rarely departed from routine empiricism – the sale of remedies and traditional internal medicine and surgery, singly or in combination. In a few places the reports allude to mystical healing, amulettes, exorcism, and magical practices. A certain Blassing in the Lutheran village of Durstel even used "so-called witchcraft" and aroused "implacable hatreds in the communes," presumably by accusing their inhabitants of casting spells on his patients.[157] But such cases were unusual.

Table 3 summarizes the findings of the 1813 survey. The total number of known irregulars in the surviving lists, which cover about a third of the department's cantons, is 71. (The reports did not systematically count *matrones*.[158] If all women practicing midwifery illegally could somehow be included, the number would be significantly higher; if those on the list are eliminated, it falls to 47.) A very crude comparison can be made with the number of authorized practitioners. The roster from the previous year (1812) included 98 first-order practitioners, 269 second-order practitioners (367 medical personnel in all), and 529 midwives.[159] Even these figures, although they do cover the entire department, are not entirely reliable; other statistics from the previous decade show some curious discrepancies.[160] But it appears that the number of irregulars was significantly smaller than the number of licensed personnel: even supposing that the missing cantons had, on the average, twice as many empirics as those for which we have reports, and including the *matrones* counted in 1813, we would arrive at a total of 355, slightly less than the number of licensed practitioners exclusive of midwives. Two caveats should be added, however. First, the profession was overrepresented in the arrondissement of Strasbourg, and particularly in the town itself, where perhaps a quarter of the official medical personnel practiced. The 1813 reports do not suggest a comparable concentration of empirics: the surviving lists for the arrondissement of Strasbourg, which include the *chef-lieu*, mention only 10. Second, the cantonal physicians undoubtedly omitted some unknown number of inconspicuous occasional practitioners, in Strasbourg and everywhere else. Complete information would probably bring the totals for regulars and irregulars closer to parity, particularly in the more rural districts.

What conclusions can be drawn from these very imperfect data? One tentative generalization suggests itself as a hypothesis that could be tested through further research. Outside Paris, the number of major empirics in the early nineteenth century – those whom the profession might seriously consider rivals – did not exceed that of licensed practitioners and may well have been substantially smaller. Even in the detailed rural list for the canton of Orpierre, the number of *officiers de santé* was slightly greater than that of local empirics. The French experience in the early years of the Ventôse regime would appear to differ from that of England in the same period or Germany in the era of medical freedom (*Kurierfreiheit*) in the late nineteenth and early twentieth centuries, when in some places the number of full-time professional "healers" greatly exceeded that of physicians.[161]

The paucity of information makes it still more difficult to discern trends. One physician of Lille wrote at midcentury that over the previous thirty or forty years, the number of "medicasters" in his region had declined from somewhere in the thousands to a few hundred, but we have no way of testing this assertion or judging how well it might apply to France as a whole. The survey conducted by the Association Générale des Médecins de France in 1861 listed 853 individuals in some thirty departments, but this information is very incomplete; two years earlier, a regional survey by the medical society of Ille-et-Vilaine alone had counted more than 150 (mostly nuns).[162] Without better data it is impossible to say more.

SEDENTARY EMPIRICISM: A SOCIAL AND ECONOMIC ANALYSIS

Like itinerant charlatanism, sedentary empiricism must be understood not only as a form of medical practice but also as an economic activity with social implications. Though rudimentary medicine and surgery remained an integral part of charitable assistance to the poor, empirics typically relied on their practice for a livelihood.

To the extent that sedentary practitioners were mobile at all, they often served, like the itinerants, as direct links between town and countryside. One response to the Comité de Salubrité's survey described a pattern in which empirics worked in the countryside on feast days and Sundays and in towns during fairs and markets.[163] In other cases, local empirics simply worked from their homes; they might extend their practice by bringing patients to them, like the Milfort woman (see Map 3) or *la demoiselle* Ribière in Poitou, who made a specialty of curing eye disorders (leucoma, "redness") and lodged her patients *en pension*.[164]

The catchment area of the most successful practitioners reached for tens of miles. One of the most celebrated rural empirics of the late seventeenth and early eighteenth centuries, a peasant of the Mantes region named Christophe Ozanne (1633–1713), gained such a reputation that special facilities had to be built to accommodate his patients, and a coach service established between his village and Paris; at the height of his vogue, he received 200 to 300 visitors a week.[165] The Lany woman, who practiced in Champagne at the end of the Old Regime, was said to draw patients from 10 leagues around.[166] And a correspondent of the Société Royale de Médecine reported in 1782 that *uromantes* might have a range of 10, 15, or 20 leagues.[167] In the nineteenth century, improved roads and then the railroad facilitated access to the major empirics. A practitioner at Dunkirk nicknamed "Guérit-Tout" was called to Bourbourg, the countryside around Saint-Omer and Dunkirk, and Belgian villages from Les Moëres to Roesbrugge; and Vignes (1830–1906), a celebrated healer at Vialas (Lozère) treated thirty to thirty-five patients a day from the Lozère, the Cantal, and even foreign countries.[168] All these practitioners stimulated local trade. The empiric who came into town to see patients presumably shopped there, as did his clients; *pensionnaires* had to be fed, and the money was spent in local shops. Empiricism, like professional medicine, belonged to the market economy.

But if there are some obvious economic similarities, there are also some important social differences between itinerant and sedentary practice. Ambulatory empiricism implied a more radical commitment. If the would-be empiric was not already living on the road, or part of a rural subculture for which seasonal migrations were the norm, he had to break with family and community. Sedentary practice could be entered more casually and more gradually, starting perhaps with the sale of a few boxes of a secret remedy. In part for this reason, it attracted persons from a broad spectrum of social backgrounds – marginals at one end, members of respectable bourgeois or noble families on the other, who turned to medical practice because of sudden financial need, or out of fascination with the field, or occasionally as an expression of what appears to have been some form of mental illness.

The Angevin physician Contoly, for example, considered a charlatan by the Angers faculty, had lived for eighteen years on his wife's fortune and, while she was alive, confined himself to such harmless activities as putting on magic lantern shows. When his income declined following his wife's death, he announced himself as a doctor and began to treat venereal disease.[169] In Brittany, the barely literate operator Lahaye, a former officer of the merchant marine, was the black sheep of a respectable bourgeois family, who sought unsuccessfully to keep him from practicing.[170] And in the little village of Armentières-sur-Avre, in the Perche region, a minor noble (*hobereau*) named Gabriel de Moucheron, who was descended from "ancient nobility" but lacked financial resources and had a family to support, resorted to selling a salve that he manufactured.[171] Sedentary empiricism also appears to have been considerably more attractive to single women than was life on the road, so long as they had a roof over their heads. The most striking distinction, though, is that local medical practice could easily be a part-time supplement to some regular occupation. Peripatetic empirics may have moved in and out of various trades, but the only one that they commonly joined to ambulatory medicine was peddling; a few were itinerant craftsmen.

Empirics' occupations

Although medicine was a field in which almost anyone could make a little money, few empirics relied solely upon it as a source of income. Most pursued another calling as well, even if they may periodically have neglected it when medicine promised a better reward. (Of the 45 empirics reported in the Bas-Rhin survey, excluding midwives, 17 were barbers or artisans and 10 more had some other known occupation: 27 in all, as opposed to 18 for whom no other occupation is mentioned.) As has been seen, the nicknames of occasional practitioners sometimes referred to their regular trade ("Pfeifenschneider," "Weber Jockel"), just as the primary occupation of full-time empirics was sometimes indicated by sobriquets like "Dr. Hans" or "Dr. Johann." In rural regions, a seasonal alternation is apparent; Dr. Nicolas noted in Dauphiné, for example, that popular practitioners were most active from November until spring – that is, between the last harvest and autumn sowing and the first new planting.[172] In towns, the two businesses would normally be conducted simultaneously; the legal occupation might provide a convenient cover for clandestine medical activities. A woman named Lapresle, for example, a chairmaker in the Deux-Sèvres during the latter nineteenth century, could be approached with an offer to buy chairs or sell cane; her work as a somnambulist was carried out discreetly, behind closed doors.[173]

Some trades or callings had long been associated with empiricism; often their practitioners had a recognized role on the fringes of the old medical network but stepped outside it as their ambitions grew. The clergy were the most conspicuous of these groups; religious treated patients at their convent pharmacies, and a priest's medical practice could extend well beyond routine charitable care. A few ecclesiastics emerged as full-fledged empirics, like Nicolas Mercénier, former assistant priest of La Madeleine in Luxemburg, whose therapies ranged from olive oil, plasters, and ointments to prayers and exorcism (1828).[174] More modest practice by priests and nuns was widespread and in parts of France (notably the West) constituted the "medical abuse" about which nineteenth-century physicians most often complained.[175] Similarly, the executioner's practice could include more than the "restoration" of broken and dislocated limbs, as allowed by tradition and some legal decisions in the Old Regime. During the First Empire, for example, the executioner of Grenoble boasted that with the help of relatives and "enlightened colleagues," he could cure leprosy, scabies, tinea, and scrofula; he had recipes unknown to the surgeons, including pomades for "*enchilosse*" (*ankylose* or ankylosis, immobility and fixation of a joint) and for rheumatism, as well as thirty-two different balms.[176] So, too, empirics could regularly be found among members of the various ancillary trades; thus Ugard, an herbalist at Paris around 1820, treated venereal disease and liver conditions.[177] Other callings, minor trades that could not usually produce an adequate income in themselves, were often associated with medical practice, especially those that called for a knowledge of practical "secrets": "Père" Liard, for example, an exterminator of rats and moles at Brinon-sur-Sauldre in the mid-nineteenth century, was also a well-known healer.[178]

Practitioners of veterinary medicine often dabbled in the treatment of human patients, sometimes offering annual contracts to treat man and beast.[179] Indeed, empirics were likely to be found among all those who worked with animals: shepherds, cattle dealers, gelders, farriers. (One word for gelder, "*mégeyeur*," commonly used in the province of Maine, may well have derived from "*mége*" or "*maige*.")[180] Rural empirics, and especially *rebouteurs*, were often described as shepherds.[181] One shepherd-empiric in the Marne, with an eye to the future, entered his daughter in a midwifery course at Reims; she would carry on the family tradition, but legally. A certain Bourdin, who came to Niort (Deux-Sèvres) in the late nineteenth century to castrate sheep, also practiced human medicine in the countryside.[182] It might be supposed that such empirics simply applied the mechanical skills they had acquired in caring for injured animals or gelding sound ones, but this was not always the case. In the late eighteenth century, a medical man in the Gironde suggested that an animal trader-cum-empiric might use magic words and topical remedies to treat ganglions, whitlows, and intermittent fever in humans.[183]

But it was probably the blacksmith-farrier who most often practiced as an empiric in the French village. In an instructive essay on the village forge, based on a questionnaire distributed to local informants, Lucien Febvre evoked the social role and multiple functions of the *maréchal* before World War I.[184] One informant recalled that drinks were sold next to the blacksmith's house, where a food store, draper's shop, and bread depot were also established. The blacksmith naturally saw everyone in the village. He practiced veterinary medicine, bleeding animals and applying setons (cords or strips inserted under the animal's hide to help drain an infection), and performed quasi-official services for the inhabitants, such as appraising furniture. He also treated human patients, pulling teeth, curing neuralgia – he had the patient inhale the vapor from two "*pierres de tonnerre*" (literally, "thunder stones"; probably prehistoric stone artifacts) rubbed together – and distributing herbs and simples. This image, naturally, is colored by nostalgia. Local authorities might take a dimmer view of the blacksmith's medical activities, like a mayor in the Loire who in 1812 denounced the smith at Saint-Cyr-les-Vignes, saying that the man had acquired a reputation as an accoucheur, physician, and even sorcerer.[185]

In addition to the empirics whose occupations were traditionally associated with medicine, a wide variety of shopkeepers, artisans, or even simple laborers might practice a little medicine on the side. Appendix D lists some cases from the late eighteenth and early nineteenth centuries; such a "sample" has no statistical value but does suggest the diversity of occupations, comparable to the range for remedy sellers listed in Appendix C. The practitioners include present and former farmers, agricultural laborers, and artisans. (The notary is one of a small number of "clerks" who turn up among the occasional practitioners, recalling a time when almost anyone in the countryside who could read and write might practice a little medicine, drawing on compendia like *Les Remèdes de Mme Fouquet*.) If we add the occupations from Appendix C and from other cases discussed earlier, they yield a diverse group: shoemakers, joiners, weavers, carders, laborers, and farm workers, as well as a miscellany of other callings: stonecutter, sabot maker, tanner, roofer, winegrower, cooper, mason, handkerchief maker, chair bottomer. Peddlers and small shopkeepers are also well represented.

Although the sources are too scattered and fragmentary to make any precise computation meaningful, they strongly suggest that among empirics who left a trace in the archives, craftsmen outnumbered peasants actually working the land. This group deserves further study. In rural society, craftsmen were often those who had been deemed unqualified for the rigors of agricultural labor; the weak boy who could not farm was much likelier to become a tailor than, say, a priest. He may also have been likelier than his sturdier brother to become an empiric; practitioners of sedentary callings often had a reputation as healers.[186]

As has been seen, some empirical medicine actually involved a transfer of knowledge, skills, or materials from a trade or craft. Shepherds knew something of poisonous herbs; a shoemaker might possess both manual dexterity and some acquaintance with emollients. But this was far from the rule; if empiricism involved some apparent special skill, it was usually acquired separately. Urine scanning is perhaps the best illustration. A random roundup of *uromantes* includes a former shepherd turned herbalist, who chiefly sold artemisia;[187] another shepherd who once threshed grain and now came to an apothecary's shop each market Thursday to inspect urine;[188] a winegrower;[189] a weaver who practiced urinoscopy during the Revolution;[190] a bargeman at Nantes named Piloquet, whose medical career spanned at least the years from 1812 to 1826;[191] gelders;[192] and a former tailor in a cavalry regiment named Jean Raget, who claimed to have inspected urine since the age of twelve, and who applied in 1804 to become an *officier de santé*.[193]

Patterns of careers in empiricism

It has been seen that empiricism commonly served as a supplement to some other trade that gave the practitioner a more or less fixed place in the community. This was not, however, the only pattern. Different practitioners followed divergent trajectories, as in all forms of parallel medicine. For some, empiricism offered a vehicle for upward mobility. A major entrepreneur might carve out a lucrative practice, like *le grand* Thomas of Paris, who left a fortune of 55,900 livres when he died in 1757, or a former executioner of Nîmes, said in the last years of the Old Regime to have earned 15,000–20,000 écus.[194] In the early nineteenth century, a urinoscopist at Paris reputedly earned 20,000 francs per annum.[195] Even more modest practices could represent a form of social advancement. A report from Serres-en-Gapençais in the late eighteenth century, for example, described how a "coarse peasant" had become in turn a lord's huntsman, a *valet de chambre*, and then an empiric.[196] An unqualified surgeon, Bafferne, blamed for numerous deaths in 1817, had begun more modestly as the domestic of an orvietan vendor.[197] Other practitioners, though, appear to have been unhappy floaters or marginals of the sort encountered in the discussion of itinerants. Marx placed the street charlatans of Paris, with some justification, among the *Lumpenproletariat*:

> Alongside decayed *roués* with dubious means of subsistence and of dubious origin, alongside ruined and adventurous offshoots of the bourgeoisie, were vagabonds, discharged soldiers, discharged jailbirds, escaped galley slaves, swindlers, mountebanks, *lazzaroni*, pickpockets, tricksters, gamblers, *maquereaus*, brothel keepers, porters, *literati*, organ grinders, ragpickers, knife grinders, tinkers, beggars.[198]

Indeed, for the least fortunate, medical practice could be only one of several stages in a checkered career. An Alsatian *dormeuse*, according to one physician's report, might have been a seamstress at Strasbourg, a prostitute in Paris, mistress of a medical student (from whom she might have acquired a rudimentary knowledge of medicine), and a singer and dancer in a popular music hall.[199] Among more conventional empirics, a typical case was that of the Hungarian Martin Bocot, who used a secret for ulcers and cancers (apparently a caustic) in the Loire, around 1819–1820. The son of a tradesman, Bocot served in the French army and then found work as a laborer at Roanne; later he was employed by a potter.[200]

A new pattern emerges: rather than a supplement to a primary source of income, empiricism might sometimes be a response to the loss of regular work. At Caylus, blindness forced a joiner to abandon his craft and make a living by bleeding patients, an operation that seemingly required less acute vision. At Vanves, an interdicted priest fell back on empiricism, telling his patients, "Do as I do, take medicine and drink snail syrup." One could even cite, at Montivilliers in the Seine-Inférieure, the case of an English prisoner of war under Napoleon who earned an income by practicing medicine and surgery.[201] A less obscure example is that of Laurent Mourguet, one of the celebrated *canuts* (silk weavers) of Lyons, who, when the depression in the silk industry forced him out of work during the Revolution, turned to tooth pulling and developed the enormously successful Guignol puppet show to draw a crowd.[202]

Many empirics, then, practiced medicine and surgery not because they were ambitious but because they were needy. The victims of economic dislocation, they had little to offer the market. Employment was unsteady, and to eke out their income they might turn to peddling; possibly to various forms of cottage industry, such as weaving; and finally to medical practice, which was perhaps the simplest recourse of all, though the return was highly uncertain.

Women

In any discussion of careers in medical empiricism, the role of women deserves special comment, not only because women contributed to popular health care but also because medicine afforded economic opportunities for them. The exclusion of women from professional medicine, and their entry into the field in the last decades of the nineteenth century, have been relatively well studied;[203] their earlier medical activities, except for midwifery, have received less attention. In general, the older works have focused on a small number of licensed "doctoresses" or perhaps on the witch-midwives celebrated by Michelet in *La Sorcière*, who (it is sometimes said) may have possessed valuable empirical lore lost to the male-dominated medical profession.[204] In fact there was a large middle ground, and the range of medical practice by women empirics largely resembled that of their male counterparts.[205]

Many women empirics practiced all branches of popular medicine and surgery, like the Thévenet woman in the Nièvre who bled and purged patients and set broken bones, acting (it was said) like "the boldest of men."[206] Some won reputations as skilled *uromantes*; at the end of the Old Regime, for example, a successful woman urinoscopist practiced in the Breton parish of Péaule (where her daughter performed phlebotomies).[207] Another *uromante*, at Durtal in Anjou, treated all medical and surgical conditions, visited patients, bled them, applied bandages, and sold drugs. The Société Royale's informant called her "*syrenne*," "*méges[s]e*," and "*coureuse*" (woman of loose morals). In one place, he said, she passed for a *magicienne*.[208] At the beginning of the Restoration, a woman urinoscopist sold drugs and practiced medicine at Seignelay in the Yonne; a Pole, she had married a native of the town, whom she had met in Russia (presumably during the Napoleonic wars).[209] Other women, like Barbe Richert, who was encountered earlier in this book, worked as somnambulists.[210] Some of these practitioners developed their own versions of physiology and pathology, like Marguerite Lany, an empiric who worked at Troyes toward the end of the Old Regime. In disease conditions, she argued, the liver became white; to make it "bright red" again, she bled the patient from the foot. She also used emetics and jalaps and sold drugs at prices ranging from 5 to 10 livres.[211]

Other women practiced as surgeons – a well-established usage, although after 1755 they were no longer legally entitled to do so, even if they were widows of surgeons.[212] The exception for widows was a widely accepted guild tradition, however, and it remained a conventional legitimating device for women empirics. (It may or may not have been true, for example, that *la dame* Collin-Chevrel, who sold the balm of life of the widow Lelièvre around Montauban in the late eighteenth century, had once been the wife of a surgeon, as she maintained;[213] but she undoubtedly believed that this claim would boost her sales and protect her against harassment.) Some practitioners simply called themselves *chirurgiennes*, like Lucie-Magdeleine Maitze, who also took the title of *officier de santé* (and wound up in the house of detention at Tours in September 1797).[214]

Among the women surgeons can be found all the traditional experts, including dentists and herniotomists.[215] In the early nineteenth century, the Norman Catherine Houssaye worked as an itinerant dentist, and a dentist's widow at Limoges named Delpeuth (or Delpeuch) carried on her husband's profession. Delpeuth dressed as a man, wore a false beard, and took to smoking a pipe, all, as she said, in order to "escape the males." (It was her trial for illegal practice that led the Cour de Cassation to decide in 1827 that dentistry was a free profession open to all, including women.)[216] Despite a widespread belief that bonesetting required great muscular strength and was unsuitable for women, the field also included successful *rhabilleuses*.[217] They may have won a clientele in part by charging lower fees than their male counterparts. The practitioner Jourdane from Séchilienne (near Vizille, in Dauphiné), who treated the nuns of the house of Prémol from 1693 to 1742, charged 12 sous for a visit; a surgeon-bonesetter summoned in 1742 and 1743 received 6 livres.[218] In some places, bonesetting by women appears to have been a well-established tradition. Two *rebouteuses* were reported in the Nantes region shortly after the promulgation of the legislation of Ventôse. The husband of one of them wrote to the prefect to defend her practice, explaining that she had been raised by an aunt skilled in bonesetting and had worked for fourteen years.[219] Perhaps in some families the art was transmitted in the female line.

Women sometimes worked in tandem with a male partner who was himself an irregular practitioner; if a couple split up, or the man died, the woman might carry on independently. At Chavagne in Brittany, for example, a butcher practiced medicine while his wife worked as an *accoucheuse*. Sometimes a father shared his methods with his daughter. In the Île de Bréhat, a certain Morice and his daughter formed a team;[220] and at Lagrand in Dauphiné, Magdeleine Barjavel carried on her father's work during the Revolution, using the operations and remedies he had passed on to her. Under the Consulate she won a certain notoriety when she attempted to cure a patient suffering from what sounds like a bipolar depression – "mellancholic vapors" that "sometimes resembled mania" – by having him immersed under a waterfall, where he unfortunately drowned.[221]

How many women empirics worked with male colleagues in France, and how many on their own, is a question that may never be answered satisfactorily in the absence of reliable censuses. (Where better lists were kept, as in parts of Switzerland in the latter eighteenth century, greater precision may be possible. At Lausanne, for example, a list of seven major empirics practicing in 1766 included four women, of whom three were widows.)[222] One is struck, however, by the names of widowed or unmarried women that are scattered throughout the French reports on illegal practice. Consider a few cases from the Loire-Inférieure in the early nineteenth century. The notorious *demoiselles* Mazureau made a comfortable living from medical practice in Nantes, though it involved them in some scrapes with the law: in 1829, for example, they were accused of killing the daughter of a local baker through injudicious use of violent purgatives.[223] A less prosperous empiric was the widow Bayard, who had been forced to sell remedies for fever to the inhabitants of the countryside since the death of her husband, a surgeon; her sister, the widow Ploteau, sold horse remedies and syrup of althaea. The widow Lancelotte, described earlier in this chapter, asked the prefect for permission to sell a remedy for rheumatism, claiming that two years earlier she had cured a woman who was unable to walk. She also administered remedies for cancers – provided, she said, that they had not become open wounds.[224]

Despite the occasional success story, women empirics were typically distinguished by their special economic vulnerability in an economy that offered the unattached woman only the most limited opportunities. Those who could write sometimes poured out their feelings of distress in letters to the authorities, hoping for official approval or perhaps for some sort of recompense for their services to the community.[225] One will have to speak for the rest: Madame Le Plénier, the self-proclaimed charitable healer encountered in Chapter 2, who sent a petition in bad French to Napoleon, invoking her services to the poor of her region and lamenting that she had lost her resources during the Revolution in the inflation of the *assignats* (the paper currency issued by the revolutionary government).

Votre majesté voudra bien permetre que je vous expeause le besoin des peauvres de la comune de bouchemenne et depiné [Bouchemaine and Épiné, Maine-et-Loire], que jay soin depuis pres de 40 an ayant perdu ma petite fortune en papié monaye, je ne puis plue leur rendre les mêmes service dans leurs maladies. il menque des bouïllon de pin blanc de vin et des remede il implore votre Secour pour leurs besoins pressant, j'ay eu l'honneur d'en prevenir Monsieur le prefete il à eu la bonté d'en charger notere mère [i.e. maire]. . . . *je nay d'autre bien que mon etat de chirurgie, pour les peauvres, et rien de fixe* [italics added].

Madame Le Plénier, who seems to have ministered to most of her patients' medical needs, had found a position on the fringes of the system of charitable relief, of which she herself was a beneficiary.[226]

Medicine could indeed be a precious resource in the economy of makeshifts. Future studies of women and medicine might give more attention to the social significance of medicine as an economic activity, and less perhaps to the now familiar story of their suppression at the hands of a male-dominated profession or the problematic notion that *guérisseuses* possessed valid healing secrets unknown to the doctors.

Empirics and their patients

Medical practice obviously implied not only an economic transaction but also a healer–patient relationship. The same sorts of questions asked earlier about physicians and their clientele apply to empirics as well, though the answers are far more elusive. Who consulted them and why? If they did not simply fill gaps where no physicians were available, what was the basis for their success? One facile response, much favored by commentators of the eighteenth and nineteenth centuries, was that uneducated people were excessively foolish, and that many suffering or moribund patients were desperate enough to try anything at least once. This observation was sometimes true, but not always; not all patients were so obtuse, or so willing to clutch at straws, or uneducated, for that matter.

Social explanations of popular resistance to official medicine have stressed the profession's high fees and its distance from the popular classes, especially the peasantry. Empirics' fees, however, were sometimes equal to or greater than those of physicians, and yet at least some patients paid them willingly. As for social status, the evidence is inconsistent. Some empirics do appear to have succeeded because they had (or adopted) the manners of the people. The bonesetter of Le Val-d'Ajol who flourished in revolutionary Paris, for example, was said (by his critics in the profession) to owe his following in part to his style: he said *"tu"* to everyone, swore, abused people in word and gesture, "and has long adopted in his conduct the principle of equality among men."[227] Other empirics, however, sought to awe their prospective clients by taking noble titles, wearing official-looking decorations (ribbons, crosses, medals), and displaying as much finery as possible – an approach that, for obvious reasons, was particularly characteristic of itinerants traveling far from their place of origin.[228]

Nor did empirics necessarily dissociate themselves from the medical profession and official medicine, though they might boast of being able to cure cases abandoned as hopeless by the physicians and surgeons. As has been seen, some called themselves physicians; at Vendôme, one empiric, the executioner, actually took the name of a local member of the profession.[229] Others adopted different but equally imposing titles, like Capelle de Vermant, who advertised himself in the *Affiches chartraines* in 1788 as a *physicien-botaniste*, boasting of credentials as a demonstrator (assistant) in a course on urines at Paris and Versailles and as "the author [sic] of a collection of 1,200 plants."[230] Many invoked supposed endorsements from members of the profession, or perhaps some past association with an official practitioner. Not only surgeons' widows but other relatives might capitalize on their connection and dabble in medicine, like *la demoiselle* Pépin, sister of a master surgeon in Poitou, who undertook to treat epilepsy, lachrymal fistulas, whitlow, furuncles, cancers, and skin disorders (1775).[231] Joseph Novarrino, a cooper who practiced medicine in the Hautes-Alpes, cited an uncle in Italy who was a physician.[232] Still other empirics claimed to have acquired a smattering of medicine from a more casual contact with a regular practitioner. In mid-nineteenth-century Brittany, for example, a man who regularly applied unguents to patients' sores and tumors said that he had acquired these remedies and others for whitlow, scabies, dartre, and specks on the eye in 1817 from a physician of Tours; the medical man had been treating him, he said, for a discharge of bile that occurred while he was in the rhetoric class of the *collège* at Vannes.[233]

One also hears (less frequently) of practitioners who had been endorsed or trained by established empirics. Such training did in fact take place. At the end of the eighteenth century, for example, in the Yonne, the widow of Étienne Hersin was dispatched by her curé and a member of the local nobility to study at Noyers with a man who treated tinea.[234] But this was not a clear alternative form of legitimation, any more than empirics were the product of a coherent radical counterculture hostile to doctors.

The main source of the empiric's appeal lay elsewhere, in experience and successful outcomes. Testimonials from satisfied customers filled flyers, newspaper publicity, and even the occasional medical books published by empirics, like the *Traité de médecine pratique*, which Larréa, curé of Varaignes, brought out in 1822. Though the authenticity of such endorsements may be doubted, their concrete specificity appears to have impressed the public. What is more, they cannot have been entirely fabricated; very similar endorsements appear in more trustworthy sources, such as the legal depositions drawn up to be used in trials for illegal practice or, better yet, transcripts of viva voce testimony. In the case of the German empiric Michel, for example, who was arrested at Saint-Malo in 1782, an illiterate woman dictated a statement saying that she

attests, certifies, and would repeat under oath, that about six weeks ago I developed a cancer on the upper lip whose root extended as far as the forehead and other parts of the face; [and] that having consulted several surgeons, they could not identify the disease. Having learned that *sieur* Michel, held in the prison, had cured several persons, using secrets, I obtained permission to go see him and begged him to take me on, which he did, using his internal and external remedies. He cured me perfectly and radically, in witness whereof I have delivered the present [document] to him ... [signed with a cross].[235]

Here are all the conventional elements of the testimonial: the surgeons failed; the patient begged the practitioner to provide his services; he succumbed to her entreaties and worked a cure. (The motif of the empiric who persists in practicing while in jail recurs frequently.) Or consider the testimony offered when the empiric Lacombe was tried in the Var in 1813. Five witnesses appeared, each of whom was paid 4 francs to give evidence. Four of the five statements were, in effect, endorsements.

1. A thirty-two-year-old woman was cured of "pleuripneumonia" and charged 24 livres; friends had urged Lacombe to help her.
2. A sixty-one-year-old widow was treated for a "torn" arm and leg; she paid Lacombe 100 francs – a modest sum, she said, considering the aid he had provided.
3. A tenant farmer testified that Lacombe had cured his wife for a modest payment.
4. A linen weaver received Lacombe's services for the "slim salary" of 24 livres.

The one unfavorable outcome was not particularly damning. A farmer testified that he had met Lacombe at an inn and brought him to see his wife, who had been sick for several years; Lacombe gave her a spoonful of liqueur and received 15 francs for remedies and medical services. The woman died a few days later. The husband gave no indication that the remedy might have poisoned her, and Lacombe could still have argued that a more extensive course of treatment would have have saved her life.[236] Testimony on the witness stand could also pay tribute to an empiric's special skills. One witness in the case of "Dame Blanche," for example, affirmed that she was good at treating *les nerfs tressaillis* ("dislocated" ligaments) and that she had arranged the ligaments in the shoulder of a patient at Bas-Meudon; indeed, she was "very clever" when it came to dislocated ligaments.[237]

Certificates of endorsement and trial testimony suggest a high level of satisfaction among at least some patients – perhaps enough to keep an empiric in business through word of mouth alone. These results are not surprising, given the placebo effect and the tendency of most illnesses to improve even without treatment. But it is important to add that not all patients were satisfied, despite what courtroom depositions might suggest. As physicians were quick to point out, clients whose expectations had not been met, or who had actually been injured, may have hesitated to disclose their gullibility in public; perhaps for similar reasons, relatives of patients who had died, despite or even because of taking empirics' remedies, rarely appeared as witnesses. Some disappointed patients did speak out, though, and they were inclined, like their happier counterparts, to judge the treatment simply by the outcome. One such client, the comte de Saint-Léger, who had been treated with smoke for deafness, complained to to the Société Royale de Médecine and asked to get some of his money back; the smoke, he said, had made him ill and "turned me into a very smelly caporal." In the case of Dame Blanche, a certain Balin recounted that he had suffered from a pain in his leg, which she unsuccessfully attempted to heal by tying a blue ribbon around it. Another witness, a woman, told of the treatment of one of her eyes, which had been "as red as a Siamese blouse." Dame Blanche told her, "I am going to cure you; give me your baptismal and family names; I will glue them in the chimney, and in nine days, after a novena, you will have good news to tell me." Eight days later the eye was even redder, and the patient had to go to "an *oculisse* [sic] to get my poor eye back."[238] A sufficient number of such accounts could dim an empiric's prestige, though he usually retained a number of true believers, however much evidence accumulated against him.

More generally, it is a mistake to suppose that empirics were universally revered among the populace. The line between the marvelous and the ridiculous was easily crossed; the less skillful charlatans could become the butt of public mockery, as happened at a festival in the Haute-Vienne in the early nineteenth century, where an empiric hawking a universal elixir lost his audience to a group of young *collégiens*, who put on a rival show with bread pills and packets of hay.[239] Skepticism also appeared in popular humor, which was particularly rich in anecdotes on urine casting. The practice of transporting the patient's water to the *uromante* opened up the possibility of witting and unwitting substitutions, with all the attendant *quiproquos*. The servant, for example, who accidentally spills the contents of a flask and unthinkingly replaces them with cow urine is told that his mistress eats too much grass.

The certificates of endorsement and trial testimony also provide some clues to the social composition of the empiric's clientele. Olivier, a spurious *officier de santé* at Nantes, produced certificates from the daughter of a sabot maker; a tobacconist; a cabaret keeper; a domestic servant; a miller; a rentier; a property owner; a flour merchant; the daughter of a woman innkeeper; the wife of a weaver; and a seamstress.[240] In the Aube, the empiric Blanc treated a winegrower-wet cooper and several women identified by their husbands' occupations: the wife of the mayor of Colombé-le-Sec and the wives of a weaver, two winegrowers, a herdsman, and a farmer.[241] The patients were drawn mainly, but not exclusively, from a milieu of artisans and small tradespeople.

This sort of material can be supplemented by the occasional report or denunciation that includes information on an empiric's clients. One communication to the Société Royale, for example, enumerated the "victims" of one of two prominent empirics (both "self-styled apothecaries") at Saint-Paul-Trois-Châteaux in Dauphiné. The list, which covered a period of three or four years in a town of some 2,000 inhabitants, named 26 individuals. (Fifteen of them were said to have died, including five who summoned a physician after being treated by the empiric.) Among the patients were the wives of four agricultural workers; the wives of two joiners; the wives of a procureur, a mason, an innkeeper, a miller, a wool carder, a shoemaker, and an otherwise unidentified artisan; another woman; "a respectable lady who was weak enough to listen to *les bonnes femmes*"; two children of agricultural workers, the child of a farmer (*laboureur*), and the child of an innkeeper; three agricultural workers, a skate maker, an innkeeper, an abbé, and a man for whom no occupation is given. Among the adults, women outnumbered men by about two to one; the crafts and agriculture predominate among the occupations of the patients or their husbands, though we must not forget the procureur, the abbé, and the respectable lady.[242]

It should indeed be emphasized that empirics did not find their patients solely among the poor, the uneducated, and those of low social status. In early modern Europe, empirics and *maiges* were routinely summoned to the bedsides of the great when the doctors had failed. A letter by the physician Gui Patin on Richelieu's death describes how, on the fourth day

of the cardinal's illness, his retainers, "despairing of the physicians," brought
to him a woman who made him swallow horse dung in white wine, and
three hours later an empiric who gave him a laudanum pill. Louis XIV, in
his last illness, was treated by a "Provençal yokel" with a remedy for
gangrene, and more than a half century later the owners of a supposed cure
for smallpox were summoned to treat the dying Louis XV.[243] Even for
more trivial ills, a fashionable charlatan like Cagliostro could draw an
equally fashionable clientele, and patients from all social backgrounds consulted more modest healers, like the old woman who, according to Casanova's highly colored account of his childhood, cured him of nosebleed in
Murano.[244] In more recent times, unqualified practitioners continued to find
patients among social groups that (in the physicians' view) should long ago
have been weaned away from them. In the early nineteenth century, the
prefect of the Deux-Sèvres noted that a *rebouteur* was sometimes consulted
by "educated persons" in the countryside, having demonstrated his superiority over surgeons.[245] This reputation for empirical skill is understandable
enough, but even more mystical healers retained some of their appeal. The
author of a nineteenth-century essay on vulgar errors in medicine cited a
magistrate cured by a *devin de village* (village cunning man), an outcome he
attributed to the patient's strong confidence in the practitioner.[246] Weber's
Entzauberung der Welt was incomplete, even for the bourgeoisie.

Though anecdote could be piled on anecdote, it is difficult to say with
any certainty how widespread such behavior was among educated people,
or even whether, as is sometimes suggested or implied, the patients were
mainly women and children. Clearly, it required a high tolerance for cognitive dissonance and, in some cases, the will to resist the deeply rooted
skepticism of relatives and friends. In 1775, for example, a woman suffering
from a presumably chronic chest disease decided, against her father's will,
to follow an elaborate and expensive course of treatment recommended by
the wife of a Paris bourgeois. It required eight bottles of a secret drink,
two and a quarter bottles of syrup, a jelly, and a pomade for the chest, at
a total cost of 790 livres.[247] And in 1785, the son of a Languedocian nobleman
sought treatment from a merchant's widow who possessed a secret remedy;
when the father, the marquis Delort, asked her to reveal its composition
to a qualified physician, she refused. The son nevertheless sent his valet to
obtain the remedy, after the woman had declined to come to him, because
(it was said) she could not make herself clear in French; in the end he took
it without his parents' consent.[248]

No doubt desperation accounts for at least some of this behavior. But
patients of whatever class who consulted empirics were not trying literally
anything; they placed their confidence in practitioners who had been recommended as sometimes offering hope when others had failed.

Sedentary practitioners who were known "to do good" could engender powerful loyalties, often enough to interfere seriously with the prosecution of illegal practice. Patients sometimes refused to testify against respected empirics, or even paid their fines after they had been convicted. According to an account in the *Gazette des tribunaux*, the empiric Auda appeared at his trial in 1827 surrounded by his "dupes," who called him their "liberator."[249] The healer sometimes figured in popular mythology as a folk hero, whose special powers or success in medicine allowed him to defy or win over the authorities. Père Proust, convicted of illegal practice in Baugé, was said to have escaped from prison through magic.[250] And a widely known story in the Hautes-Alpes related how the immensely popular curé of Sigoyer dealt with a gendarme sent to arrest him: he diagnosed a worm in the man's gut, hung the patient upside-down from a hook above a bowl of warm milk, and seized the worm when it attempted to drink the milk. So triumphed popular medicine; the good curé, it was said, was never molested again.[251] It is not surprising that in such cases an empiric's prestige could eclipse that of the official personnel.

5

Folk healers: *maiges* and witches

In his celebrated medical handbook, *L'Avis au peuple sur sa santé*, the eighteenth-century Swiss physician Samuel-Auguste-André-David Tissot distinguished between ambulatory charlatans and "*maîges*," or "spurious village doctors, both male and female."[1] "*Maige*" (also spelled *meige* and *mége* or *mège*) is related to "*mire*," an old word for a physician; Littré defines it as "[the] name given in several provinces and in Switzerland to medicasters."[2] In dialect, the related verb "*mégir*" means to heal or cure (by magical means). "I m'a mégi mon charbon" signifies "he cured my carbuncle."[3] In the eighteenth century, the term had greater currency than it does today, and although its meaning was somewhat elastic, it usually had a more precise sense than "medicaster." As the quotation from Tissot suggests, it generally referred to sedentary local healers, especially in the countryside. This usage appears, for example, in a report to the recently chartered Société Royale de Médecine from a physician of Caylus in Quercy, a region of southwestern France: "It is not so much empirics, charlatans and vendors of mithridatum [a traditional antidotal compound] who, in passing through, most greatly ravage this region, but rather the *maiges*, that is, peasants who do not know how to read or write, who set themselves up as physicians." Beginning with the veterinary art, these peasants progressed to human medicine, but they persisted in seeing all illness as *le mauvais mal* or *louvet* – a tumor-producing disease of livestock, resembling anthrax. (The three most prominent *maiges*, though, sound like typical empirics: a farmer and innkeeper who administered "incendiary remedies"; a former joiner who bled more than 500 patients; and another healer who "practiced the same trade.")[4] At the beginning of the nineteenth century, in an "Observation . . . on the practice of charlatans and *maÿges*," an *officier de santé* in the Hautes-Alpes set up the same dichotomy and presented similar views on the relative dangerousness of the two types of practitioner.[5]

"*Maige*" could also convey a still narrower meaning. The physician Jean-Emmanuel Gilibert, for example, in his treatise on "medical anarchy," spoke of peasant practitioners who exploited popular superstition, claiming that they had learned nothing from their fellow men, that their talents came directly from God, and, more specifically, that their cures were due to a special divine "gift." Their hold over the population seemed to Gilibert to be proportional to their distance from the city. Within 1 league from town, three sorts of practitioners competed: *le grand médecin*, the medical doctor; the "simple physician," or surgeon; and "the physician of God," or *maige*. At 2 leagues or more, the physician was unknown, and the *maige* increasingly displaced the surgeon.[6] Gilibert seems to have lumped together all unauthorized practitioners in the countryside, but his discussion adumbrates a useful conceptual category; it is possible to distinguish a group of mostly small-time, rural practitioners, who did not ape the physicians but instead based their practice on popular beliefs ("superstitions" or "errors," as the men of the Enlightenment almost invariably called them) shared by their peasant neighbors.

THE FOLK PRACTITIONER: CONCEPTS AND APPROACHES

The category and the term *"maige"* will be retained here, but they raise troubling questions of interpretation and method. Gilibert's physician of God represents but one stage in the long transformation of popular healers in the imagination of educated Europeans, from demonic agents to colorful folk characters. Whatever name we give them, we now almost unavoidably see such practitioners through the filter of successive layers of interpretation, particularly the conception of the typical folk healer developed in the late nineteenth and the twentieth centuries by several generations of ethnographers. To avoid misunderstanding, it may help to review the evolution of the concept, the main outlines of the ethnological model, and the special difficulties encountered by the historian who attempts to apply to the study of the past a modern interpretive schema that contemporary observers have developed on the basis of field work.

Folk healing in historical perspective

Long before the eighteenth century, the elites of western Europe had considered popular medical practice from two points of view. On the one hand, the mere fact of unauthorized practice violated the monopolies claimed by the medical corporations. In the Middle Ages, such cases were prosecuted by the Church, which had chartered the faculties and could excommunicate offenders. (Responsibility for trying empirics subsequently passed into the hands of the secular courts.)[7] On the other hand, certain forms of healing (many of which might not be taken seriously as unauthorized practice if they occurred outside a corporate seat) were believed to involve sacrilege or witchcraft. These cases came within the purview of either ecclesiastical or royal justice, until Colbert's edict of 1682 ended secular trials for witchcraft. In its sweeping attack on superstition, the Counter Reformation singled out several forms of popular healing that concerned the Church as the mere fact of unqualified practice did not. The secular arm, in its own campaigns against witchcraft, also sought out and punished certain forms of "superstitious" medical practice.[8]

In his major treatise on demonology and witchcraft, Pierre de Lancre, the councillor of the Parlement of Bordeaux charged by Henri IV with a special mission against witches in the Southwest, distinguished four types of healers whose work was independent of the art and science of medicine. Two were perfectly innocent. Some individuals, through special divine grace, truly enjoyed the gift of healing; others, distinguished by their extraordinary sanctity, might have an exceptional capacity to obtain the cure of disease through prayer. Very different were two other groups: impostors, who blasphemously feigned a divine healing gift; and magicians, enchanters, and witches, whose remedies, Lancre suggested, should be suspect to every good Christian. They used spells and incantations, rather than simple prayers, and their formulas were marked by "superstitions," such as numerological prescriptions: a ritual would have to be performed for a certain number of days, or so many tapers burned, or so many pater nosters said, or alms given to so many beggars. These charms did sometimes work or appear to work, but only through the power of the Devil.[9] (A similar belief in the demonic efficacy of medical superstitions can be seen in abbé Thiers's work on popular errors, published later in the seventeenth century; as a safeguard, he sometimes omitted part of a recipe or the name of the disease for which the remedy was used.)[10] Such an interpretation made little or no distinction between a magician and a witch in the narrower sense of a person who has entered into a compact with the Devil. It is not surprising that large numbers of healers were swept up in the early modern witchcraft prosecutions simply because they were said to have worked cures that they could not explain.[11]

It was a commonplace, then, of the literature on witchcraft to distinguish this large category of unauthorized practitioners from ordinary empirics who used drugs and surgery (and even from some who used methods that to us seem occult, such as astrology and alchemy, though the line between *magia naturalis*, or natural magic, and *goetia*, or necromancy, was difficult to draw). These healers were mainly, though not exclusively, peasants and rural artisans; the chief target of the campaign against medical superstition was popular culture in the countryside. A similar distinction appeared in sixteenth- and seventeenth-century treatises on the medical field – for example, in André Du Breil's *Police de l'art et science de médecine*, which ascribed many medical abuses to deficient faith in God.[12]

The Enlightenment inherited and retained these basic categories, though they now assumed a different form. The *philosophes* denied both the real efficacy of the demon and (usually) the special providence of God; they rejected the possibility of an inborn healing gift, whatever the source. Where the magistrates and theologians of the early seventeenth century had seen a variety of practices as evidence of either witchcraft or a saintly vocation, they saw tricksters who exploited "popular superstition." (They lacked, though, a single comprehensive term for the healers who worked in this tradition, using *"thaumaturge," "conjureur," "sorcier,"* and sometimes *"maige"* almost interchangeably.) Even more than their predecessors, they saw these practices as characteristic of the peasantry, particularly the peasantry of the most isolated and backward regions of France; pagan practices flourished among the *pagani*, the rustics.

The importance of popular medicine as a subject of study increased during the Romantic era, stimulated in part by physicians and administrators concerned about rural health care, in part by antiquarians who saw in popular practices the remnants of a distant pagan way of life – survivals, perhaps, of the Celts and Druidism. Treatises on rural medicine or vulgar medical errors (a popular subject for M.D. theses in the nineteenth century) reveal a marked fascination with *devins*, sorcerers, or magicians who "charmed" injuries, burns, and animal bites, purported to heal tumors by touch, prescribed such "ridiculous" remedies as making certain signs or gestures, burning old shoes, or sticking pins into a calf's heart, or specialized in "destroying the work of another magician."[13] By the standards of the present day, these works betray a lack of ethnographic consciousness. Like the *philosophes*, the nineteenth-century physicians tended to see the healers as unscrupulous frauds who preyed on their less clever peasant neighbors; they associated magic more with the gimmickry of charlatans, who gulled a credulous populace, than with a preexistent set of popular beliefs shared by healer and patient.[14] But they did see such practices as a distinctive cultural phenomenon, and its very otherness captivated them.

The ethnological model

In the last century, a vast literature has accumulated on "medical folklore" of all kinds, the work first of amateur and then of professional ethnographers.[15] Where earlier generations had studied "superstitions" or "antiquities," the new folklorists took a broad interest in traditional popular culture as it survived in peasant life. (The scholarly investigation of "urban folklore" has been a comparatively recent development.) From their work has emerged a rough and not entirely consistent notion of what in English is called a "folk healer." This expression has no precise equivalent in French; perhaps the commonest term is simply "*guérisseur*" (healer), although the same word can be applied to almost any unlicensed practitioner. A variety of other terms are in current use: "*panseur*" or "*panseur de secret,*" "*barreur*" (especially a healer of burns), "*toucheur*" (in the North), *brèish* in Occitanie. Dialectal variants are legion: "*peinsour*" (masculine) or "*peinserie*" (feminine) in the Confolentais, "*soinheur*" or "*garissoux*" in the Angoumois and Saintonge, "*persigneux*" in Berry, "*gogneux*" and "*charmeux*" in Morvan and the Nivernais, "*gougneurs*" or "*gougnoux*" in the Forez region. In the Basque-speaking region of the Southwest, magicians and healers possessing a special gift are called "*aztiak*"; particularly celebrated healers receive the title of "*yainko-ttipiak.*" Some of these terms denote special functions. A number are related to "*devin*" (diviner or soothsayer): "*endevinaire*" in Languedoc, for example. Healers through prayer take the name of "*pregandé*" or "*pregandare*" in the Béarnais, "*saludador*" or "*seynador*" in Roussillon. (In Spanish, "*saludador*" refers to one who salutes, or to a healer; "*salutación*" [salutation] can mean a Hail Mary, and the *saludador* is characteristically supposed to be able to heal through prayer alone.) In Corsica, healers known as "*signadori*" cure with signs or gestures. Experts in "disenchanting" the victims of witches are called (in standard French) "*désensorceleurs*" or "*leveurs de sorts.*"[16]

But whatever he (or she) is called, the healer of the folklore literature is a rural practitioner who is an established member of a village community and whose practice depends on a set of values and beliefs shared with that community.[17] He is to be distinguished from such modern bourgeois parallel practitioners as faith healers, magnetizers, and unlicensed homeopaths or osteopaths (though some peasant magnetizers and *radiesthésistes* do exist). Unlike them, and unlike the old itinerant charlatan, the healer is not an outsider, although he may sometimes be seen as different because of eccentric behavior or a physical abnormality. Unlike the empiric, he does not ask for a fee, although he accepts gifts (occasionally substantial ones) in money or kind.

The techniques of the characteristic folk healer further set his work apart from routine empiricism or domestic practice – from all the families with medical recipes, from the *bonnes femmes* who know a remedy or two for headache or fever. The healer's inherited formulas are quite literally secrets: he is pledged not to reveal them, and they may lose their efficacy if disclosed. His therapies, moreover, depend not only on simples and other "empirical" remedies from the vegetable, animal, and (sometimes) mineral kingdoms but also on rituals that mingle religion and magic – although these categories are not so sharply defined for him as they are for us. A healer typically requires that patients be baptized Christians. Catholic practitioners punctuate their incantations with signs of the cross; they recommend novenas and invoke healing saints. Protestants may use the Bible to arrive at a diagnosis and heal through prayer and laying on of hands.[18]

Other rituals depend on sympathetic magic or magical transfer. An object may be touched to the affected part and then discarded; as it decays, the disease will wither away. Or the disease may be passed on, through physical contact and magic formulas, to some other person, an animal, or an inanimate object. In some cases the healer may have to obtain a remedy through a special ordeal, imbuing very ordinary objects with the power to cure. Near Lyons, for example, the healer who wishes to treat warts may have to gather the wood of nine nonfruit trees in the same morning; in lower Brittany, until the end of the nineteenth century, he might attempt to cure eye disease by tracing the sign of the cross nine times on each lid, using each of nine grains of wheat begged from as many different houses. Even seemingly empirical remedies may depend for their effect on a special ritual. A *rebouteur* may mutter charms as he manipulates a patient's sprained ankle; herbs may have to be gathered on a special occasion, usually the eve of the feast of Saint John the Baptist (24 June); a water against warts may be prepared (as the old handbooks of domestic medicine recommended) by boiling red slugs with a little salt, but the *maige* may then throw the slugs into running water to help carry away the warts.[19]

At least some of these procedures are common knowledge in the countryside, but the true healer adds something more: his personal efficacy. Only he has *le don*, the gift, which is perhaps his crucial defining characteristic. A few empirics advertised that special powers inhered in their minds or bodies, but it was in folk medicine that the idea of the indwelling healing virtue flourished.

The healer's gift must be understood in its social context. Its exercise depends on the consensus of the community. The false healer runs the risk of public ridicule; the true healer is revered, and great healers of the past who worked miraculous cures were sometimes called "saint." The healer endowed with the gift, moreover, is obligated to heal others (for if he does not, according to one informant in the Cévennes, the gift will "avenge itself," making the healer or his family suffer). He must, as it were, make a gift of his person to the community, which is the prime beneficiary of his powers. Indeed, according to one study of folklore in Languedoc, the healer has no power to cure himself or members of his family.[20] And when the gift, in accordance with a widely established custom, is transmitted to a member of a younger generation, it cannot be passed to just anyone – unlike the formula of a proprietary remedy or knowledge of medical theory. It normally goes to another member of the community (though it may sometimes be transmitted to a passing stranger out of gratitude for a service rendered).

As the folklorists see it, these practices form part of a largely autonomous, if now rapidly dwindling, popular culture, which is rooted in a highly traditional agrarian society.[21] Not that a completely independent "folk culture" can be isolated, comparable to the indigenous cultures of, say, sub-Saharan Africa. In a classic study of peasant society and culture, the anthropologist Robert Redfield has argued that the world of the peasantry is a "part society," in which "there are long-established relations with an elite whose culture is that of the peasant carried to another level of development." So, too, peasant culture reflects both the "great tradition of the reflective few" and the "little tradition of the largely unreflective many."[22] Or, as Henri Mendras has put it, a peasant society enjoys only relative autonomy within a larger society; it is not itself a "global society."[23] These general observations apply specifically to the medical culture of the peasantry. Redfield cites the pervasive influence of the humoral pathology of Hippocrates and Galen, which he suggests may derive in turn from earlier, more primitive notions of physiology.[24] Some healers who use charms and incantations are literate and have drawn many of their formulas from published *grimoires* (magic books) like the *Grand Albert* and the *Petit Albert*, which came out of the learned print tradition. Nevertheless (according to the prevalent ethnological interpretation), the peasantry have incorporated such borrowings into a distinctive outlook and way of life radically different from those of the educated elites and incompatible with modern science.

Tied as it is to a preindustrial past, this rural popular culture maintains beliefs and usages centuries old. Some are more durable than others, and folk medicine more than most; in certain rural communities, folk healers may coexist with such symbols of modernity as television sets, farm machinery, and well-equipped hospitals.[25] But they have survived in the greatest numbers in the most rural, most isolated, and least modernized regions of France – the Armoricain Massif (which stretches from the Paris basin west into Brittany, up into Normandy, and down into the Vendean bocage), Rouergue, and the Basque country, or the economically stagnant regions of Berry recently studied by François Laplantine. Such backwaters are virtual ethnographic museums, preserving exceptionally high concentrations of both tangible and intangible artifacts from "the world we have lost," a world already vanishing as the folklore movement gathered momentum in the last decades of the nineteenth century; they suggest what life may have been like in the greater part of early modern France.

This ethnological model of contemporary folk medicine offers, by implication, a way of looking at the earlier history of popular practices. But one important difference of context must be stressed. It is understandable that the folklorists should have distinguished folk healers, the product of a traditional popular culture embedded in a local *Gemeinschaft*, or community (to borrow the classic terminology of the sociologist Ferdinand Tönnies);

modern-style healers, the product of mass culture and a national *Gesellschaft* (society); and professionals, the exponents of a scientific discipline (usually considered one among a variety of elite subcultures). In the eighteenth century, however, these distinctions were far less clear. Just how blurred the boundary was between regular and irregular practice has already been seen. It can be equally difficult to sort out folk healers and rural sedentary empirics. Marginal barber-surgeons, nonreceived surgical specialists, and urinoscopists who bled and purged their patients presumably do not count as folk healers (though some *rebouteurs* conceivably might). But what of the local herbalist or owner of a few special remedies, who were just as much integrated into their local communities as the most prestigious *devin-guérisseur*? Or the blacksmith who might be thought to enjoy certain special healing powers, as well as skill in pulling teeth and restoring dislocated joints? Then, too, some village healers seem quite mercenary, and some major charlatans used forms of conjuring, touching, and religious healing in the countryside or exploited beliefs in witchcraft. It is not surprising that the term *"maige"* should have covered a multitude of sins.

Still, no typology can describe all individuals; it is merely an analytic tool. Even for the eighteenth and early nineteenth centuries, it is useful to distinguish *maiges* in the narrower sense of the term: rural healers who were not primarily entrepreneurs; who resided in villages rather than bourgs; and who were recognized by their communities as specially gifted or versed in medicine in ways that doctors, nostrum peddlers, and ordinary urine scanners were not. Their expertise might include knowledge of the hidden properties of local flora and fauna, as well as more mysterious "secrets." Contemporaries recognized these practitioners as a special category and treated them differently from other medicasters. By and large they were not direct rivals of the professionals, though they might discourage patients from consulting them; insecure surgeons and *officiers de santé* had fewer motives to put them out of business than in the case of the major empirics. Since they were relatively obscure, the authorities typically ignored or over-looked them. Moreover, their practice did not often inflict direct harm on patients (though some of the plants they used contained potent toxins); the informants who denounced *maiges* as more dangerous than the charlatans had in mind sedentary empirics who relied on phlebotomy and drastic remedies and inevitably did more damage than the itinerants, because they were available year round. The healers' main offense, in the view of the profession, was to delay proper medical attention.

Folk medical practice as a historical problem

The present chapter, then, concerns this special group of rural practitioners. A separate section deals with the problem of witchcraft and *leveurs de sorts*, since it involves a discrete set of beliefs and practices extending beyond the medical field. But any attempt to study this group for the period before modern ethnography immediately encounters difficulties of another order. Although contemporary sources suggest that *maiges* abounded in the late eighteenth and early nineteenth centuries, they provide only sporadic glimpses of actual healers. Comments on popular medicine (as, for example, in the responses to the abbé Grégoire's questionnaire of 1790 on patois, or the investigation of popular usages conducted under the First Empire by the Académie Celtique) focus more on superstitious beliefs and practices than on healers; they usually refer to practitioners in general terms and very briefly – often, one suspects, because the informant knew of them only through rumor.[26] Almost no one systematically gathered information on them, as was done, after a fashion, for charlatans. Not surprisingly, *maiges* occupy a small place in the medical and police archives. Cases not involving dangerous drugs or significant sums of money were less likely than large-scale empiricism to draw attention from the authorities or the profession and thus leave a record for future historians. Those *maiges* who do appear often bear a family resemblance to the empirics who were under police surveillance as *mauvais sujets*, or who aroused the doctors' ire when they extracted exorbitant sums from their patients or crippled or killed them. Nowhere in the government archives can the researcher find documentation as rich as the minutes of the seventeenth-century witchcraft investigations. (No doubt some detailed descriptions of healers exist in the records of pastoral visits, which were not used for this study, but they would appear to be a low-density source.)[27]

In order to fill out our sketch of the *maiges*, it is therefore necessary to fall back on an approach much like the regressive method that Marc Bloch applied to French agrarian history,[28] and draw on the rich corpus of materials collected by the folklorists in the late nineteenth and twentieth centuries. Though unavoidable, this procedure entails some risks. It is obviously open, first of all, to the charge of ahistoricism – a criticism commonly leveled at the folklorists themselves, who have sometimes written as if traditional popular culture were an immobile block. Arnold Van Gennep, usually considered the founding father of modern French folklore studies, treated the period from the late Middle Ages to the present as a "temporal unity" and intermingled observations from recent fieldwork with material taken from printed sources centuries old (although at the same time he attached an exaggerated importance to specifying the locale where a belief or practice was recorded).[29] Marcelle Bouteiller, whose *Médecine populaire d'hier et d'aujourd'hui* at least attempts (as its title indicates) to talk about popular medicine as having a past and a present, has been chided for describing traditional practices as they survived in the nineteenth century without consulting sources from the Old Regime.[30] Clearly, it is dangerous to assume that folklore has existed since time immemorial. As the recent work of Emmanuel Le Roy Ladurie has shown in concrete detail, popular beliefs, customs, and stories are not outside history; folklore was in many ways profoundly transformed between the late Middle Ages and the nineteenth century.[31]

This study, though, reaches back only to the last decades of the Old Regime – not the late Middle Ages. Nor does it claim that even the late eighteenth century and the late nineteenth century can be considered as a single block; the significance of very similar practices may have been quite different in the two periods, if only because the context had changed. The peasant who consulted healers, empirics, and surgeons and very occasionally saw a *médecin des épidémies* is not the same as a peasant who consults physicians, sometimes uses a hospital, and very occasionally sees a healer. The argument here is simply that the elements of what the folklorists described as traditional popular healing had their counterparts a century or a century and a half earlier. Comparisons of the folklore corpus with, say, the early modern works on popular errors and superstitions show striking continuities, not just over generations but over centuries. François Lebrun, who carried out a brief comparison of Thiers and Van Gennep in an attempt to historicize the study of popular culture, was driven to conclude that "virtually all" the superstitions denounced by Thiers were widely attested in the nineteenth century and the first half of the twentieth.[32] This finding does not, of course, prove the converse – that virtually all the practices considered traditional by later observers had remote antecedents; but the continuities are great enough to justify using the more recent materials to flesh out the skeleton provided by earlier sources.

A second objection to the regressive approach calls attention to the limitations of the folklore corpus itself, which have been blamed on the collectors' lack of qualifications (many were enthusiastic but untrained amateurs), their biases, or their half-conscious presuppositions. Thus "folk healer" was a category created by the folklorists, who, like any researchers, tended to find what they were looking for. Not that folk healing is simply an artifact, but the folklorist may have given undue prominence to exotic-seeming beliefs and practices, and to those that supported the notion of the survival of an autonomous precapitalist way of life in the countryside.

No doubt the picture of the "folk" world has been overdrawn and overcolored; *guérisseurs* were probably more prosaic figures than some of the accounts in *Mélusine* or the *Revue des traditions populaires* would suggest, and during hard times some of them may have seen their work more as a source of much needed income than as a divine mission. But it is unlikely that the pioneer folklorists and ethnologists exaggerated the incidence of folk healing; careful recent field work suggests, if anything, that it is more widespread than has been commonly supposed.[33] It can be assumed that such practices were at least as prevalent in earlier periods, even if they usually went unnoticed or at least unreported by the medical profession and the authorities.

The discussion that follows begins, then, by sketching an overview of the *maiges*, relying heavily on the folklore literature. This general picture then provides a framework for examining and interpreting some of the fuller accounts of *maiges* and *maige*-like practitioners from the late eighteenth and early nineteenth centuries, and particularly the reports that give information (as published works on popular medicine rarely did) on the activities of specific individuals. The section on witchcraft follows a similar plan.

MAIGES

To understand the place of the *maige* in the medical network, it is important first of all to recognize that he or she was not a sort of unlettered family doctor offering routine medical care to the other inhabitants of the village. Families provided most of their own health care, with the help of neighbors; a patient would consult a *maige* for a specific problem, usually when home remedies had failed. Each healer was known to cure certain conditions. Some (like most empirics) treated a variety of conditions. A *panseur* living at Clémont in Sologne toward the end of the Old Regime claimed to be able to cure colics, bites, fever, pleurisy, and other disorders.[34] Often, however, the folk healer limited himself to a narrower specialty or even a single disease or disorder. The specialties of twentieth-century *panseurs de secret* near Châteauroux (Hautes-Alpes), for example, included chill, "fallen stomach," burns and sprains, warts, erysipelas, whitlow, nosebleed, bee stings and snake bite, and horse colic.[35] One nineteenth-century physician and student of medical folklore suggested that the peasants' distrust of the official practitioner was due in part to his not being a specialist.[36] This theme appeared explicitly in one of the *cahiers de doléances* of 1789, from Jagny (Paris-hors-les-murs), which complained that practitioners treated disorders they did not understand,

it being scarcely possible for a physician to be universal. It would be appropriate to establish a certain number for each kind of disease, who would have only a small number of diseases to study; they would become very adept at it. . . . So that afterwards one would be almost certain, whatever disease one might have, to be cured of it, unless Providence or other circumstances were adverse.[37]

In popular medicine the elaborate division of labor extended even to distinctions between human practitioners and healing saints, so that in lower Brittany, for example, furuncles were cured by a saint, whereas in Poitou they were the responsibility of *toucheurs*.[38]

Popular specialties embraced many disorders that were also in the domain of local empirics and surgical experts. Folk *rebouteurs,* who were often considered to enjoy the healing gift, treated sprains and dislocations.[39] Like the farrier Lasseneuve, cited in a 1779 report to the Société Royale de Médecine, they typically murmured a few charms over the injury.[40] In some regions, old women treated cataract; a child with an eye disorder might be taken to a sorcerer *qui lui dit la maille* (literally, who tells his leucoma [a dense white opacity in the cornea]).[41] Hernia, which empirics treated with surgical operations, bandages, or even herbs, might also be "healed" by women who danced around an oak, muttering prayers.[42] Similarly, toothache might be healed by a dentist such as Henri Blanchet (1823–1907) in Berry, who touched the ailing tooth with a nail, which he then drove into wood.[43] Poisonous bites, including the bites of mad dogs, were the province of various *guérisseurs de venin et de rage* (healers of venom and rabies). In a treatise on rabies, the physician Andry, a member of the Société Royale de Médecine, cited a report on a healer at Autignac in Languedoc, who made an incision in the victim's ear, expressed a few drops of blood, murmured some unintelligible words, and then dispatched the patient to bathe in the sea (thalassotherapy being an ancient remedy for rabies, together with omelettes containing powdered oyster shell).[44] *Saludadors* were also credited with the power to cure rabies, according to Pierre de Lancre (who cited Antonio de Torquemada as his authority).[45] Around the beginning of the present century, a woman in the commune of Chaumont-d'Anjou (Maine-et-Loire) specialized in the treatment of rabies. She possessed an old iron key – presumably a Saint Hubert's key – used in the healing rite; it had once belonged to two old noble families of the region.[46] Many other such specialties could be cited; there were even special *panseurs* for worms.[47]

Other popular specialists treated conditions that corresponded only loosely, if at all, to disorders in the official nosology. *Rebouteurs* might rehang a "fallen stomach" or treat a twisted liver, rotated kidneys, or forked lungs; special *accrocheurs de coeur* were supposed to be able to resuspend a heart that had been dislodged from its "hook" on the sternum.[48] *L'estomac ouvert* (dilation of the stomach) was treated in the early twentieth century at Villemoirieu (Isère) by an old woman who bound the abdomen and recited magic formulae.[49] For sunken ribs one might call in a skilled *frotteur,* or "rubber."[50] Other healers knew how to *accacher la mère* (restore an errant uterus), if necessary by kneeling on the patient. (Some *accacheurs* also treated more mundane complaints, such as colics.)[51] Similar practices were well attested in the eighteenth century; a correspondent of the Société Royale at Chambon-en-Combraille, for example, reported a carder with surgical pretensions who healed disturbances of the womb and spleen, restored the collapsed "fabric" of the abdomen, and so on.[52]

Other disorders from the popular nosology that might be treated by specialists included *le carreau* (an intestinal complaint – the word covers a number of conditions) and *la luette tombée* (literally, a fallen uvula, which was popularly believed to be responsible for sore throats and their complications). *Le carreau* was often treated with plasters. *La luette tombée* was in some places the province of specialists who treated it by pulling a certain hair from the top of the patient's head, but in some regions the baker passed a hot oven peel between the patient's legs. Cramp might also be healed by bleeding the patient under the tongue – another specialty; in Brittany, the *coupau de corde* treated quinsy by "cutting" an imaginary filament in the throat.[53] In Morvan, a vague condition called *"cautère"* or *"catère"* (dyspnea, with dryness of the mucoids, or convulsions in a child) was treated by a *diseur de cautère*, usually an old beggar.[54] In western France, *les hunes* or *les hules*, one of the most ill-defined of popular disorders (which Bouteiller identifies with rheumatism but which often sounds simply like nervous fatigue), was in the hands of specialists who observed the patient's tongue to confirm the diagnosis and then treated the condition with scarification and conjuration; a *coupeur de hunes* (*hunes* cutter) might make an incision on the palate of a child who was not talking, or the ham of a child who was not walking.[55] And in eighteenth-century Provence, a disease of neonates known as *les crinons* (comedones) or, in dialect, *ceès* (a corruption of the Provençal *ceddès*, or bristle) was treated by women who massaged the baby to "bring out" the illness. (The characteristic symptoms of the disease included itching, agitation, hoarseness or complete loss of the voice, and inability to suckle; if left untreated it might lead to diarrhea, convulsions, and wasting. Following successful treatment, the *crinons* "emerged" in the form of hairs, sometimes black and very stiff, sometimes fine and reddish, with a little ball at the end.)[56]

Other healers exploited the popular belief that disease might be caused by animals that invaded the body – not microbes or even worms, but a creature that one could hold in one's hand. In the early nineteenth century, for example, a shepherd at Saint-Aubin in the Eure was said to have received 200 francs for extracting a beast from the stomach of an epileptic farmer, using drugs and spells. He instructed the patient to have novenas said and to go to a certain wood during the celebration of the Mass. If at that time he heard an animal's cry, he was cured; if not, he would have to start over again.[57] (Some folklorists would argue, though, that neither this particular healing role nor the substantial fee was sanctioned by popular tradition, and that the shepherd is better seen as an enterprising rural empiric.)

Some specialists, finally, provided certain ritual services associated in popular tradition with the care of invalids or with childbirth. In regions where parturient mothers were expected to engage in sexual intercourse immediately after the first labor pains, a specialist sometimes took the place of the husband; one such practitioner was still active in a mountain village of the Cévennes in 1925. After the delivery, a *tétaïre* ("suckler") might help stimulate lactation, taking the place of the infant.[58]

The question of therapeutic methods cannot be considered here in any detail, but it should be noted that each specialty had its particular procedures; indeed the technique often defined the specialty. Whereas some healers were in effect possessors of secret remedies or were learned in local botanical lore,[59] others used magical techniques to expel or arrest the malady: spells and incantations; signs and gestures; the laying on of hands. Commentators referred to users of magical healing formulae as *"rebouteurs mystiques"* and sometimes *"charmeurs,"* although the word was not in general use.[60] (In Alsace, the word *"schormer"* – probably a cognate of *"charmeur"* – was applied to Jewish healers, consulted by Jews and Gentiles alike, who used charms to treat sprains and eye disorders.)[61] Other healers relied on gestures, like the *signeuses* of the nineteenth-century Hautes-Alpes, who divined from seeds cast on water the number and nature of a patient's fractures and then "operated" using signs of the cross.[62]

Still other practitioners were best known for their healing touch (though, like the rest, they typically combined several techniques). In popular usage they were generally called *"toucheurs"* (Brittany, Norman bocage, Poitou, Cévennes, and elsewhere); by extension the term often became a loose synonym for "healer." *Toucheurs* were supposed to conjure away sprains, burns, wounds, sores, ulcers, and other external disorders.[63] Some concentrated on the treatment of warts, which occupied a prominent place in folk medicine.[64] Others took on abscesses, so-called scrofula (strictly, tuberculosis of the lymph nodes, especially in the neck, but in popular parlance the equivalent of "swollen glands"), and throat disorders.[65] Normally the *toucheur* passed his hands over the affected part. One occasional healer (more empiric than *maige*), a joiner who practiced at Paris for more than twenty years at the end of the eighteenth century, cured toothache by touching the patient's hand.[66] A number of healers touched with the big toe or tongue, rather than the hand; one specialist in throat disorders used his foot, which between treatments he kept wrapped in a badger skin, presumably to contain and preserve its marvelous curative powers.[67] Others interposed an object between their body and the patient; one practitioner in Poitou used a branch.[68] Unlike *toucheurs*, *souffleurs* did not rely on direct contact, but used their breath to treat eye disorders and sometimes other conditions as well. In eighteenth-century Roussillon, the *saludadors de santa Quiteria* (so called after a saint invoked in southern France and northern Spain against the bite of a mad dog) used insufflation to treat rabies. In the twentieth century, a healer of the Baugé region, a deaf old man, was said to cure with his glance alone.[69] In all of these cases the power of curing was thought to reside in the healer; he or she expressed it through direct or indirect contact with the patient.

A very different role was played by specialists who acted as intermediaries in religious healing and were known by various regional names – "*croyants*" and "*croyantes*" in the Angoumois, for example, and "*récoumandeuso*" and "*récoumandèries*" in the Confolentais. A diviner might identify the saint to whom a patient could pray for relief (by observing, for example, whether a bit of fabric, straw, or charcoal floated or sank in a basin of water) – a practice known as "*le tirage des saints*" in French ("*viré lou devars*" in the Confolentais).[70] In Laplantine's experience (mainly in Berry), this ritual is always performed by old women.[71] A *voyageuse* (or, sometimes, *voyageur*) not only diagnosed *le mal de saint* (the saint's illness) but also undertook the necessary pilgrimage as a proxy for the patient. Travelers often exacted a substantial charge for this service, and among them can be found some of the occasional practitioners encountered in the previous chapter, who relied on their medical work as a supplementary resource; in the middle of the nineteenth century, for example, a farrier and his wife charged 30 to 50 francs for making pilgrimages to the chapel of Sainte-Suzanne-du-Désert in the middle of the forest of Breteuil.[72]

The popular version of medical specialization, then, contrasts strikingly to the professional specialties. The healer had a secret or a gift for treating a condition or several not necessarily related conditions. His field was not a branch of some more general medical art, nor did he necessarily claim any particular understanding of a body part or bodily function. In many cases (though not all), the specialty was so narrowly defined that it left the healer completely unprepared to help victims of other diseases. At the beginning of the present century, for example, Linières-Bouton (Maine-et-Loire) had a healer for colic (an old woman who was said to have empowered her hands to cure by suffocating a toad while still young enough to be nursing from a bottle) and others for snakebite, dartre, and burns.[73] Modern folklore studies have even described a system of regional specialization, possibly the result of an uneven decline in the old network. On the *causse* (plateau) of Blandas, in the Gard, there was no healer for intestinal worms or liver attacks; hence it was necessary to travel to Peyregrosse, Le Mazel, and the area around Alès. At Saint-Ambroix a *bonne femme* healed simple cases of *les estouris* (jaundice) with a little sac of red cloth containing a nut, to be worn on the stomach for nine days and then burned; but for serious cases it was necessary to travel to a neighboring region.[74]

Nor could these specialties be considered occupations in themselves, even if the work provided some income in money or goods. Any one village had only so many cases of *carreau*; only a few practitioners had far-reaching reputations. Most of the time the healers were engaged in something else

– usually agriculture, a craft, or domestic work. Medicine was, at most, a sideline.

The gift and how to get it

The healer's therapeutic efficacy in his specialty was believed to depend on the possession of secrets (recipes, charms, knowledge of unusual plants, and so on), a personal gift, or both. In Languedoc, one says of such healers *"sap fa"* (*il sait faire*; he knows how to go about it).[75] It was the acquisition of such a privilege that determined the healer's vocation; one did not decide to become a healer and then cast about for a suitable specialty.

Secrets were not invented; they had to be bestowed by someone who already possessed them. According to a widespread belief, the owner was obligated to disclose them to someone before dying; failure to do so meant that he would suffer a protracted final agony. Secrets might be traded among *guérisseurs*, or occasionally transmitted to a stranger, but typically they stayed within the family; healing became a hereditary vocation. In the early nineteenth century, for example, one family in the Haute-Vienne had a long-established reputation for preventing rabies with a special stone (caustic potash, most likely), which they touched to the wounds of people bitten by mad dogs.[76] A twentieth-century unlicensed practitioner, who won a fashionable Paris clientele and whose publications have probably made him the best-known *guérisseur* in France, recalls that a familial tradition had made his forebears healers in the Gers for generations.[77] Secrets might be transmitted to the eldest child, or from father to son and mother to daughter (though sometimes to alternate genders).[78] The secrets of *rebouteurs* usually stayed in the male line; it was widely believed that the father could reveal them only on his deathbed.[79] Some healers wrote their formulas down in little notebooks, which they bequeathed to their successor; these *carnets* could not be used by just anyone.[80] The transmission of secrets involved more than imparting knowledge. It was an initiation, often marked by a little ritual, sealed by a kiss or a handshake; the neophyte swore to observe certain rules and maintain the tradition of which he was now a part. (In some places, social conventions dictated the terms of the ceremony; in contemporary Corsica, the ritual takes place at midnight on Christmas eve, often in a specially laid out magic square.)[81] The initiate in effect joined a confraternity.

In popular belief the most powerful healers were not simply initiates; they possessed an immanent healing virtue – *le sang fort* ("strong blood"), *le regard perçant* (a piercing glance), *la main heureuse* (a lucky hand).[82] (They might also enjoy other special powers. Some were thought able to foresee the future; *saludadors* and certain other healers were believed to be invulnerable to fire.)[83] In the extreme case, the healer himself was the remedy.

In seventeenth-century France, a young girl with jaundice might have been told to drink the urine of a *magicienne*; this procedure follows from the old homeopathic principle of *similia similibus curantur*, or like cures like, but the urine is also the vehicle of the healer's personal power. Magical healing or effective action of a counterspell may depend on the personal strength (*sang fort*) of the agent who undertakes the cure. Marc Leproux cites a twentieth-century case (1945) in which a healer found that he could not cure a patient who had a "stronger" temperament.[84] In the course of therapy, the malady may pass through (*traverser*) the healer, who displays every sign of great effort and even suffering and emerges exhausted from his ordeal. When he succeeds, the event confirms his powers and enhances his local prestige, which refers to his person rather than his remedies.

Typically the healer had the power, or simply the talent or knack, to cure a certain disease or diseases; this inherent virtue was known as "*le don*" (the gift) in French and by various names in dialect (e.g., "*poder*" [power] in Provençal and Languedocian).[85] In some cases the gift simply enhanced an empirical skill or a medical secret; a family, for example, might have a talent for setting fractures, like the eponymous Bailleul dynasty in the seventeenth century.[86] One such case from the end of the Restoration involved a former *maige* turned active empiric. Ignace Auda, a Piedmontese farmer who practiced medicine for two months at Toulon, said that his family had a gift from God, passed on from father to son. His secret for headaches was to apply a 5-franc piece to the patient (three pieces, if necessary); he also claimed to be able to cure the blind.[87] Certain therapies were believed not to work at all unless the healer possessed the necessary gift; this was particularly true of conjuration and healing by touch.

How was the gift acquired? Hereditary transmission since time immemorial was a common explanation, though it was thought that God might originally have conferred the power on a particular ancestor. Often the gift accompanied a healing secret when it was passed on to the next generation, but some families were believed to have the ability, as members of their "race," to cure certain diseases.[88] A Provençal gardener cited by abbé Thiers as healing corns on the foot through his touch said that his family and a few others in the province enjoyed this privilege.[89] Certain families with the gift were thought to belong to the lines of saints – Martin for healers of epilepsy, Catherine, Mark, Paul, and Roch for healers of various disorders. As was seen in Chapter 4, descendants of Saint Hubert were said to enjoy the power to cure rabies; in the Montois region of Champagne, healers of burns were considered descendants of Saint Catherine (although she was supposed to have died a virgin); and in Normandy, specialized healers of *le carreau* claimed descent from Saint Martin.[90] Other healers belonged to noble lineages. The house of Coutance in the Vendômois was said to be able to cure *le carreau* by touch; the eldest sons of the house of the baron d'Aumont, comté de Châteauroux, were reputed to have the power to cure scrofula not with their touch but with consecrated bread.[91] Ernest Renan, in his memoirs, recalled his mother's story of an impoverished member of another noble line, Kermelle, who supported himself as a flax grinder:

It was believed that as head [of his family] he was the depositary of the force of his blood, that he possessed to an eminent degree the gifts of his race, and that he could, with his saliva and touch, raise [a patient's strength] when it was weakened. People believed that in order to perform cures of this sort, it was necessary to have an enormous number of quarters of nobility, and that he alone had them. His house was surrounded, on certain days, by people who had come from twenty leagues around. When a child was walking late and had weak legs, it was brought to him. He dipped his finger in his saliva [and] traced unctions on the small of the child's back, which was thereby strengthened. He did all this seriously, and with gravity.

The nobles of the town mocked him for it.[92] The healing gift of the kings of France is a related phenomenon, though among all the members of his dynasty, only the anointed monarch, from the moment of his sacring, was thought to enjoy the power of the royal touch.[93]

Some gifts, however, were not hereditary. The date and circumstances of a child's birth, for example, might confer healing powers on it for life. A good healer should be born on Good Friday, according to testimony offered in witchcraft trials at the end of the sixteenth century.[94] In Flanders, abbé Thiers reported, children born on Good Friday were supposed to be able to cure tertian and quartan fevers and other diseases;[95] in Normandy, at the beginning of the twentieth century, they were said to have the power to cure twenty-two diseases by touch.[96] Other birthdates also conferred *le don*. In Brittany, a healer could cure burns if born on 31 December, the feast of Saint Sylvester, who, according to the *Golden Legend*, had sealed the mouth of a dragon breathing flames. Operators born on that day or on the feast of Saint Matthew (21 September) could touch for venomous bites. So could healers born on 25 January, the date of the conversion of Saint Paul, for Paul had then become immune to the bites of snakes and spiders.[97] Those born on 24 June, the feast of Saint John the Baptist, had various powers according to different regional traditions. In Roussillon they and persons born on Christmas were marked with a little cross on the palate and might become *saludadors*.[98]

A widespread popular belief concerned the privilege conferred by order of birth. Exceptional healing powers inhered in a fifth, seventh, or ninth son (especially in an uninterrupted succession of sons), generally known as a *"marcou"* (*"setou"* in Gascony, *"seté"* in Roussillon, in the case of the seventh-born).[99] The *marcou* was most closely associated with the treatment of scrofula; indeed, the word almost surely derives from the name of the minor saint invoked to heal the disease, Saint Marcoul, whose feast is

observed on the first of May. (The saint's medical specialty probably originated, like that of many healing saints, in a pun: *mar* = *mauvais* = bad;
coul = *cou* = neck.) As Marc Bloch has shown in his history of the royal
touch, popular beliefs and practices involving the three healers for scrofula
– Marcoul, the king, and seventh sons – have become curiously tangled.[100]
The monarchs, whose power to cure "the king's evil" was originally un-
connected to Marcoul, touched patients after the coronation ceremony,
during a pilgrimage to the saint's tomb at Corbeny, about 25 kilometers
northwest of Reims. Moreover, some patients believed that the saint was
the ultimate source of the healing power, and that a novena at his tomb
was still necessary even after contact with the king. (The independent prestige of the royal touch died hard, though, despite the mixed results of
Charles X's revival of the custom in 1825; when Louis-Napolean Bonaparte
made an official visit to Sologne as President of the Republic in April 1852,
some peasants saw in him a healer for scrofula.)[101] As for the *marcous*, they
often invoked the saint and played a special role in religious observances.
Nérée, a nineteenth-century *marcou* in the hamlet of Vovettes, near Theuville
(Eure-et-Loir), prayed with his patients before a statue of Saint Marcoul
and had them join his confraternity at Saint-Pierre of Chartres and pledge
themselves to a lifelong regimen whose conditions included eating no heads
of animals or fish.[102] But *marcous* were associated with the monarchy as
well. Like many born healers, they were believed to bear on their persons
a special stigma (just as healers of the race of Saint Catherine were marked
with a Catherine wheel – a sign from the Devil, according to Torquemada,
that they deserved to be broken on the wheel – and those of the race of
Saint Paul with a serpent); in the case of the *marcou*, it was often a fleur-
de-lys, and ambitious parents sometimes named a seventh son Louis for
good measure.[103]

The old works on vulgar errors stipulated certain conditions (usually
some form of asceticism) that the *marcou* had to observe if he were to realize
his inborn powers. Laurent Joubert says that according to popular belief he
must remain a virgin;[104] Thiers specifies that he must be born of a legitimate
marriage and must fast for three to nine days before touching the patients.[105]
Modern folklorists have reported other restrictions. At Riaillé in the Loire-
Atlantique, for example, it was said that a seventh son could cure scrofula
only on Good Friday and during the Quatre Temps (ember days, the
Wednesday, Friday, and Saturday of the first week of each season, set aside
for fasting and prayer).[106]

Though scrofula was the great specialty of the seventh son, his powers
were not always confined to it. In Poitou, the *touchou* (*toucheur*), who was
supposed to be a seventh son, could cure thrush, skin diseases, tumors, and
rheumatism.[107] Other diseases treated by *marcous* included malaria and hy-
pertrophy of the spleen (in the Landes).[108] In the Côtes-du-Nord, the *marcou*
(in this case a seventh child preceded by six siblings of the opposite sex)

was believed to have the power to cure madness by using the magic procedure of counting backwards.[109] And the *saludadors* who treated rabies in Roussillon and Catalonia were supposed to be *setés*, seventh sons; as has been seen, however, they were devoted to Saint Quiteria rather than Marcoul.[110]

Less common than the belief in the seventh son, but well attested since the seventeenth century, is the power attributed to the fifth, seventh, or ninth daughter to heal scrofula and other diseases.[111] According to Thiers, the seventh daughter has the privilege of curing chilblain on the heel.[112] Charles Perrault (of Mother Goose fame) mentions the belief that she can cure tinea, and an anonymous manuscript compendium from the late seventeenth or early eighteenth century notes that any seventh-born daughter "helps childbirth wonderfully, it is said."[113] In Sologne, according to a modern folklore study, the youngest of seven daughters was a somnambulist – a nineteenth-century graft onto an older stock.[114]

The healing power of the seventh-born has been one of the most widely diffused popular medical beliefs in Europe and America – although the association with scrofula has been prevalent only in England and France, the two countries with the tradition of the royal touch. Marc Bloch suggests that the tradition may have originated in the early modern period, owing perhaps to the diffusion of popular books on magic and numerology.[115] Whether (as seems likely) it derived in this way from the print culture or belongs to an older oral tradition not reported in the documents that Bloch examined, it is undoubtedly misleading to label it simply a "folk" belief. In the seventeenth and eighteenth centuries, empirics seeking to legitimate their medical practice sometimes called themselves seventh sons or daughters.[116] In the nineteenth century, the tradition appears to have declined, except in the countryside; there, however, it took firm hold and has persisted into recent times. In 1959, for example, at Saint-Viâtre (Loir-et-Cher), a twelve-year-old *marcou* was said to have healed a six-month-old baby by laying on of hands.[117]

The posthumous child might also enjoy a reputation as a local *guéritout* – for *carreau*; *longs-coeurs* (described as a sort of abscess with a purplish-blue color); goiter; *vertaupe* (furuncle), *verteau* (in lower Brittany, a boil on the neck), and "scrofula"; and wens (a privilege shared with the executioner freshly returned from dispatching a victim, according to Thiers).[118] Marcelle Bouteiller suggests a possible interpretation: the healing power thus transferred is a kind of mystical compensation for secrets that the father might otherwise have taught the child. Perhaps for a related reason, the mother of twins – neither of whom could inherit a gift through primogeniture – acquired the privilege of healing (sprains, bruises, and wens).[119]

Even the accidents of childbirth could yield a healing gift. A breech-birth baby acquired the power to cure sprains or, according to one report, the deformities of rickets (Plougastel-Daoulas, Finistère).[120] When an infant was born *"coiffé"* or with a caul (that is, with the amniotic sac over the head and shoulders), magical powers were thought to reside in the child and the caul itself.[121]

An alternative source of curative power might be the healer's principal occupation, especially if it involved "handling an axe." Loggers, *flotteurs* (raftsmen who guided floated timber), and, above all, carpenters could cure diseases such as *le carreau*. The carpenters' power was said to come from Joseph, their patron saint; it was also said that the man whose trade it was to cut wood could "cut" diseases.[122] In Morvan, the carpenter had to be the son of another carpenter; in Brittany, a carpenter descended from another carpenter could heal *chaple* (meaning variously an abscess, swollen lymph nodes in the neck or groin, and a painful condition of the tendons known in nineteenth-century standard French as *"l'aï,"* a word said to be derived onomatopoetically from the sound of the patient's screams).[123] The tools of the trade played an essential role in the healing ritual. In the mid-nineteenth century, a carpenter at Gallardon (Eure-et-Loir) worked cures with the "wind" of his axe; at Raon (Vosges), the axe was used to cut a cross of straws placed over a *fourchotte* (a painful phlegmon on the hand).[124] Elsewhere, carpenters were believed able to cure carbuncle or induce an abortion by making signs of the cross with the same instrument; a tumor could be healed by feigning to strike it.[125] When apprentices were taught how to use the tools of carpentry, they often learned how to apply them in healing.[126]

Millers, too, were commonly believed to enjoy *le don* as successors of their patron, Saint Martin. They could cure *enchappes* (adenitis, abscesses, or "humors") with simulated blows from the hammer used to dress the millstone (*le marteau à chapeler*).[127] One nineteenth-century collection of magical medical formulae says that to cure *enchappe* (here used to mean rheumatism), a miller who is the son and grandson (or daughter and granddaughter) of millers must strike three blows with a mill hammer near the patient and say a pater noster.[128] A work on popular errors of the same period says that millers were believed to cure quinsy by scraping the windpipe with a brush inpregnated with river water.[129] In some cases the miller's mysterious prestige overlapped that of the conjurors; one magic healer in twentieth-century Brittany went by the name of Meilla Ru (*le meunier rouge*, or red miller).[130]

We have already seen that blacksmiths and farriers played a major role as local empirics; many were believed to enjoy *le don*, associated in part with the patronage of Saint Éloi, and perhaps also with the magic of fire.[131] In the Corrèze, *metzes* had the power to cure stomach disorders by "ham-

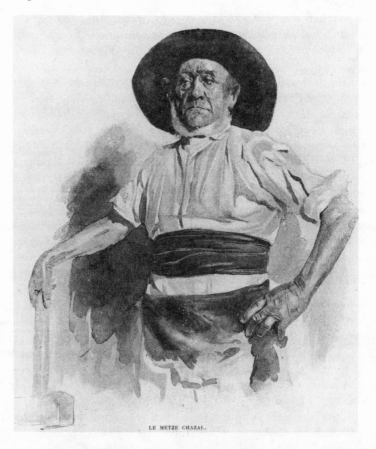

LE METZE CHAZAL.

The *metze* Chazal: a romantic vision of a blacksmith-healer from the classic era of the French folklorists. (From E. Vuillier, "Chez les magiciens et sorciers de la Corrèze," *Le Tour du monde* [1899]; photograph courtesy of the Musée National des Arts et Traditions Populaires, © Musées Nationaux.)

mering the spleen" if they were the son and grandson of a blacksmith.[132] The technique usually combined feigned blows to the abdomen with real, resounding blows to the anvil.

Members of other occupations who used magical healing techniques, notably shepherds, were sometimes believed to possess the gift.[133] The executioner, even if he did not enjoy a permanent gift, was magically endowed when returning from an execution.[134] The weaver, who made shrouds, was another traditional healer whose prowess putatively derived from his *métier*.[135] A form of gift was of course attributed to members of religious orders; *convers* (lay brothers and sisters) were often believed to have special healing powers, as was the secular clergy.[136]

Though such healers were typically established members of a local community, mysterious and even sinister powers were sometimes attributed to groups whose work kept them on the margins of rural communities (seasonal workers, loggers, wood splitters) and to wanderers (tramps, gypsies). Bouteiller cites the case (from about 1850) of a farmer of Déols (Indre) cured of an open sore on his arm by a vagrant to whom he had given alms.[137]

In other cases the gift derived from neither birth nor occupation, but was believed to have been divinely conferred. A work on vulgar errors written in the last decade of the Old Regime mentions an illiterate peasant healer near Versailles who became a physician the day of his first communion, which he took "much later than one usually does," the author noted, "because of his imbecility."[138] (The idiot favored with the healing gift also illustrates the widely attested association between abnormality and supernatural powers.) Often the healer had received a reward for a signal act of piety. According to a legend of Limousin, for example, one family acquired the gift of healing as *rebouteurs* in 1793, when an ancestor put together a mutilated effigy of Christ that he had found in a field.[139] Similarly, a *rebouteuse* in Berry said that her gift derived from that of an ancestor who had received it from God during the revolutionary Terror, when he restored a cross knocked down by a storm.[140] At Nasbinals in the nineteenth-century Lozère, a road mender named Pierre Brioude, known as Pierrounel, reassembled a broken crucifix that he noticed while watching sheep; as a result, it was said, his fingers received the healing gift.[141] Another *rebouteur*, Michel Waris, known as "Père Joyeux," who worked during the first half of the century at Berig, 55 kilometers southwest of Metz, supposedly received his *don* directly from the Virgin after he had restored a crucifix and saved a Marian image.[142]

One might also attempt to acquire the healing gift without divine intervention through a magic ritual. Almost invariably, this called for manipulating a special plant or animal. The would-be healer might cut a cross on the first day of May in the bark of an apple tree that had never borne fruit. Passing his thumb and index finger into the incision, he would say, "Tree, give me the power to cure every witlow, fever, and every disease that I touch." The power that flowed from the tree was supposed to retain its force for a lifetime.[143] In the bocage, he might go on the morning of the feast of Saint John the Baptist to find a certain cotton-like excrescence that appears on the dog rose and crush the "worm" that it contains between thumb and index finger. These two digits would then have the power, for a year, of curing ailing teeth.[144] A related belief required the healer to crush the larva found in fuller's teasel.[145]

The source of the gift was often an animal with an ancient place in pagan medical lore. A healer, it was believed, could empower his hand to cure by placing it in the mouth of a she-wolf not yet fed meat; or a newborn baby might be made a universal healer by passing its left arm into a wolf's mouth.[146] The more specific gift of conjuring viper venom might be acquired by staring at the first viper met during the year and saying "*le bel oiseau, qu'il est beau*" (how beautiful is the beautiful bird).[147] A more common procedure was to strangle a certain animal – a snake, a toad, or (most often) a mole. In France the belief rested in part on the linguistic association between the word for mole, "*taupe*," and the popular word for furuncle, "*vertaupe*." The future operator had to suffocate one or more moles under specified conditions. The mole must be enclosed in a small linen sac or in the child's swaddling clothes; or the child must crush it "before the age of understanding," before weaning, before eating soup with grease, or before losing his virginity. In Berry, the technique was said to work only for *laboureux* who were sons of *laboureux* (usually the third generation). One version required the child to strangle seven moles and eat their grease; in Maine a young man – who had to be a virgin – took a live mole, opened its belly, and immersed his finger for one night. In addition to furuncles, the diseases that *vertaupiers* were supposed to cure, according to various accounts, included adenitis, "scrofula," cancer, erysipelas, and even colic in horses.[148]

A form of healing gift might also be acquired incidentally – not by following a prescribed ritual, but in the course of some other activity. Bouteiller cites, for example, the powers attributed to the women who kept vigil over the dead.[149]

Finally, the healing gift could be obtained through voluntary transmission – as opposed to automatic inheritance from an ancestor, through the blood. In the Ariège, the populace attributed a *rebouteur*'s gift to a favor conferred by the Russians who arrived in 1814; and a farmer, Laurent Odouard, known as "Père Saint-Sabin" (1815–1886), was said to have received the power to heal from a priest whom his family had sheltered during the Revolution and who said, when leaving, "I cannot do anything to thank you, but I leave the gift I have to this child in the cradle."[150] A healer in the early nineteenth century had the power from his forest warden, who had himself inherited it from his father and grandfather. As the servant lay apparently dying, the master asked for the gift and received it; when the man recovered, he found that he could not get it back again.[151] This form of gift could inhere in only one person and usually had to be transmitted according to set rules – normally to a younger person, if possible to a member of the family.[152]

Although the acquired healing gift would seem in principle to be open to anyone, in practice it was limited to those who could play a defined role in the village community and whose prestige could be reinforced by com-

Table 4. *Types of practitioners*

	Source of legitimation	Mode of healing
Physician	Official approbation	Medical art
Empiric	Experience, results	Secret
Maige	Gift	Personal power

mon approval. Some empirics boasted of having indwelling healing powers, but we are not likely to run across itinerants who had, say, strangled moles and eaten their grease when they were children. Moreover, some sources suggest that the gift could be deliberately acquired only in exceptional cases, and that even then the curative power might be only temporary.[153]

Table 4 indicates in highly simplified form some distinctions between the types of practitioners considered so far.

The social position of the healer

Information on the various techniques employed by *maiges* is relatively plentiful; it is far harder to write a social history of their practice, especially for the period before the late nineteenth century. What, for example, was the density of folk healers in the old medical network? Of all the categories of practitioners considered in this study, this one is the most refractory to quantitative analysis, for obvious reasons. Contemporary observers often said that each village had at least one *maige*; during the Restoration, one treatise on popular medicine suggested that each canton had its "miracle worker," especially for rabies.[154] These estimates (if they can even be called that) are vague, and we have no way to test them, though it does seem safe to assume that nearly every inhabitant of rural France in the Old Regime had access to a folk healer. Modern ethnographic studies, some of which give lists of known healers by village of residence, show that the services of *guérisseurs* remained widely accessible in twentieth-century rural France.[155] Some particularly prestigious healers acquired reputations extending well beyond their own villages. In Morvan, for example, at the end of the nineteenth century, a *gougneux* drew clients from as far as 40 or 50 kilometers around Saint-Honoré.[156]

In this population of healers, what was the place of women, *les bonnes femmes guérisseuses*, who figure so prominently in the conventional image of popular healing? Here again, no objective assessment is possible for the period prior to the modern folklore studies. The *maigesse*, however, clearly fascinated physicians and others who wrote on medical "superstitions";

they almost invariably mentioned women as one important category of peasant practitioners.[157] Twentieth-century field work suggests that the actual proportion of women healers varies considerably from region to region. A 1961 investigation of Angevin healers revealed that almost three-quarters were men. But Adelin Moulis's study of the Ariège found that most magicians and healers were women.[158] Studies of other regions show widely divergent ratios of women to men: 1:2 in Aubrac; 3:2 in the canton of Huriel (Bourbonnais); 3:1 in Corsica; about 1:1 in Berry.[159] Certainly the world of popular healing was not exclusively the province of women; the evidence for the earlier period suggests that many of the more prestigious healers were men. But without better data, it is impossible to be more precise.

What was the healer's place in the community? The historical evidence is fragmentary. If we turn for assistance to ethnological studies of contemporary France, we encounter a paradox: the healer is both an active member of the community and perhaps set a bit apart from it.[160] (But he is *not*, François Laplantine insists, a psychopath or a deviant, except perhaps in the eyes of the professionals.)[161] Healers are often marked as different. In Forez, for example, they are commonly *bichounis* (old bachelors); as an emblem of their practice (and their oddness), they nail crows or owls to their door.[162] In a study comparing the *panseur à secret* and the shaman, Marcelle Bouteiller notes the simultaneous "attraction and repulsion" of the healer. Yet the healer is generally recognized as contributing to an essential function, which he shares with the local saints and perhaps with the curé: he helps protect the welfare of the village, its households, livestock, and harvests. His role is cemented by what Bouteiller calls a "double contract" with society and the supernatural. In her model, the *conjureur* must be a Christian and can heal only Christians and animals belonging to them. The morality of the client must complement the personal asceticism and morality of the healer if the medical ritual is to work.[163]

The folklorists and ethnographers stress that folk healers have no *esprit de lucre* (greed for profit); their relationship to the community is not the relationship of an occupation to the market.[164] At most, Marcelle Bouteiller explains, the healer will accept a gift as an expression of gratitude, rather than as compensation for a service performed.[165] Charlatans who ask for payment, especially when they resort to publicity and self-promotion, are seen as city people and as inauthentic healers; theirs is not the true vocation. Healing typically appears as an act of Christian charity. A highly successful practitioner at Vialas in the Cévennes, according to an account of 1904, always refused payment, saying that "the good Lord will pay for all that."[166] The principle of charitable healing is taught, in less conventional form, in a curious prayer formula for erysipelas from nineteenth-century Flanders; it says that the Virgin Mary asked Saint Rose how much she owed her for curing *la rose* (erysipelas), to which the saint replied: "That must be in honor of Christ and out of fraternal charity."[167]

Healing, then, would not normally be a primary source of income. How did healers make a living? Concrete information on their occupations in the earlier periods is extremely thin, despite the occasional references to the special role of carpenters, farriers, and, above all, shepherds. Modern ethnographic studies, despite their emphasis on these privileged callings, suggest that many, perhaps most, healers worked the land, like most of their patients. A survey conducted in Anjou in 1961 confirmed that healing was usually a secondary activity (the number of *guérisseurs installés* was small) and involved predominantly *cultivateurs* (about 60 percent of the practitioners). Some 7 percent were gelders and only about 9 percent artisans – in obvious contrast to the estimates suggested for empirics in Chapter 4.[168] One would expect that the majority of healers in the Old Regime were peasants, but again, the hard data are lacking.

Who consulted folk healers, and what did patients and their fellow villagers think of them? Once more, there is little direct evidence; even modern field work may be suspect, because informants usually hesitate to show sympathy for a form of medical practice that is technically illegal and is also reproved as backward. The ethnographers suggest that the healers once were almost universally accepted and widely used among the peasantry, even those who were not practicing Catholics. Certainly the most successful developed an extraordinary bond with their patients, as can be seen in the latter's loyal adherence to healers unlucky enough to be prosecuted for illegal medical practice. One indirect indication of acceptance: popular humor and proverbs do not poke fun at healers as they do at doctors and, occasionally, quacks. An argument *ex silentio* seems justified. Acceptance, though, does not necessarily extend to deep conviction; no doubt many who turned to healers had in mind the old peasant platitude: "if it doesn't do any good, at least it doesn't do any harm."

Studies of twentieth-century *panseurs* suggest that the peasants who make up the great bulk of their practice include both the poor and the comfortably off, and that the most respected among them attract patients from a variety of social classes.[169] Specific evidence for earlier periods is very scarce. But the existence of rural nobles claiming a healing gift points to the pervasiveness of the folk medical belief system. Moreover, as writers on vulgar errors repeatedly indicated, many educated people, even in towns, gave credence to medical superstitions. In the mid-eighteenth century, a notary at Arreau in the Pyrenees had a formula against worms that called for writing a Latin charm around a basin, saying the Lord's Prayer and Hail Mary three times, pouring in water (some of which was used to erase the inscription), and giving it to the patient to drink.[170] In 1794, a justice of the peace in

Poitou took his child to bathe in the sea after it had been bitten by a mad dog.[171] Many other such cases could be cited. They mostly involve the use of personal recipe collections and other forms of self-help. Although they bespeak an outlook that might have made patients receptive to the work of *panseurs*, they do not prove that the rural elites actually consulted them.

Indeed, one senses at times that when the notables had their own magical remedies, they did not feel it necessary to turn to a peasant *maige* unless he was reputed to have extraordinary powers. Consider the case of the lord of the manor of Granchamp in Maine at the end of the Old Regime, who was in the habit of treating not only his own dependents but also patients sent to him by the curés of the surrounding communities, who had great confidence in his abilities. In June 1777, the curé of Moncé-en-Saosnois wrote to him concerning his nephew, apparently a victim of epilepsy:

Monsieur, concerning the remedies which you were good enough to prescribe for my nephew: he began by taking the cold baths for two weeks, in the evening and morning. I waited until the moment when his attack occurred yesterday to have him take [the remedy made from] the shirt he had worn continuously for a month, burned [and mixed] in wine.... I ask you, Monsieur, to indicate whether it is appropriate to have the frogs applied to him immediately, and to be kind enough to tell me for how many days, the quantity, the places where they should be applied, and the length of time they should be there.[172]

This procedure of course involves a medical secret, rather than a personal healing gift or power. (Nor does it make use of prayer or of magico-religious formulas.) The curé did not consider it superstitious. And yet it clearly offered a mysterious and conceivably powerful alternative to the phlebotomies and clysters of the physicians, much like what a *maige* might have furnished.

In the end, the ethnologists might insist that social or economic status mattered less than participation in a cultural system that included the local patois, the religious and agricultural cycles, various other festivities, rites, and rituals, and much more besides. According to this view, the relationship between healer and patient must be seen as part of a whole, not simply as a class-specific form of medical practice or a manifestation of a prescientific world view.

Maiges: the record before the folklore movement

With the ethnological model in mind, let us return to the late eighteenth and early nineteenth centuries. What can we learn about actual *maiges* from contemporary observers?

The sources, it must be stressed once more, are very sparse. Occasional references do appear to types of practitioners or specific individuals who are recognizable folk healers. One correspondent of the Société Royale de Médecine at Sauvé-en-Cévennes complained of peasants with hereditary secrets who were *rhabilleurs* of dislocated stomachs or *coupeurs de la ratte* (*rate*, or spleen).[173] In late-eighteenth-century Brittany, a weaver named Jean Fouquet, called Le Breton, a native of the parish of Lécousse near Fougères, claimed to be a seventh son with the power to cure scrofula; he was said to have a mark on his chin shaped like a fleur-de-lys. As payment he accepted stockings, shoes, and shirts.[174] In the nineteenth-century Marne, a farmer at Coligny was a "visionary" healer (according to the contemporary description) who purportedly worked cures with magic words; he never asked for a fee and accepted gifts only with difficulty.[175]

The ethnologically inclined historian seizes on these examples, thinking (as a colleague once put it), "*Voilà un vrai!*" But these are at best isolated instances of what presumably was an extremely common phenomenon. The more systematic surveys, which were of some value in studying empirics, generally ignored them. *Maiges* are almost entirely absent from the Bas-Rhin survey. In the Comité de Salubrité investigation, only a handful of respondents mentioned practitioners who might be classed as *maiges*. A letter from Ploërmel (Morbihan) noted that few parishes did not have a "thaumaturge, urinoscopist, *rebouteur*, witch, etc." Dourdan (Seine-et-Oise) mentioned urinoscopists and scrofula surgeons (possibly *marcous*; more likely operators who lanced boils); the report from Ustaritz (Basses-Pyrénées) complained of spiritual and magical medicine. The response from Cognac (Charente) provided somewhat more detail. In addition to *rebouteurs*, the department had certain *gens à secret*, specialists who treated the conditions popularly known as "*chaple*" and "*vertaupe.*" A correspondent at Saint-Sever (Landes) noted the activities of shepherds who came "down from the mountains." Finally, at Hyères in the Var, the physician Bataillez wrote that although charlatans were not a source of concern, since the people were learning to distrust them, *gens à secret*, especially those who passed for witches, were nonetheless a problem.[176]

A few documents give substantially more information. Three will be examined here: an exceptionally full account of the activities of one *maige*-like practitioner, a *devin* of Guyenne; a list of unauthorized practitioners in a district of the Mediterranean coast near the Spanish border, which gives unusual prominence to *maige*-like healers; and a detailed account, by a careful observer, of the work of one type of healer, the specialist for *les hunes*, in the region around Dol (Ille-et-Vilaine).

1. The *devin* was named Louis Cugnat; we learn of his practice from a report by his parish priest, Father Vacle, curé of the church of Notre-Dame at Bazas, a small town a little more than 10 kilometers south of the Garonne River. Vacle forwarded his observations to the Société Royale de Médecine

in the hope that the Society might use its connections with the government to have Cugnat expelled from his parish, after his own efforts to dislodge him had failed.[177] The curé appears to have had little contact with Cugnat; he and his *vicaire* recorded the testimony of their parishioners, including several of the *devin*'s patients (though part of it was simply hearsay). Vacle was understandably hostile to Cugnat, especially since the *devin* seemingly wished to usurp some of his own functions in the community. He appears, though, to have set down a literal record of what he learned, even when, as in the case of an obscene charm, the words embarrassed or offended him, "my duty being to report with greatest fidelity what was said to me." The curé would have made a good inquisitor.

Clearly, Cugnat was no modest *panseur*; he was a panacean healer, exploiting a mixture of magico-religious and empirical remedies. If he was supposed to have a specialty or a healing gift, the curé was unaware of it, though Cugnat does seem to have had a reputation as a witch; Vacle believed, without being absolutely sure, that Cugnat claimed to be able to make a person sick simply by touching him. And unlike the stereotypical folk healer, Cugnat accepted substantial gifts and at least in some cases charged money fees.

The curé's first witness, a landowner named Bisme, reported that a *laboureur* had given three hogsheads of wine to Cugnat to cure his mentally disturbed son, who after a long treatment was more insane than before. Jean Case, a tailor suffering from an unspecified ailment in his arm, testified that he had consulted Cugnat, who applied herbs to his arm. When he returned to discuss the progress of his case with Cugnat, the *devin*, as the tailor was talking to him, read in a parchment-covered book that was "small, like an almanac," at the same time making several signs of the cross; he promised Case a complete cure. He then asked the tailor to accompany him to Lignan, a village about 5 kilometers from Bazas, where he treated a child, reading in the same book and crossing himself. Cugnat had another patient, Jean Ferrand the elder, swallow three little pills wrapped in paper. Catherine Cabanes, wife of Michel Lagroua, testified that Cugnat had "written the name" of her son Jean and had wanted him to take herbs for an unspecified disease; the child, however, refused. Anne Guerre, wife of Jean Espargnet, testified that she saw Cugnat write on little pieces of paper, which he then rolled in his hands, wet in holy water blessed on Easter day, and gave to patients to swallow. Jean Mansecal, a parishioner of the chapel of ease of Tontolon, said that Cugnat had attended him for a throat disease, once with his "wife" and once alone. The healer rubbed the affected area, said some unintelligible words, made signs of the cross, held a little book, and finally asked for the sum of 6 livres, 15 sous, which Mansecal paid immediately. On another occasion, Cugnat, returning from Le Nizan (again a village about 5 kilometers from Bazas), where he had gone to see a patient, entered the residence of the sacristan of Tontolon, whose daughter was ill, and said that he wished to cure her. In this case he offered pills, which he said she should take for the three following days. The wife of Montpierre, whose older son walked in his sleep, turned to Cugnat only after having first consulted the curé. Vacle told her that the child was a somnambulist, urged her to wake him in the future if he started talking in his sleep, and recommended fastening all doors and windows; if she took this precaution, he added in jest, her son would not be able to attend the sabbath any more. The priest's facetious allusion to the witches' sabbath only heightened the mother's anxiety; disappointed by his refusal to offer more potent countermeasures, she resorted to the *devin*, who did not fail her. Cugnat provided an amulet, a little sac for the boy to wear on his chest, and it seemed to work to her satisfaction. The irritated priest opened the sac and found half a sheet of paper on which had been written the opening lines of the Gospel according to John in Latin; there followed a cross and then some "barbarous" words, concluding with the formula, "I exorcise and conjure you in the name of the Father, the Son, and the Holy Ghost." (Jeanne Noguée the elder testified that Cugnat had had her write out the biblical passage two or three times, without telling her what he planned to do with the copies.) The Montpierre woman seems to have become a firm believer in Cugnat's powers and even a sort of agent.

Cugnat's woman companion, Marianne, appears to have practiced both in collaboration with him and on her own. Cécile Audignan testified that Montpierre's wife had sent Bisme's daughter to invite her to visit, and that when she arrived the Montpierre woman informed her that Marianne would cure her eye disorder. Marianne told her to wash her eyes nine times each evening with Easter holy water and the crumb (*mie*) from a loaf of bread, saying each time a Hail Mary and another prayer; for good measure, she was to say the words "devil's shit" three times a day for a week. According to Bisme's wife, Marianne also spread allegations of witchcraft, saying that if one met such-and-such a woman or girl, it was necessary to say *"et verbum caro"* (and the Word [has become] flesh) as a preservative.

In the course of their medical activities, Cugnat and his consort delivered a populist message openly hostile to the professional elites. Not only did he discourage his patients from seeing physicians; he was also said to boast that he had as much power as the priests, and that he could remove a disease from any patient and give it to any of the gentlemen of Bazas that he wished. Marianne had been heard to say in the presence of Lasserre, the farrier, that she did not give a damn about the *messieurs* of Bazas and about the curé. Nevertheless, the couple coveted the clergy's sacerdotal instruments and emblems. Cugnat, with Montpierre, asked the sacristan to lend him his ritual book, which he agreed to do, thinking it was for a sick parishioner; and Montpierre's wife, presumably acting as an intermediary, told the sacristan's wife that she would like to ask one day for the loan of a stole (though in this case she met with a refusal).

By the standards of the folklorists, Cugnat should perhaps not be counted as a true healer. For one thing, he was not a native of Bazas; rumor had it that he and his companion had been expelled from Casteljaloux, which is more than 25 kilometers away. He never became an established, integral part of the community. The town appeared divided on his case. Bisme seemingly turned against him after a much-hoped-for cure failed to materialize, whereas the Montpierre woman became a virtual accomplice. Moreover, Cugnat traveled about, like many empirics; he used a variety of remedies to treat a variety of diseases; and he accepted fees as well as gifts (indeed, he seems to have had no other source of income). Perhaps, then, he should be seen as a minor entrepreneur cynically exploiting popular beliefs. One last feature of this case deserves to be stressed: the overlapping powers attributed to the healer, the *désensorceleur*, and the witch.

2. The list of unauthorized practitioners was prepared in 1811 by Ramonet, an *officier de santé* at Elne, a small town in the old province of Roussillon (now in the Pyrénées-Orientales), about midway between Perpignan and the Spanish border, and a few miles from the sea.[178] Ramonet identified six "disenchanters, *rhabilleurs*, [and] charlatans" living in Elne, in Perpignan, in Palau-del-Vidre, a town a few kilometers south of Elne, in the coastal town of Banyuls-sur-Mer, the center of a celebrated wine-producing district some 20 kilometers southeast of Elne, and in the inland town of Baixas, more than 20 kilometers northwest of Elne, on the other side of Perpignan. According to Ramonet (whose descriptions are summarized or paraphrased here):

> François Puy, called "Manut," is a *désensorceleur* at Baixas. A treatment with fumigants killed a woman after childbirth, and he was responsible for another death as well. He receives patients in his house and also visits several communes.
>
> Joseph Cortade, a weaver at Perpignan, is also a *désensorceleur* who teaches the technique of turning a sieve to discover witches; he criticizes the remedies of the physicians and surgeons.
>
> Marguerite Mallot, known as "Palaille," residing in the commune of Banyuls-sur-Mer, practices as a *désensorceleuse* of humans and livestock in several communes. It is said that those who wish to ask for her services must seek her on a white horse.
>
> The wife of Mathieu, pharmacist at Elne, gives emetics and purgatives, and also treats wounds and ulcers. (In general, rural apothecaries dispense remedies without prescriptions.)
>
> Baille, a bonesetter at Banyuls-sur-Mer, says that he possesses a hereditary healing gift.
>
> Fabre, another *rhabilleur*, is a shepherd at Palau-del-Vidre; he once removed a dressing applied by a surgeon of Elne and is said to have quarreled with another surgeon.

Bouche, a *mangonnier* (dealer in vamped goods) at Elne, calls himself a healer of cancers. He undertook to cure a breast cancer being treated by a surgeon; the patient died of a hemorrhage caused (according to Ramonet) by a caustic that the empiric had applied.

De Colioure, at Perpignan, is a *saluant* or *saludador*. He has made his fortune from subscriptions guaranteeing treatment in the event of a bite from a rabid dog.

Ramonet also mentions a dubious *officier de santé* at Elne who has made only 300 francs in that capacity, although he had an opportunity to replace a surgeon at Sorède who made 1,100; two priests who lift spells; and an ex-Capuchin, a priest who sells Ailhaud's powders, which have caused a death.

The list of popular healers includes three *désensorceleurs* (or five, counting the priests); two *rhabilleurs* (one of whom boasts of having a hereditary healing gift); and a *saludador*. As in the case of Cugnat, popular medicine and countersorcery overlap. These practitioners seem to be unusually prominent healers, some of whom have quarreled with the professionals or have been accused of maiming or killing patients. They live in the cluster of towns surrounding the old provincial capital, now the departmental seat, or, in one case, in Perpignan itself – rather than in the isolated villages of the hinterland. All appear to have extensive reputations; one travels around several communes. Although there is no way to gauge the completeness of this list, the more modest healers have evidently been overlooked or omitted.

3. In 1827, the Académie Royale de Médecine and the Société Médicale d'Émulation de Paris received a communication from J. Lecourt de Cantilly on healers in the region around the Breton town of Dol, near the bay of Mont Saint-Michel in the northern extremity of the department of Ille-et-Vilaine.[179] Lecourt briefly alluded to a wide range of illegal practitioners, both itinerants and various local healers, some of whom he believed were fairly well educated and prosperous enough not to need the income from their medical work. One group had secret ointments and other miraculous recipes for ulcers, dartre, scabies, and ophthalmia, inherited from their ancestors; *rebouteurs* treated supposedly dislocated ribs; so-called thaumaturges used prayers to treat fevers and purportedly raised fallen stomachs. His principal subject, though, was the treatment of that "so-called malady [known as *les hunes*], said to be very common in the greater part of the province of Brittany." This term intrigued the members of the Academy's Commission on Medical Police, who had been delegated to read and report on Dr. Lecourt's manuscript; they wished to know what objective disorder it might actually designate. Turning for help to a Breton dictionary, they found no entry for "*hunes*"; they did, however, find "*hun*" (sleep or dream), "*honoë*" (to sleep), and "*à hun dy hunet*" (disturbed sleep), which they spec-

ulated might be the crucial manifestation of the disease, whose symptoms were redundantly identified as lassitude, fatigue, and sluggishness.[180]

When an enervated patient suspected the awful truth that he suffered from *les hunes*, the first course of action was to rub him with a little *beurre de rouvraison* (butter containing a secret mixture of aromatic plants, prepared during the three Rogation days; from an old word for Rogation); prayers accompanied this massage. If the symptoms persisted (as they almost invariably did), the patient went to consult *celui qui panse des hunes,* either at his home or in some other agreed-upon house. "This man," wrote Lecourt, made his diagnosis by observing the patient's tongue. (The phrase implies that all such *panseurs* were men; but only a month before Lecourt wrote his memoir, the health council of Nantes reported a woman named Huchon with a well-established medical practice that consisted of incising the palate with a "bad razor" – the classic treatment, as will be seen, for *les hunes.*)[181] If the region under the tip of the tongue appeared red or bluish (its normal color), the healer announced that *les hunes* were "*éprises*" (a word that in current French means enamored or overcome by emotion, but here seems to have the old sense of kindled or perhaps inflamed) and that they were red, blue, violet, and so on. Taking a rusty razor, he made cuts on the wrists, the back of the hands, the fingers, the gastrocnemius (the large muscle of the calf of the leg), and other parts of the body. Sometimes he made two or three razor cuts on the palate, or opened the ranine veins and even arteries, using a lancet in place of the razor. The patient would be given a little water with which to rinse his mouth, but the *panseur* never bandaged the wounds; in this popular version of phlebotomy, the more blood that flowed, the better.[182] The scarifications would be repeated one or more times during propitious periods, when the moon was waning, for a year or two, if the patient did not recover sooner. Good Friday was considered to be the best day for treatment, and on that occasion it was not unusual for more than a hundred persons to come to Dol to see a *panseur*. But all year long, during the waning moon, one or two healers came to town each Saturday (market day) and received patients at a private house.

Lecourt blamed the treatment for debilitating and, in some cases, maiming the patient; one child, with deep horizontal cuts in his gastrocnemius muscles, was unable to stand. (The physician's own preferred treatment called for antiphlogistics, or anti-inflammatory agents – essentially a pharmacological alternative to bloodletting in patients believed to suffer from "plethora.") He urged the patients not to return to the *panseur*, but they replied that physicians did not understand this disease and that they would be dead if they had not submitted to treatment. The population seemed to Lecourt to have a deep and unshakable faith in the procedure, which he thought might be a survival of an old religious scarification ritual practiced by the Druids. As for the healers, although he supposed that a very few might be fatuous enough to believe in all sincerity that they were acting out of charity, he saw the majority as opportunists preying on the "blind confidence" of the people.

Clearly, the *panseur* who treated *les hunes* was not simply another surgical "expert." The treatment strangely conflated some sort of scarification ritual, astrology, and the bloodletting of humoralist therapeutics. The *panseur*, who might or might not enjoy a special gift (the manuscript is silent on this question), appears to have possessed more than routine empirical skills; although the actual operation was fairly straightforward (as compared with, say, couching a cataract), not just anyone could perform it. Moreover, the healer's practice depended on a deeply rooted popular conception, which had no real counterpart in official medicine. This belief explained chronic fatigue arising from anxiety, depression, overwork, or possibly a latent organic illness; although it represented the disease as a potential threat to life, it also held out hope for a radical cure. The condition could almost have been designed to respond to a placebo.

In other respects, though, the *panseur* for *les hunes* seems less like the classic traditional healer. His methods, apart from the initial remedy of massage and prayer, were only tenuously connected to nineteenth-century popular religion and magic. And although Lecourt never mentioned money, he implied that the *panseurs*, whatever their deepest motive, derived an income from their practice by coming on market days to Dol, which was not a village or even a bourg, but a *petite ville* with a population (including the outlying districts) of 3,800, according to Lecourt.

By drawing on the work of the ethnographers, it would no doubt be possible to produce a "thick description" of the practices reported in this manuscript of 1827 and the other documents and perhaps to improve on Dr. Lecourt's amateur antiquarianism (which led him to add an archeological postscript to his description of the *panseurs*). But all three documents also raise another question of a different sort; they point to the existence of practitioners whose work seemingly linked them to the world of folk medicine, but who may have had major practices, lived in towns, charged fees, and in other ways behaved like empirics. Whether they genuinely shared their patients' belief system or simply exploited it is almost impossible to say; here the historian is at a sad disadvantage compared with the ethnographers, particularly those who, like François Laplantine, grew up in the very culture on which they are now conducting field research. One could argue at some length about whether such practitioners should be classed among the minority of highly successful folk healers, whom nearly all the folklorists mention, or some subspecies of sedentary empiric; the label is not particularly significant in itself. But their existence is important, and their place in the medical network, as well as their relations with patients – particularly the peasants who might have come to market towns to consult them – deserve further study.

The conclusion of this chapter will return to the questions raised by trying to classify such nondescripts. First, though, it is important to turn to another problem that has emerged in documents 1 and 2: the relationship between sorcery and healing.

WITCHES AND DEVINS-GUÉRISSEURS

The contemporary sources refer to a number of healers as *sorciers*, *devins*, or *désensorceleurs*. How did they differ from ordinary *maiges*?

Witchcraft and healing: concepts and approaches

The terminology used in the eighteenth- and nineteenth-century sources is at best a confusing guide to the world of medical witchcraft, for in the thinking of many educated observers, witches and magical healers were interchangeable. The same was often true of popular discourse: local healers were sometimes called witches if they were believed to possess extraordinary powers, and witches might be called *maiges*; the usual word for a sorcerer in the Corrèze and Haute-Vienne, for example, was *"metze."*[183] Healers known as witches practiced a wide range of magical and empirical medicine, like the "so-called witch of Pontorson," an illiterate sabot seller and servant of a country priest, denounced to the Société Royale by the physician Jean-Guillaume Chifoliau.[184] An account from the Gironde (1797) describes the local *sorcière* who "raises the fallen stomach [and] who repositions the child in the mother's belly, when it is displaced," using bandages and topical remedies.[185] A woman called Menuet, better known as "the witch of the three mills," who practiced for ten years near the hamlet of Pont-Rousseau (Loire-Inférieure) in the early nineteenth century, was probably just an empiric.[186] Some witches may have induced abortions;[187] others simply sold secret remedies.[188] A twentieth-century work on rural medicine even notes a distinction between "red sorcerers," who heal with simples they have gathered following a certain ritual, and "white sorcerers," who use an electric battery (an indication, too, that popular medicine is not immune to the influences of changing technology).[189]

Yet one category of healers can be distinguished from the rest – those who purported to treat not only natural illnesses but also maladies attributed to evil spells or (occasionally) demonic possession. Their work can be understood only in the context of popular witchcraft beliefs.

This world is not an easy one to penetrate. No extensive sources exist for our period comparable to the records of witchcraft trials from the sixteenth and seventeenth centuries (and in those trials, testimony often reflected the inquisitors' expectations more than popular practices and beliefs). Modern folklore studies that deal with witchcraft generally provide only fragmentary information; as Van Gennep confessed, for example, in his study of the folklore of Dauphiné, "my informants have unanimously declared that belief in witches has disappeared almost everywhere, and that it is very difficult nowadays to discern traces of it."[190]

A sense of the limitations of Van Gennep's method (questionnaires distributed to local inhabitants) and the more general difficulties of research on this subject can be gained from the recent work of the ethnologist Jeanne Favret-Saada on contemporary witchcraft in the bocage of western France.[191] Even the most sensitive investigator in the field works under the severe constraints imposed by the peasants' distrust and fear: distrust of established institutions (school, Church, and state), which ridicule witchcraft beliefs; fear of dangers within the witchcraft system itself, in which words have magical significance, speech is a powerful act, and a verbal exchange may set terrifying forces in motion. Peasants are likely to have two discourses on magic and witchcraft, one for outsiders – "oh, only a few old women believe such superstitions" – and another for themselves. A fortiori, healers who have a reputation as a witch disavow it. (Some comparable reactions appear in accounts from the period covered by this book. When the healer known as Dame Blanche, for example, who was tried for illegal medical practice at the end of the Restoration, heard a witness say that she passed for a witch, she laughed and exclaimed, "Witch? Me a witch? That's a good one!" When the prosecutor admonished the defendant to show respect for justice, she replied, "Well, if I laugh, it's because it's funny.... Witches! It makes you laugh. Have you ever seen any witches?")[192] After more than thirty months of residence in the bocage, Favret-Saada established the existence of a system of witchcraft beliefs and practices far more extensive than her informants had suggested during initial interviews – more extensive, indeed, than most ethnographers would have predicted. Her investigation succeeded after she had, in effect, entered the witchcraft system herself. Despite the candid explanation she gave of her research, her informants came to believe that she herself was either a witchcraft victim or an unwitcher (to whom one must "tell all"); eventually she became a sort of assistant to "Madame Flora," a *désorceleuse*, as a *désensorceleuse* is called in the Mayenne.[193]

The historian cannot of course enter into this sort of interaction with his subjects. With the evidence available from the periods when social norms sanctioned public accusations of witchcraft, it is possible to reconstruct roughly how the belief system worked and to elaborate social or psychological explanations of why some individuals were identified as witches and others as witchcraft victims;[194] but it simply is not possible to gauge the full depth and range of the phenomenon.

The term "witchcraft" has been used to cover a wide range of beliefs and practices, from pacts with the Devil, demonic possession, and goety, or black magic, to "white" sorcery and popular dabblings in the occult. Most students of the subject have distinguished sharply, as Keith Thomas does in his study of magic and religion in early modern England, between witches who do harm, and cunning men, or white witches, who are consulted as healers, unwitchers, and diviners. A white witch might occasionally be accused of casting spells, and in the eyes of the law all uses of sorcery were equally damnable; but "in England, as on the Continent, the blurring together of black and white witchcraft was fundamentally alien to popular beliefs."[195]

Such a distinction has been challenged, most recently by Robert Muchembled, who sees it as the creation of cultural elites.[196] For the peasant, in his view, all forms of magic were fundamentally ambiguous, possessing the dual potential for protection and harm. Muchembled's own work on early modern witchcraft in northern France suggests that the same witches who were feared as a sinister force by those within their own village may have been consulted – and praised for doing good – by outsiders. (In the twentieth-century bocage, according to Favret-Saada, peasants choose to consult distant *devins*, preferably from outside their diocese or department.)[197] Similarly, the popular image of the witch in the materials collected by French folklorists often combines elements of black and white witchcraft. For example, at Vaujany in Dauphiné, according to Van Gennep, witches were seen as people with an uncanny look who predict the future and help find lost objects; although they provide a useful service, one has to be very submissive to them, or they will cast spells.[198] In the witchcraft system studied by Favret-Saada, the unwitcher typically must use a counterspell to disenchant the patient, and in so doing is believed to injure and even kill the suspected witch. Indeed, the relations are strictly reversible, and the witch attacked by the unwitcher may see himself as the victim of witchcraft.[199] Laplantine notes, too, that the unwitcher may be willing in some cases to initiate hostilities at a client's behest – for example by using *le nouage de l'aiguillette* to induce impotence. ("*Aiguillette*" is an old word for a cord used to fasten a man's breeches, and to tie [*nouer*] *l'aiguillette* is to use a charm, generally by knotting a string, to rob a man of his sexual powers.)[200]

Nevertheless, the distinction between black and white witchcraft appears to have sufficient validity to justify retaining it here. Although the *devins* may have been feared figures, consulted only with trepidation, they were not regularly accused by their neighbors of using their powers maliciously (although they may have been swept up in some of the great witch hunts); nor were the people accused of casting spells ordinarily recognized as consultants. More work is needed, however, to adjudicate decisively between the Thomas and Muchembled interpretations.

The study of black witchcraft primarily concerns discourse *about* witches. It is a commonplace of the literature that the absent figure in the witchcraft system is the witch; if one probes deeply enough, one finds believers, victims, accused witches, and unwitchers, but no one who says "I am a witch" – except in the old trials, when many of the accused confessed, yielding to psychological pressure and often torture.[201] (Some recent studies have plausibly argued that not all confessions were coerced, and that a number of the accused may actually have thought that they consorted with the demon or used black magic; they perhaps applied witches' salve, which contains plant alkaloids said to be capable of inducing dream states accompanied by bizarre hallucinations and sensations of flying.[202] The prevalence of such actual witches, however, remains a matter of speculation.) Among educated people on the Continent, from the late Middle Ages until the triumph of skepticism, witchcraft was believed to consist basically in an alliance with the Devil; it was a form of heresy. This concept, and the related notion of the witches' sabbath at which Satan was worshipped, has its counterparts in French popular culture (as the story of one of the *devin* Cugnat's patients illustrates); but in France, as in England, the popular conception of the witch remained essentially that of someone who used sorcery to do harm.

Students of European black witchcraft have sometimes borrowed from anthropology a distinction, introduced by E. E. Evans-Pritchard in his work on the Zande, between *witchcraft* as such, which is an innate involuntary power in some individuals (physically residing in their stomachs, in the case of the Zande), and *sorcery*, or the illicit use of medicine to hurt others.[203] The actual terminology cannot be directly translated into French, which has only the word "*sorcellerie*"; but in his study of Berry, for example, François Laplantine distinguishes "born" witches, comparable to possessors of the evil eye, from "voluntary witches," who have learned how to cast a spell by means of thought or physical contact, how to inflict a *charge* through a specially treated object hidden in the victim's house, or how to practice *l'enclouage*, which consists in driving a nail or nails into, say, the victim's footprint while uttering a curse.[204] In practice, though, as Favret-Saada argues, the distinction breaks down. Witchcraft almost always appears to be voluntary, and witches are believed, like the *maiges*, both to use magic rituals and to possess a special personal power.[205] The key distinction in most folklore studies is between the ordinary *sorcier*, a fairly benign magician-healer, and the witch who casts spells and who is often called by a special name – "*masc*" in Languedoc, "*enjomineur*" in Anjou, "*jeteux de sorts*" in Maine and elsewhere.[206]

In contrast to the black witches, it is relatively easy to identify self-professed white witches or "cunning men," as they were called in English, for they generally had established reputations as consultants.[207] In their capacity as counterwitches they were known as *leveurs de sorts* (spell lifters) or *désensorceleurs* (unwitchers) in standard French, and by a variety of regional names (*désenjomineur* in Anjou, *escounuyrayre* in Béarn).[208] Typically they also practiced divination and healing, hence the common French dyadic term *devin-guérisseur*.[209] The *devin* dealt with a great diversity of actual or potential human misfortunes. He might practice cartomancy and prophecy, undertaking to obtain a favorable lottery number for conscripts; to find lost objects, hidden treasure, or lost persons; and to identify thieves.[210] Josué Rochat, *le Devin de la Pièce* at Mont-la-Ville in eighteenth-century Vaud (Switzerland), was consulted by the commune of Vaulion about a girl lost in the snow.[211] Michel Cauveau of Chetigné, arrondissement of Saumur (Maine-et-Loire), a *devin*, animal doctor, and *guérisseur de secret*, was involved at the beginning of the nineteenth century in a search for hidden treasure.[212] René Houssant, a sorcerer and *devin* in the nineteenth-century Aube, practiced cartomancy and probably helped conscripts escape military service.[213] In the medical domain, the *devin* might be consulted for *le tirage des saints*, the magic procedure for identifying the saint "responsible" for a patient's illness.[214] The *devin-guérisseur*, then, was a healer but also much more.

Individual illnesses or other misfortunes were rarely attributed to witchcraft, except when there was something mysterious about them (such as a patient's unaccountably wasting away while consuming huge quantities of food), or when they followed immediately after an angry encounter with a likely witch. In the system of witchcraft beliefs, human misfortunes were seen as interlinked; Favret-Saada's first publication on the subject deals, significantly, with the *repetition* of biological misfortune. A cow might become sterile, a crop might fail, family members might suffer from skin eruptions. The popular explanation attributed the pattern to a single maleficent agent; treating the individual misfortunes separately would have been, to this way of thinking, what treating the various manifestations of syphilis as different diseases would be for official medicine.

If witchcraft were thought to be at work, the family might first resort to self-help; rituals such as pricking an ox's heart with pins or placing nails in boiling water seem to have been commonly known, together with a wide range of prophylactic measures against evil influences.[215] If the misfortunes persisted, the curé might sometimes be persuaded to perform the rites of exorcism. The Church made a strict distinction between the influence of evil spirits, which called for exorcism, and witchcraft, which required proceeding against the witch, but these two concepts largely merged in the popular imagination. In the contemporary bocage, the curé (who generally does not cooperate) is considered a minor unwitcher *pour le bon* – that is, he can lift spells without returning them to the sender – but he is considered to be ineffective in serious cases.[216] Some popular medical practitioners had a reputation as lay exorcists, like Jean-Michel Fritsch, who worked at Geis-polsheim (Bas-Rhin) in the early nineteenth century.[217]

If misfortunes persisted, a *désensorceleur* might be called in. His first task was to discover the identity of the witch. Some *devins* claimed to have an inborn gift for knowing witches.[218] Others relied on rituals of divination; the purpose of these proceedings was usually to elicit from the victim the name of the person he already suspected of tormenting him. The next step was normally the counterspell, to force the witch to desist, and, if necessary, to inflict slow agony and death; for, as Favret-Saada explains, the witch must not only be prevented from preying on the victim but must also be made to yield up the vital force already stolen from him. In the end, though, not all misfortunes were necessarily ascribed to witchcraft, and the *devin-guérisseur* had to come equipped for all eventualities; he needed to be ma-gician, veterinarian, and physician, as well as counterwitch. At La Boissière in Anjou, for example, at the end of the Old Regime, the farrier Martin doctored man and beast, bewitching and unbewitching "according to cir-cumstances"; during epizootics (in which misfortune was too widely shared to be attributed to a specific personal animus), he recommended burying dead animals under living ones to attract all the "poison."[219]

As described by Favret-Saada, the counterwitch is the healer for whom the immanent power to cure is the most important, in contrast to the physician, who applies techniques external to his person. He may already possess a gift as a *toucheur*; but beyond that he possesses a magical personal force, with which he can oppose the force that the witch uses to rob the patient of his vital energy. Without *le sang fort*, the *désorceleur* is nothing, and magic formulas or rituals would be worthless. Unwitchers "take it all on themselves"; in the conflict of forces, they say, "either he dies or I do" – although in practice, if the unwitcher's endowment proves insufficient, he simply withdraws, saying that the patient is too strongly "taken."[220] Just how well this model applies to witchcraft in other periods or places cannot be said with certainty, but it is clear that both the witch and the counterwitch were believed to possess not just information or knowledge, but special power.

In addition to analyzing belief systems, historians of witchcraft have spilled much ink in attempts to analyze what Keith Thomas has called its "social environment." By and large, they have focused on the social position of accused witches and their relationship with the accuser. Witches lacked a comfortable social niche; the archetypal witch was, as the popular stereotype suggests, elderly, poor, and female. Keith Thomas has argued that the accused in early modern England was very likely someone who had been refused charity by a more established member of the community (an in-dividualist who rejected traditional paternalistic obligations) and then cursed him for his hardheartedness. Alan Macfarlane's study of Essex and Muchembled's work on northern France point to a comparable relationship between accuser and accused. In Salem, according to Paul Boyer and Stephen Nissembaum, similar tensions were at work, although here the pattern was reversed: the accusations originated in Salem village, a declining agricultural community, and were directed against people associated with Salem town, a seaport whose elite was growing in power.[221]

These analyses, which were all produced by historians studying the sixteenth and seventeenth centuries, attempt to show how social change accounts for the chronology of witchcraft prosecutions and the identities of accuser and accused. Ethnographers have developed more static models to account for what might be thought of as endemic, as opposed to epidemic, witchcraft. The typical witch is to some extent an outsider and is marked as other because he or she deviates in various ways from social and biological norms. (One major exception: Favret-Saada finds no consensus that anyone is the village witch. The relationship exists between two families, usually of similar socioeconomic status, rather than between an individual and the community.)[222] Witches are marked by exceptional poverty (or, occasionally, exceptional and unexplained wealth), senility, physical deformity, and neurological disorders. In the Charente, it was believed that witches were likely to be found among those "marked with a 'B' " – *les boiteux, les bègues, les bigles,* and *les borgnes* (the lame, the stammerers, the squint-eyed, and the blind).[223] Witches might also be associated with some vaguely understood outside enemy. In the Charente, they have been confused with Free Masons. In the Mayenne, according to Favret-Saada, the chain of personal forces connecting them is believed to lead ultimately to a network of superwitches in Paris, the distrusted headquarters of the outsiders, of the people peasants think of simply as "them."[224]

For ethnologists, two possible structural interpretations suggest how the witch may be seen as disturbingly other. In the dualist cosmology that defines one peasant view of the natural world, God's creation and the Devil's creation coexist, and each work of God has its diabolical counterpart: sheep/goat, dog/cat, vine/ivy, sun/moon, and so on.[225] In such a context, it makes sense that "if the priest is the vicar of God on earth, the sorcerer remains the Devil's."[226] Alternatively, following a line of argument developed by Mary Douglas, the witch may be seen as the misfit who falls outside familiar structures, becoming the focus of "the fears and dislikes which other ambiguities and contradictions attract in other thought structures."[227] The witch is outsider/insider, male/female, impotent/superpotent, decrepit/debauched, and so on.

The social position of the *devin-guérisseur/leveur de sorts* has received considerably less attention. Muchembled sees the healers as interchangeable with the witches; they are marginal figures whose status follows from the fundamental ambiguity of their powers. Most are female because of the "primordial" role of women in transmitting popular culture.[228] The folklorists note that unwitchers tend to come from outside the group of farmers who make up the rural majority, from among shepherds, loggers, even tramps.[229] In another sense, though, the *devin/désorceleur* is neither misfit nor outsider; he plays a crucial social role as defined by a widely shared belief system. This system is so powerful that a phenomenon described by the anthropologist W. B. Cannon as "voodoo death" can occasionally occur when a person supposes himself to be the victim of a spell.[230] So, too, the intervention of the counterwitch can bring real relief to troubled clients, thanks to the same sort of "symbolic efficacy" that Claude Lévi-Strauss has attributed to the shaman and the psychoanalyst.[231] He may also serve an integrative function by helping to resolve the social conflicts that manifest themselves as suspicions of witchcraft (although, as Favret-Saada observes, the conflict of personal forces may never be definitively resolved, so that popular measures may be less effective at easing social tensions than the trials of an earlier era).

There are some obvious dangers, however, in treating the witch-healer of a complex peasant society as a shaman-like figure in a village culture that is autonomous, stable, uniform, and fundamentally different from our own. As Favret-Saada stresses, peasant attitudes toward unwitchers are neither uniform nor unambivalent.[232] As for the practitioners themselves, they can be found along a gamut ranging from blacksmiths, at the center of the community, to poachers, on the margins;[233] their ranks even include a few landowners like Vignes, the celebrated Calvinist empiric and *sorcier-guérisseur* (1830–1906), who practiced at Vialas (Lozère).[234] The extent of their activities varied widely; the most successful seem quite different from the stereotyped local folk healer. Helped perhaps by the prejudice against consulting a neighbor, they developed practices reaching well beyond their residences – for example, 10 leagues in the case of the witch of La Trinité-Surzur in the Morbihan.[235] An extensive practice is suggested by a list of "condemnations" found among the papers of a *leveur de sorts* in the Châteauroux region of the Indre:

There came during the months of March and April [1845] 132 men, condemned [bewitched] for from 24 hours to 5 years, and 96 women [condemned for various intervals]. . . . They came every day. Most of all they came a lot from Valençay [about 40 kilometers from Châteauroux]; the greatest number are from Levroux [about midway between Valençay and Châteauroux].[236]

In the twentieth century, according to a study of Charentais folklore, clients used modern transportation to reach the best sorcerers.[237] The *devin-guérisseur* Vignes had such an extraordinary following that in 1895 special direct trains were put in service from Geneva to Genolhac (the station nearest his residence in Vialas), so that Swiss and Germans could come to consult him.[238] Some consultants with established reputations, moreover, charged substantial fees; an exorcist near Dunkirk at the end of the nineteenth century, for example, required a retainer of 70 to 100 francs.[239] And some made use of magic books and other paraphernalia borrowed from the occult tradition of high culture. They may seem, in fact, like minor entrepreneurs, although it is now virtually impossible to settle the question of their sincerity.

Witches in the contemporary sources

It has proved more difficult to paint a composite portrait of the witch-healer than of the *maige*; there is no general agreement among ethnologists and historians on the relation of black and white witchcraft or on the exact connections between unwitching, divining, and healing. In the eighteenth and early nineteenth centuries, however, educated observers had a clearer conception of the witch than of the *maige*, despite the looseness with which they often applied the term. This conception might take one of two forms.

Some descriptions recall the popular notion of the witch-healer as essentially a magician who boasts of having special powers to protect or harm. For example, a topographical description of the Vendée published during the First Empire singles out those persons (whom it identifies, curiously, with the storytellers at rural *veillées* – fireside gatherings, on winter evenings, for work or amusement) who are believed to be "beings privileged by nature, who divine the past and read the future; who, with a gesture, a word, or a single act of will, cure sick men and animals, or visit death on them; find lost belongings; excite love or hatred between two lovers; practice, in a word, the fearful ministry of the sorcerer. And these people are not rare, especially at Chambretaud."[240]

Other writers, like Jean-Luc d'Iharce, in his late-eighteenth-century treatise on popular medical errors, introduced the compact with Satan. One group of healers, he wrote,

pretend that there are wicked people capable of inflicting diseases, through a power that they have received from the evil spirit, by virtue of a pact made with him; they call this casting a spell, or bewitching; the wicked people endowed with this power they call witches, and the illnesses they give are known as *maléfices*, *sortilèges*, or *ensorcèlements* [all words for spells]. They go to nocturnal assemblies, which they call the sabbath; women take part in these gatherings, and they always outnumber the men. These so-called physicians take care not to say that they, too, like the witches, have a pact with the evil spirit, in order to discover the authors of the spells that they wish to cure, and to force them to indicate the remedies to them (for they would not be able to do it themselves) – but they make every effort to suggest it, and never fail to accomplish this; as a result, people call them magicians or *devins*.[241]

Iharce saw the *devins* as unscrupulous frauds who might at best know a few simples and, on rare occasions, do some good.

Although the concepts are fairly straightforward, it has been seen that the vocabulary in which they were expressed could be ambiguous. As in popular speech, "*sorcier*" could refer simply to a magical healer; it is often essential to know the context. Even so, it is not hard to find references to identifiable witches and counterwitches in contemporary records. Although by the eighteenth century witchcraft was merely a superstition rather than a crime, physicians sometimes complained about the medical activities of sorcerers in their region, and individual counterwitches sometimes came to the attention of the police when their efforts were blamed for injury or loss of life or when a dissatisfied client decided to denounce them for swindling.

In 1776, for example, Dumereau, a peasant of Beauvoir in Poitou, was accused of prescribing a treatment for a girl said to be ill from witchcraft. The patient was to attach a rooster to the foot of her bed and deprive it of food and water; as the bird declined, she would improve. But the girl died, hence the degree of official interest in the affair.[242] In a notorious case of 1783, Jean Gallifier, a beggar and reputed *devin* in the diocese of Sens, was blamed for a far greater catastrophe. Marie Semaine, the wife of a *laboureur* at Cerisiers, suffered from attacks of "vapors," which she attributed to witchcraft. The husband was persuaded to seek out Gallifier, in the parish of Les Bordes; the old man (sixty-five to eighty years old, the report says) looked every bit the sorcerer, and his techniques fulfilled the family's expectations. The events, as they were reconstructed, involved classic counterwitchcraft rituals. Gallifier recommended that the family have a few masses said, but he also bought an earthen pot, an ox's heart, and slat nails (without haggling for them, out of respect for a magical prohibition). After closing up the chimney in Marie Semaine's house to prevent the demon from penetrating and the suspected witch from hearing or seeing the proceedings, he lit coals and grilled the heart, which he then pricked with ninety-five nails. In the morning, when all the participants were found dead of carbon monoxide poisoning, the neighbors concluded that the demon had taken his revenge.[243]

Many such cases involved members of occupations that traditionally provided magical healers: gelders and lay veterinarians, farriers, carpenters. For some of them, healing and unbewitching seem to have been a regular sideline and source of supplementary income.

In 1814, for example, a laborer and animal doctor from the commune of Neuvy-Deux-Clochers (Cher), a bachelor named Bedu, undertook "magical operations" in the house of Simon Migeon, in the commune of Crézancy, to discover, with the aid of a book and a bucket full of water, who had cast spells on the household. He accused the mayor of Crézancy and two inhabitants of his own commune. Next he threw three cart nails into the fire, attached with thread and hairs from Migeon's head. He would leave the nails, he said, if the patient wished the witches to die suddenly; if he preferred them to die a lingering death, one nail should be removed. In any event, Migeon would be well within two weeks. As payment, Bedu received 36 francs in three installments.[244]

A farrier living at Meung-sur-Loire in the last years of the Old Regime inspected urine and prescribed the same remedy for all – an ounce of jalap, which was said to cause miscarriages. In one case, when a miller from Tavers brought his wife's urine for examination, the farrier pronounced her bewitched and offered to cure her by means of a magical procedure for 100 écus.[245]

At the beginning of the nineteenth century, a carpenter at Villeneuve-sur-Yonne, named Martin, was known as a *devin*; the mayor of Vaudeurs blamed him for the death of Étienne Rallu, from the hamlet of Brisault, who in his opinion had suffered from only a neglected cold.[246] In the Nevers region, another carpenter, François Antoine, known as Desormeaux, and his wife, Julie Raquin, won an extraordinary reputation as magical healers toward the end of the First Empire; the husband was supposed to be able to lift spells, and his wife was consulted as a *devineresse*. In June 1814, they used what officials described as "illicit means" to convince a landowner, Nicolas Camus, that he and his livestock were bewitched and that his wife would be too if she did not come to consult them. The wife duly went to see Raquin for a session of cartomancy and learned that a "foreign Mason" had bewitched her husband. She accepted a remedy made of rat droppings for her husband and another for the livestock. To ensure the efficacy of the treatment, she had to furnish a capon and a duck, which Raquin took away, going out backward. Raquin subsequently required unwashed butter; the breeches that the patient was wearing when he took to his bed; the featherbed on which he lay; several hanks of flax; wool; a sack of flour; salt; chickens; and bread. The wife was also to prepare and place at the foot of a cross a sacrificial offering of milk, cream, eggs, bran, and straw. Finally, she was to wash the Desormeaux laundry for two months, since "it was not appropriate that magicians should put their hands in water so long as they were treating a patient." The spell was eventually lifted; according to one account, Raquin's father uttered horrible cries that supposedly issued from the tormented demon and released a bat to suggest its departure from the patient's body. The healers then required a further payment of 120 francs. In this case, the confidence game was said to extend to extortion; the local justice of the peace observed that "the reputation of the Raquin woman is such that by means of a simple threat, [she and her husband] have the capacity to terrorize the credulous inhabitants of the countryside."[247]

Still other *devins* combined unwitching with unsteady employment in rural industry. Jean-Baptiste-Casimir Louchon, for example, worked as a wool carder at Saint-Maximin in the Var, where he might have remained happily unnoticed had he not in 1823 crippled a patient named Blanc after persuading him that he was bewitched.[248]

Apart from specialized *désensorceleurs*, the ranks of the unwitchers included active empirics who took on a witchcraft case now and again. Thus, in 1827, a certain Roger of the Indre, who called himself a "great physician," treated an unmarried woman who had been in poor health for several years and who attributed her illness to a spell. Roger provided packets to throw on the fire and instructions for carrying out a ritual using candles and holy water. He asked at first for 25 francs; the following day he requested the same amount for the candles used in the rites, which he fetched at night (he said) from the "Grand Devin de Châteauroux."[249] Sibenaler, nephew of a former prior of Amilly, combined occasional treatment of witchcraft cases with his work as an "operator-dentist" in the commune of Saint-Georges-de-Noisné (Deux-Sèvres). He told a patient, Giblot, who was gravely ill, that he could determine who had bewitched him and deliver a prognosis. His technique mingled folk magic and a quackish trick. Two stone-colored pellets (possibly containing phosphorus) were put in a glass of water; if the patient was lost, the pellets would sink, whereas if he could be saved, they would rise. They rose and burst into flames. The healer gave the couple a few bottles of pectoral water, a package of powder to sprinkle in the stables to preserve the livestock from illness, and a cross, which the wife was to place in the cupboard among her linens.[250]

Some entrepreneurial sorcerer-empirics established vast practices. In the early nineteenth century, members of two "clans" in the Vosges mountains achieved great notoriety, especially two brothers, the "great" and "lesser" sorcerers of Saint-Dié, whose reputation in the 1820's extended throughout the department of the Vosges and into the Meurthe, Haute-Saône, Haute-Marne, and Bas-Rhin. *Le grand sorcier* was in effect an itinerant charlatan who traveled around the countryside inspecting urine, healing with his breath, cupping patients, and treating livestock; in the game sack that he carried constantly, he kept a sort of portable pharmacy. The authorities noted as an indication of his prestige that he continued his consultations while in prison.[251]

As in the case of the *maiges*, it is hard to differentiate sharply between the *devins* or sorcerers who figure in documents from the late eighteenth and early nineteenth centuries and other categories of popular practitioners mentioned in the same sources. The ethnological models of folk healing and witchcraft do not account for the significant body of practitioners for whom magical medicine and unbewitching may have been one source of income among others, who may or may not have fully believed in their methods,[252] and who did not necessarily play a generally sanctioned role as integral members of a village community. To say this is not to deny the widespread existence of obscure folk healers much like those described by the ethnologists. The police records give disproportionate attention to the exceptional deviant; and contemporary observations do confirm, in a general way, that much rural health care was in the hands of anonymous local healers. But neither is the group described here an artifact of the judicial records; any social interpretation of popular healing must take it into account. Such practitioners were doubly obnoxious to the professionals, who saw in them both economic rivals and fomenters of popular superstition.

Indeed, it may be misleading to present traditional popular medicine as the remnants of a once purer, more coherent, and vastly more widespread popular medical system that dominated health care in the largely isolated village communities of preindustrial Europe. With the modernization of the countryside, according to this view, folk medicine has generally disintegrated, giving way to professional medicine, on the one hand, and new-fangled forms of parallel medicine, on the other; it lingers on in the more stagnant rural backwaters. As Marcelle Bouteiller characteristically puts it, "the vogue of popular medicine, in full flower in the eighteenth and nineteenth centuries, grew progressively weaker during the first quarter of our century. At the present moment [mid–1960's], the prestige of the magnetizer and radiesthesist is competing more and more with that of the healer using the old secrets."[253] But the old medical network, as has been seen, was enormously various; between the classic folk healer and the physician there flourished a wide range of practitioners, who formed a continuum rather than a set of radically incompatible alternatives. Although folk healing was undoubtedly more widespread two hundred years ago than it has been in the last century, it was less sharply differentiated from other forms of medical practice than the usages studied by the folklorists, and popular medicine was less of a coherent whole than it may now appear.

The present status of folk healing is in part the result of an often unacknowledged historical process. For it is not just traditional popular medicine that has declined; the profession's old rivals in the rural medical market, from half-trained barber-surgeons to urinoscopists and itinerant sorcerers, have disappeared or assumed new guises. Some remnants of the old system survive – precisely those that are furthest removed from entrepreneurship. But they do not represent all of popular medical practice as it existed two centuries ago. To suppose otherwise is to yield to a certain nostalgia for the good old days.

PART III

Toward a social interpretation

6

The structure of medical practice:
an overview

Each of the preceding chapters has developed a partial view of the old medical network: the changing varieties of authorized practitioners; itinerant and sedentary empirics; *maiges* and witches. It is time now to stand back and consider the social world of medical practice as a whole. The analysis that follows falls into three main parts. The first considers the old network as a global health-care system, in which patients and practitioners, with their divergent clinical assumptions and expectations, interacted in complex and sometimes surprising ways. The discussion turns next to the practitioners' relation to the market for medical services; we cannot understand the social significance of medical practice unless we first understand it as an economic activity. But medical practice is more than the art of healing and a livelihood; it is also a social role. The third part considers the place of the practitioners in the society in which they worked, giving special attention to the relation of popular practitioners to their local communities and to the dominant national culture represented by doctors and government officials. A brief concluding section explores some of the broader implications of this analysis for the social interpretation of medical practice in general and popular healing in particular.

RIVALRY AND COOPERATION

As many licensed practitioners and other educated observers saw it, France was divided into two medical worlds. An enlightened fraction of the population consulted the minority of practitioners who had been formally trained and officially certified; the rest turned to quacks. The Lyons physician Gilibert, in his *Anarchie médicinale* of 1772, suggested that only a quarter of *les personnes du peuple* (members of the populace) whom he knew took advice from a physician. The medical faculty of Angers similarly estimated that about three-quarters of the population consulted empirics. The author of an 1825 work on abuses in medicine calculated that unqualified practitioners outnumbered physicians by about two-thirds, and that perhaps two-thirds of the population consulted them. (He defined the first category broadly, though, including ignorant *officiers de santé* and midwives and pharmacists who encroached on the medical field, as well as full-fledged charlatans.)[1]

Several reasons accounted for this apparent division of labor. The empiric was close at hand; the regular practitioner might be inaccessible. Even when a surgeon or physician was available, his education placed him in an alien and forbidding social sphere. One observer in Anjou at the end of the Old Regime, for example, noted that despite a sufficient number of surgeons, "the people" preferred to consult empirics, who by birth were closer to their own station; and in 1810, the municipal health council of Laval regretfully concluded that "man naturally likes to encounter, in those who come near him, his way of thinking, his way of being and feeling," from which it followed that peasants would always choose the farrier, the gelder, and the mole catcher over the *officier de santé*.[2] In addition, licensed practitioners' fees were generally too high. One report from the department of the Loire in the early nineteenth century suggested that the physicians could hardly expect a popular clientele when they sometimes charged a poor patient 20 francs or more.[3] Most observers also suggested that members of the lower classes were gullible and superstitious and were therefore more likely to succumb to the blandishments or threats of a charlatan. A healer in the Aube named Blanc, for example, was said to have made a patient "lose her head by announcing to her that she would die promptly if she did not take his remedies."[4] Then, too, the medical men themselves sometimes accepted and thereby encouraged a dualist system of health care. One report on a pair of empirics in eighteenth-century Brittany noted, for example, that the local surgeons connived at their activities, "since none of them can be bothered to go out and contend with them for their clients."[5]

It is misleading, however, to treat popular and official medicine as completely separate spheres, each with its own exponents and clientele. Self-medication and regular and irregular medical practice coexisted and overlapped. It has been seen that not all empirics' clients were lower-class. One typical case involved a housekeeper who practiced medicine in Touraine at the end of the Old Regime; when she was brought before a judge, more than half of the patients who testified in her behalf were well-off farmers and innkeepers who, it was said, could have paid for the services of physicians or surgeons.[6] Nor did consultation with one type of practitioner necessarily exclude calling in another. A popular healer might see a patient before, during, or after treatment by a physician or (more likely) a surgeon or *officier de santé*. According to Gilibert, every patient was treated by neighborhood women before being examined by a doctor, and even then they often continued to see unqualified practitioners. As a result, he suggested, they were subject to a "double action" in which the physician might order one thing and the *femmelettes* (literally, "little women") another, often directly opposed to what the medical man had recommended.[7] A patient would first try self-treatment, perhaps dosing himself with cinnamon-flavored wine to encourage sweating if he had a fever; next he might try a local healer – or a passing empiric, if one were available. Only afterward, and then only in serious cases, would he summon a regular practitioner. As a result, the physicians constantly complained, they generally arrived too late to provide effective assistance. Nor did the patient's fickleness always end here. One correspondent of the Société Royale de Médecine suggested that a peasant might return to the empiric if the physician's first treatment did not work; but then if he were still dissatisfied, or if he suffered an injury at the hands of the unqualified practitioner, he would return to the licensed medical man and demand an instant cure.[8]

The most common pattern, then, was to bring in a physician as a last resort. But it also happened, particularly among better-educated patients, that an empiric or *maige* might be consulted as a final desperate recourse; indeed, some healers specialized in the treatment of patients who had been abandoned by the physicians. At Blanc's trial in the Aube, a farmer's wife described how, when her husband first suffered an attack of fever, he was treated by an *officier de santé*; when the results proved disappointing, she took his urine to the empiric, who confidently informed her that her husband had a liver disease with "glairs" (mucous secretions) and that, as he could plainly read in the urine, the unfortunate man had languished a long time.

As official medical personnel settled in the countryside, a third pattern sometimes appeared: an informal division of labor. Popular practitioners were in some cases preferred for special operations or the treatment of minor injuries. At Fressies (Nord), for example, in the mid-nineteenth century, the physician was rarely consulted for burns, sprains, and fractures; instead the patient sought out an old woman who blew on the injuries, made the sign of the cross, and recited fragments of Scripture.[9] In general, the nineteenth-century physician was less likely to be asked to procure an abortion, treat impotence, or help a recruit escape military service. In more recent times, the official practitioner's function might be to serve as a link with the social security system.[10] Popular and licensed practitioners met different needs.

Often, however, licensed and unlicensed practitioners found themselves competing for the same patients. In the Old Regime, this theme appeared repeatedly in the correspondence of the Société Royale de Médecine and in the reports of the epidemic physicians dispatched to the countryside by the royal intendants. When, for example, the curé of Moncé-en-Belin asked for help during an epidemic in 1767–8, the intendant sent a physician from Le

Mans, who tried to administer free bouillon, bread, and wine; the patients, however, refused his ministrations and maintained their confidence in the local empirics.[11] During an outbreak of dysentery at Saint-Ouen-de-Mimbré, peasants refused physicians' remedies in favor of the empirics' or sometimes took both.[12]

Many empirics, indeed, actively discouraged patients from consulting physicians or interfered with treatments prescribed by official personnel. They might play upon an old and widespread magical belief, which held that either the Christian sacraments or the intervention of official medicine could hinder the working of magical remedies; at the end of the Old Regime, the "witch of Pontorson," in Normandy, "absolutely [forbade] bleeding and purging," according to a contemporary account.[13] More typically they sought (much like the licensed practitioner) to frighten patients away from their rivals. In 1785, during an outbreak of typhus in Brittany, the healer Pellerin alarmed the peasants of Langourla by describing the bad treatment they would receive at the hands of the physicians and by predicting that their cadavers would be opened after their death; they refused to have anything to do with the official personnel.[14] In the 1780's, at Bréal-sous-Montfort, also in Brittany, a urinoscopist opposed to the use of phlebotomy told patients that bleeding would be fatal in their case and suggested that the surgeons might cut their throats.[15] In the early nineteenth century, public health campaigns provoked similar resistance. Vaccination, for example, was opposed not only by some members of the clergy, who saw in it an affront to Providence, but also by empirics, who boasted of having the sole means of preserving the population from the scourge of smallpox.[16]

In some such cases, empirics succeeded in disrupting and even cutting off treatment by official personnel. In the 1780's, at Vieux-Pont in Normandy, a practitioner complained that witches, as he called them, substituted their remedies for his after he had left and inflamed the suspicions of the peasantry.[17] The Comité de Salubrité's questionnaire of 1790 brought a response from Auch denouncing a charlatan who, several years earlier, had arrived at a house where six patients were suffering from mushroom poisoning and had persuaded them to throw out all the remedies provided by a physician.[18] A surgeon who treated an external injury might return for a follow-up visit only to discover that an unlicensed rival had removed his dressing. Thus, in 1818, a Dr. Forlenze, who had been sent into the provinces by the Minister of the Interior to treat eye diseases, found that an oculist named Guibert was following in his wake and interfering with his treatments.[19]

In these encounters, the unlicensed practitioners predictably adopted a hostile stance toward the profession. True, they often called on official medicine to legitimate their own activities and adopted official-sounding titles. Some sought to work under the cover of a licensed practitioner; at the end of the Old Regime, an empiric at Saint-Ouen-de-Mimbré in Brittany even had his son study surgery and then used him as a front for his own practice of urinoscopy.[20] But persisting conflict with the profession forced many healers to follow a different principle: if you can't join them, beat them. And so the empiric claimed to know more than physicians; he might even say, like the celebrated "great sorcerer" of Saint-Dié in the Vosges, that physicians knew absolutely nothing about medicine.[21] The professionals found the invective "venomous," as one health officer put it.[22] One example will suggest the flavor of the criticisms. It comes from a tirade against the medical profession that a woman named Boucher pronounced before her trial at the Royal Court in Paris in 1828:

Who are these tyrants who are crushing me? They have a diploma and that's all; with that they cut, clip, and kill; there is no jail or [charge of] homicide for them. Provided that the cloven hoof does not show, they say *victoria* [a cry of "victory," in Latin], which in plain French means "hee-haw." [Here she imitated the sound of an ass braying.][23]

The healers' defensive sarcasm fairly permeates these trial reports and similar documents; the reader cannot help but be struck by their willingness to dispute with the doctors, point by point, on questions of diagnosis and therapeutics. Consider, for example, the case of Mademoiselle Blanc, an early-nineteenth-century empiric who practiced midwifery and administered a secret remedy (a liqueur of gum benzoin) but also served occasionally as a medical auxiliary. Accused of disobeying a doctor's orders, she impugned the wisdom of the profession. A physician testified that if Blanc was asked to apply leeches to a patient's nose, she put them on the legs. Ordered to place ice on the patient's head, the "female doctor" had placed a bonnet there instead, covered the patient with heavy blankets, administered fumigants, dosed him with her special *liqueur Benjoin*, and then surrounded him with bones and chicken carcasses in order, she said, to purify the air and "remove the putridity." Blanc gave a cocky reply. Ice on the patient's head would have made him consumptive; bathing him, as the doctors recommended, would have killed him.[24]

Empirics invariably ascribed the physicians' animadversions to jealousy and cupidity – much the same motives that the regular practitioners attributed to them. In the early-nineteenth-century Eure, a woman sentenced for illegal practice to several months in jail (where she continued her work undaunted by the authorities) characteristically said that the physicians had had her punished because she took away their patients.[25] In one extreme case, in Paris during the early 1790's, the bonesetter who called himself Valdajou accused the city's surgeons of planning to assassinate him. When he visited his most distinguished patient, the duchesse de Luynes, he took along a bodyguard; and he went so far as to hang conspicuously in his waiting room a suit of clothing that had been pierced by a knife.[26]

Much like the empirics, the professionals evinced an ambivalent attitude toward their rivals. For many, mounting a frontal attack on popular medicine was out of the question, for to do so might alienate the clientele they shared with the empirics. A few physicians were actually said to send patients to healers.[27] More often they simply tolerated popular practices or looked the other way. In the name of calming a patient's anxieties, for example, they might accept that a person bitten by a possibly rabid dog would make a pilgrimage to the shrine of Saint Hubert in the Ardennes.[28] Other practitioners, as has been seen, adopted or pretended to adopt the empirics' methods in order to win a larger following, out of self-interest or perhaps with the sense that the end (public health) justified the means (deception). The surgeon- or apothecary-urinoscopist was not unknown in the Old Regime, and similar cases could be cited for the first half of the nineteenth century.[29] Indeed, physicians who wrote on "abuses in medicine" sometimes counseled practitioners who could not overcome popular beliefs to give the impression of conforming to them in order to win the confidence of uneducated patients – though some stricter colleagues treated this practice as an abuse.[30] François-Emmanuel Fodéré's widely respected treatise on legal medicine enumerated the various advantages enjoyed by charlatans in the competition for a popular clientele (exotic and supposedly infallible remedies, the promise of quick cures, the claims to a healing gift, the willingness to make diagnoses from the inspection of urine without seeing the patient, the use of extravagant and popular language, etc.) and concluded that physicians should imitate not the ignorance of charlatans but their way of sustaining illusions – what we would now call their charisma. Practitioners, he said, needed savoir faire as well as *le savoir* (knowledge, science).[31]

How to read such recommendations? Though they might suggest that the profession could learn something positive from empirics about the healer–patient relationship, an undercurrent of resentment runs not far beneath the surface. With perfect sincerity, the licensed practitioners saw in the business skills of their unlicensed rivals an equal threat to the public weal and to their own livelihood. They believed that the fees they had paid for training and licensure gave them a legal property in medical practice, which empirics degraded or even stole from them. Nor was it simply a matter of principle. So fierce was the unauthorized competition that some regular practitioners were said to have been reduced to indigence.[32]

THE MARKET FOR MEDICAL SERVICES

The physicians' complaints had an objective foundation. In the late eighteenth and early nineteenth centuries, a growing number of practitioners competed in an inelastic market for medical services. Only in the latter nineteenth century did the development of third-party payment schemes (mutual aid societies, insurance, government assistance, and the like), bolstered by rising real salaries, begin to increase substantially the effective demand.

One major question this study has addressed (and a promising topic for future monographic studies) is the relationship of the various types of medical practitioners to the market. The preceding chapters have stressed that although some unauthorized healers practiced out of philanthropy, a great many others – almost certainly the majority of the most active practitioners – relied on medicine as at least an occasional source of income. They typically accepted charity cases as a way of legitimating their activities (even Mesmer had his special tub for the indigent). Thus a woman named Parent, wife of an engineer in Poitou, announced a remedy that was to be available gratis to the poor but would cost 3 francs a pill for people who were well off.[33] Pierre Richard, the "saint" of Savières, distributed remedies with a more liberal hand, maintaining that when he made up a new batch of his ointment, the first patient to use it paid, whereas everyone who followed received it without charge.[34]

By all accounts, though, few empirics had anything like a regular fee schedule. Some, like the joiner Druau, who practiced dentistry, had their own version of a sliding scale: they simply accepted what was offered. The operator Boulogne, after working on a fistula or wen, would say, "Give me what you like." In one case he reportedly received about 100 francs; in another, 48. Falot, the Grand Chevalier de Saint Hubert, used a similar approach; in one recorded case, the patients paid 20 sous apiece.[35] Testimony was sometimes contradictory, suggesting that a practitioner may have asked for or accepted money inconsistently. In the case of Dame Blanche, some witnesses said that she took money and others not; a few stated that she requested money for her horse.[36]

Some healers were paid only in kind, presumably because many of their peasant patients had nothing else to offer (in the countryside, even a regular practitioner might have to accept gifts of produce or butter in lieu of money), and perhaps also in some cases because a stigma was attached to cash remuneration.[37] A practitioner reported in 1786 at "Cheveigné" (Chavagne?) in Brittany collected his fees in the form of pots of cider.[38] The noble Kermelle, mentioned in Ernest Renan's memoirs of his childhood, did not wish to be paid for his medical services but freely accepted various small offerings: a dozen eggs, a piece of lard, a handful of flax, butter, potatoes, or fruit. Some practitioners asked directly for such a fee. It is reported, for example, that one healer in the Sologne region, after treating a patient, would simply announce, "ce s'ra quatre p'tits gâtiaux" (that will be four little cakes).[39] The most exigent could empty a household of a sizable part of a family's belongings. It was said at Mende (Lozère) in the 1790's that "the value of the goods that one is obliged to bring to [empirics] would more than pay for consultations with good physicians and surgeons."[40]

Other practitioners, though, and not just itinerant mountebanks, asked for fees in money. The charges varied widely, but they were usually less than the sums that licensed practitioners required. Toward the end of the Old Regime, Nicolas Clément, a knight of Saint Hubert, asked 9 livres, 10 sous, for treating four patients.[41] In the mid-nineteenth century, a woman at Fressies (Nord) asked 10 francs for blowing on sprains and fractures. Pierron of Orist (Landes), who prescribed remedies against witchcraft spells, charged the same.[42]

If the popular practitioners had simply undersold the profession, physicians might have been able to understand and even accept them (as occasionally happened) as a cut-rate service providing inferior medical care to the lower classes. But their charges sometimes ran much higher. A *désensorceleur* might play on his clients' intense fears of witchcraft to extract substantial sums, warning that if his services were not accepted, the entire family might fall ill and perish. At the end of the eighteenth century, a farrier at Beaugency in the Loiret asked 100 écus for treating a miller's supposedly bewitched wife.[43] In the early nineteenth century, a shepherd-*devin* in the department of the Eure received 200 francs for "healing" a farmer by supposedly extracting a sinister beast from his stomach.[44] Transactions with rural healers and counterwitches could involve hardheaded negotiations, in which a client would have to bargain as he might for the purchase of a draft animal, a piece of land, or the services of a hired hand. The old works on popular healers that stress their mercenary activities contain a large element of truth.

Special operators and empirics could also exact high fees. In the 1770's, for example, hernia operators in Languedoc asked 30 livres for their services, and a Madame Vacherot submitted a bill for 790 livres after treating the daughter of a modest noble (*écuyer*). Some of the lieutenants of the King's First Surgeon who responded in the survey of 1790–1791 also commented on what they considered the high cost of empirical healing under the Old Regime. At the beginning of the new century, an itinerant empiric at Caen sold his remedies at 710 francs a pound; and in the early years of the Restoration, a girl suffering from scrofula who lodged *en pension* at the establishment of a Parisian empiric named Gérard accumulated a bill of 605 francs, of which her family could pay only somewhat more than half.[45]

Clearly, charges of this magnitude could cause serious hardship. According to one of the informants of the Comité de Salubrité, the fees of the farrier at Beaugency were so high that patients were forced to go into debt in order to pay him.[46] In eighteenth-century Dauphiné, a peasant suffering from difficulty in urinating was persuaded by an empiric to sell a piece of land in order to purchase his very expensive remedy. Similarly, it was reported that the Mazureau sisters, who practiced medicine at Nantes in the early nineteenth century and demanded a major financial commitment from their patients, forced some of them to sell their furniture to pay the bill.[47] One empiric active at Paris in the early years of the Restoration even threatened to send the bailiff when his patients neglected to make the exorbitant payment that he required.[48] Somehow, empirics were able to screw money fees out of artisans, laborers, sharecroppers, and others of very modest means, many of whom appeared to contemporary observers to be almost dying of hunger to begin with.[49] The result of these depredations, according to one regular practitioner, was that the patients could not pay their taxes or meet "the most pressing needs of their family."[50]

Why did patients, including members of social groups notorious for their stinginess and reluctance to pay physicians, willingly part with such large sums of money? Desperation may explain a good deal. But it is worth stressing one major feature that often distinguished the economic transaction between empiric and client from the usual doctor–patient relationship. The physician charged for visits and other professional services, whatever the outcome. The sedentary empiric's patient typically paid for a cure. The two parties sometimes drew up a formal contract, often including a money-back guarantee, and it was the failure to honor such a compact that got some empirics into trouble with the law.[51] In 1806 a laborer at Bléneau (Yonne) named Cheuillot struck a bargain with Marguerite Satiat, wife of Jean Bernard, a farrier from the hamlet of Tricotets, to heal her ailing husband for a fee of 66 francs, agreeing to return 27 francs if he failed. Cheuillot practically extorted the payment, warning the woman that if she did not deliver the money, her husband would soon die and the same illness would afflict other members of the household. The negotiations started at an inn and continued at the home of another laborer, until eventually Satiat paid over 37 francs 80 centimes and agreed to remit the remaining 28 francs 20 centimes on her first return trip. Cheuillot, for his part, was obliged to treat her husband until a "perfect cure" was obtained and promised to return 27 francs if he failed.[52]

In popular medicine, the contract and the exchange of money could also have more than economic significance. The healer might, for example, magically link the payment to the patient by fixing the fee at the same number of money units as the patient's age in years; thus the empiric Sibenaler charged 57 francs in one case and 34 in another. In the second case the money was to be wrapped in linen and put in Sibenaler's magic book without his seeing it – a procedure suggesting the fear that money might contaminate the healing ritual.[53]

Such payments might amount to a comfortable income; it has been seen that the successful empiric could live from his practice and even, in exceptional cases, grow rich, like the urinoscopist Schmitt, or the empiric Hey-rauld, who became so prosperous that a neighbor asked that his assessment for the *taille* be increased. In the mid-nineteenth century, a traveling charlatan visiting the Hautes-Alpes was said to have earned 900 francs in eight days.[54] Even a local *maige* could make a decent living if he was enterprising. A *saludador* in the Pyrénées-Orientales prospered by selling subscriptions around the department to persons who wished to receive his services in the event of an attack by a rabid wolf or dog.[55] Later in the nineteenth century, a *toucheur* in Normandy, whose income as a worker was small, was able to earn 2,000 francs a year from his medical practice.[56]

In the moral economy of the medical old regime, a healer was entitled to a just recompense for his services; his claim may have been even more compelling than that of the qualified practitioner, because his need was so much greater. When the owner of a secret remedy against epilepsy, a peasant of Beaulieu near Parthenay in Poitou, advertised his specific in 1775, he announced that he was "flattered to be able to help humanity in this way," but that he also required "something, a very little something," for his efforts.[57] For many practitioners and remedy sellers, medicine provided an indispensable supplement to an otherwise inadequate income. The empiric Suzov, appealing to the Minister of the Interior for official approbation within a week of the adoption of the law of Ventôse, argued that medical practice was all he had left to support his family. A farrier made a similar plea to the Société Royale de Médecine in 1782: his costs were much higher than before the war of American independence, and yet he was lucky to get the old price for his work.[58] Many other such examples could be cited.

That medical practice met an economic need was recognized by all; in the debate over professional monopoly, even hardened opponents of empiricism stopped to consider whether the very real plight of some occasional healers could override the interests of public health. A surgeon at Gacé in Normandy complained to the Société Royale in 1789 about Martin d'A-vrigny, who he said practiced quack medicine; and yet he was willing to allow him to continue selling topical (external) remedies, since this trade was comparatively safe and "each individual must have a livelihood."[59] Similarly the mayor of Seignelay in the Yonne, who in 1818 reported a Polish woman who had been practicing urinoscopy, did not wish to prevent her from finding a means of support.[60] The argument that poor people should not be prevented from earning a living remained an obstacle to the repression of illegal medical practice well into the nineteenth century.[61] Too often, no ready alternative was available. As one respondent to the Comité de Salubrité's survey noted, there were those "who have no other resource for living than the knowledge of a few medicaments or secrets suitable for curing a number of illnesses."[62]

Clearly, not all practitioners were involved in the market for medical services in the same way or to the same degree. For many contemporary observers, just as for later historians and sociologists of medicine, a particular relationship to the market helped define the typical physician, charlatan, and folk healer. At least in principle, the physician's corporate privileges in the Old Regime, or the profession's postrevolutionary legal monopoly, should have placed licensed practitioners outside the frenzied competition of the open market. The professional ethos required that a physician live respectably from his legal property in his practice, like a sort of rentier; the immediate object of his practice was to provide a service to suffering humanity, rather than to increase his wealth. This normative characterization of the professional role has informed many modern definitions of the professions.[63]

The charlatan, in contrast, was an entrepreneur. His tricks might seem like an elaborate confidence game, which of course in a way they were; but these were the marketing techniques used by tradesmen in the Old Regime who operated outside the restrictions (and protection) of the guilds. The charlatan had to find ways to extract money from a clientele that had little cash and did not part with it easily. In both eighteenth- and nineteenth-century rhetoric on medical empiricism, quacks were sometimes described, appropriately, as *industriels*.[64] The term carried unsavory connotations. An old expression, "*vivre d'industrie*," meant to live by one's wits, and *chevaliers d'industrie* were essentially charlatans: people without property who made a living by practicing dishonest skills. Littré's dictionary cites a line from Jean-François Regnard, the seventeenth-century comic playwright: "Faute de revenu, je vis de l'industrie" (for lack of income, I live by my wits).[65] (From the French, this term passed into English. The swindlers in Herman Melville's *Confidence Man* are "chevaliers" – that is, *chevaliers d'industrie*, among them an herb doctor who in Melville's allegory stands for the Devil.) It is perhaps this sense of the word that the prefect of the Escaut, a department carved out of annexed Belgian territory, had in mind when he spoke in 1810 of police surveillance established to prevent empirics from "practicing their fatal industry."[66] But "*industriel*" could also mean industrialist, and nineteenth-century observers recognized medical empiricism as a form of entrepreneurship; thus the author of a thesis on charlatanism published in 1868 expressed the hope that with widespread education, "industrial genius will shift its activity to a less fatal terrain than public health."[67]

The activities of many local healers, finally, fell into the domain of what contemporary observers called *l'économie domestique*, the daily management of the household in a traditional society.[68] The paterfamilias healed his own family and perhaps a few neighbors. The gifted folk healer worked among a wider circle, but he did not solicit custom; to borrow another expression

from the nineteenth-century rhetoric, he was not *entreprenant* (enterprising).
As in the case of charitable healing by local notables, his activities may have
owed more to considerations of tradition and prestige than to economic
need. This would appear to be a case in which, as Karl Polanyi has put it,
"man's economy . . . is submerged in his social relationships"; self-treatment
is of course a still better illustration of the place of medicine in Polanyi's
oeconomia.[69] The anthropologist Robert Redfield's conception of the "folk
society" may also come to mind: an economically independent culture in
which economic activity is pursued primarily in order to gain social
recognition.[70]

According to this way of thinking, then, the relation of the various
practitioners to the market may be simplified as follows:

Traditional economy	Corporatism	Market economy
Folk healers	Physicians	Empirics

But for reasons that should by now be apparent, this model is not entirely
satisfactory. Recent work in the sociology of the professions has pointed
to the discrepancy between the physicians' service ideal and the objective
effect of their legal privileges, which is not to place them outside the market
for medical services, but to enable them to secure control over it, the better
to exploit it.[71] This contention has proved controversial, as indeed it deserves
to be if it ignores the dedication of most physicians to their patients and
the degree to which their authority derives from their real power to alleviate
human suffering. But the point is one that many French physicians would
have understood, and probably accepted, in the early nineteenth century.
They saw themselves as competing with unqualified practitioners for a
limited medical market; what they demanded was a monopoly of "this sort
of industrial property," as the health council of Laval wrote in 1810, "which
the law grants us as a just recompense for licenses and the tax on business
[the *patente*, which physicians, unlike salaried workers, had to pay]."[72] As
for the folk healers, the last chapter has suggested just how ambiguous a
category that is. In truth, the village was not completely dissociated from
the market, and no pure folk society existed in eighteenth-century France.

Moreover the tripartite model cannot easily accommodate those occasional practitioners who were neither full-time empirics nor neighborly old
wives who knew some traditional lore. For most of them, medicine was
simply a source of supplementary income; some were victims of severe
economic dislocation and found themselves with no secure niche in either
the traditional or more modern economic sectors. Often unsuccessful artisans, the occasionals might mix various *petits métiers*, from peddling to
music teaching; the least successful were floaters and drifters. Even the ranks
of the itinerant charlatans and unlicensed surgeons included practitioners

who were less entrepreneurs than displaced persons, like the foreigners who roamed France peddling drugs and housewares, or the half-trained army surgeons from the Napoleonic wars who tried to establish themselves as health officers.

The following hypothesis is worth exploring: if the successful empirics exploited the possibilities available to those willing and able to take risks in early capitalist societies, linking the hinterland to the mercantile centers where they bought their drugs, many of the part-time practitioners were victims of economic change, overwhelmed by the same tides that raised their happier brethren to prosperity. The fluctuations of the market economy accentuated these trends. In good times, the entrepreneurs grew fat on the wealth of the land; in hard times, the number of marginal practitioners multiplied as the poor sought a source of income in one makeshift after another.

MEDICAL PRACTITIONERS AND SOCIETY

The tripartite schema of folk healer, quack, and physician implies a set of social as well as economic relationships. The folk healer belongs to the local community, and his prestige depends on a body of shared assumptions and values in popular culture; the quack is almost by definition an outsider, whose prestige depends on his exoticism; and the physician, though he may reside in the countryside and may even have been born there, is identified with the urban-bourgeois values of the university where he trained. The preceding chapters have suggested some of the limitations of such a model; it has no room for *maige*-like healers who are clearly outsiders, for local empirics with established reputations, or for surgeons and *officiers de santé* who shared the speech, manners, and some of the outlook of their peasant patients.

In one sense, then, the model is too simple. But in another sense, it is not simple enough. Whatever their legal status, the medical practitioners' occupation placed them at a fault line where local communities in a still predominantly rural society met an emerging national culture dominated by urban elites. Most were in some respect outsiders. If the university graduate who practiced in the countryside often remained a distrusted foreigner, so did the active irregular practitioner in the eyes of the authorities and the enlightened elites, who branded him (or her) a deviant or even a savage. Curiously, some of the physicians shared with their rivals (who might hold quite dissimilar views of health and disease and of medicine as an occupation) the sense that they were not fully accepted and that they had implacably hostile enemies. These practitioners seem to have suffered the pain and inner conflict that come from a failure of integration, in the sense of harmonious coordination of behavior and personality with the environment. How could it have been otherwise when their environment transmitted such contradictory messages?

For obvious reasons, rural physicians were better able than their unlicensed counterparts to articulate their sense of dislocation. We have virtually no records of the inner feelings of empirics and healers in the era before ethnographic interviews. What does emerge from many contemporary descriptions by educated observers is a common perception of empirics as misfits and people out of place. Even allowing for exaggeration by hostile witnesses, their ranks included a disproportionate number of social marginals and deviants – though it was not always clear whether their medical practice contributed to making them eccentrics or whether (as seems more probable) an established pattern of nonconformity made them likelier candidates for unauthorized medical practice. It was not only that they typically lacked a recognized *état* (station/occupation) or that they were guilty of unauthorized medical practice, which might include such associated crimes as procuring abortions or castrating hernia victims. From the point of view of the authorities and the social elites, the healer was often a *mauvais sujet* or even a threat to "law and order" (a term of ancient provenance).

Active empirics were commonly described as drunkards, like Deschamp in eighteenth-century Brittany, who was said to be "drunk night and day," or a self-styled baron at Écury-le-Repos in the nineteenth-century Marne, who reportedly was constantly intoxicated. Corbiot, a practitioner denounced as a charlatan at Saint-Sauvant (Charente-Maritime), was not only "drunk from morning to evening" (according to a local health officer), but also had the bad taste to keep company with the executioner of the town of Saintes.[73] An empiric named Noël, tried for illegal medical practice in 1827, was an ecclesiastic who had been interdicted for drunkenness.[74] In one mid-nineteenth-century case, a village schoolteacher who had been fired because (among other things) he healed with magic formulas, was accused of contributing to drunkenness in others by selling cheap brandy and inciting his pupils to drink.[75] (Characteristically, popular thinking sometimes inverted these values; a healer might have the reputation of being effective only, or especially, when drunk.)[76]

Some prominent healers notoriously compounded drunkenness with sexual dissipation. The Lany woman in Champagne, according to the report of the intendant's subdelegate at Troyes, was not merely given to drink, sometimes tippling with her patients. She had also "been debauched as much as her age and face allowed and prostitutes her little girl who lives with her."[77] (This last practice, it need hardly be added, was another example of an economic makeshift.) A healer's "debauchery" or sexual deviance could bring him or her into conflict with the Church, as well as the secular authorities. In 1784, for example, the Société Royale de Médecine received a complaint from the curé of Saint-Georges-de-Rouelley, near Domfront in Normandy, passed on by the Superior General of the Eudists, accusing Jean Haurée, an illegal practitioner of surgery, of having abandoned his wife and living in concubinage with a woman named Madeleine Heusé, who had borne him four children.[78]

Other deviant healers were thought insane, like Bichat Potin of the Cher, an interdicted priest who lived in destitution and whose "mental exaltation had become close to madness."[79] Similar cases, like that of the empiric and sanatorium manager Tissot, have appeared in earlier chapters. As one leafs through the police records on unauthorized medical practice, or the petitions sent to the government and to medical bodies by private individuals convinced that they had discovered a radical new treatment for previously incurable diseases, it is impossible to escape the impression that something in medicine irresistibly attracted people who would now be labeled paranoid schizophrenics, manic-depressives, or borderline personalities. All shared to some degree delusions of grandeur and persecution. One seemingly paranoid hat finisher from Montpellier submitted this communication to the revolutionary National Convention (2 Floréal Year II or 21 April 1794):

I am sending to the National Convention the addresses that I delivered at Montpellier on the 20th Nivôse and 20th Ventôse in the temple of reason and truth, and following [that] a supplement on the quackeries, impostures, and the way in which the great trickster [enguseur = engueuseur], the late [Pope] Clement XIII, tricked me, and how his agents deceived me and despised me, and how the late Manoël Pinto Gram, Master of Malta, with his followers, detained me and robbed me with impunity of what I had won with sword in hand and by the sweat of my labors.

And on the discovery of remedies to cure perfectly and promptly, at little expense, wounds and other illnesses, with which I have had a long and successful experience. Remedies are ready. I ask to [be allowed to] act in the hospitals, with the choice of doctors and others whom I know to be honest and pure patriots, who will be witnesses of the experiment. You will find there a part of my naval and military talents, which I offer with my life to the Fatherland.

Salut et fraternité[80]

It is not clear how successfully the mad hatter of Montpellier practiced empirical medicine, but the medical activities of many similar practitioners enjoyed popular toleration and even a reputation for inspiration. It was accepted that healers were sometimes odd; their medical practice, although it compounded their delinquency in the authorities' view, seems paradoxically to have helped reintegrate them into the community. The same may have been true of practitioners who suffered from physical abnormalities and handicaps; medical practice could serve, for example, to increase the self-sufficiency of the blind.[81] Empirical medicine had room for the misfits and the outcasts – even for such unfortunates as the pseudohermaphrodite Marie-Madeline Lefort (d. 1864), well known in nineteenth-century Paris medical circles, who, despite a long experience of menstruation, adopted a masculine identity and earned a living as a charlatan.[82]

It usually took more than odd or unusual behavior to make a *mauvais sujet*. Many of the economic makeshifts associated with popular medicine were illegal or at least frowned upon by the authorities. An empiric denounced in the 1770's by a practitioner at Saint-Quentin was a former smuggler; the sometime domestic of an orvietan peddler who set himself up as a surgeon in the Haute-Loire in 1817 supported himself in part by poaching. In the Ardèche, an empiric named Antoine Dury was convicted of vagrancy and carrying prohibited weapons, and Pierre Abel, convicted of illegal medical practice, was also charged with peddling without a license, violating the passport law, poaching, and insulting and resisting the authority of the police. (Abel was also said to be a deserter.)[83] Swindling and petty thievery were still more common. No doubt many occasional practitioners did not get into trouble with the law, but the behavior of their more disreputable colleagues did much to give the world of popular medicine its distinctive atmosphere.

In the minds of the ever suspicious local authorities, petty criminality always threatened to spill over into some more serious threat to public order. When the Italian Saqui appeared in the Eure-et-Loire in 1797 with a troupe of sixteen persons, the local commissioner of the Directory observed: "Considering that the numerous retinue of Monsieur Saqui . . . makes it hard to believe that the sale of his drugs alone could suffice for his support, he may reasonably be suspected of having some mission foreign to his apparent profession."[84] Crime? Fomenting unrest? During the Restoration, the empiric Boulogne in the Var was rumored to have attacked the government and was suspected of being an "emissary of ill will."[85] At Toucy in the Yonne, a band of charlatans who visited the town in 1821 aroused suspicions by spreading absurd and "criminal" political rumors.[86] The seemingly most innocuous healer could become politically suspect; thus the curé of Givry in the Yonne, who (according to his own account at least) had treated patients free of charge for forty years, found himself incriminated under the Restoration by a forged laudatory certificate, which supposedly came from the mayor of Blannay, but which he had in fact acquired from a certain Lappertot – a revolutionary and notorious schemer who claimed to be attached to the Order of Malta, the subprefect of Avallon reported.[87]

Government officials expressed particular concern over the influence of popular healers on military recruitment. One source of income for a small-time entrepreneur in the early nineteenth century was to find substitutes (*remplaçants*) for young men who had been called for military service; under this perfectly legal arrangement, the substitute received a fee, and the agent who arranged the contract would pocket a commission. But the authorities feared that unscrupulous agents might defraud their clients or the army itself, and the prefects looked askance at empirics who diversified their activities and began recruiting substitutes.[88] Worse yet, a popular healer might sell a spurious medical certificate exempting the conscript from service, or even help him simulate a disease in order to obtain a medical discharge. The empiric Sibenaler, for example, was prosecuted at Rochefort (Maine-et-Loire) for having told a young man called up for military service to swallow sheep's blood mixed with milk, so that he might spit it up at his medical examination and appear consumptive.[89]

In this last case, the popular practitioners and their clientele clearly formed a deviant community, united in their opposition to conscription. This was only one of a number of ways in which a healer's delinquent behavior may have enhanced his appeal and paradoxically reinforced the ties that bound him to his neighbors. Not just drunkards but also ex-convicts were said to enjoy special prestige as healers, together with marginals whose eccentric behavior might lead to rumors of witchcraft and commerce with demons.[90] "In the countryside," wrote Victor Hugo, "the more suspect the physician is, the more certain the remedy is."[91]

Still, no simple model can adequately encompass the extraordinary social diversity of popular medical practice. If for some healers medicine represented a traditionally sanctioned role in a seemingly stable village culture, perhaps reinforced by collective resistance to outsiders, for others it was a response to stress, to dislocation, and to loss. If some healers won a large following, other healing careers ended – usually sooner rather than later – in failure.

The archives have little to say about the experience of the failures, although the literate ones and those who could manage to hire the services of a scrivener sometimes had their say. They painted themselves as pathetic figures, victims of change; loss of a job, depressed earnings, widowhood, or old age might have driven them to practice medicine. They left a trace of their existence precisely because they did not receive adequate support from their communities and turned elsewhere for help. These people have not received much attention; when they appear in the literature, it has typically been their role to divert the reader, like the charlatans whose encounters with the criminal justice system the *Gazette des tribunaux* so sardonically recounted. To be sure, their petitions were self-serving, larded with conventional phrases meant to win the reader's sympathy; no doubt they contained many lies. They nevertheless deserve sympathetic historical consideration. Not that we should celebrate their healing powers or call for a return to the good old days of domestic and amateur medicine; if that myth still needs discrediting, this book surely contributes to the task. But if popular medicine unquestionably had its victims, the popular healers might often be called victims themselves.

MEDICAL PRACTICE AND SOCIAL CHANGE

The social interpretation of popular healing outlined here can be generalized and extended over time and space. The old literature on charlatanism held that quacks are always with us. Some men and women will always be deceivers; the populace wishes to be deceived (*vulgus vult decipi*); and so charlatanism always flourishes. No doubt it does. And yet the forms and incidence of irregular medical practice have not remained constant. Why did empirics thrive when and where they did, and why in particular was the early modern period in Europe a "golden age of quackery," as it has sometimes been called?

In its broadest terms, the analysis developed here suggests that medical empiricism has been a liminal phenomenon: charlatans prospered in what we now see as a transition stage between an older agricultural society (in which the medical market was virtually nonexistent) and contemporary industrial societies with their modern medical marketplace, which, thanks to government subsidies, includes practically everyone. Classic charlatanism arose in an era of mercantile capitalism in the commercial centers, market towns, and fairs of the Old Regime. Quackery, moreover, has always drawn much of its strength from the imperfect contact of city and country, from the existence of a frontier. In the nineteenth century, in France and elsewhere, empirics regularly turned up at the urban–rural interface – in the American West, for example, or the Russian steppes. The itinerant shuttled back and forth between city and town, town and village, bringing the medical market to the countryside. His patients became accustomed to paying for specialized health care; in a sense, illegal medical practice was, as Jacques Léonard has put it, "an advanced post of medicalization."[92]

In western Europe, the old-style mountebank slowly declined in the nineteenth century, though other remedy vendors increasingly exploited the periodical press to promote patent medicines. In an era of mass marketing, the old itinerant became obsolete; the repression of illegal practice, the greater accessibility of official medicine, and perhaps also increasing popular skepticism hastened his passing from the scene. It is also possible that those who might earlier have supported themselves as empirics found other careers in a diversified regional or national economy with improved opportunities for both entrepreneurship and salaried labor.

Folk medicine, predictably, continued to flourish longest in isolated and economically backward regions such as Brittany or Appalachia in America, although (as ethnographic studies have confirmed) traditional medicine can be imported to the city, together with other folkways, and prosper there so long as immigrant groups maintain their cultural identity.[93] But even rural society changes, and the status of the folk healer, despite some striking survivals, has become increasingly marginal.[94] This transition deserves further study. Some evidence suggests, for example, that the trend did not proceed irreversibly in one direction. Several ethnographic investigations carried out in France during the first half of the present century indicate that in certain regions healers became more numerous and more active after World War I – in lower Maine, for example, and in Berry.[95] Such findings cannot now be verified, but they are not implausible or inexplicable; whatever their numbers, healers may well have become more visible and more accessible both to patients and to outside observers. Modern technologies in communication and transportation that in the long run contributed to eradicating traditional medicine may have had the paradoxical short-term effect of making its adepts easier to reach.

Although the discussion here has been largely restricted to France, the analysis could apply to other Western societies and probably to many non-Western ones as well. The extensive literature on American frontier doctors, snake oil peddlers, and "powwow" and "yarb" doctors is generally more anecdotal than analytic; and yet, if one fits the pieces together, a consistent pattern emerges, comprising folk healers, urban empirics, and itinerants who passed from an urban economy where they bought their drugs to a rural society in which they hawked their wares and practiced medicine.[96] It is more difficult to generalize about non-Western cases, but broadly speaking, the more urbanized agricultural societies developed elaborate medical systems, whereas less developed village cultures did not. The Zande witch doctor described in Evans-Pritchard's famous study was not a medical specialist or even a figure of great prestige.[97] But a medical network resembling that of Old Regime France can be found, for example, in modern Nigeria. In Ibadan, Hausa barber-surgeons, who practice bloodletting and cupping and other operations, are organized into a guild. "Native doctors" offer to cure disorders ranging from ruptures to witches' spells; vendors hawk proprietary remedies in the streets. Yoruba materia medica – sea sand, chameleons, "fairy bones," and much more – are sold at the principal markets, where jugglers attract customers, as in early modern Europe. Medical practice also provides a livelihood for traditional healers – *onishegun* (mainly herbalists) and *babalawo* (priests of the Ifa cult, who rely on divination). Slightly more than half of these practitioners are outsiders, somewhat resembling our displaced healers. Northern India, too, has its quacks, barbers, and bonesetters, and medical practitioners in Imperial China included soothsayers, geomancers, fortune tellers, oculists, aurists, dentists, herbalists, cuppers, barber-masseurs, and various species of empirics.[98] Many of these trades still flourish in contemporary Taiwan, where the government tolerated them until 1975.[99] Moreover, in China and India, together with a number of Islamic countries that follow the Yunani (Arabic-Persian) medical tradition, learned practitioners of classical medicine professionalized their calling in ways that paralleled the experience of their Western counterparts.[100] More work needs to be done along these lines; the comparative study of medicine as an occupation remains largely undeveloped, in contrast to the increasingly sophisticated work that ethnologists and others have produced on health care as a cultural system.[101]

Analogies between Western and non-Western medical systems, however, should not be pressed too far. Even very similar medical practices can take on very different meanings, depending on the context in which they occur and the range of alternatives available to the patient. The witch doctor and the *maige* are not interchangeable; one of the defining characteristics of the latter was that he or she was not a physician. Nor is the European physician the exact equivalent of the learned practitioner in regions where the Chinese, Ayurvedic, or Yunani medical traditions remain strong, whether the latter practices indigenous or modern medicine or some combination of the two. It is important, too, to beware of the temptation to see all societies as passing ineluctably by stages from *maige* to empiric to physician, as Europe might appear to have done; China is one obvious counterexample.[102] The point of the comparison is not to suggest that all medical systems have followed the same path to modernity, but rather that both their similarities and their differences say something about the societies, economies, and polities in which they evolved. The exercise will have served its purpose if it reminds us that the various forms of popular medicine are products not simply of a universal human willingness to be deceived but also of specific historical conditions; and that what we need in the end is not a new model of popular medicine but a comparative social history of healing in all its forms.

AFTERWORD: MEDICALIZATION AND SOCIAL THEORY

If one takes the long view of the changes described in this book – the consolidation of a new medical profession, the redefinition of the boundaries between official and popular medicine, and the slow decline of old forms of popular healing (together with the rise of new ones, such as patent remedies advertised in mass-circulation newspapers) – it is tempting to conclude that the development of the medical profession and what the French call "medicalization" (the increasing use of professional medical services) should be considered epiphenomena of something much more fundamental: the modernization of traditional society. The discussion in Chapter 6 emphasized urbanization and the growth of the market economy; other accounts of professionalism have associated it with the social and economic processes that accompanied the Industrial Revolution[1] or pointed to such indices of modernity as role specialization and scientific rationality. In traditional society (according to this last view), healing was one of several diffuse roles that almost anyone could adopt; in modern society, consultants provide highly specialized services in return for cash payment. In traditional society, the healer's status as practitioner depended on personal prestige and the sanction of the local community; in modern society, it depends on objective criteria of competence. (In Talcott Parsons's parlance, the physician's role has shifted from "particularistic ascribed" structuring to "universalistic achievement.")[2] A double dynamic is at work here. The same forces that promoted the rise of professionalism simultaneously doomed the traditional roles and practices that it replaced. In nineteenth-century rural France, schools, roads, railroads, military service – indeed, anything that promoted contact between the village and the outside world – helped break down traditional patterns of behavior among the peasantry, while introducing more modern urban values and facilitating access to new goods and services. We might even speculate that as economic development provided greater opportunities for salaried employment, occasional medical practice became less attractive as a way to eke out an otherwise meager income.

Such an interpretation is suggestive. But is it adequate? In recent years, modernization theory, already the target of serious criticism among social theorists,[3] has come under fire from historians of nineteenth-century France. As a global description, it slights the distinctive experiences of the various regions. The pace of development was not everywhere the same; clearly the industrial department of the Nord was not the Morbihan.[4] Moreover, the strongest versions of the theory suggest that modern economic, cultural, and political phenomena (industry, scientific rationalism, democracy) develop in tandem; but in nineteenth-century France, which, despite the emergence of industry, was still primarily a society of peasants and artisans, the partners were out of step with each other. As one historian has put it, "the Republic of the future appealed to the society of the past."[5] Any theory, finally, that presents political, cultural, and social development as flowing naturally from technological and economic change tends to discount or even trivialize politics, depreciating the role of human choice and conflict in historical change.[6]

Clearly, these objections apply to any simple model of the rise of modern medicine. On the first point: to trace the medicalization of the population of France would require detailed local investigations of patients' use of hospitals and physicians' services, particularly in the latter nineteenth century. The experience of, say, a company town with physicians practicing under contract would obviously be radically different from that of a region like the rural Seine-et-Oise.[7] Nor is it hard to find examples in medicine of the coexistence of tradition and modernity; thus prescientific views of the body and disease seem almost ineradicable even in contemporary society. More important, profession and society did not evolve pari passu. The medical profession emerged in a still mainly traditional and rural society; modernization generated medical careers far faster than it swelled the demand for medical services. In response, the physicians, with government support, undertook a "civilizing mission" among the French population that strikingly resembled the efforts of their colleagues who worked as colonial medical officers overseas.[8] This observation brings us to the final point: a medical network based on universalistic achievement did not evolve without conflict, and any account of its development must embrace politics. Physicians battled unqualified practitioners for the limited resources of a popular clientele.

Indeed, the most conspicuous mutations in the relationship of popular and official medicine in France during the latter eighteenth and early nineteenth centuries were essentially political: they produced an ideology of professional power and new laws and institutions that promoted professional monopoly. These changes were not in themselves sufficient to bring about the medicalization of the population, which owed more to later developments, such as mass education, urbanization, and economic growth (together with new systems of third-party payments to physicians and hospitals), but they determined the shape that the future medical network would take. The changing conceptions of the medical field and the profession's struggle to control it will form the subject of another book.

APPENDIX A: DENSITY OF FRENCH MEDICAL PERSONNEL IN THE NINETEENTH CENTURY

Calculating the density of medical personnel in nineteenth-century France is an enterprise fraught with difficulty. In theory it should have been much easier than in the Old Regime to say how many practitioners France had, since, under title 4 of the law of Ventôse, each medical man was required to register his credentials with both the tribunal of his arrondissement and his subprefecture. The *commissaire du gouvernement* of the tribunal would then compile a list of practitioners and send it to the Minister of Justice; the subprefect, for his part, would transmit the data he received to the prefect, who would draw up and publish a list for the department and send a copy to the Minister of the Interior.[1] But no penalty was attached to failure to register, and in fact this material is both incomplete and unreliable (credentials were not necessarily correctly reported); the documentation for the period of the Restoration is particularly thin. To compound the problem, even the quinquennial censuses of the total French population, which began in 1801, are not entirely reliable.[2]

Starting in the second third of the century, the picture becomes somewhat brighter. The national census improved from 1831 on, and under the July Monarchy, the government made several efforts to count medical practitioners more systematically. The first successful attempt to compile data for the entire country came in 1847, the work of the Minister of Public Instruction, Salvandy, who was preparing a bill on medical practice; this material has been analyzed by George Sussman.[3] Even these figures, however, leave much to be desired. Better (though still imperfect) statistics are available for the second half of the century, when regular lists of practitioners were drawn up every five years to coincide with the quinquennial census.[4]

Given the inadequacies of the data, particularly for the earlier part of the century, the only way to arrive at a fully accurate count would be to reconstruct lists of practitioners through a painstaking comparison of the official registration reports with a great variety of other sources, such as registers of professional *patentes* and reports by departmental medical juries.

With the help of a computer, Jacques Léonard has compiled and analyzed such lists for six departments of western France (Côtes-du-Nord, Finistère, Ille-et-Vilaine, Loire-Inférieure, Mayenne, and Morbihan).[5] Although a few other studies have considered the density of medical personnel in individual departments or districts, no work of comparable scope, detail, and rigor exists for other parts of France.

With these caveats in mind, it is still possible, by using the quinquennial census reports and the statistics of the Ministry of the Interior and the prefects, to get a sense of how widely the density of medical personnel varied from one part of France to another. Table 5, which is based primarily on an early and incomplete national survey of medical practitioners (1834), gives the densities of practitioners by department in the 1830's and confirms the familiar pattern of low levels of medicalization in the West and high levels in the South; it should be compared with the findings of Léonard for the West and Sussman for the mid–1840's. The source does not allow a systematic comparison of all the various types of practitioner in the different departments. (Most responses broke practitioners down into Old Regime physicians; surgeons who had been licensed under the Old Regime to practice anywhere; surgeons who had been licensed to practice locally by a lieutenant or community; new medical doctors; new doctors of surgery; health officers licensed under article 23; and health officers received by a jury. Others, however, simply counted physicians and health officers, and a few introduced other variations.) The contrasts are nonetheless striking. Health officers licensed under the law of Ventôse, who nationwide made up about half of medical practitioners, constituted more than two-thirds in at least 11 out of the 86 French departments, but less than a third in another 10. The two departments with the highest proportion of health officers (the Hautes-Pyrénées and the Gers, with 77.3 and 76.1 percent, respectively) had unusually high overall densities of practitioners – though the Oise, with 74.3 percent, and the Pas-de-Calais, with 73.7, did not. Exceptionally low percentages appeared in the Seine (10.7) and the Aveyron (12.7, though another 10.4 percent were described simply as surgeons).

Table 5. *Densities of French medical practitioners by department, 1830's*

Department	Density[a]	Department	Density[a]
Ain	n.a.	Loir-et-Cher	3.83
Aisne	4.95[b]	Lot	n.a.
Allier	5.14	Lot-et-Garonne	7.73
Alpes (Basses-)	6.73	Lozère	3.33
Alpes (Hautes-)	2.69[c]	Maine-et-Loire	5.23
Ardèche	2.64[d]	Manche	4.00[n]
Ardennes	4.22	Marne	5.28
Ariège	5.68	Marne (Haute-)	4.98
Aube	6.12	Mayenne	3.00[o]
Aude	8.16	Meurthe	3.67
Aveyron	6.05	Meuse	5.54
Bouches-du-Rhône	7.18[e]	Morbihan	2.20[p]
Calvados	4.98[f]	Moselle	2.35
Cantal	4.72	Nièvre	3.97
Charente	6.11[g]	Nord	4.64[q]
Charente-Inférieure	4.58	Oise	4.80
Cher	3.79	Orne	3.27
Corrèze	5.09	Pas-de-Calais	6.11
Corse	9.46	Puy-de-Dôme	3.61
Côte-d'Or	n.a.	Pyrénées (Basses-)	6.89[r]
Côtes-du-Nord	2.46[h]	Pyrénées (Hautes-)	14.38
Creuse	4.36	Pyrénées-Orientales	14.13
Dordogne	n.a.	Rhin (Bas-)	4.81
Doubs	6.35	Rhin (Haut-)	3.28
Drôme	3.47[i]	Rhône	5.17
Eure	3.70	Saône (Haute-)	4.05
Eure-et-Loir	3.80	Saône-et-Loire	3.37
Finistère	1.62[j]	Sarthe	3.09
Gard	n.a.	Seine	10.68[s]
Garonne (Haute-)	8.82	Seine-et-Marne	5.08
Gers	10.72	Seine-et-Oise	5.19
Gironde	7.71	Seine-Inférieure	4.26
Hérault	11.22	Sèvres (Deux-)	4.71
Ille-et-Vilaine	4.39[k]	Somme	6.22
Indre	3.90	Tarn	6.45
Indre-et-Loire	4.39	Tarn-et-Garonne	6.36
Isère	2.94	Var	9.96[t]
Jura	4.91	Vaucluse	8.86
Landes	9.11	Vendée	3.25
Loire	3.63	Vienne	4.98
Loire (Haute-)	2.66[l]	Vienne (Haute-)	4.06[u]
Loire-Inférieure	5.91[m]	Vosges	2.82
Loiret	4.70	Yonne	5.67[v]

Notes to Table 5

[a]"All densities are expressed as the number of practitioners per 10,000 inhabitants. Except as indicated in the notes, the source for the number of medical men is AN F^{17} 4536 (lists or reports on numbers of medical personnel, mainly from a survey of 1834); unless otherwise specified, the data are for 1833 or 1834. In the case of material from 1833–34, the density was computed using the mean of the population totals from the censuses of 1831 and 1836; in other cases, the nearest quinquennial census was used (source: *Statistique de la France*, ser. 1, vol. 2 [1837], pp. 200–14).
[b]Report for 1829.
[c]The information is clearly incomplete. John Spears gives a density of 2.7 for the arrondissements of Gap and Embrun in 1831 (Spears and Diane Sydenham, "The Evolution of Medical Practice in Two Marginal Areas of the Western World, 1750–1830," *Historical Reflections/Réflexions historiques* 9 [1982]: 199).
[d]AD Ardèche, ms. list, 1832. The statistics in Michel Boyer, "L'Encadrement médical en Ardèche au XIXe siècle," master's thesis, University of Lyons II, 1977, p. 139, table 1, would give a density of 2.76.
[e]AD Bouches-du-Rhône 14 J, printed list, 1836–37.
[f]AD Calvados M 83, ms. lists for arrondissements of Bayeux, Lisieux, Vire (all 1836), and Falaise (1835), and lists by town for the arrondissement of Caen (1836); does not include arrondissement of Pont-l'Évêque.
[g]AD Charente, ms. list, 1837.
[h]Léonard, *Les Médecins de l'Ouest* (1978), table 3B, gives 1 physician for 3,626 inhabitants in 1831, for a density of 2.76.
[i]AD Drôme, printed list, 1835.
[j]Léonard: 2.08 in 1836.
[k]Report for 1833. Léonard: 4.66 in 1831.
[l]AD Haute-Loire 7 M, ms. list, 1828.
[m]Based on Léonard's count for 1836.
[n]Does not include physicians attached to navy and hospitals.
[o]Léonard: 3.65 in 1836.
[p]Léonard: 2.33 in 1836.
[q]Statistics on medical personnel from *Annuaire statistique du département du Nord*, 1830, p. 288.
[r]Report for 1828.
[s]Report for 1833, listing 1,091 practitioners: 23 physicians and 15 surgeons (including 1 dentist) licensed under the Old Regime; 900 doctors of medicine licensed under the law of Ventôse; 36 doctors of surgery; and 117 health officers. The *Almanach royal et national* for the same year lists 878 doctors of medicine and 77 doctors of surgery (pp. 925–34); cf. the 1831 edition, which lists 1,080 doctors of medicine and 237 doctors of surgery (pp. 889–902).
[t]Report for 1835.
[u]AD Haute-Vienne, ms. lists by arrondissement (and by canton for arrondissement of Limoges), 1829.
[v]Report for 1829.

APPENDIX B: SOME ITINERANT
EMPIRICS, 1802–1844

1802 Bas-Rhin. The Traber brothers, natives of Mutzig, practice medicine and surgery; they travel through the region accompanied by a harlequin and sell drugs in the public squares.[1]

1806 Loire. Villechèze, mayor of a local commune, peddles remedies from door to door.[2]

1807 Roer. Reappearance, at Aix-la-Chapelle (Aachen), of one of the Traber brothers.[3]

1810 Mont-Tonnerre. Reappearance, at Speyer, of one of the Traber brothers, now identified as from the Bas-Rhin. He "not only called himself a dentist and oculist, but traveling on horseback through the villages where he stopped, he called himself the owner of a miraculous specific to cure chronic illnesses in twenty-four hours and straighten deformed legs, make goiters disappear, etc., and was followed by a buffoon who distributed his flagons."[4]

1811 Bas-Rhin.
(1) Jean Propheter, a native of Germany, known as Dr. Johann.
(2) Jean Volk, or Volck, known as Dr. Hans and sometimes confused with Propheter, practices medicine in the countryside.[5]

1813 Bas-Rhin. Justin Breit, known as "Justul," practices medicine; he has no other known profession and no fixed abode.[6]

1817 Vaucluse. Jean-Martin Michel practices as a specialist in dartre and ulcers; he left his native town of Suze-la-Rousse, arrondissement of Montélimar (Drôme), at an early age.[7]

1819 Hautes-Alpes. A Piedmontese nicknamed "Brochet" (pike, i.e., the fish – but also slang for "belly") travels through the villages around La Saulce. According to his police record, his name is Joseph Novarrino; he is forty years old and a native of the Swiss canton of Valais. A wet cooper by profession, he claims to be traveling in France to find work in his trade and adds that his occasional practice of medicine is financially disinterested. (Novarrino settled in the Hautes-Alpes and enjoyed a long career there, despite being prosecuted for illegal medical practice.)[8]

1821 Yonne. A certain Léger appears at Toucy and announces himself as a tooth puller and seller of panaceas. And a man named Lauffin, calling himself a dentist, arrives with "seven individuals, adults and children, men and women, French and foreign, whites and Negroes, nimble-footed and with wooden legs, mounted on an enormous ramshackle old vehicle, which serves them as a conveyance and as a display [for their wares]."[9]

Bas-Rhin. Clementz, an inhabitant of Eschwiller (canton of Sarrebourg) travels around the countryside in the department and practices medicine.[10]

1822 Aube. A troupe of charlatans appears at Bar-sur-Seine; they have been traveling around the local towns selling an "American balm." According to the report of the subprefect, the group consists of "ten persons and seven horses." The leader, a native of the Aveyron, claims to have been a junior assistant medical officer in the army; his aide calls himself an *officier de santé*. The troupe also comprises their families and "five other individuals, including one of color, who are domestics or musicians." Their expenses seem to exceed their revenues, but they insist that they enjoy an independent fortune and that they travel more "out of habit than pecuniary interest."[11]

1823 Loire-Inférieure. According to an anonymous denunciation, the former itinerant Piloquet, known as Pilate, sees peasants in his apartment at Nantes for medical consultations, since he is "too old and too fat" to travel around the environs. The same informant charges that Mérigot, a former soldier and son of a surgeon, whose means of support are unknown, practices as a charlatan in the countryside under Pilate's name.[12]

1826 Paris. A Genoese charlatan named Boozzo, who claims descent from King David, is put on trial; he has been charged with the theft of a watch as well as illegal medical practice.[13]

1829 Yonne. A band of four charlatans appears at Toucy in two "elegant cabriolets"; they claim to be pensioned and authorized "*privilégièrement*" by the king of France, in return for services rendered in Spain during a "highly murderous epidemic" (presumably yellow fever). Mounted on the cabriolets, they draw a crowd with the sound of fanfares and sell both internal and external remedies.[14]

Paris. The Baulard woman, known as "la dame Blanche," appears before a session of the *tribunal de police correctionnelle* (court for lesser criminal cases). Forty-five years old, she rides around Meudon, Clamart, and their environs on a small horse; she carries a sac with amulettes, prayers for earaches, an earthen balm for all illnesses, and many conjuring tricks. She also passes as a witch.[15]

1841 Bas-Rhin. A charlatan known as Frère Martin travels around the arrondissement of Schlestadt (Sélestat) practicing medicine and surgery; he has patients as far away as Strasbourg. Son of a farrier at Hirsingue (Haut-Rhin), he lived as a hermit in different parts of the arrondissement and then at a shrine near Dambach, where the inhabitants, according to the subprefect, expelled him for misconduct. He specializes in disorders of vision and hearing.[16]

1844 Bas-Rhin. An itinerant charlatan dressed as a Chinaman circulates in the villages around Strasbourg, selling medicines to the sound of drum and trumpets. "Standing in a carriage to which two horses are hitched, and covered by an enormous umbrella, he tells the astonished spectators that he has a fortune of a million," writes the cantonal physician at Schiltigheim. "He has not come to make money [he says], since he has chests full of the stuff; as proof, he shows the basket full of gold at his feet. [He says that he] has traveled 3,000 leagues to France solely to relieve the sufferings of humanity." In four villages around Strasbourg, he sells 400 flagons of a greenish liquid advertised as a "universal panacea" at 1 franc and 1.50 francs.[17]

APPENDIX C: SOME FRENCH REMEDY SELLERS, 1773–1830

1773 Oudin, employee of the tobacco monopoly at Poitiers, has a miraculous water for eye diseases and inflammation.[1]

1774 *La dame* Parent, wife of an engineer in Poitou, has an ointment for cancer.[2]

c. 1780 André Pelletier, a tailor of Baugé, has a remedy for ringworm. He is willing to pay his way to Paris to present it to the Société Royale de Médecine, although he "is not rich."[3]

1780 Wahart, a farrier at Glaire (near the border of Champagne and Lorraine), has a remedy for polyps; he presents a certificate signed by a physician named Pierre.[4]

1782 Bonfils, a farrier at Marignane in Provence, has three secret remedies; he pleads that he needs the income derived from them.[5]

Loches, a tanner from Verneuil in Normandy, has a water for eye diseases, whose ingredients include dog dung. He obtained the recipe from a regimental drummer who lodged with him. For the last two years he has resided at Paris.[6]

A certain Dor in Paris distributes a universal medicine. He has a master's diploma (*maître-ès-arts*) but is actually illiterate; his real name is Dol, and he was originally a joiner and clockmaker.[7]

1783 Sadier, a *laboureur* at Nérondes in the diocese of Bourges, has a powder said to be effective against the bite of reptiles and venomous insects. In Luzy, diocese of Nevers, a poor tailor has a recipe against rabies.[8]

1784 At Coltainville, the wife of Jean Robillard, gamekeeper of the abbess and nuns of Jouarre, has a remedy against rabies.

Legrand, former farrier and horse doctor in Beauce, on the road from Chartres to Dreux, has a secret against carbuncles, scrofula, and cancers.[9]

1797 A weaver from the Gironde has a caustic for cancers and fistulas.[10]

1803 Pierre Bellouin, a carpenter at Goupillières, near Beaumont-le-Roger (Eure), administers a remedy composed of Glauber's salt, turpentine, etc.[11]

Jacques Serin, a shoemaker, sells medicine in the Loire-Inférieure.[12]

1807 Désiré Audase, joiner, is denounced by a surgeon at Oudon (Loire-Inférieure); he has a shop where he not only sells drugs but also compounds various remedies.[13]

1808 Moreau, a tailor at Saint-Sauveur in the Yonne, has a remedy for scrofula.[14]

1820 Schirvel, a shoemaker at Aix-la-Chapelle (Aachen), has a remedy for scabies; he seeks the approbation of the French government.[15]

1830 Couet, a handkerchief maker at Nantes, is accused of having poisoned a patient with a remedy.[16]

1830 A farrier at Bourbon-Vendée claims to have an empirical cure for cancer; he produces seven certificates.[17]

APPENDIX D: SOME EMPIRICS AND
THEIR OCCUPATIONS, 1775–1838

1775 Jean Fouquet, a weaver from Lécousse, near Fougères in Brittany, is a *marcou* marked with a fleur-de-lys on his chin (see Chapter 5). Fouquet (known as Le Breton) prefers cash payment but also accepts goods – stockings, shoes, shirts. In a letter to the Intendant of Brittany, Malesherbes notes that although Fouquet knows a trade, he "prefers idleness."[1]

1779 At Angers, a day laborer named Vau or Veau gives consultations and claims to have a specific.[2]

    During an epidemic in Poitou, a wine grower and a shoemaker practice medicine.[3]

1786 Deschamp, a butcher at "Cheveigné" (Chavagne?) in Brittany, practices medicine, attracting patients from far away; his wife is an unauthorized midwife. Saint-Lau or Saint-Laurent, formerly town crier at Guingamp, practices medicine in the *subdélégation* of Lannion (Brittany).[4]

1788 At Montréjeau in Gascony, a *marchand de liqueurs* who claims to own farms in Béarn works as an empiric and uses corrosive sublimate.[5]

1800 A chair bottomer of Montargis (Loiret) who cannot live from his regular trade has practiced as a surgeon for two or three years.[6]

1803 Pierre Bellouin, a carpenter from Goupillières, near Beaumont-le-Roger (Eure), treats the widow of Nicolas Morin for the venereal disease that killed her husband. He protests that he is a carpenter, not a physician, but he admits giving her a "water," which he says helped others.[7]

    At Évreux, Georges-Jean Yronnet, a needle maker, practices medicine.[8]

1805 At Strasbourg, the notary Kiechel (or Küchel) practices medicine and distributes an elixir.[9]

1806 In the Yonne, Cheuillot, a laborer (*manoeuvre*), signs a contract for his medical services.[10]

    At Saint-Jean-de-Bournay in the Isère, André Orgeolet, a wool carder, practices medicine and maintains a pharmacy.[11]

1808 At Chauvé, 9 leagues from Nantes, the two Renaud brothers, farm workers (*valets de ferme*) practice medicine; the peasants think they are sorcerers.[12]

    Radais, a weaver in the Orne, practices surgery.[13]

1810 At Boynes, in the arrondissement of Pithiviers (Loiret), Audineau, a former sabot maker, practices medicine.[14]

1811 Vincent writes to the Minister of the Interior that he has a remedy for hernias and wounds; he used to be a court clerk, but the post was eliminated.[15]

1819–

38 An Italian wet cooper, Novarrino, practices medicine at Ventavon (Hautes-Alpes).[16]

1823 The widow of a farmer (*laboureur*) at Beausoleil (Loire-Inférieure) treats patients in an inn run by another widow.[17]

NOTES

ABBREVIATIONS

AC   *archives communales*
AD   *archives départementales*
AM   Académie Nationale de Médecine, Paris (manuscript collection; archives
              of the Académie Royale de Médecine)
AN   Archives Nationales, Paris
Annales E.S.C.   *Annales: Économies, sociétés, civilisations*
AP   Archives de la Préfecture de Police, Paris
ARC   Archives de l'Académie Royale de Chirurgie, in the library of the Académie
              Nationale de Médecine, Paris
BM   *bibliothèque municipale*
BN   Bibliothèque Nationale, Paris
d.   *dossier*
FM   *faculté de médecine*
FP   Archives de la Faculté de Pharmacie, Bibliothèque Interuniversitaire de
              Pharmacie, Paris
l.   *liasse*
reg.   register
SRM   Archives de la Société Royale de Médecine, in the library of the Académie
              Nationale de Médecine, Paris

OTHER CONVENTIONS

Unless otherwise indicated in the citations, the place of publication is Paris.

As an aid in locating published French theses, the citations give the faculty and year in which the thesis was accepted and its number (when known); the year and place of publication, if different, are given in parentheses.

In quotations from the French, the original punctuation and spelling have been retained, but the accent marks (rarely used with any consistency in the eighteenth century) have in most cases been silently modernized.

PREFACE

1 On the use of the egg (from the journal of a barrister in Angers), see François Lebrun, *Les Hommes et la mort en Anjou aux 17ᵉ et 18ᵉ siècles: Essai de démographie et de psychologie historiques* (1971), p. 394.
2 Despite (or perhaps because of) the great wealth of available materials, the history

of popular medicine can be an alluring but ultimately elusive *ignis fatuus*: the further afield one pursues it, the more one has the sense of standing in the same place. For one thing, folk healing is less remarkable for its occasionally interesting regional variations than for the wide dissemination of its basic notions and usages (see, for example, Oskar von Hovorka and Adolf Kronfeld, *Vergleichende Volksmedizin*, 2 vols. [Stuttgart, 1908–09]). Healing formulas have also proved remarkably persistent over time: many of the examples recorded by field workers in the late nineteenth and twentieth centuries appeared in the seventeenth-century work on popular superstitions by the abbé Thiers, and it is not hard to find parallels in compendia from classical antiquity, such as Pliny's *Natural History* (see François Lebrun, "Le *Traité des superstitions* de Jean-Baptiste Thiers: Contribution à l'ethnographie de la France du XVIIe siècle," *Annales de Bretagne* 83 [1976]: 443–65). No doubt, as Robert Mandrou once argued, popular medicine does have a history, and it is wrong simply to accept it as having existed since time immemorial. (See his review of Marcelle Bouteiller's *Médecine populaire d'hier et d'aujourd'hui* in *Revue historique* 238 (1967): 214–17; and cf. Eugen Weber's review of several folklore studies in the *Times Literary Supplement*, 14 July 1978, pp. 801–02.) But this history occupies, in Fernand Braudel's parlance, *la longue durée*, and much of it, as Mandrou himself implies, concerns not the evolution of the popular medical corpus but the changes within learned medicine that slowly distanced it from its popular counterpart. Moreover, concrete evidence of the influence of these new ideas on the thinking of ordinary men and women is hard to come by; physicians did not collect it the way antiquarians collected medical folklore. (The fragmentary information that is available suggests a surprising acceptance of popular medicine and healers even among middle-class Frenchmen in the nineteenth century.) I hope, however, to pursue some of these problems, and to provide fuller documentation, in subsequent studies.

3 This interpretation appears, for example, in the classic sociological study of the modern profession, Eliot Freidson, *Profession of Medicine: A Study of the Sociology of Applied Knowledge* (New York, 1970). Cf. Paul Starr, *The Social Transformation of American Medicine* (New York, 1982), bk 1, chap. 3, "The Consolidation of Professional Authority, 1850–1930."

INTRODUCTION: *Professionalization and popular culture*

1 Keith Thomas, *Religion and the Decline of Magic* (New York, 1971), p. 663.

2 Peter Burke, *Popular Culture in Early Modern Europe* (New York, 1978), pp. 280–81 and passim.

3 Eugen Weber, *Peasants into Frenchmen: The Modernization of Rural France, 1870–1914* (Stanford, Calif., 1976), p. 495 and passim.

4 See, however, Gerald L. Geison, ed., *Professions and the French State, 1700–1900* (Philadelphia, 1984), a collection of papers from the 1978–80 seminar on the history of the professions at the Shelby Cullom Davis Center for Historical Studies, Princeton University. This seminar followed not long after a seminar devoted to the history of popular culture; the reader interested in academic meteorology may plot the shifting fronts for himself.

5 The observations that follow are drawn from a fuller discussion in Matthew Ramsey, "History of a Profession, *Annales* Style: The Work of Jacques Léonard," *Journal of Social History* 17 (1983–84): 319–38, esp. pp. 319–21.

6 See, for example, Harold Perkin, *The Origins of Modern English Society, 1780–1880* (London, 1969), which underscores the importance of the "non-capitalist or professional middle class" (p. 252); Theodore Zeldin, *France, 1848–1945*, vol. 1, *Ambition, Love, and Politics* (Oxford, 1973), which takes the history of the physicians as a model success story, illustrating how "each section of [the bourgeoisie] raised itself up by a monopoly which gave them power and enemies at the same time" (p. 42); or Burton Bledstein's book-length essay on the middle class in nineteenth-century America, which suggests that the "culture of professionalism" came to dominate a

society suspicious of European class ideologies (*The Culture of Professionalism: The Middle Class and the Development of Higher Education in America* [New York, 1976]).

7 See, for example, Daniel Bell, *The Coming of Post-Industrial Society: A Venture in Social Forecasting* (New York, 1973); Alvin Gouldner, *The Future of Intellectuals and the Rise of the New Class* (New York, 1979); and, for a neo-Marxist variant, Alain Touraine, *The Post-industrial society: Tomorrow's Social History: Classes, Conflicts, and Culture in the Programmed Society*, tr. Leonard F. X. Mayhew (New York, 1971). Krishnan Kumar gives a lucid review of the literature in *Prophecy and Progress: The Sociology of Industrial and Post-industrial Society* (New York, 1978).

8 This view informs a number of otherwise disparate studies, from Ivan Illich's anarcho-libertarian indictment of technological medicine (*Medical Nemesis* [London, 1975]) to Christopher Lasch's neo-Marxist critique of the professions and state agencies that impinge on the lives of families, thereby extending "capitalist control" (*Haven in a Heartless World: The Family Besieged* [New York, 1977], p. 191, n. 3, and passim).

9 See Roger Chartier, "Culture as Appropriation: Popular Cultural Uses in Early Modern France," in Steven L. Kaplan, ed., *Understanding Popular Culture: Europe from the Middle Ages to the Nineteenth Century* (Berlin, 1984), pp. 229–53. For a case study, see Robert M. Isherwood, *Farce and Fantasy: Popular Entertainment in Eighteenth-Century Paris* (New York and Oxford, 1986), which stresses the presence in the audience of members of *le beau monde*. He has outlined his argument in "Entertainment in the Parisian Fairs in the Eighteenth Century," *Journal of Modern History* 53 (1981): 24–48, esp. pp. 29–32.

10 On the changing status of the clergy and attitudes toward popular superstition, see Jean Delumeau, *Le Catholicisme entre Luther et Voltaire* (1971), pt. 3, chap. 4.

11 Howard M. Vollmer and Donald L. Mills, eds., *Professionalization* (Englewood Cliffs, N.J., 1966), Introduction, pp. vii–viii.

12 For attempts to define the characteristic traits of a profession, see Ernest Greenwood, "Attributes of a Profession," *Social Work*, vol. 2, no. 3 (July 1957): 45–55; William J. Goode, "Encroachment, Charlatanism, and the Emerging Profession: Psychology, Sociology, and Medicine," *American Sociological Review* 25 (1960): 903; and Geoffrey Millerson, *The Qualifying Associations: A Study in Professionalization* (London, 1964), pp. 4–5. For a critique of the traits model, see Terence J. Johnson, *Professions and Power* (London, 1972), pp. 22–37. Eliot Freidson reviews the controversy (and reasserts the need to develop a working definition of a profession) in *Professional Powers: A Study of the Institutionalization of Formal Knowledge* (Chicago, 1986), chap. 2.

13 This argument is cogently developed in Martin S. Pernick, *A Calculus of Suffering: Pain, Professionalism, and Anesthesia in Nineteenth-Century America* (New York, 1985), "Afterword: Professionalism and Change: History and Social Theory."

14 For a lucid exposition of this distinction, see William H. Sewell, Jr., *Work and Revolution in France: The Language of Labor from the Old Regime to 1848* (Cambridge, 1980), pp. 19–25.

15 Toby Gelfand, *Professionalizing Modern Medicine: Paris Surgeons and Medical Science and Institutions in the Eighteenth Century* (Westport, Conn., 1980).

16 Gelfand, "The Decline of the Ordinary Practitioner and the Rise of a Modern Medical Profession," in Martin S. Staum and Donald E. Larsen, eds., *Doctors, Patients and Society: Power and Authority in Medical Care* (Waterloo, Ont., 1981), pp. 105–29.

17 Magali Sarfatti Larson, *The Rise of Professionalism: A Sociological Analysis* (Berkeley and Los Angeles, 1977), p. xvi; italics in the original. She continues: "because marketable expertise is a crucial element in the structure of modern inequality, professionalization appears *also* as a collective assertion of special social status and as a collective process of upward social mobility." Enhanced social and economic status is part of what we understand by "the rise of professionalism," but as Larson herself points out (p. xvii), upward mobility is best considered an "outcome" of professionalization.

18 Eliot Freidson, *Profession of Medicine: A Study of the Sociology of Applied Knowledge* (New York, 1970), p. 42. Freidson argues that "what is generic to the professional is control over his technique or skill, monopoly over its practice"; even in the Soviet Union, he suggests, physicians, as experts, enjoy considerable control over technical decisions and a monopoly vis-à-vis laymen.

19 I. D. P. M. O. D. R. [Jean de Gorris; also attributed to Jean Duret], *Discours de l'origine, des moeurs, fraudes et impostures des ciarlatans, avec leur découverte* (1622), p. 48. This work is largely taken from Girolamo Mercurio, *De gli errori popolari d'Italia . . .*, 2 vols. (Venice, 1603), bk. 4, chaps. 1–8.

20 Pierre Darmon, *La Longue Traque de la variole: Les Pionniers de la médecine préventive* (1986). Bercé, *Le Chaudron et la lancette: Croyances populaires et médecine préventive, 1798–1830* (1984).

21 See G. Jeanton and E. Mauriange, "Les Archives ecclésiastiques de l'Ancien Régime, source de folklore," *Revue de folklore français* 11 (1940): 97–122, and 12 (1941): 185–218; J. Gadille, D. Julia, and M. Venard, "Pour un répertoire des visites pastorales," *Annales E.S.C.* 25 (1970): 561–66; and for an overview of the ecclesiastical sources, Delumeau, *Catholicisme*, pt. 3, chap. 2.

22 "Medical History without Medicine," unsigned editorial, *Journal of the History of Medicine and Allied Sciences* 35 (1980): 5–7; Lloyd G. Stevenson, "A Second Opinion," *Bulletin of the History of Medicine* 54 (1980): 139–40.

23 Illich, *Medical Nemesis*, p. 12 and passim.

24 Clifford Geertz, review of *Discipline and Punish*, *New York Review of Books*, 26 January 1978, pp. 3–6.

25 Freidson, *Profession of Medicine*, p. 381.

26 See, for example, the otherwise brilliant chapter on doctors in Zeldin, *France*, especially the caricatural portrait of Broussais.

27 It is an encouraging sign, though, that a new literature has begun to emerge on "fringe" medicine in England. See W. F. Bynum and Roy Porter, eds., *Medical Fringe and Medical Orthodoxy, 1750–1850* (London, 1986); Roy Porter, "The Language of Quackery in England, 1660–1800," in Porter and Peter Burke, eds., *The Social History of Language* (Cambridge: Cambridge University Press, forthcoming); and Roger Cooter, ed., *Alternatives: Essays in the Social History of Irregular Medicine* (London: Macmillan, forthcoming).

CHAPTER 1   *The regular medical network at the end of the Old Regime*

1 Eliot Freidson, *Profession of Medicine: A Study of the Sociology of Applied Knowledge* (New York, 1970), chap. 1 (quotation, p. 11).

2 See, for example, Magali Sarfatti Larson, *The Rise of Professionalism: A Sociological Analysis* (Berkeley and Los Angeles, 1977), chap. 1.

3 The importance of considering physicians as one element in a broad range of medical practitioners has been underscored by several perceptive studies of English medicine. For the sixteenth, seventeenth, and eighteenth centuries, see, respectively, Margaret Pelling and Charles Webster, "Medical Practitioners," in Webster, ed., *Health, Medicine and Mortality in the Sixteenth Century* (Cambridge, 1979), pp. 165–235; Harold J. Cook, *The Decline of the Old Medical Regime in Stuart London* (Ithaca, N.Y., 1986), chap. 1, "The Medical Marketplace of London"; and Irvine Loudun, "The Nature of Provincial Medical Practice in Eighteenth-Century England," *Medical History* 29 (1985): 1–32. Cf. Loudun, *Medical Care and the General Practitioner, 1750–1850* (Oxford, 1986), chap. 1.

4 This is particularly true of studies of colonial America, where licensing legislation was the exception rather than the rule. See, for example, Whitfield J. Bell, Jr., "Medical Practice in Colonial America," *Bulletin of the History of Medicine* 31 (1957): 442–53.

5 On French corporatism, see François-Jean-Marie Olivier-Martin, *L'Organisation corporative de la France d'Ancien Régime* (1938); Émile Coornaert, *Les Corporations en France avant 1789* (1941); William H. Sewell, Jr., "État, Corps, and Ordre: Some

Notes on the Social Vocabulary of the Old Regime," in Hans-Ulrich Wehler, ed., *Sozialgeschichte Heute: Festschrift für Hans Rosenberg zum 70. Geburtstag*, Kritische Studien zur Geschichtswissenschaft, 11 (Göttingen, 1974), pp. 49–68; and idem, *Work and Revolution in France: The Language of Labor from the Old Regime to 1848* (Cambridge, 1980), esp. chap. 2, "Mechanical Arts and the Corporate Idiom." See also Roland Mousnier, *Les Institutions de la France sous la monarchie absolue, 1598–1789*, vol. 1, *Société et État* (1974), esp. pp. 356–60, "Les Corps de la santé publique."

For the history of the three *corps*, their legal status, and their relations with one another, the best guides are a series of works by Jean Verdier (1735–1820), who was both a medical doctor and a barrister at the Parlement of Paris. Verdier projected a six-volume work that would deal first with problems common to the three *corps* and then with each individually. He published the synthetic section, *La Jurisprudence de la médecine en France, ou Traité historique et juridique des établissemens, règlemens, police, devoirs, fonctions, honneurs, droits et privilèges des trois corps de médecine...*, *Première partie, commune à toutes les professions de la médecine*, 2 vols. (Alençon, 1762–63); the section on surgery, *La Jurisprudence particulière de la chirurgie en France...*, 2 vols. (1764); and a further volume that provided a conspectus of the whole enterprise, *Essai sur la jurisprudence de la médecine en France, ou Abrégé historique et juridique des établissemens, règlemens, police, devoirs, fonctions, récompenses, honneurs, droits et privilèges des trois corps de médecine...* (Alençon, 1763).

6 There is unfortunately no major recent published study of the Old Regime medical profession, either monographic or synthetic, though some good work is now in progress or has resulted in informative unpublished theses (e.g., Catherine Maillé-Virole, "Médecins et chirurgiens parisiens à la fin de l'Ancien Régime," master's thesis [*mémoire de maîtrise*], University of Paris I, 1977]. The best current introduction to the medical world of the Old Regime, François Lebrun's *Se soigner autrefois: Médecins, saints et sorciers aux 17ᵉ et 18ᵉ siècles* (1983), contains a chapter on medical knowledge and training. Among the older works, two books by the physician-historian Paul Delaunay are useful: *La Vie médicale aux XVIᵉ, XVIIᵉ, et XVIIIᵉ siècles* (1935); and *Le Monde médical parisien au dix-huitième siècle* (1906). See also Alfred Franklin, *La Vie privée d'autrefois: Arts et métiers, modes, moeurs, usages des Parisiens du XIIᵉ au XVIIIᵉ siècle d'après des documents originaux ou inédits*, vol. 11, *Les Médecins* (1892); and Joseph Lévy-Valensi, *La Médecine et les médecins français au XVIIᵉ siècle* (1933); and a newer but chatty overview of the seventeenth-century profession: François Millepierres, *La Vie quotidienne des médecins au temps de Molière* (1964). In the more recent literature, two regional demographic studies contain valuable accounts of local medical personnel: François Lebrun, *Les Hommes et la mort en Anjou aux 17ᵉ et 18ᵉ siècles: Essai de démographie et de psychologie historiques* (1971), chap. 6; and Jean-Pierre Goubert, *Malades et médecins en Bretagne, 1770–1790* (Rennes, 1974), pt. 2, chap. 1.

7 "Édit portant règlement pour l'étude et l'exercice de la médecine dans le royaume," March 1707, in Athanase-Jean-Léger Jourdan, Decrusy, and François Isambert, comps., *Recueil général des anciennes lois françaises, depuis 420 jusqu'à la Révolution de 1789*, 29 vols. (1821–33), 20: 508–17, art. 26; Jacques Léonard, *Les Médecins de l'Ouest au XIXᵉ siècle*, state doctoral thesis, University of Paris IV, 1976 (1978), pp. 9, 161–62. In the French pontifical states, a bachelor's degree in medicine sufficed, although in difficult cases the *bacheliers* were required, like the *officiers de santé* in the nineteenth century, to summon a doctor (Victorin Laval, *Histoire de la Faculté de Médecine d'Avignon: Ses Origines, son organisation et son enseignement, 1303–1791* [Avignon, 1889], p. 136).

8 Lebrun, *Les Hommes et la mort*, p. 199; Goubert, *Malades et médecins*, p. 132.

9 *L'Anarchie médicinale, ou La Médecine considérée comme nuisible à la société*, 3 vols. (Neuchâtel, 1772), 2: 3–4.

10 The discussion that follows is based mainly on Toby Gelfand, *Professionalizing Modern Medicine: Paris Surgeons and Medical Science and Institutions in the Eighteenth Century* (Westport, Conn., 1980); he summarizes his argument on the changing status of surgeons in "From Guild to Profession: The Surgeons of France in the

Eighteenth Century," *Texas Reports on Biology and Medicine* 32 (1974): 121–34. See also Alfred Franklin, *Vie privée*, vol. 12, *Les Chirurgiens* (1893); and Marie-José Imbault-Huart, "Les Chirurgiens et l'esprit chirurgical en France au XVIIIᵉ siècle," *Clio Medica* 15 (1981): 143–57.

11 Pierre L. Thillaud, *Les Maladies et la médecine en pays basque nord à la fin de l'Ancien Régime, 1690–1789*, École Pratique des Hautes Études, IVᵉ Section (Sciences historiques et philologiques), ser. 5, Hautes études médiévales et modernes, no. 50 (Geneva, 1983), p. 97.

12 Verdier, *Jurisprudence particulière*, 2: 13, 49–50.

13 On surgery as a model for medicine: Oswei Temkin, "The Role of Surgery in the Rise of Modern Medical Thought," *Bulletin of the History of Medicine* 25 (1951): 248–59; Gelfand, *Professionalizing Modern Medicine*, pt. 3; idem, "The Hospice of the Paris College of Surgery (1774–1793): 'A Unique and Valuable Institution,'" *Bulletin of the History of Medicine* 47 (1973): 375–93.

14 Verdier, *Jurisprudence particulière*, 1:88, 102, 103–04 (on the Bordeaux statutes); *Statuts et règlemens pour les chirurgiens des provinces . . .* (1735), art. 7 (p. 4).

15 On the persistence of the barber-surgeons, see two articles by Toby Gelfand: "Deux cultures, une profession: Les Chirurgiens français au XVIIIᵉ siècle," *Revue d'histoire moderne et contemporaine* 27 (1980): 168–84; and "The Decline of the Ordinary Practitioner and the Rise of a Modern Medical Profession," in Martin S. Staum and Donald E. Larsen, eds., *Doctors, Patients, and Society: Power and Authority in Medical Care* (Waterloo, Ont., 1981), pp. 105–29. For the German barber-surgeon model and its influence in Alsace: Alfons Fischer, *Geschichte des deutschen Gesundheitswesens*, 2 vols. (Berlin, 1933), 1: 323, 2: 57–58, and Robert Boeglin, *L'Évolution historique de la pharmacie en Alsace* (Strasbourg, 1939), p. 98. For the Southwest: Toby Gelfand, "Public Medicine and Medical Careers in France during the Reign of Louis XV," in Andrew W. Russell, ed., *The Town and State Physician in Europe from the Middle Ages to the Enlightenment*, Wolfenbütteler Forschungen, 17 (Wolfenbüttel, 1981), pp. 99–122, esp. pp. 109–16. On *empiétement* by the barber-wigmakers, see (for example) Maurice Mével, *Chirurgiens dijonnais au XVIIIᵉ siècle*, Lyons medical thesis, 1901–02 (Lyons, 1902), p. 7.

16 For an example of a denunciation: SRM 107, 25 August 1782, on a barber at Soultz in Alsace who treated a woman's tumor for eight months, using mainly corrosive plasters.

17 *Statuts*, tit. 6–7 (pp. 16–19). See Gelfand, "Deux cultures," on the structure of the profession.

18 Goubert, *Malades et médecins*, pp. 134–36; Goubert and François Lebrun, "Médecins et chirurgiens dans la société française du XVIIIᵉ siècle," *Annales cisalpines d'histoire sociale*, no. 4 (1973): 130–32. For the ban on selling remedies: decree of 12 April 1749, art. 10, cited in Jean-Baptiste Denisart, *Collection de décisions nouvelles et de notions relatives à la jurisprudence actuelle*, 6th ed., 3 vols. (1768), 1: 92. There is no general work on provincial surgeons comparable to Gelfand's work on Paris. Among the local and regional studies (mostly older and anecdotal): Paul Delaunay, *Les Chirurgiens du Haut-Maine sous l'Ancien Régime* (Le Mans, 1933); Mével, *Chirurgiens lyonnais*; and Albert Puech, *Les Chirurgiens d'autrefois à Nîmes: Étude historique d'après des documents inédits* (1880). On country practice, see also Edna Hindie Lemay, "Thomas Hérier, A Country Surgeon Outside Angoulême at the End of the XVIIIth Century: A Contribution to Social History," *Journal of Social History* 10 (1976–77): 524–37.

19 See, for example, R. Auvigné, J.-P. Kernéis, and L. Rouzeau, "Les 'Chirurgiens navigans' civils de jadis: Leur multitude oubliée, ou l'aspect naval des études médicales pratiques aux XVIIᵉ et XVIIIᵉ siècles," *Comptes rendus du 87ᵉ Congrès National des Sociétés Savantes, section des sciences* (1963), pp. 47–57.

20 On unlicensed surgeons: AN F¹⁷ 2276, d. 2, no. 277, report of lieutenant of the King's First Surgeon at Saint-Gaudens (Haute-Garonne), complaining that it has never been possible to oblige them to have themselves formally received (1790). See Gelfand, "Deux cultures," pp. 477, 480, and idem, "Medical Professionals and

Charlatans: The *Comité de Salubrité Enquête* of 1790–91", *Histoire sociale–Social History* 11 (1978): 62–97 (p. 72 on surgeons who practice without reception).

21 Erwin H. Ackerknecht, *Medicine at the Paris Hospital, 1794–1848* (Baltimore, 1967), p. 163; George M. Rosen, *The Specialization of Medicine, With Particular Reference to Ophthalmology* (New York, 1944), pp. 2, 50, and passim; quotation, p. 50. See also Toby Gelfand, "The Origins of the Modern Concept of Medical Specialization: John Morgan's *Discourse* of 1765," *Bulletin of the History of Medicine* 50 (1976): 511–35. (Not all physicians in early modern France shared a confidence in special operators. Laurent Joubert, for example, condemned it as a popular error. See his *Seconde partie des erreurs populaires et propos vulgaires touchant la médecine et le régime de santé . . .* [1587], p. 115: "Contre ceux qui ont opinion, que les chirurgiës ne sont propres à remettre les desnoüeures, & veulent des renoüeurs empiriques, comme y estans plus heureux.")

22 On the midwife's ecclesiastical function, see Joseph-Antoine-Toussaint Dinouart, *Abrégé de l'embryologie sacrée, ou du traité du devoir des prêtres, des médecins et autres, sur le salut éternel des enfans qui sont dans le ventre de leur mère* (1762), bk. 4, chap. 4; on licensure, Richard L. Petrelli, "The Regulation of French Midwifery during the Ancien Régime," *Journal of the History of Medicine and Allied Sciences* 26 (1971): 276–92

I have not been able to consult what promises to be a massive thesis by Jacques Gélis on midwifery and obstetrics in the Old Regime. Parts of his work have appeared in a number of key articles, notably "Sages-femmes et accoucheurs: L'Obstétrique populaire aux XVIIᵉ et XVIIIᵉ siècles," *Annales E.S.C.*, vol. 32 (1977), no. 5, special number: *Médecins, médecine et société en France aux XVIIIᵉ et XIXᵉ siècles,* pp. 927–57. See also "La Formation des accoucheurs et des sages-femmes aux XVIIᵉ et XVIIIᵉ siècles: Évolution d'un matériel et d'une pédagogie," *Annales de démographie historique,* 1977, pp. 153–80; "Regards sur l'Europe médicale des Lumières: La Collaboration internationale des accoucheurs et la formation des sages-femmes au XVIIIᵉ siècle," in Arthur E. Imhof, ed., *Mensch und Gesundheit in der Geschichte* (Husum, 1980), pp. 279–99; and "L'Accoucheuse rurale au XVIIIᵉ siècle: Transformations du rôle d'un intermédiaire entre culture rurale et culture urbaine," in *Les Intermédiaires culturels: Actes du Colloque du Centre Méridional d'Histoire Sociale, des Mentalités, et des Cultures, 1978* (Aix-en-Provence, 1981), pp. 127–37); and on the role of the surgeon-accoucheurs, "La Pratique obstétricale dans la France moderne: Les Carnets du chirurgien-accoucheur Pierre Robin (1770–1797)," *Annales de Bretagne et des Pays de l'Ouest,* vol. 86 (1979), no. 3, special number: *La Médicalisation en France du XVIIIᵉ au début du XXᵉ siècle,* pp. 191–210; and "Obstétrique et classes sociales en milieu urbain aux XVIIᵉ et XVIIIᵉ siècles: Évolution d'une pratique," *Histoire des sciences médicales* 14 (1980): 425–33. (His substantial volume, *L'Arbre et le fruit: La Naissance dans l'Occident moderne, XVIᵉ–XIXᵉ siècle* [1984] is an anthropological study of the history of childbirth and is not directly concerned with midwifery.)

In addition to the work of Gélis, see Alfred Franklin, *Vie privée,* vol. 14, *Variétés chirurgicales* (1894), pp. 57–120; Mireille Laget, "La Naissance aux siècles classiques: Pratique des accouchements et attitudes collectives en France aux XVIIᵉ et XVIIIᵉ siècles," *Annales E.S.C.*, vol. 32, no. 5, pp. 958–92; idem, *Naissances: L'Accouchement avant l'âge de la clinique* (1982); and, for a radical feminist perspective, Yvonne Knibiehler and Catherine Fouquet, *La Femme et les médecins: Analyse historique* (1983), pp. 177–84. An English version of the Laget article has appeared in Robert Forster and Orest Ranum, eds., *Medicine and Society in France,* Selections from the *Annales,* vol. 6, trans. Elborg Forster and Patricia M. Ranum (Baltimore, 1980), pp. 137–76. Among the useful regional studies: Goubert, *Malades et médecins,* pp. 161–72; and Paul Delaunay, *Les Sages-femmes dans le Maine à la fin de l'Ancien Régime: Communication faite au 1ᵉʳ Congrès de l'Histoire de l'Art de Guérir* (Antwerp, 1921).

23 Franklin, *Variétés chirurgicales,* pp. 121–225, passim; Bernard Jacquet, *Empiriques et charlatans troyens du XVᵉ au XIXᵉ siècle,* Paris medical thesis, 1960, no. 458, p. 61.

24 Franklin, *Variétés chirurgicales,* pp. 207–08; Louis-Alexandre de Cézan and Guillaume-René Le Fébure de Saint-Ildephont, *État de médecine, chirurgie, et pharmacie en Europe*

pour l'année 1776 (1776), pp. 122–26; *Almanach royal* (1787), p. 627. The lithotomists specialized in the *petit appareil* and the *grand appareil*. The *petit appareil*, used especially for children, involving bringing the stone to the neck of the bladder, from which the surgeon could remove it through the perineal ureter; the *grand appareil* entailed making an incision in the ureter and searching for the stone in the bladder. A third technique, the *haut appareil*, called for the surgeon to approach the site through the abdomen (Lévy-Valensi, *Médecine*, p. 181).

25 *Almanach royal* (1787), p. 627; ARC 4, report, 29 May 1793; M.-J. Guillaume, ed., *Procès-verbaux du Comité d'Instruction de la Convention Nationale*, 6 vols. (1891–1907), 3: 229.

26 Verdier, *Essai*, pp. 278–79; Dr. Charpignon, "Rebouteurs, bandagistes, secours aux indigents malades avant 1800," *Mémoires de la Société d'Agriculture, Sciences, Belles-Lettres et Arts d'Orléans*, 4th ser., 21 (1879): 246–47; Guillaume Péry, *Histoire de la Faculté de Médecine de Bordeaux et de l'enseignement médical dans cette ville, 1441–1888* (1888), p. 228.

27 Nicolas Jadelot, Report of the Faculty of Medicine of Nancy to Comité de Salubrité, Assemblée Nationale Constituante (October, 1790), in AD Meurthe-et-Moselle D 82, Registre des délibérations de la Faculté de Médecine de l'Université de Nancy, depuis sa translation à Nancy, fol. 84v.

28 Raymond Petit, "La Science et l'art de guérir en Bretagne," *Annales de Bretagne* 2 (1886): 268 (on restrictions at Rennes). Arthur Bordier, *La Médecine à Grenoble: Notes pour servir à l'histoire de l'École de Médecine et de Pharmacie* (Grenoble, 1896), p. 109, n. 3; p. 111.

29 Franklin, *Variétés chirurgicales*, p. 212.

30 Paul Delaunay, "Les Guérisseurs ambulants dans le Maine sous l'Ancien Régime," *Deuxième Congrès International d'Histoire de la Médecine* (Évreux, 1922), pp. 211–23.

31 SRM 199, d. 9, nos. 25–26, Tadiny complaining of charlatans (9–19 December 1780), and nos. 27–29, self-justification. Cf. SRM 104, d. 39; the Society allowed Tadiny to apply his eye remedies, but not to sell them to the public.

32 See Balthasar-Anthelme Richerand, *Des Erreurs populaires relatives à la médecine*, 2d ed. (1812), pp. 156–57.

33 François-Paul-Lyon Poulletier de la Salle, Charles-Louis-François Andry, and Félix Vicq d'Azyr, "Rapport sur les inconvéniens de l'opération de la castration, pratiquée pour obtenir la cure radicale des hernies," *Mémoires de la Société Royale de Médecine*, 1 (1776): 291.

34 Delaunay, "Guérisseurs ambulants," p. 216, quoting *Affiches du Mans*, 5 September 1785. All these techniques should be contrasted with the traditional popular treatments in the form of cataplasms, internal remedies, and special diets. See, for example, FM Paris ms. 5389, recipe for a cataplasm made from lamb's droppings and cow's milk, to be maintained in place with a bandage for forty days – though the poultice might be changed if it should "spoil."

35 AN F^{15} 228/2, no. 7, lieutenant of the King's First Surgeon, report to Comité de Salubrité, Assemblée Nationale Constituante, 2 December 1790.

36 Philippe Macquer, "Bailleul," *Dictionnaire raisonné universel des arts et métiers, contenant l'histoire, la description, la police des fabriques et manufactures de France et des pays étrangers . . .*, new ed., revised by abbé Jaubert, 4 vols. (1773), 1: 190.

37 Charpignon, "Rebouteurs," p. 246.

38 Pierre-François Percy, article "Déboîtement," *Dictionnaire des sciences médicales, par une société de médecins et de chirurgiens*, 60 vols. (1812–22), 8: 107; Nicolas-François-Joseph Éloy, "Hommes du Valdajol," *Dictionnaire historique de la médecine ancienne et moderne. . .*, 4 vols. (Mons, 1778), 4: 454–55.

39 P. S. Goffin, *Un Coin de haute montagne: La Vallouise*, 2d ed. (Grenoble, 1959), cited by Marcelle Bouteiller, *Médecine populaire d'hier et d'aujourd'hui* (1966), p. 104. Hereditary vocations could be found in other surgical specialties as well; in the region between Plombières and Luxueil, for example, the Nardin family specialized in trepanation for two hundred years (Bordier, *Médecine à Grenoble*, p. 109, n. 1).

40 See, for example, Paul Delaunay, "La Médecine populaire: Ses origines religieuses,

dogmatiques et empiriques," *La Médecine internationale illustrée*, 1930, p. 421; and J.-M.-C. Naville, *Lettres bourguignonnes, ou Aperçu philosophique et critique sur les causes des difficultés dans l'exercice de l'art de guérir.* . . (1822), p. 141. On the executioner's expertise: Pierre-Jean-Jacques-Guillaume Guyot, *Répertoire universel et raisonnée de jurisprudence civile, criminelle, canonique et bénéficiale* . . . , 64 vols. (1775–83), 10: 540: "Le vulgaire s'imagine que parce qu'ils sont au fait de rompre les os à un malheureux, ils doivent avoir plus d'habileté qu'un chirurgien pour les remettre, & par ce moyen ils cherchent à faire illusion & à s'accréditer."

41 SRM 136, d. 11, no. 13, complaint by Baumes, physician at Nîmes, 4 June 1787.

42 Delaunay, "Médecine populaire: Ses origines," p. 421.

43 M.-A. Saint-Léger, "Conflit entre le corps des chirurgiens et le bourreau de Lille en 1768," *Revue du Nord* 2 (1911): 49–54.

44 See, for example, AN F^{17} 2276, d. 2, no. 293, on Poitiers, and a report in ibid., no. 266 (Angoulême).

45 AD Vendée B 1140, 1145 (1677 and 1697), quoted in Prosper-Marie Boissonnade, *Essai sur l'organisation du travail en Poitou, depuis le XIe siècle jusqu'à la Révolution*, vols. 21–22 of *Mémoires de la Société des Antiquaires de l'Ouest*, 2d ser. (1898–99), 21: 517–18.

46 Franklin, *Variétés chirurgicales*, pp. 141, 184–85; Cézan and Le Fébure de Saint-Ildephont, *État de médecine* . . . *1776*, p. 123; Naville, *Lettres bourguignonnes*, p. 122.

47 AC Nantes FF 249.

48 Gelfand, "Medical Professionals," pp. 72-73.

49 On the Paris apothecaries: Charles C. Gillispie, *Science and Polity in France at the End of the Old Regime* (Princeton, N.J., 1980), pp. 207–12; and Bénédicte Dehillerin and Jean-Pierre Goubert, "A la conquête du monopole pharmaceutique: Le Collège de Pharmacie de Paris (1776–1796)," *Historical Reflections/Réflexions historiques*, vol. 9, nos. 1–2, special number, *La Médicalisation de la société française, 1770–1830*, ed. Jean-Pierre Goubert, pp. 233–48. For the declaration of 1777, see Adolphe Trébuchet, *Jurisprudence de la médecine, de la chirurgie, et de la pharmacie en France* . . . (1834), p. 319. For an overview of the history of French pharmacy: L. André-Pontier, *Histoire de la pharmacie: Origines, Moyen Âge, temps modernes* (1900); Maurice Bouvet, *Histoire de la pharmacie en France des origines à nos jours* (1937); and Louis Reutter de Rosemont, *Histoire de la pharmacie à travers les âges*, 2 vols. (1931), vol. 2, *Du XVIIe siècle à nos jours*. See also Alfred Franklin, *Vie privée*, vol. 9, *Les Médicaments* (1891).

50 For provincial pharmacy, which varied widely from place to place, it is necessary to turn to a series of local and regional studies, among them: A. Baudot, *Études historiques sur la pharmacie en Bourgogne avant 1803* (1905); Paul Delaunay, "Les Apothicaires du Haut-Maine et du Maine angevin sous l'Ancien Régime," serialized in *Revue d'histoire de la pharmacie* 6–7 (1938–39); Jean Doucet, *Les Apothicaires nantais sous l'Ancien Régime* (Fontenay-le-Comte, 1959); Alexandre-Charles Germain, *L'Apothicairerie à Montpellier sous l'ancien régime universitaire: Étude historique d'après les documents originaux* (Montpellier, 1882). For the Academy of Dijon: Baudot, *Études historiques*, "Cinquième période," chap. 2, esp. pp. 506–11. On pharmaceutical instruction in the provinces, see also Charles Bedel, "L'Enseignement des sciences pharmaceutiques," in René Taton, ed., *Enseignement et diffusion des sciences en France au XVIIIe siècle* (1964), pp. 252–55.

51 Delaunay, "Apothicaires du Haut-Maine," 6: 404 (on the relationship with *l'épicerie*); Victor Dauphin, "La Corporation des apothicaires d'Angers, de ses origines à sa suppression en 1791," *Mémoires de la Société Nationale d'Agriculture, Sciences, et Arts d'Angers* 6 (1931): 5–46 (p. 16 on Latin).

52 AD Ille-et-Vilaine C 347, quoted in Dupuy, "Épidémies," *Annales de Bretagne* 2 (1886–87): 200.

53 On the statutes governing the apothecaries, see François Prévet, *Histoire de l'organisation sociale en pharmacie* (1940).

54 Delaunay, "Apothicaires du Haut-Maine," 6: 291.

55 See Joseph F. Kett, "Provincial Medical Practice in England, 1730–1815," *Journal of the History of Medicine and Allied Sciences* 19 (1964): 17–29; and S. W. F. Holloway,

"The Apothecaries' Act, 1815: A Reinterpretation," *Medical History* 10 (1966): 107–29, 221–36.

56 On the decline of the apothecaries: Baudot, *Études historiques*, p. 437; Pierre Rambaud, *La Pharmacie en Poitou jusqu'à l'an XI, Mémoires de la Société des Antiquaires de l'Ouest*, 2d ser., 30 (1906): 43. On the role of the clergy and religious: M. Fosseyeux, "Les Apothicaireries des couvents sous l'Ancien Régime," *Bulletin de la Société de l'Histoire de Paris et de l'Île-de-France* 46 (1919): 42–59; and Joseph-Lucien-Victor Tournier, *Le Clergé et la pharmacie: Essai sur le rôle du clergé, et plus particulièrement des congrégations religieuses, dans la préparation et la distribution des remèdes avant la Révolution* (1938). The text of the statute of 25 April 1777 is reprinted in P. Dorveaux, "Procès-verbaux du Collège de Pharmacie de Paris," *Revue d'histoire de la pharmacie*, no. 24 (1935): III–14: "Déclaration du Roy portant règlement pour les professions de la pharmacie et de l'épicerie à Paris"; see art. 8. On an unsuccessful attempt to enforce art. 8 in the provinces, see Delaunay, "Apothicaires du Haut-Maine," 6: 300–01.

57 Baudot, *Études historiques*, p. 520.

58 Bibliothèque de l'Arsenal, ms. 6772, quoted in Rambaud, *Pharmacie en Poitou*, p. 567.

59 See, for example, Verdier, *Essai*, "Du commerce des drogues," pp. 341–52, which traces the corporate boundaries.

60 Ibid., p. 339.

61 Raoul Mercier, *Le Monde médical de Touraine sous la Révolution* (Tours, 1936), p. 207; *Gazette de Hollande*, 1 August 1766, quoted in Franklin, *Variétés chirurgicales*, p. 213.

62 Gelfand, *Professionalizing Modern Medicine*, pp. 137, 152–53; Léonard, *Médecins de l'Ouest*, pp. 177-78.

63 Gelfand, "Decline of the Ordinary Practitioner"; cf. Ivan Waddington, "General Practitioners and Consultants in Early Nineteenth-Century England: The Sociology of an Intra-Professional Conflict," in John Woodward and David Richards, eds., *Health Care and Popular Medicine in Nineteenth-Century England: Essays in the Social History of Medicine* (New York, 1977), pp. 164–88.

64 On the privileges of the royal physicians and surgeons, see Pierre-Jean-Jacques-Guillaume Guyot, *Traité des droits, fonctions, franchises, exemptions, prérogatives et privilèges annexés en France à chaque dignité, à chaque office, & à chaque état . . .* , 4 vols. (1786–87), vol. 1, bk. 1, chap. 31, "Des officiers de santé," esp. pp. 546–47, 561–67.

65 Edict of Marly, art. 24. Philippe-Antoine Merlin, comp., *Répertoire universel et raisonné de jurisprudence . . .* , 5th ed., 15 vols. (Brussels, 1825–28), 2: 664.

66 AN F^{17} 2276, d. 2, no. 329.

67 SRM 199, d. 6, no. 1, report from physician at Le Blanc, 16 October 1779; AN F^{15} 228/2, no. 3, Montdidier, 30 November 1790; AN F^{17} 2276, d. 2, no. 301, Villeneuve-de-Berg (Ardèche). On the trade in privileges, see Gelfand, "Medical Professionals," pp. 72-73; on the reception of charlatans: Jean-Pierre Goubert, "L'Art de guérir: Médecine savante et médecine populaire dans la France de 1790," *Annales E.S.C.* 32 (1977): 910–11. See also SRM 199, d. 22, no. 4, Terrède at L'Aigle, 18 November 1780, complaining of quacks practicing urinoscopy who have been received as master surgeons.

68 SRM 199, d. 3, no. 1, 30 June 1779.

69 Pierre Lunel, "Pouvoir royal et santé publique," *Annales du Midi*, no. 119 (1974): 349, citing AD Pyrénées-Orientales C 1967.

70 Jean-Gabriel Gallot, *Essai sur la topographie médicale du Poitou, Annuaire de la Société d'Émulation de la Vendée* 18 (1871): 128.

71 *Almanach*, p. 121, quoted in Paul Delaunay, *Études sur l'hygiène, l'assistance, et les secours publics dans le Maine sous l'Ancien Régime*, 1st ser. (Le Mans, 1920), p. 87, n. 2; AD Indre-et-Loire 407, Roche case, cited by Delaunay, *Études sur l'hygiène*, 2d ser., fasc. 3 (Le Mans, 1923), p. 227.

72 Caroline C. Hannaway, "Veterinary Medicine and Rural Health Care in Pre-Rev-

olutionary France," *Bulletin of the History of Medicine* 51 (1977): 431–47.
73 See, for example, Léonard, *Médecins de l'Ouest*, p. 140, on nomadic surgeons in Brittany who obtained authorizations from the local *sénéchal*; and AD Yonne 5 M 7/1, no. 95, petition from François-Antoine Maillet, an ambulatory surgeon born in 1757 and struggling to survive in postrevolutionary France.
74 On the history of orvietan in France, see Claude-Stephen Le Paulmier, *L'Orviétan: Histoire d'une famille de charlatans du Pont-Neuf aux XVIIe et XVIIIe siècles* (1893).
75 On permissions at the national level, see, e.g., the manuscript memoirs on charlatanism in AN 154 AP II (177 Mi 159), 1775–76.
76 See, for example, Paul Delaunay, "Guérisseurs ambulants," pp. 211–25. In 1738 the College of Physicians of Le Mans resolved that it would no longer give attestations to drug vendors who lacked warrants conforming to the royal edicts of 25 October 1728 and 17 March 1731 and imposed a payment of 3 livres (Delaunay, pp. 219–21). See also Jacquet, *Empiriques troyens*, chap. 5, on orvietan vendors and, for texts of permissions, Marie-Claire Gandrille-Oursel, *La Médecine populaire en Bourgogne* (1957), pp. 26–27.
77 AC Angers FF 39, 16 April 1776; a certain Rubini, however, was *refused* an authorization by the Commission Royale de Médecine in Paris (BN ms. Joly de Fleury 499, fol. 218v) – though the Commission may simply have deemed his remedy unoriginal. Cf. AD Côtes-du-Nord B 576, petition of de Bluche, orvietan merchant, 1732, given in Paul Aubry, *Notes sur l'exercice illégal de la médecine et les charlatans en Bretagne avant la Révolution* (Lyons, 1895), pp. 14–15.
78 Rambaud, *Pharmacie en Poitou*, p. 536, citing Greffe de Châtellerault 1.424. Technically, an *apothecary* might "administer" a drug, but this claim clearly took the empiric beyond mere remedy vending. On the sale of orvietan as a pretext for peddling other remedies, see, for example, SRM 199, d. 24, no. 14, copy of a letter concerning an empiric, from Beaussieu de la Bouchardière, physician at Vendôme; and cf. Louis Lépecq de la Cloture, *Collection d'observations sur les maladies et constitutions épidémiques . . .* (Rouen, 1778), p. 542, note on charlatans: "non-seulement ces Charlatans & Vendeurs de Spécifiques, vendent & débitent tous autres remèdes que ceux pour lesquels ils ont obtenu des Brevets, mais . . . ils reçoivent des Consultations & voient des Malades dans nos Villes."
79 "Copie de l'ordonnance de Monseigneur le Procureur Général mise en marge d'un placet présenté par le sieur Guillaume Graulau, docteur en médecine et médecin pensionné de la présente ville, contre les sieurs Leherr, médecin, et le sieur Hilmer, oculiste," published by Durand (no forename given) under the title "L'Exercice de la médecine au XVIIIe siècle," *Paris médical* 32 (1919): 158–59; Delaunay, "Guérisseurs ambulants," pp. 214–15; Jacquet, *Empiriques troyens*, p. 57.
80 For an illuminating study of a sixteenth-century example, see Claude Blanguernon, *Gilles de Gouberville: Gentilhomme du Cotentin, 1522–1578* (Coutances, 1969), "La Médecine de Gilles," pp. 109–15. Gilles had read the old medical treatises and played the physician on his estate. Upon examining a man who had injured himself falling out of a tree, he diagnosed pleurisy and advised bleeding and applying plasters. To the wife of a man whose knee was painfully swollen, he sent goose grease, beer, and cider as panaceas.
81 Paul Delaunay, "Gentilshommes du XVIIIe siècle: La Médecine au château," *La France médicale* 57 (1910): 405–06.
82 Rambaud, *Pharmacie en Poitou*, p. 39 (and cf. other examples on pp. 38–40); Pierre-Jean-Baptiste Legrand d'Aussy, *Voyage fait en 1787 et 1788, dans la ci-devant Haute et Basse Auvergne . . .*, 3 vols. (Year III), 3: 316–17.
83 Paul Delaunay, "La Médecine populaire dans le Maine à la fin de l'Ancien Régime: La Médecine illégale, les charlatans," *Premier Congrès de l'Histoire de l'Art de Guérir* (Antwerp, 1921), p. 84.
84 AD Ille-et-Vilaine C 1346, quoted in Dupuy, "Épidémies en Bretagne," *Annales de Bretagne*, 2: 197.
85 Legrand d'Aussy, *Voyage*, 3: 316.

86 AD Ille-et-Vilaine C 4934, Delucenay to Premier Conseiller des États de Bretagne, 19 May 1774.

87 See, for example, the discussion of relations between the Academy of Sciences and "self-acclaimed geniuses" in Roger Hahn, *The Anatomy of a Scientific Institution: The Paris Academy of Sciences, 1666–1803* (Berkeley and Los Angeles, 1971), chap. 5.

88 See Camille Bloch, *L'Assistance et l'État en France à la veille de la Révolution (généralités de Paris, Rouen, Alençon, Orléans, Châlons, Soissons, Amiens, 1764–1790)* (1908), pp. 242–46; Léon Le Grand, "Remèdes fournis gratuitement dans les généralités par les soins des Intendants, au XVIIIᵉ siècle," *La France médicale* 57 (1910): 341–44; and Louis Lafond, *La Dynastie des Helvétius: Les Remèdes du roi* (1926). For a local example: Baudot, *Études historiques*, p. 402.

89 J. Denais, *Portefeuille d'un curieux*, p. 230, quoted in Dauphin, "Corporation des apothicaires d'Angers," p. 13.

90 AD Seine-Maritime C 132, cited in Gelfand, "Public Medicine," p. 103.

91 Marie de Maupeou, Mme. François Fouquet: *Recueil de receptes choisies, expérimentées et approuvées. . .* (Villefranche, 1675 and later editions); *Recueil de remèdes faciles et domestiques. . .* (Dijon and Paris, 1678 and later editions); *Les Remèdes charitables de Mme Fouquet* (Lyons, 1681, and later editions).

92 *Le Chirurgien des pauvres*, 2d ed. (1671), pp. iii–iv: "Non, ie ne crains pas, MESDAMES, en vous offrant ce Traité fait en faveur des Pauvres, de vous demander, que vous vous approchiez d'eux, quoy que puans d'apostèmes, de playes & d'ulcères, puisque ie suis persuadé que suivant les démarches d'un Dieu-homme, qui a visité les lépreux & les malades vivant sur la Terre, vous voulez encores imiter les Reynes & Princesses Chrestiennes, qui ont préparé les remèdes des Pauvres avec les mesmes mains qui portoient le Sceptre & n'ont point estimé indigne de leur Grandeur, d'appliquer les appareils aux playes & aux ulcères, sans que l'odeur cadavreuse ait pû arrester cette divine ferveur qui les portoit à un si saint ministère."

93 Victor Dauphin, "La Corporation des chirurgiens d'Angers, de ses origines à sa suppression en 1791," *Mémoires de la Société Nationale d'Agriculture, Sciences, et Arts d'Angers* 5 (1930): 30.

94 On the general question of the medical activities of the Church, see Paul Delaunay, *La Médecine et l'Église: Contribution à l'histoire de l'exercice médical* (1948).

95 AD Ille-et-Vilaine C 1357, quoted in Dupuy, "Épidémies en Bretagne," *Annales de Bretagne*, 2: 199–200.

96 Boissonnade, *Essai*, *Mémoires de la Société des Antiquaires de l'Ouest*, 21: 486, on Poitiers statutes; Denisart, *Collection*, 1: 94; *Statuts*, p. 3; Gelfand, *Professionalizing Modern Medicine*, p. 106.

97 Jadelot, report to Comité de Salubrité (cited in n. 27), fol. 88r.

98 Marie-France Morel, "Les Curés, les paysans: Un même langage," *Autrement*, no. 15 (September 1978), special number: *Panseurs de secrets et de douleurs*, p. 70.

99 Robert Heller, " 'Priest-Doctors' as a Rural Health Service in the Age of Enlightenment," *Medical History* 20 (1976): 361–83; and cf. idem, "Johann Christian Reil's Training Scheme for Medical Auxiliaries," *Medical History* 19 (1975): 321–32. For a proposal submitted to the Société Royale de Médecine calling for training priests in medicine, see Lindsay Blake Wilson, "*Les Maladies des femmes*: Women, Charlatanry, and Professional Medicine in Eighteenth-Century France," Ph.D. dissertation, Stanford University, 1982, p. 380, quoting SRM 132ᴮᴵˢ, no. 55, Dr. Empercier.

100 Jadelot, report to Comité de Salubrité, fol. 88r.

101 Delaunay, "Médecine populaire dans le Maine," p. 91, n. 2. The ointment was prepared by the abbey of Saint Vincent in Le Mans.

102 See, for example, AD Hautes-Alpes 141 M, no. 2, denunciation addressed to Minister of the Interior, 13 Nivôse IX/3 January 1801: "Plusieurs prêtres . . . ne trouvant plus dans les produits de leur état les mêmes ressources qu'autrefois se mêlent aussi d'exercer l'art de guérir . . . ."

103 Morel, "Curés," p. 70.

104 AN F¹⁷ 2276, d. 2, no. 273, report from Mende (Lozère).

105 Boissonnade, *Essai sur l'organisation du travail, Mémoires de la Société des Antiquaires de l'Ouest,* 21: 508; Étienne Dupont, "Les Lettres de cachet et l'exercice illégal de la médecine en Bretagne au XVIIIe siècle," *Chronique médicale* 30 (1923): 261, citing AD Ille-et-Vilaine C 204.

106 See Mousnier, *Institutions,* 1: 335–36.

107 Bordier, *Médecine à Grenoble,* pp. 56–57; Olivier-Martin, *Organisation corporative,* p. 369.

108 Maurice Bouvet, "Les Commissions de contrôle des spécialités pharmaceutiques au 18e siècle," *Bulletin de la Société d'Histoire de la Pharmacie* 3 (1922): 88–94, 119–24.

109 On the faculties and colleges, see Delaunay, *Monde médical,* chap. 1; Louis Liard, *L'Enseignement supérieur en France, 1789–1893,* 2 vols. (1888–94), 1: 4–11; J. Bodinaud, *Contribution à l'étude de l'enseignement médico-chirurgical en France au XVIIIe siècle,* Rennes medical thesis, 1963; and Charles Coury, "The Teaching of Medicine in France from the Beginning of the Seventeenth Century," in C. D. O'Malley, ed., *The History of Medical Education* (Berkeley and Los Angeles, 1970), pp. 121–72. On the various constitutions of the medical faculties, see Jules Barbot, *Les Chroniques de la Faculté de Médecine de Toulouse du treizième au vingtième siècle,* 2 vols. (Toulouse, 1905), 1: 192. On Montpellier: Alexandre-Charles Germain, *L'École de Médecine de Montpellier: Ses origines, sa constitution, son enseignement . . .* (Montpellier, 1880). On Nancy: P. Pillemont, "L'Ancienne Faculté de Médecine de Nancy (1768–1793)," serialized in *La France médicale* 57 (1910).

110 Delaunay, *Vie médicale,* p. 294.

111 AD Meurthe-et-Moselle D 82, Jadelot memoir, fol. 82r, on purposes of the Collège Royal de Médecine; ibid., fol. 6v, "Délibération de la Faculté contre son association avec le Collège Royal de Médecine de Nancy," 22 May 1769; fols. 37r-v, exchange with Vicq d'Azyr. See also SRM 110, d. 20, no. 1, faculty to Société Royale, 11 June 1778.

112 Delaunay, *Vie médicale,* p. 291; Edict of Marly, arts. 30–33.

113 Edict of Marly, art. 35; AD Meurthe-et-Moselle D 82, fols. 65v ff.; Pillemont, "L'Ancienne Faculté de Médecine de Nancy," p. 58.

114 Cézan and Le Fébure de Saint-Ildephont, *État de médecine . . . 1776,* p. 282. André Boquel, *La Faculté de médecine de l'Université d'Angers, 1433–1792: Son évolution au cours des XVIIe et XVIIIe siècles . . .* (Angers, 1951), pp. 134–36; cf. chap. 13 on the Chartier case. See also Léonard, *Médecins de l'Ouest,* p. 137, on the successful campaign by Guillaume Laennec (the uncle of the more celebrated René Laennec, inventor of the stethescope) to obtain his *agrégation* at Nantes for 150 livres rather than the 2,000 required by the faculty.

115 On Nancy: Pillemont, "L'Ancienne Faculté de Médecine de Nancy," p. 36; on Brittany: Goubert, *Malades et médecins,* p. 132.

116 Germain, *École de médecine,* p. 34; Maurice Raynaud, *Les Médecins au temps de Molière,* new ed. (1866), p. 227; Delaunay, *Vie médicale,* p. 381.

117 Auguste Corlieu, *L'Ancienne Faculté de Médecine de Paris* (1877), pp. 211–14; Raynaud, *Médecins au temps de Molière,* pp. 274–77 (emphasizing the ambiguous legal status and checkered career of the Chambre Royale); and Delaunay, *Vie médicale,* pp. 306, 309. For the royal declaration of 3 May 1694, see Jourdan et al., *Recueil général,* 20: 223–25.

118 On medicine and the state (in the context of a more general study of state scientific institutions), see Gillispie, *Science and Polity,* chap. 3 (pt. 2 for the Société Royale de Médecine).

119 Delaunay, *Vie médicale,* p. 290. See also Guyot, *Traité des droits,* bk. 1, chap. 31.

120 [Jean Goulin, Jacques de Horne, and Pierre de la Servolle], *État de médecine, chirurgie et pharmacie en Europe et principalement en France pour l'année 1777* (1777), pp. 251–52.

121 SRM 199, d. 13, no. 22, Bellon, physician at Valence, to Vicq d'Azyr, 23 September 1777.

122 Delaunay, *Vie médicale,* p. 284; Lunel, "Pouvoir royal," pp. 350–51.

123 On Germany, see, for example, Reinhold August Dorwart, *The Prussian Welfare*

State *before 1740* (Cambridge, Mass., 1971), chap. 16. On Italy: Carlo M. Cipolla, *Public Health and the Medical Profession in the Renaissance* (Cambridge, 1976), chap. 1. On Switzerland: Eugène Olivier, *Médecine et santé dans le pays de Vaud au XVIIIe siècle, 1675–1798* (Lausanne, 1939), pt. 1.

124 See, for example, Jeanne Rigal, *La Communauté des maîtres-chirurgiens jurés de Paris au XVIIe et au XVIIIe siècle, 1675–1798* (1936); Dauphin, "Corporation des chirurgiens d'Angers"; and Édouard Isambard, *La Communauté des chirurgiens de Pacy-sur-Eure aux XVIIe et XVIIIe siècles* (Pacy-sur-Eure, 1894).

125 Gelfand, "Medical Professionals," pp. 67–71.

126 Cited in Raymond Petit, "La Science et l'art de guérir en Bretagne," *Annales de Bretagne* 2 (1886): 268.

127 Gelfand, *Professionalizing Modern Medicine*, pp. 6–7; and idem, "Deux cultures," p. 473; Goulin et al., *État de médecine...1777*, p. 253.

128 Jean-Baptiste Denisart, *Collection de décisions nouvelles et de notions relatives à la jurisprudence, donnée par Me Denisart, mise dans un nouvel ordre...et augmentée par MM. Camus et Bayard*, 14 vols. (1783–1807), 4: 539; Saint-Brieuc, community of surgeons to royal judge, 29 January 1777, registers of the Greffe Royal de Saint-Brieuc, quoted by Aubry, *Notes sur l'exercice illégal*, pp. 2–3.

129 Verdier, *Jurisprudence particulière*, vol. 1, chap. 5, art. 3; Lunel, "Pouvoir royal," pp. 350–51. In principle, the first article of the 1730 statutes for provincial surgery gave the First Surgeon jurisdiction over all provinces and colonies without exception (*Statuts*, p. 5).

130 Gillispie, *Science and Polity*, p. 206.

131 See Caroline C. Hannaway, "Medicine, Public Welfare and the State in Eighteenth-Century France: The Société Royale de Médecine of Paris (1776–1793)," Ph.D. dissertation, The Johns Hopkins University, 1974, chap. 7.

132 On the provincial communities, see, for example, Dauphin, "Corporation des apothicaires d'Angers"; and Ernest-Joseph Laruelle, *Contribution à l'histoire de la pharmacie en Normandie: Les Apothicaires rouennais: Histoire de la corporation du Moyen-Âge à la Révolution* (Rouen, 1920). On the rights of the First Physician: SRM 114, d. 13, "Observations du chirurgien du Roi sur le projet de suppression de la Commission Royale de Médecine et de sa réunion à la Société Royale de Médecine."

133 Delaunay, "Apothicaires du Haut-Maine," pp. 291–95; Gillispie, *Science and Polity*, pp. 207–12.

134 See, for example, Guy Williams, *The Age of Agony: The Art of Healing, c. 1700–1800* (London, 1975).

135 For a succinct statement of the argument that medicine had a negligible influence on demographic trends, see Thomas McKeown, R. G. Brown, and R. G. Record, "An Interpretation of the Modern Rise of Population in Europe," *Population Studies* 26 (1972): 345–82. On other possible social functions of therapeutics, notably meeting the patient's cultural expectations and producing visible results: Charles E. Rosenberg, "The Therapeutic Revolution: Medicine, Meaning, and Social Change in Nineteenth-Century America," in Rosenberg and Morris J. Vogel, eds., *The Therapeutic Revolution: Essays in the Social History of American Medicine* (Philadelphia, 1979), pp. 3–25. On placebos: Arthur K. Shapiro, "A Contribution to the History of the Placebo Effect," *Behavioral Science* 5 (1960): 109–35.

136 Antoine-François de Fourcroy, "Rapport et projet de décret sur l'établissement d'une école centrale de santé à Paris..." (7 Frimaire III/27 November 1794), in Alfred de Beauchamp, comp., *Médecine et pharmacie: Projets de loi*, 5 vols. (1888–95), vol. 1 [covering the period 1789–1803], pp. 200–01.

137 AN F¹⁷ 2276, d. 2, no. 301, Villeneuve-de-Berg (Ardèche).

138 One example among many: SRM 199, d. 13, no. 23, Bellon (*médecin du roi* at Valence), 25 October 1780.

139 François-Emmanuel Fodéré, *Voyage aux Alpes-Maritimes, ou Histoire naturelle, agraire, civile et médicale du comté de Nice et pays limitrophes...*, 2 vols. (1821), 2: 293.

140 SRM 145, Du Boueix, report on dysentery in the arrondissement of Clisson in 1779 (1780).

141 AD Ille-et-Vilaine C 58, quoted by Dupuy, "Épidémies en Bretagne," *Annales de Bretagne* 2: 197–98.

142 AN F[17] 2276, d. 2, no. 277.

143 See, for example, the list of victims of *empiétement* by surgeons and apothecaries sent by the physicians of Nevers and the Nivernais to the intendant at Moulins in 1787: ms. from a private collection, quoted in Mercier, *Monde médical de Touraine*, pp. 201–02.

144 François-Emmanuel Fodéré, *Traité de médecine légale et d'hygiène publique, ou de police de santé, adapté aux codes de l'Empire Français, et aux connaissances actuelles . . .* , 6 vols. (1813), 6: 405–06.

145 Gallot, *Essai*, p. 129.

146 Marc Bouloiseau, ed., *Cahiers de doléances du tiers état du bailliage de Rouen pour les États-Généraux de 1789*, 2 vols. (1957–60), 1: 31.

147 Marcel Marion, *Dictionnaire des institutions de la France aux XVIIe et XVIIIe siècles* (1923), p. 369, on Cloyes and Courson. See also Pierre Goubert and Michel Denis, eds., *1789: Les Français ont la parole* (1964), pp. 222–23.

148 A. Le Moy, ed., *Cahiers de doléances des corporations de la ville d'Angers et des paroisses de la sénéchaussée particulière d'Angers pour les États-Généraux de 1789*, 2 vols. (Angers, 1915–16), 1: cliii, 2: 441, and passim. See Dauphin, "Corporation des chirurgiens d'Angers," pp. 31–33.

149 See, for example, Pierre Huard, "L'Enseignement médico-chirurgical," in Taton, *Enseignement*, pp. 171–236; Delaunay, *Vie médicale*, pp. 329–31; and Léonard, *Médecins de l'Ouest*, pp. 145–48. On surgical training: Gelfand, *Professionalizing Modern Medicine*, pt. 2, and, on teaching in hospitals, idem, "Gestation of the Clinic," *Medical History* 25 (1981): 169–80, and " 'Invite the Philosopher as Well as the Charitable': Hospital Teaching as Private Enterprise in Hunterian London," in W. F. Bynum and Roy Porter, eds., *William Hunter and the Eighteenth-Century Medical World* (Cambridge, 1985), pp. 129–52 (131–35 concern Paris). See also Marie-José Imbault-Huart, *L'École pratique de dissection de Paris de 1750 à 1822, ou L'Influence du concept de médecine pratique et de médecine d'observation dans l'enseignement médico-chirurgical au XVIIIe siècle et au début du XIXe siècle* (Lille, 1975), and, on the development of clinical instruction in various parts of Europe (including France), Othmar Keel, "The Politics of Health and the Institutionalisation of Clinical Practices in Europe in the Second Half of the Eighteenth Century," in Bynum and Porter, *William Hunter*, pp. 207–56.

150 Lemay, "Thomas Hérier."

151 Le Paulmier, *Orviétan* pp. 95–107; Mittié, *A l'Assemblée Nationale*, 25 June 1789, p. 5; SRM 199, d. 14, no. 16, Saladin, 8 August 1783, with copy of flyer distributed by Le Cerf; ibid., d. 18, no. 11, report from physician at Boulogne, 3 December 1785. For the Society's views of Mittié, see AM ms. 15, pp. 91–96; and cf. BN ms. Joly de Fleury 513, fol. 22r, complaint by Dr. Michel Laugier of Marseilles, who says that the Société Royale has harassed him for promoting his remedy against jaundice.

152 SRM 199, d. 5, no. 3, 13 October 1783; AD Indre-et-Loire C 354, Le Mans, 1786, quoted in Goubert, "Art de guérir," p. 910.

153 AN F[17] 2276, d. 2, no. 307, Domfront, 5 January 1791.

154 Gillispie, *Science and Polity*, pp. 258–61; Péry, *Histoire*, pp. 66–67; Delaunay, *Vie médicale*, p. 303. For the details of the Préval case, see Mathieu-François Pidanzat de Mairobert, *L'Espion anglois, ou Correspondance secrète entre Milord All'eye et Milord All'ear*, 10 vols. (London, 1777–86), 6: 260–307.

155 Delaunay, *Vie médicale*, pp. 16, 346–50. On the Nancy case: Pillemont, "L'Ancienne Faculté de Médecine de Nancy," p. 259. On the exclusion of Protestants: Jean-Baptiste Denisart, *Collection de décisions nouvelles et de notions relatives à la jurisprudence*, 6th ed., 3 vols. (1768), 2: 184, and G. Robert, "La Révocation de l'édit de Nantes et les professions de santé," *Histoire des sciences médicales* 17 (1983): 181–87. Even before the revocation of the Edict of Nantes (in October 1685), a royal declaration of 6 August 1685 barred the reception of Protestants as physicians; a declaration of

20 February 1680 and a decree of 15 September 1685 prohibited them from working as midwives and then as surgeons and apothecaries. Earlier, corporate statutes and decisions by parlements and local authorities had excluded Protestants from the medical professions or restricted their numbers. But cf. Arie Theodorus van Deursen, *Professions et métiers interdits: Un Aspect de l'histoire de la révocation de l'Édit de Nantes* (Groningen, 1960), chap. 3 (on physicians, surgeons, and apothecaries) and chap. 4 (on midwives). Van Deursen suggests that there were few real interdictions after 1685 (p. 132) and that "en général le médecin protestant du dix-huitième siècle a pu exercer sa profession tranquillement" (p. 148). On the Edict of Toleration, see Armand Lods, ed., *La législation des cultes protestantes, 1787–1887* (1887), p. 3, and Burdette Poland, *French Protestantism and the French Revolution: A Study in Church and State, Thought and Religion, 1685–1815* (Princeton, N.J., 1957), pp. 80–81.

156 On women in medicine, see Mélanie Lipinksa, *Histoire des femmes médecins, depuis l'antiquité jusqu'à nos jours* (1900). On women surgeons at the end of the Old Regime: Gelfand, "Medical Professionals," pp. 83–84.

157 Edict of Marly, arts. 9, 13–15, 18–19. On Nancy: Pillemont, "L'Ancienne Faculté de Médecine de Nancy," pp. 39, 57.

158 Léonard, *Médecins de l'Ouest*, pp. 143–44. Cf. Corlieu, *L'Ancienne Faculté de Médecine de Paris*, chaps. 2–5, on the stages of medical study.

159 Delaunay, *Vie médicale*, p. 37.

160 On Orange: SRM 199, d. 13, no. 2, Ricavy, at Digne, 25 July 1779; ibid., no. 1, Ricavy, 23 March 1779 (on Bignau).

161 Péry, *Histoire de la Faculté de Médecine de Bordeaux*, p. 4; Léonard, *Médecins de l'Ouest*, p. 137.

162 Fees for the baccalaureate, *licence*, and doctorate are given in Liard, *Enseignement supérieur*, I: 19–21. See also Delaunay, *Vie médicale*, pp. 37–38; idem, *Monde médical parisien*, pp. 7–8; and Léonard, *Médecins de l'Ouest*, pp. 154, 158, 160.

163 Corlieu, *L'Ancienne Faculté de Médecine de Paris*, p. 263; Delaunay, *Vie médicale*, pp. 41–42; *Arrest de la cour du Parlement, du 13 aoust 1764, qui homologue un acte, portant établissement en la Faculté de Médecine de Paris, d'un concours, pour procurer, gratis tous les deux ans, à un candidat, le bonnet de docteur, & l'acte de régence* (1764).

164 Léonard, *Médecins de l'Ouest*, p. 137.

165 Gelfand, *Professionalizing Modern Medicine*, chaps. 3, 5, 6; Léonard, *Médecins de l'Ouest*, p. 128. Delaunay, *Vie médicale*, p. 335.

166 Léonard, *Médecins de l'Ouest*, pp. 178–79; Gelfand, *Professionalizing Modern Medicine*, pp. 92–93; Goubert, *Malades et médecins*, p. 130.

167 Gelfand, "Public Medicine and Medical Careers," p. 114.

168 Léonard, *Médecins de l'Ouest*, pp. 164–65; Gelfand, *Professionalizing Modern Medicine*, pp. 77–78; Goubert, *Malades et médecins*, pp. 134–35.

169 *Statuts*, pp. 16–19; see Gelfand, "Medical Professionals," p. 71.

170 Dr. Patay, "Résumé des statuts & règlements des maîtres chirurgiens d'Orléans au XVIIIᵉ siècle," *Mémoires de la Société d'Agriculture, Sciences, Belles-Lettres et Arts d'Orléans*, 4th ser., 21 (1879): 265; Léonard, *Médecins de l'Ouest*, p. 169; Catherine Maillé-Virole, "La Naissance d'un personnage: Le Médecin parisien à la fin de l'Ancien Régime," *Historical Reflections/Réflexions historiques* 9 (1982): 164 (on the cost of the Paris mastership); Pierre-Jean Darracq, "Les Chirurgiens à Bordeaux au XVIIIᵉ siècle," *Histoire des sciences médicales*, 15 (1981): 300.

171 Léonard, *Médecins de l'Ouest*, p. 177; Gelfand, "Public Medicine," p. 114.

172 Lebrun, *Médecins, saints et sorciers*, pp. 46–50. For a regional study of obstetrical training: Olivier Couffon, *Les Cours d'accouchement en Anjou à la fin du XVIIIᵉ siècle* (Angers, 1913). On Le Vigan: Laget, *Naissances*, p. 206.

173 Laget, *Naissances*, p. 205.

174 François-Yves Besnard, *Souvenirs d'un nonagénaire* (1880), I: 124, quoted in Lebrun, *Les Hommes et la mort*, p. 220.

175 On manual trades: Guy Godlewski, *Des Médecins et des hommes...* (1972), p. 27; Germain, *École de Médecine de Montpellier*, p. 50, citing art. 28 of the 1634 statutes.

176 Samuel-Auguste-André-David Tissot, *Essai sur les moyens de perfectionner les études*

de médecine (Lausanne, 1785), p. 15.

177 François Aubin, *Histoire de la Faculté de Médecine à Nantes au XVIIIe siècle*, Paris medical thesis, 1947, p. 125.

178 Lebrun, *Les Hommes et la mort*, pp. 219–20. On dynasties, cf. Goubert, *Malades et médecins*, pp. 145–55; and Léonard, *Médecins de l'Ouest*, p. 127.

179 L. Montariol, *Sur l'étude et l'exercice de la médecine depuis le XIVe siècle jusqu'à la Révolution Française . . .*, Toulouse medical thesis, 1912, p. 23. Raynaud, *Médecins au temps de Molière* pp. 75–79; Laval, *Histoire de la Faculté de Médecine d'Avignon*, p. 158.

180 *Vues de législation médicale adressées aux États-Généraux assemblés par ordre de Sa Majesté, par le Docteur Sabarot de L'Avernière, correspondant de la Société Royale de Médecine de Paris* (1789), p. 6.

181 On nobles practicing medicine and the problem of *dérogeance*, see Gilles André de La Roque, *Traité de la noblesse*, new ed. (Rouen, 1710), pp. 527–28; cf. Edmond Locard, *Le XVIIe siècle médico-judiciaire* (Lyons, 1902), pp. 42–43.

182 Nobles practicing as physicians were more common in regions of Roman law than elsewhere, but even there nobles more often chose the law as a profession. On noble and ennobled physicians, see Guy Chaussinand-Nogaret, "Nobles médecins et médecins de cour au XVIIIe siècle," *Annales E.S.C.* 32 (1977): 851–57, and François de Vaux de Foletier, "Anoblissements de médecins et chirurgiens de Louis XIV à Louis XVI," *Histoire des sciences médicales*, 16 (1982): 163–6.

183 Marion, *Dictionnaire des institutions*, s.v. "médecins"; quotation, p. 369. Delaunay, *Vie médicale*, p. 258.

184 SRM 107, letter from a certain Perreau, detailing a long list of grievances.

185 Daniel Roche, *Le Siècle des Lumières en province: Académies et académiciens provinciaux, 1680–1789*, 2 vols. (1978), 1: 235.

186 Chaussinand-Nogaret, "Nobles médecins," p. 856.

187 Jean Meyer, "Le Personnel médical en Bretagne à la fin du XVIIIe siècle," pt. 2, chap. 1 of J.-P. Desaive et al., *Médecins, climat et épidémies à la fin du XVIIIe siècle* (1972), p. 184.

188 Delaunay, *Vie médicale*, p. 190.

189 Maillé-Virole, "Naissance d'un personnage," p. 175; Delaunay, *Vie médicale*, p. 189; Jean-Pierre Goubert, "The Medicalization of French Society at the End of the Ancien Régime," in Lloyd G. Stevenson, ed., *A Celebration of Medical History: The Fiftieth Anniversary of the Johns Hopkins Institute of the History of Medicine and the Welch Medical Library* (Baltimore, 1982), pp. 157–72 (p. 164 on Paris incomes).

190 Dupuy, "Épidémies en Bretagne," *Annales de Bretagne*, 2: 194; Goubert and Lebrun, "Médecins et chirurgiens," pp. 119–36 (p. 133 on capitation).

191 SRM 132, d. 64, n.d., anon. paper from Poitou on abuses and need for reform in the medical field, p. 16.

192 AC Le Croisic BB fol. 108r; AD Ille-et-Vilaine C 718, C 728. Quoted in Dupuy, "Épidémies en Bretagne," *Annales de Bretagne*, 2: 192–93.

193 Goubert, *Malades et médecins*, p. 129; Lebrun, *Les Hommes et la mort*, p. 226. For the legislation of 10 August 1756, see Denisart, *Collection*, 8th ed., 14 vols. (1783–1807), 4: 540: "Les chirurgiens qui exercent uniquement leur profession, sans faire ni faire faire par leurs femmes d'autre trafic, sont réputés notables bourgeois, & comme tels, peuvent être revêtus d'offices municipaux, sont exempts de toute taxe d'industrie, de la collecte de la taille, de guet et garde, de corvées, & de toutes autres charges de ville & publiques, dont sont exempts, suivant les usages observés en chaque province, les notables bourgeois."

194 AN D XXXVIII 3, d. 45, Nicolas *le cadet* to the National Assembly, 27 June 1790.

195 Gelfand, "Decline of the Ordinary Practitioner," p. 112. Gelfand also notes the importance of a regional tradition in the Southwest, especially in Gascony. Auch natives at the Paris College of Surgery represented about 2% of the males who could have been expected to survive to that age – a figure that rose to 7.5% in the case of the village of Saint-Mont (Gelfand, "Public Medicine," p. 116).

196 Goubert, "Medicalization," p. 164.

197 Lebrun, *Les Hommes et la mort*, p. 222. On one example of social ascension, the Sorbier family, see Toby Gelfand, "From Guild to Profession: The Surgeons of France in the Eighteenth Century," *Texas Reports on Biology and Medicine* 32 (1974): 128–29.

198 Meyer, "Personnel médical," p. 183. At Rennes in 1789, 8 out of 18 surgeons paid over 30 livres (Goubert and Lebrun, "Médecins et chirurgiens," p. 134).

199 Goubert, "Medicalization," pp. 163 and 171, n. 23. The provincial towns include 11 in Brittany, plus Lyons and Angers.

200 AN F^{17} 2276, d. 2, no. 319, Seurre (Côte-d'Or); AN D XXXVIII 3, d. 45, Nicolas letter. See Lemay, "Thomas Hérier," on a surgeon who could not support his family on his professional earnings and depended on his income as the owner of a *métairie*.

201 Gillispie, *Science and Polity*, p. 242, n. 196, guesses 3,000–5,000. Hard evidence is difficult to come by. Surveys of authorized practitioners were carried out sporadically at the local level throughout the eighteenth century (usually lists of the members of the *communautés*). See, for example, *Inventaire-sommaire*, AD Hérault, series 2: 412 (C 2276, 1737). Later lists were often restricted to fully qualified physicians, surgeons, and apothecaries; see, for example, AC Nantes I 5 7, d. 1 (1791).

At the national level, we know of three attempts to compile censuses of practitioners, including two in the first half of the century (1726 and 1737). Jean-Pierre Goubert and François Lebrun characterize the first as a total failure and the second as a beginning; the last survey, carried out at Calonne's instigation in 1786, they consider a partial success. Records survive, scattered in the *archives départementales*, for a third of the thirty-odd *généralités* that existed in France at the end of the Old Regime, mostly in the northern half of the country; they list 832 physicians and 2,721 surgeons. (Midwives were belatedly included in the survey; see Jacques Gélis, "L'Enquête de 1786 sur les sages-femmes du Royaume," *Annales de démographie historique*, 1980, pp. 299–343.) These materials may be supplemented with data from an investigation of hospitals carried out by Jacques Necker as minister of finance in 1779 and from some of the lists prepared after 1803, which identify physicians and surgeons admitted to practice under the Old Régime "according to the old procedures." (See Goubert and Lebrun, "Médecins et chirurgiens," pp. 119–36.) Finally, the survey conducted by the Comité de Salubrité in 1790–91 gives estimates of the number of surgeons in the various jurisdictions overseen by the lieutenants of the King's First Surgeon. (Similar surveys were to have covered medicine and pharmacy, but few responses have survived.) In the case of the survey on surgery, the replies are dispersed: the major part of those at the Archives Nationales are in box F^{17} 2276. See Marie-José Imbault-Huart, "Sources de l'histoire de la médecine aux Archives Nationales de 1750 à 1822," *Revue d'histoire des sciences* 25 (1972): 45–53.

Local almanacs and directories can fill some of the gaps for individual provinces. On the national level, an undated ms. prepared about a decade before the Revolution, probably at the instigation of the Société Royale de Médecine, lists 1,881 physicians and 2,029 surgeons, with their place of residence ("État des médecins et chirurgiens de la province, par ordre alphabétique des lieux," FM Paris, ms. 221). We may also turn to four *états*, or directories, of practitioners, published in the 1770's by various authors: Cézan and Le Fébure de Saint-Ildephont, *État de médecine . . . 1776*; Goulin et al., *État de médecine . . . 1777*; *L'État des médecins et chirurgiens de France* (Bouillon, 1772); and Trécourt [physician (c. 1716–c. 1785)], *L'État de la médecine et de la chirurgie en France* (1773).

202 See Gelfand. "Medical Professionals," p. 76, and "Deux cultures," p. 468. The duc de Luynes estimated that France had 30,000–40,000 "barbers or surgeons" in the second third of the century; in 1789, François Chaussier, a physician of Dijon, put the figure at 45,000.

203 Goubert, "Medicalization," p. 162.

204 Gelfand suggests 10/10,000 for surgeons alone ("Deux cultures," p. 469). Goubert, however, proposes an average density of 4.5/10,000 (physicians and surgeons) for the regions covered in the 1786 investigation, only about a third of the present level:

"Réseau médical et médicalisation en France à la fin du XVIIIe siècle," *Annales de Bretagne et des pays de l'Ouest* 86 (1979): 223.
205 Lebrun, *Les Hommes et la mort*, p. 218.
206 See the calculations in Goubert, *Réseau médical*, p. 226.
207 Based on the figures given in Arnold Chaplin, *Medicine in England during the Reign of George III* (London, 1919), p. 8. The principal source for such calculations is the last edition of the London physician Samuel Foart Simmons's directory of British and foreign medical practitioners, *The Medical Register for the Year 1783* (London, 1783). See Joan Lane, "The Medical Practitioners of Provincial England in 1783," *Medical History* 28 (1984): 353-71.
208 But cf. Goubert, "Réseau médical," pp. 226–27. See also his calculations for Brittany as a whole (2.7/10,000, raised to 3/10,000 by marine and naval surgeons, suggesting that 12% of the population was medicalized) in "Die Medikalisierung der französischen Gesellschaft am Ende des Ancien Régime: Die Bretagne als Beispiel," *Medizinhistorisches Journal* 17 (1982): 95, 105.
209 Goubert, "Medicalization," p. 162; "Réseau médical," p. 224; and idem, "The Extent of Medical Practice in France around 1780," *Journal of Social History* 10 (1976–77): 414–17.
210 Goubert, "Réseau médical," p. 224. On Brittany, see also Goubert, "Topographie médicale de la Bretagne à la fin du XVIIIe siècle," *Bulletin du Centre d'Histoire Économique et Sociale de la Région Lyonnaise*, 1973, no. 2, pp. 52–53, and his *Malades et médecins*, pp. 52–119; also Meyer, "Personnel médical."
211 For this comparison, see Goubert and Lebrun, "Médecins et chirurgiens," pp. 132–34; and see also Goubert, "Topographie," p. 53. On Anjou: Lebrun, *Les Hommes et la mort*, pp. 217–35; and Robert Favreau et al., *Atlas historique française: Anjou*, 2 vols. (1973), text vol., p. 83.
212 Dupuy, "Épidémies en Bretagne," *Annales de Bretagne*, 2: 193; Goubert, *Malades et médecins*, p. 89, and "Topographie médicale," p. 53; Meyer, "Personnel médical," p. 174.
213 Maillé-Virole, "Naissance d'un personnage," p. 155. Cf. the somewhat lower figures in Corlieu, *L'Ancienne Faculté de Médecine de Paris*, p. 87; and Lebrun, *Médecins, saints et sorciers*, p. 88.
214 Based on figures given in Chaplin, *Medicine in England*, pp. 8–9: 149 physicians, 274 surgeons, and 351 apothecaries. Somewhat different densities can be derived from W. F. Bynum, "Physicians, Hospitals, and Career Structures in Eighteenth-Century London," in Bynum and Roy Porter, eds., *William Hunter and the Eighteenth-Century Medical World* (Cambridge, 1985), pp. 106–07. Bynum suggests totals of 148 physicians and about 960 medical men in all, for a population of 800,000 (higher than Chaplin's figure); the densities would be 11.76 practitioners and 1.85 physicians per 10,000 inhabitants.
215 Goubert, "Extent," passim; see esp. table 3, p. 422. Félix Laffe, "Médecins et société à Saint-Rémy-de-Provence au XVIIIe siècle," *Provence historique*, fasc. 134 (1983): 462–63.
216 Keith Thomas, *Religion and the Decline of Magic* (New York, 1971), p. 10.
217 See Jean-Pierre Goubert and Bernard Lepetit, "Les Niveaux de médicalisation des villes françaises à la fin de l'Ancien Régime," *Historical Reflections/Réflexions historiques* 9 (1982): 45–67. Daniel Roche gives densities for 32 provincial towns in *Le Siècle des Lumières*, 2: 348.
218 Gelfand, "Deux cultures," p. 472.
219 Goubert and Lebrun, "Médecins et chirurgiens," pp. 125–26.
220 Gelfand, "Public Medicine," pp. 109–11. On Italy, see Carlo Cipolla, *Public Health and the Medical Profession in the Renaissance* (Cambridge, 1976), chap. 2.
221 See Dupuy, "Épidémies en Bretagne," *Annales de Bretagne*, 2: 193; Delaunay, *Vie médicale*, pp. 183–91; Jean-Pierre Goubert, "La Pénétration du médecin dans le corps social en France, 1770–1850," *Histoire des sciences médicales* 14 (1980): 435–38 (p. 437 on Loudéac); Léonard, *Médecins de l'Ouest*, p. 193; Maillé-Virole, "Naissance d'un

personnage," p. 175 (on Paris). On the plight of the rural poor, see, for example, AN D XXXVIII 3, d. 45, Nicolas *le cadet* at Auch to National Assembly, 27 June 1790.

222 AD Vienne D 7, "Règlement des droits et honoraires des médecins de Poitiers," 14 July 1734, and 1748 statutes, both cited in Boissonnade, *Essai sur l'organisation du travail*, p. 476.

223 Thillaud, *Maladies*, pp. 95–96. In the 1740's, at a small town called Bardos, 41 families paid a physician 160 livres per annum plus 10 sous for each visit (pp. 82, 112).

224 AD Vosges 1 C 43, quoted in Goubert, "Pénétration," p. 435.

225 Goubert, "Pénétration," pp. 436–37 (citing AN Y 1905–1906 on nonpayment by rich patients in Paris and the Île-de-France, 1781–1791).

226 AD Ille-et-Vilaine C 1327, quoted in Dupuy, "Épidémies en Bretagne," *Annales de Bretagne*, 3: 183–84. Cf. p. 185, C 1329, subdelegate of Châteaubriant, on peasants' greater confidence in *matrones*.

227 Jules Lecoeur [Louis-Jules Tirard], *Esquisses du bocage normand*, 2 vols. (Condé-sur-Noireau, 1883–87), 2: 98–99.

228 AD Ille-et-Vilaine C 1390, quoted in Paul Delaunay, *Études sur l'hygiène, l'assistance publique et les secours publics dans le Maine sous l'Ancien Régime*, 2d ser. fasc. 3 (Le Mans, 1923), p. 226.

229 AD Ille-et-Vilaine C 1365, quoted in Dupuy, "Épidémies en Bretagne," *Annales de Bretagne* 2: 213.

230 Denis Diderot, *Supplément au voyage de Bougainville*, 1st pub. 1774, in *Oeuvres* (1951), p. 1020.

231 Delaunay, *Vie médicale*, p. 185.

232 Gelfand, "Public Medicine," p. 102, citing Georges Frêche, *Toulouse et la région Midi-Pyrénées au siècle des Lumières, vers 1690–1789* (1974), p. 112. The *généralité* of Soissons at the end of the Old Regime had a physician-in-chief for the province, a *médecin ordinaire* for each *élection*, and a surgeon for each subdelegation, according to AM 228, Chevallier, "Abus dans l'exercice de la médecine dans les campagnes" (1819), but these officials could not have done much more than oversee public hygiene and health care. For a comparative perspective, see the essays in Russell, *Town and State Physician*, esp. Richard Palmer, "Physicians and the State in Post-Medieval Italy," and Manfred Stürzbecher, "The Physici in German-Speaking Countries from the Middle-Age [sic] to the Enlightenment." See also Cipolla, *Public Health*, pp. 84–92, 113, 118–23.

233 AD Vienne D 6, deliberations of the Faculty of Medicine of Poitiers, cited in Boissonnade, *Organisation du travail*, p. 479; Edict of Marly, art. 36.

234 The petitions are in the "C" series of the *archives départementales*. The proposal: SRM 124, Dufour at Noyon, 17 March 1777, cited in Wilson, "*Maladies des femmes*," p. 392.

235 Muriel Jeorger, "La Structure hospitalière de la France sous l'Ancien Régime," *Annales E.S.C.* 32 (1977): 1025–51. Cf. Gelfand, "Public Medicine," and Lebrun, *Médecins, saints et sorciers*, p. 83.

236 On government assistance, two older works are still useful: Shelby Thomas McCloy, *Government Assistance in Eighteenth-Century France* (Durham, N.C., 1946); and Bloch, *L'Assistance et l'État*, esp. bk. 2, chap. 5, "Le Service de santé et d'hygiène publiques sous Turgot et Necker" (pp. 244–45 on the *médecins des épidémies*). On the remedies: Lafond, *Dynastie des Helvétius*.

237 See, for example, a report by Livré on the epidemic of dysentery at Le Mans in 1779 (SRM 145): "L'indocilité des malades est absolue; leur répugnance pour les secours que procure le gouvernement ne peut se rendre; ils croient toujours mal à propos que l'on ne les procure que pour les surcharger de nouveaux impôts." Also see Livré's report of 23 May 1780, deliberations of the Bureau d'Agriculture du Mans, reg. 6, quoted in Delaunay, *Études sur l'hygiène*, 2d ser., fasc. 3, p. 226.

238 Burton, *The Anatomy of Melancholy*, 3 vols. (London, 1926–27), 2: 240. Opinion

attributed to Hobbes by John Aubrey, *Brief Lives*, ed. A. Powell (London, 1949), p. 251, quoted in Thomas, *Religion*, p. 14.

239 Article by chevalier de Jaucourt, in *Encyclopédie, ou Dictionnaire raisonné des sciences, des arts, et des métiers*, vol. 10 (Neuchâtel [false imprint], 1765), p. 292. Moheau [probably a pseudonym for Montyon], *Recherches et considérations sur la population de la France*, ed. René Gonnard (1912; 1st pub. 1774), p. 285. See William Coleman, "L'Hygiène et l'État selon Montyon," *Dix-huitième siècle* 9 (1977): 101–08.

240 Peter Gay, *The Enlightenment: An Interpretation*, vol. 2: *The Science of Freedom* (New York, 1969), pp. 12–23.

241 Julien Offray de La Mettrie, *L'Homme-machine*, in *Oeuvres philosophiques*, 2 vols. (Berlin, 1774), 2: 283; Goubert and Lebrun quote this passage in "Médecins et chirurgiens," p. 136. Voltaire, article "Médecin," in *Dictionnaire philosophique*, *Oeuvres complètes de Voltaire*, 52 vols. (1877–85), 20: 56. On Voltaire's skepticism, see Renée Waldinger, "Voltaire and Medicine," *Studies on Voltaire and the Eighteenth Century* 58 (1967): 1777–1806.

242 It would be helpful to have investigations of medical history in France from the patient's point of view, of the sort now being carried out for England under the inspiration of Roy Porter; they have already shed much light on attitudes toward the profession, among other topics. See Porter, "The Patient's View: Doing Medical History from Below," *Theory and Society* 14 (1985): 175–98; and idem, ed., *Patients and Practitioners: Lay Perceptions of Medicine in Pre-industrial Society* (Cambridge, 1985), esp. chap. 8, Joan Lane, " 'The Doctor Scolds Me': The Diaries and Correspondence of Patients in Eighteenth-Century England," and chap. 10, Porter, "Laymen, Doctors, and Medical Knowledge in the Eighteenth Century: The Evidence of the *Gentleman's Magazine*."

243 *Corps municipal*, Moitron, quoted in Delaunay, "Médecine populaire dans le Maine," p. 80; AD Ille-et-Vilaine C 1381, quoted in Dupuy, "Épidémies en Bretagne," *Annales de Bretagne*, 2: 214.

244 At Chantonnay (Poitou); quoted in Rambaud, *Pharmacie en Poitou*, p. 64.

245 AD Ille-et-Vilaine C 1331, C 1347. Cf. Dupuy, "Épidémies en Bretagne," *Annales de Bretagne*, 2: 215, quoting C 1383, on the 1773 outbreak at Riec; C 1347 on "putrid fever" in 1774 at Bonnemain; and C 1370 on an epidemic around Moncontour in 1779.

246 SRM 124, Jean-Guillaume Chifoliau, "Préjugés opposés aux sages précautions du gouvernement, aux efforts des ministres de la santé, et à la voix de la nature," Saint-Malo, 22 March 1780; Fodéré, *Voyage aux Alpes-Maritimes*, 2: 291.

247 SRM 145, Dr. du Boueix, Report on outbreak of dysentery around Clisson in 1779 (1780).

248 Alice Taverne, *Coutumes et superstitions foréziennes*, no. 5: *Médecine populaire, sorcellerie, diables et lutins* (Ambierle, 1971), p. 6. Françoise Loux, *Le corps dans la société traditionnelle* (1979), p. 136; Loux and Philippe Richard, *Sagesses du corps: La Santé et la maladie dans les proverbes français* (1978), p. 161.

249 AD Ille-et-Vilaine C 1327, quoted in Dupuy, "Épidémies en Bretagne," *Annales de Bretagne*, 3: 178.

250 SRM 124, Chifoliau, "Préjugés." Cf. Michel-Noël-Patrice Vétillart du Ribert, *Histoire médicale des maladies dyssentériques qui affligent la province du Maine en 1779 . . .* (Le Mans, 1779), p. 21: "Les gens du Peuple, les paysans surtout, ne peuvent ajouter foi aux remèdes évacuans dans la maladie en question; ils pensent & nous disent qu'ils n'évacuent déjà que trop, qu'ils n'ont déjà que trop envie de vomir! La crainte qu'on ne leur propose des remèdes, les engage à cacher leur mal dans le commencement, & même jusqu'à ce qu'ils soient totalement abattus"; and, on the popular reaction during an outbreak of dysentery in the Netherlands in 1786, Simon-Nicolas-Henri Linguet, "Bruxelles," *Annales politiques, civiles, et littéraires du dix-huitième siècle* 7 (1779): 163: "Des vomitifs, disoient-ils, des purgations, quand la Nature nous accable déjà par des évacuations! Notre mal est précisément l'effet que l'on veut produire en nous!"

251 See Joseph Folliet, *La Médecine du docteur Gnafron* (Lyons, 1966), p. 18.
252 AD Ille-et-Vilaine C 1359, quoted in Dupuy, "Épidémies," *Annales de Bretagne*, 2: 212.
253 Lebrun, *Les Hommes et la mort*, p. 394.
254 Gaston Vuillier, "Chez les magiciens et les sorciers de la Corrèze," *Le Tour du monde*, n.s., 5 (1899): 507, and Michel Coissac, "Guérisseurs et sorciers limousins," *Aesculape* 4 (1914): 107.
255 AN CC 473, *liasse* 622, no. 252, Framinet, physician at Cerdon (Ain) to legislature, n.d. [1840's]; Framinet was in his eighties, and his recollection presumably went back to the beginning of the century. The clerk who read his communication, though, dismissed it as containing "des observations qui se refusent à l'analyse, tant elles sont incohérentes, confuses, insignifiantes."
256 Lecoeur, *Esquisses*, 2: 104; Ernest Sévrin, "Croyances populaires et médecine supranaturelle en Eure-et-Loir au XIXᵉ siècle," *Revue d'histoire de l'Église de France* 32 (1946): 282.
257 Pierre-François Letourneau, "Miscellanea" (BM Grenoble), quoted in Edmond Esmonin, *Études sur la France des XVIIᵉ et XVIIIᵉ siècles* (1964), pp. 487–88.
258 SRM 132, d. 64, anon. memoir on abuses in medicine, Poitou, n.d., p. 22.
259 AD Ille-et-Vilaine C 1376, quoted in Dupuy, "Épidémies en Bretagne," *Annales de Bretagne*, 2: 214.
260 Marc-Adrien Dollfuss, "Un Procès médical en Haute-Normandie au XVIIIᵉ siècle," *Bulletin de la Société Nationale des Antiquaires de France*, 1969, pp. 141–44.
261 Charles Tilly, *The Vendée: A Sociological Analysis of the Counterrevolution of 1793* (Cambridge, Mass., 1964), pp. 242–52.
262 *Oeuvres complètes de Voltaire*, 52 vols. (1877–1885), 19: 289.
263 On the republican critique of doctors and professional monopoly in seventeenth-century England, see Christopher Hill, *The World Turned Upside Down: Radical Ideas During the English Revolution* (New York, 1973), p. 240; and Charles Webster, *The Great Instauration: Science, Medicine, and Reform, 1626–1660* (New York, 1975), pp. 256–62. On later developments: Matthew Ramsey, "The Politics of Professional Monopoly in Nineteenth-Century Medicine: The French Model and Its Rivals," in Gerald L. Geison, ed., *Professions and the French State, 1700–1900* (Philadelphia, 1984), pp. 225–305.

CHAPTER 2 *The medical profession in the early nineteenth century*

1 The literature on medicine during the Revolution is vast. Recent general discussions include Michel Foucault, *The Birth of the Clinic: An Archaeology of Medical Perception*, tr. A. M. Sheridan Smith (New York, 1973); David M. Vess, *Medical Revolution in France, 1789–96* (Gainesville, Fla., 1975); and Pierre Huard, *Sciences, médecine, pharmacie: De la Révolution à l'Empire, 1789–1815* (1970). See also the useful précis by Huard and Marie-José Imbault-Huart, "Concepts et réalités de l'éducation et de la profession médico-chirurgicales pendant la Révolution," *Journal des savants*, 1973, pp. 126–50; and Erwin H. Ackerknecht, *Medicine at the Paris Hospital, 1794–1848* (Baltimore, 1967). For a useful corrective to the view that revolutionary France was the *fons et origo* of clinical medicine, cf. Othmar Keel, "The Politics of Health and the Institutionalisation of Clinical Practices in Europe in the Second Half of the Eighteenth Century," in W. F. Bynum and Roy Porter, eds., *William Hunter and the Eighteenth-Century Medical World* (Cambridge, 1985), pp. 207–56.
2 The notable exception is Jacques Léonard. See his state doctoral thesis, *Les Médecins de l'Ouest au XIXᵉ siècle*, University of Paris IV, 1976 (1978), pt. 1, "Situation initiale." Among older studies, Constant Saucerotte, *Les Médecins pendant la Révolution, 1789–1799* (1887), can still be read with profit.
3 See, for example, the reform proposals from the late 1770's and 1780's in SRM 115; others are scattered throughout the archives of the Société Royale.

4 See, for example, *Archives parlementaires de 1787 à 1860*, 1st ser. (1862–), 4: 20, clergy of Montargis; 6: 79, nobility of Troyes; and 6: 233, Wasigny (*bailliage* of Vitry-le-François).

5 SRM 115, d. 9–20, includes projects for medical education submitted to the Comité de Salubrité. Many are in the AN: e.g., D VI 56, d. 916, Percheron de la Galézière, "Plan de règlement sur l'exercice de la médecine et de la chirurgie dans les campagnes," 1789. It would be interesting to analyze these proposals systematically; Jean-Pierre Peter has been working along these lines. Some are relatively conservative, particularly on the question of professional organization. Claude-Marie Devaulx, for example, a physician at Roanne, attacked "medico-surgeons" and called for a rigorous separation of medicine, surgery, and pharmacy (SRM 112, "Observations et réflexions relatives aux moyens de perfectionner l'art de guérir," 1790, p. 17).

6 Foucault, *Birth of the Clinic*, p. 32.

7 Retz, *Motion d'une utilité remarquable proposée à l'Assemblée des États-Généraux* (n.p., 1789), p. 7; Michel-Augustin Thouret, memoir on cantonal surgeons, 6 August 1790, in Camille Bloch and Alexandre Tuetey, eds., *Procès-verbaux et rapports du Comité de Mendicité de la Constituante, 1790–91* (1911), pp. 107–08; La Rochefoucauld-Liancourt, *Secours à donner à la classe indigente...*, in ibid., pp. 394–95. Sabarot de l'Avernière, *Vues de législation médicale, adressées aux États-Généraux...* (1789); on the analogy with the curé, cf. Jean-Jacques Menuret de Chambaud, *Essai sur les moyens de former de bons médecins...* (1791), p. 119. See also the memoir by Pierre Rouch, former member of the Montpellier faculty, *Réflexions sur la réforme générale de la médecine* (1813), sent to the Constituent Assembly in ms. form in 1791; copy in AN F⁸ 164. On public assistance and public health in the Constituent Assembly, see Huard and Imbault-Huart, "Concepts," pp. 127–28, and Dora B. Weiner, "Le Droit de l'homme à la santé: Une Belle Idée devant l'Assemblée Constituante, 1790–1791," *Clio Medica* 5 (1970): 209–23. On the intellectual background, consult the suggestive essay by Harvey Mitchell, "Politics in the Service of Knowledge: The Debate over the Administration of Medicine and Welfare in Late Eighteenth-Century France," *Social History* 6 (1981): 185–207.

8 Gallot, *Vues générales sur la restauration de l'art de guérir...* (1790). Société Royale de Médecine, *Nouveau Plan de constitution pour la médecine en France...* (1790); reprinted in the Society's memoirs (*Histoire et mémoires de la Société Royale de Médecine*), vol. 9. On the background and composition of the *Nouveau Plan*, and especially the role of contributors other than Vicq d'Azyr, see Toby Gelfand, "A Clinical Ideal: Paris, 1789," *Bulletin of the History of Medicine* 51 (1977): 397–99.

9 For Guillotin's views, see his *Motion pour l'établissement d'un comité de santé* (1790); copy in AN AD VIII 33.

10 A general history of the committee, which functioned until the end of the Constituent Assembly (30 September 1791), may be found in Henry Ingrand, *Le Comité de Salubrité de l'Assemblée Nationale Constituante, 1790–1791*, Paris medical thesis, 1934, no. 432; see also Huard, *Sciences*, pp. 115–16. Weiner gives the details of relations between the two committees (Mendicité and Salubrité) in "Une Belle Idée"; she stresses the rivalry between La Rochefoucauld-Liancourt, with his physician ally, Thouret, and Guillotin and Gallot, who represented the interests of Vicq d'Azyr. Toby Gelfand has called attention to the exchanges between the Comité de Salubrité and the Société Royale in ARC 4 ("Medical Professionals and Charlatans: The *Comité de Salubrité* enquête of 1790–91," *Histoire sociale–Social History* 11 [1978]: 65, n. 9). The committee's archives unfortunately were not collected under the classification reserved for them at the AN; some materials can be found elsewhere (e.g., AF I* 23, *procès-verbaux*), but a part appears to have been lost.

11 On the larger debate on public assistance and hospital reform, see Foucault, *Birth of the Clinic*, pp. 18–20, 39–44; and Louis S. Greenbaum, "Health Care and Hospital Building in Eighteenth-Century France: Reform Proposals of Du Pont de Nemours and Condorcet," *Studies on Voltaire and the Eighteenth Century* 152 (1976): 895–930.

For the committee's views, see AN F^{16} 936, "Secours à donner aux pauvres dans les campagnes" (session of 6 August 1790, revised 25 August 1790), calling for cantonal physicians and surgeons.

12 See the lists in the *procès-verbaux*, AN AF I★ 23.

13 Guillotin, *Projet de décret sur l'enseignement et l'exercice de l'art de guérir* . . . (August 1791), in Alfred de Beauchamp, comp., *Médecine et pharmacie: Projets de lois*, 5 vols. (1888–95), 1: 159–89. Cf. Gallot, *Observations . . . sur le projet de décret sur l'enseignement et l'exercice de l'art de guérir, présenté par M. Guillotin* . . . (1791); and see Weiner, "Une Belle Idée," pp. 216–17.

14 For a useful overview of the Revolution's attack on the corporations, see William H. Sewell, Jr., *Work and Revolution in France: The Language of Labor from the Old Regime to 1848* (Cambridge, 1980), chap. 4.

15 ARC 4, report, 29 May 1793. M.-J. Guillaume, ed., *Procès-verbaux du Comité d'Instruction de la Convention Nationale*, 6 vols. (1891–1907), 2: 511–12, 2: 866, and 3: 229; and *Archives parlementaires*, 1st ser. (1862–), 83: 543–44.

16 Huard and Imbault-Huart, "Concepts," pp. 130–32; Marie-Élisabeth Antoine and Jean Waquet, "La Médecine civile en France à l'époque napoléonienne et le legs du XVIIIe siècle," *Revue de l'Institut Napoléon*, no. 132 (1976): 70; Foucault, *Birth of the Clinic*, pp. 67–68. On Caen: Charles Fayel-Deslongrais, *La Faculté de Médecine de Caen de 1436 à 1808* . . . (Caen, 1890), pp. 26–29; Pierre-Jean-Georges Cabanis, *Oeuvres philosophiques*, ed. Claude Lehec and Jean Cazeneuve, 2 vols. (1956), 2: 390. On Besançon: AN AF III 107, cited by Louis Liard, *L'Enseignement supérieur en France, 1789–1893*, 2 vols. (1888–94), 1: 222. On Montpellier: Alexandre-Charles Germain, *L'École de Médecine de Montpellier* . . . (Montpellier, 1880), p. 70. See also Léonard, *Médecins de l'Ouest*, pp. 198, 219–21; he cites (p. 219) AN F^{17} 2455 for the number of Caen graduates.

17 Law of 14–17 April 1791, temporarily maintaining the legislation on pharmacy in existence on March 2 (date of the antiguild measure), in *Lois et actes du gouvernement* 3 (1806): 109–10. Ministère de l'Intérieur, *Extrait des registres du Directoire Exécutif, du troisième jour du mois floréal (an IV)*, certified copy in FP A4 114. The reactions of the College of Pharmacy can be traced in its minutes, FP reg. 13. See esp. no. 147, a humble petition to the National Assembly (28 January 1792); although thanking the legislature for maintaining the old restrictions on pharmaceutical practice, the college nonetheless renounces old rights and privileges, recognizing that "leur existence actuelle forcée sous le mode de corporation, est contraire aux principes de la Constitution," and accepts the abolition of the College as a corporation that had been temporarily conserved. In the event, it endured. See Bénédicte Dehillerin and Jean-Pierre Goubert, "A la conquête du monopole pharmaceutique: Le Collège de Pharmacie de Paris, 1777–1796," *Historical Reflections/Réflexions historiques* 9 (1982): 246–48; Charles Bedel, "L'Enseignement des sciences pharmaceutiques," in René Taton, ed., *Enseignement et diffusion des sciences au XVIIIe siècle* (1964), p. 251; and Georges Dillemann and Marie-Edmée Michel, "La Réception des pharmaciens en France de la Révolution à l'application de la loi du 21 germinal an XI, 1791–1803," *Revue d'histoire de la pharmacie* 72 (1984): 42–61.

18 On the educational reforms of the Year III, see Vess, *Medical Revolution*, chaps. 9–10; Toby Gelfand, *Professionalizing Modern Medicine: Paris Surgeons and Medical Science and Institutions in the Eighteenth Century* (Westport, Conn., 1980), pp. 165–70; Huard and Imbault-Huart, "Concepts," pp. 134–37. On medical education under the new legislation: André Prévost, *Les Études médicales sous le Directoire et le Consulat* (1907).

19 Fourcroy, *Rapport et projet de décret sur l'établissement d'une école centrale de santé à Paris*, 7 Frimaire III/27 November 1794, esp. pp. 4–5, on the existing situation. Text of the law of 14 Frimaire/4 December in *Bulletin des lois*, 1st ser., Year III, no. 96, pp. 2–6.

20 Huard and Imbault-Huart, "Concepts," pp. 139–42.

21 On the debates of the Directory era, see Gelfand, *Professionalizing Modern Medicine*, pp. 168–69; and André Prévost, "Les Projets de réforme de l'enseignement médical

sous le Directoire," *La Presse médicale*, 1903, nos. 67, 81, 103. The texts of the major projects and reports are in Beauchamp, *Projets de lois*, vol. 1.

22 See, for example, Jacquinot, *Observations sur le projet de résolution, présenté au Conseil des Cinq-Cents, par Emm.* Pastoret, *au nom de la Commission d'Instruction Publique, dans la séance du 16 thermidor, an V, sur un mode provisoire d'examen pour les officiers de santé* (n.d.), pp. 19–23. Copy in AN AD VIII 33.

23 See, for example, the debates in the *Procès-verbaux du Conseil des Cinq-Cents*, 14–17 and 28–29 Germinal VI.

24 AN AD VIII 33, no. 20, *Aux représentans du peuple français: Plan général pour l'enseignement, la pratique, & la police de la médecine* (Year VI?).

25 Jules Barbot, *Les Chroniques de la Faculté de Médecine de Toulouse du treizième au vingtième siècle...*, 2 vols. (Toulouse, 1905), 2: 11. See also Liard, *L'Enseignement supérieur*, vol. 1, appendix J, on a plan for a health school in Toulouse.

26 Pierre-Jean-Georges Cabanis, *Rapport fait au Conseil des Cinq-Cents, sur l'organisation des écoles de médecine*, 29 Brumaire VII/19 November 1798, in *Oeuvres philosophiques*, 2: 409. Louis Vitet, *Rapport sur les écoles spéciales de médecine*, 17 Ventôse VI/7 March 1798.

27 *Projet de loi sur l'enseignement et la police de la médecine*, Year IX, in Beauchamp, *Projets de lois* pp. 489–97; *Projet d'arrêté concernant les écoles de médecine*, Year IX, ibid., pp. 498–504; *Projet d'arrêté sur l'organisation et la police de la pharmacie*, Year X, ibid., pp. 505–13; *Projet de loi sur le mode d'examen et de réception des médecins, des chirurgiens, et des officiers de santé* Year X, ibid., pp. 523–27. On the successful project, see AN C 617, d. 29, "Messages et motifs qui étoient annoncés au projet de loi du 7 pluviôse an XI"; Conseil d'État, extract, *registre des délibérations*, 30 Pluviôse. For the debates, see Fourcroy, "Exposé des motifs du projet de loi sur l'exercice de la médecine," in *Archives parlementaires*, 2d ser. (1862–), 4: 30–32; Thouret report, 16 Ventôse XI/7 March 1803, ibid., 4: 100–104; Carret, report of 17 Ventôse, ibid., pp. 113–14; AN C 648, d. 10, extract, *procès-verbal du Tribunat*; and, on the final session in the Corps Législatif, *Archives parlementaires*, 4: 141–46 (p. 143, Jard-Panvillier) and Corps Législatif, *Procès-verbaux*, Year XI, p. 720. See also Saucerotte, *Les Médecins*, pp. 156–57. The text of the law of Ventôse is in *Bulletin des lois*, 3d ser., 7: 567–76. See also René Roland, *Les Médecins et la loi du 19 ventôse an XI: Étude historique et juridique sur l'organisation de la profession médicale et sur ses conditions d'exercice* (1883).

28 *Archives parlementaires*, 2d ser., 4: 542–46.

29 Ibid., pp. 577–79, 606–08.

30 Jacques Léonard, *La Vie quotidienne du médecin de province au XIXᵉ siècle* (1977), p. 9.

31 Désiré, Armand, and Édouard Dalloz, *Jurisprudence générale du royaume: Répertoire méthodique et alphabétique de législation, de doctrine, et de jurisprudence...*, new ed., 44 vols. (1845–70), 31: 554.

32 Theodore Zeldin, *France, 1848–1945*, vol. 1: *Ambition, Love, and Politics* (Oxford, 1973), p. 37.

33 See Robert Heller, "*Officiers de santé*: The Second-Class Doctors of Nineteenth-Century France," *Medical History* 22 (1978): 25–43 (pp. 39–43 are an English translation of the law of Ventôse). Another useful discussion of the debate over the *officiat* can be found in an unpublished paper by Harry Marks, "French Medical Reform, 1810–1848: The Return of the Repressed."

34 For example: AN F⁸ 165, Saulé, Montpellier graduate at Castillon (Haute-Garonne) to minister, 28 Brumaire XII/20 November 1803. The law had taken effect on 1 Vendémiaire (24 September).

35 See, for example, AN F¹⁷ 2437, 9 Prairial XII/29 May 1804, protest signed by nine surgeons of the Bas-Rhin.

36 P.-J. Marie de Saint-Ursin, *Manuel populaire de santé à l'usage des personnes intelligentes vivant à la campagne...* (1808), p. v.

37 Such objections recall those voiced before the Ventôse law, as in Pierre-Jean Lioult's *Les Charlatans dévoilés, ou Réflexions sur la liberté considérée dans le rapport qu'elle a avec*

l'exercice des professions (Year VIII), which argued that following the dissolution of the hierarchy of physician, surgeon, and apothecary, everyone was a physician and needed only a 50-franc patent in order to practice (pp. 65–67).

38 AM 231, Bertrand, "Proposition sur l'organisation de l'art de guérir." *Nouveau Projet de réorganisation de la médecine, de la chirurgie, et de la pharmacie en France* (1817), pp. 44–46.

39 See, for example, AN F¹⁷ 2107, prefect of the Doubs to Fourcroy, 3 Messidor XI/ 22 June 1803, and AN F¹⁷ 2423, B. Girard, member, medical jury of the Lozère, to Minister of the Interior, 23 Prairial XII/12 June 1804.

40 *Annuaire de la Société de Médecine, Chirurgie, et Pharmacie du Département de l'Eure, pour l'année 1819*, pp. 209–11. For example: "La maladie est un vaisseaux qui doit purger tout le sang, et il doit dessendre au bas ventre qui fait bien la racine du germe et ce mauvais vaisseaux a bien dessendu jusqua dessus les reins et il a monté l'estomact et le foix qui en est enveloppé."

41 AN F⁸ 153, de S . . .[?] to minister, 30 Germinal XII/20 April 1804.

42 AN F¹⁷ 1146, d. 9, Royer to *conseiller d'état* for public instruction, covering letter, 12 Thermidor XII/31 July 1804, and memoir. Cf. the correspondence in F⁸ 164, together with his pamphlet, *Bienfaisance, ou Projet d'un code médical rural.* Royer was also the author of a three-volume *Ouvrage médicinal populaire* (Provins, 1809), and coauthor, with his son, of *Bienfaisance médicale rurale, ou Institution d'environ cent mille hospices à domicile ou dispensaires ruraux* (Troyes, 1814).

43 Édouard Lemaître, *Exposé des abus qui existent dans l'exercice de la médecine, et moyens d'y remédier* (1825), pp. 35.

44 The debates are in AN F¹⁷ 2655 and F¹⁷ 2108. See Léonard, *Médecins de l'Ouest*, pp. 387–89.

45 On this question, see Jacques Léonard, "La Restauration et la profession médicale," *Historical Reflections/Réflexions historiques* 9 (1982): 70–72.

46 Lemaître, *Exposé des abus*, p. 43; Lemaître's ability to adapt to political change is demonstrated by a pamphlet he published after the Revolution of 1848: *Catéchisme républicain, ou Code des droits du citoyen: Dialogue entre un docteur, un ouvrier et un conservateur rallié à la République* (1848). AN F⁸ 162, Plantié, "Considérations sur l'anarchie médicale en France," 1814.

47 See, for example, AN F⁸ 153, Dr. Desmares de Bonneville to Minister of the Interior, n.d.

48 AN F¹⁷ 3680, cited in George Weisz, "Constructing the Medical Elite in France: The Creation of the Royal Academy of Medicine, 1814–20," *Medical History* 30 (1986): 419–43 (citation, p. 429).

49 Marquais, *Rapport au roi sur l'état actuel de la médecine en France, et sur la nécessité d'une réforme dans l'étude . . . de cette science* (1814); and *Adresse au Roi et aux deux Chambres sur la nécessité de réorganiser les écoles de médecine et de chirurgie en France . . .* (1817), esp. pp. 35–36 on the *officiat*.

50 Marquais, *Rapport de la commission nommée par l'ordonnance du Roi du 9 novembre 1815, à l'effet de lui rendre compte de l'état actuel de l'enseignement de la médecine et de la chirurgie en France . . .* (1816). Cf. (for a defense of the continued union of medicine and surgery) a work by two professors of the Paris faculty who served on the commission: Jean-Jacques Leroux des Tillets and Guillaume Dupuytren, *Mémoire et plan d'organisation pour la médecine et la chirurgie* (1816). For the background of the debates of 1815–17, see Weisz, "Constructing the Medical Elite," pp. 428–35.

51 See, for example, Lemaître, *Exposé des abus*, pp. 35–36.

52 The discussion here follows Léonard, "La Restauration," pp. 77–80. See also *Médecins de l'Ouest*, pp. 772–77.

53 Corbière, *Projet de loi sur les écoles secondaires de médecine, les chambres de discipline, les eaux minérales artificielles . . .* (1825). For the legislative debates: *Archives parlementaires*, 2d ser., 43: 166–69, 14 February 1825; 44: 563–75, committee report, Chambre des Députés, 12 April 1825; 47: 72, 74–75, commission's report (Chaptal), Chambre des Pairs, 11 April 1826.

54 For an example of a provincial proposal, see AM 236, Gilly, pharmacist at Marseilles, 15 January 1829. On the work of a provincial commission, see, for example, *Rapport de la commission nommée par les médecins de la ville de Metz, pour l'examen des questions relatives à une nouvelle organisation médicale, proposée par le ministre de l'intérieur* (Metz, 1829), copy in AN F¹⁷ 4467, d. 2/3a.

55 On reform under the July Monarchy and Second Republic, see Léonard, *Médecins de l'Ouest*, pp. 782–822, and George Weisz, "The Politics of Medical Professionalization in France, 1845–1848," *Journal of Social History* 12 (1978–79): 3–30. Educational reform is discussed in Léonard, *Médecins de l'Ouest*, pp. 940–1002, and George Weisz, "Reform and Conflict in French Medical Education, 1870–1914," in Weisz and Robert Fox, eds., *The Organization of Science and Technology in France, 1808–1914* (Cambridge, 1980), pp. 61–94. On professional reorganization and legislation under the Second Empire and Third Republic, see Léonard, *Médecins de l'Ouest*, chap. 15; René Roland, *Les Médecins et la loi du 30 novembre 1892: Étude historique et juridique sur l'organisation de la profession médicale et sur ses conditions d'exercice* (1893); and Martha L. Hildreth, "The Foundations of the Modern Medical System in France: Physicians, Public Health Advocates, and the Medical Legislation of 1892 and 1893," *Proceedings of the Eighth Annual Meeting of the Western Society for French History* (Las Cruces, N.M., 1981), pp. 311–27. The text of the law of 1892 is in *Bulletin des lois*, 12th ser., 46 (1893): 833–40.

56 Instruction of 13 Fructidor XI/31 August 1803. Text in *Recueil des lettres circulaires, discours, et autres actes publics émanés . . . du Ministère de l'Intérieur*, 20 vols. (Year VII–1821), 4: 605–07.

57 AD Bas-Rhin 5 M 22, no. 40, 1813 list of practitioners for the canton of Brumath (and cf. no. 42, Wissembourg, another case).

58 On this point, see John V. Spears, "Peasants, Doctors and Typhoid Fever: The French Department of the High Alps, 1780–1870," Ph.D. dissertation, The Johns Hopkins University, 1978, p. 159.

59 AD Bas-Rhin 5 M 22, no. 35, report by Lion, 19 June 1813.

60 AD Loire-Atlantique 12 U 20, 5 Messidor XI/24 June 1803, cited n Léonard, *Médecins de l'Ouest*, p. 292.

61 AN F⁸ 152, Clément case.

62 J.-B. Deserin, *Observations et réflexions sur la loi du 19 ventôse an XI, relative à l'exercice de la médecine . . .* (Paris and Auxerre, 1820), p. 39.

63 AN F⁸ 153, petition from Marie Daux, *femme* Delestang.

64 Jurists pointed out that women had not been admitted by the faculties of the Old Regime and had finally been barred from practicing surgery; some, like the Dalloz team, perceived a "moral obstacle" to medical practice by women (*Répertoire*, 21: 547). See also E. Beaugrand, "Médecins (femmes)," in *Dictionnaire encyclopédique des sciences médicales*, 100 vols. (1865–1889), n.s. 5: 594–607. For the more generous construction of Chaptal's circular, see Georges-Denis Weil, *De l'Exercice illégal de la médecine et de la pharmacie: Législation pénale et jurisprudence* (1886), pp. 16–17. Weil argues that the circular concerned only persons who benefitted from article 23; since women had not been received in the Old Regime, they could not invoke the provisions of that article, but they could now be received by the new health schools.

65 On the entry of women into European medicine in the latter nineteenth century, see Caroline Schultze, *La Femme-médecin au XIXᵉ siècle*, Paris medical thesis, 1888, no. 49.

66 Serrières, *Discours sur l'influence de la Révolution française dans l'enseignement et la pratique de la médecine* (Nancy, n.d.).

67 AN F⁸ 163, Poulain to Minister of the Interior, n.d.

68 Gastellier, *Observations et réflexions relatives à l'organisation actuelle de la médecine* (Montargis, 1806), pp. 10–11.

69 Spears, "Peasants," pp. 157–58.

70 George M. Rosen, *The Specialization of Medicine, with Particular Reference to Ophthalmology* (New York, 1944), p. 53. Guénon de la Chanterie nonetheless appeared

as an oculist on the official list of doctors of medicine in the department of the Seine down to the beginning of the July Monarchy (see *Almanach royal et national*, 1831, p. 894).

71 AN F⁸ 160, prefect of the Bas-Rhin to Minister of the Interior, sending report by Lion, cantonal physician of Soultz-sous-Forêts, to subprefect at Wissembourg [after 1810], "sur les accidens fâcheux arrivés à des enfans juifs, par l'ineptie de celui qui leur a fait l'opération de la circoncision."

72 Jean-François Barailon, *Rapport . . . au nom de la Commission d'Instruction Publique . . . sur la partie de la police qui tient à la médecine*, 11 Germinal VI/31 March 1798, p. 21, n. 6; Gustave-Thomas de Closmadeuc, *Esquisse sur la médecine et la chirurgie populaires dans le département du Morbihan* (Vannes, 1861), p. 12.

73 AN F¹⁷ 2437, Bas-Rhin, printed list of practitioners for 1812.

74 *Annuaire de la Société de l'Eure . . . 1819*, p. 212; AN CC 476, l. 652, no. 48, note on petition of Nicolas Quinet (1804).

75 A. Treille, *Quelques réflexions sur les principaux abus en médecine* (Auch, 1823), pp. 10–11.

76 Léonard, *Médecins de l'Ouest*, p. 425. On popular oculists, see Paul-Abraham Pesme, *De quelques erreurs en médecine*, Paris medical thesis, 1855, no. 34, p. 90.

77 AN F⁸ 164, Minister of the Interior to prefect of the Loiret, 2 March 1811 (and other documents). On Royer, whose activities were not limited to keeping public baths, see Louis Faligot, *La Question des remèdes secrets sous la Révolution et l'Empire* (1924), pp. 62–63.

78 AC Lyons I 5 4, no. 664, prefect of the Rhône to mayor, 3 September 1820; M. Laureau, "Silvan de Lyon, bandagiste herniaire et breveté du roi," *Le Vieux Papier* 30 (1984): 145–46.

79 AN F¹⁷ 2107, prefect, Doubs, to Fourcroy, 3 Messidor XI/22 June 1803. Cf. AN BB¹ 204, *commissaire, tribunal de première instance*, Alençon (Orne), to Minister of Justice, 11 Pluviôse XII/1 February 1804, on an itinerant *dentiste-herniaire* received at Venice; despite the official's negative recommendation, the minister ruled that the practitioner could register his title.

80 AD Ille-et-Vilaine 20 Md 1, 5 Vendémiaire XII/28 September 1803, cited in Léonard, *Médecins de l'Ouest*, pp. 291–92.

81 AD Hautes-Alpes 136 M 2, cited in Spears, "Peasants," p. 104.

82 AD Loire 38 M 9, no. 9, Péricard to Emperor, 25 April 1808; no. 10, petition from mayors, 8 April; no. 8, Minister of the Interior to prefect, 13 May.

83 Léonard, *Médecins de l'Ouest*, pp. 425–27.

84 AN F¹⁷ 4470, 5 February 1848, from [illegible signature – Lagoguey?].

85 Deserin, *Observations*, p. iv.

86 Arthur Bordier, *La Médecine à Grenoble* (Grenoble, 1896), p. 109, n. 1.

87 Dr. Girard, "Guérisseurs et charlatans," *Revue médicale de Nancy* 73 (1948): 360.

88 AN F¹⁷ 2108, report by medical jury, Bordeaux, 6 June 1819; supplementary report, 14 June.

89 See Ulysse Trélat, *De la constitution du corps des médecins et de l'enseignement médical: Des réformes qu'elle devrait subir dans l'intérêt de la science et de la morale publique . . .* (1828), p. 74.

90 Dalloz, *Répertoire*, 31: 548–50.

91 AN F¹⁷ 2110, Cour de Cassation, 23 February 1827 and 15 May 1846; see Léonard, *Médecins de l'Ouest*, p. 734.

92 Ministry of Education, 3d division, 1st bureau, circular to prefects, 20 September 1837; copy in AD Meurthe-et-Moselle 5 M 18, no. 89.

93 AD Haute-Loire 13 M 18, no. 481, police commissioner at Le Puy to prefect, 19 April 1819.

94 Dalloz, *Répertoire*, 31: 551.

95 Armand Trousseau, *Conférences sur l'empirisme, faites à la Faculté de Médecine de Paris . . .* (1862), p. 49.

96 Marcelle Bouteiller, for example, in *Médecine populaire d'hier et d'aujourd'hui* (1966), p. 26, cites a case from 1960.

97 George Sand, *Histoire de ma vie*, new ed., 4 vols. (1876), 4: 63; see Léonard, *Vie quotidienne*, p. 156.

98 Closmadeuc, *Esquisse*, p. 7.

99 Léonard, *Médecins de l'Ouest*, p. 1457.

100 See Dalloz, *Répertoire*, 31: 551, and Jacques Léonard, "Femmes, religion, et médecins," *Annales E.S.C.* 32 (1977): 887–907. Decisions and decrees of 1 Nivôse IX/ 22 December 1800; 9 Pluviôse X/29 January 1802; 12 Floréal XIII/2 May 1805; 8 Vendémiaire XIV/30 September 1805; 1 November 1806; 16 April 1828. On nurses, see also Dora B. Weiner, "The French Revolution, Napoleon, and the Nursing Profession," *Bulletin of the History of Medicine* 46 (1972): 274–305. On émigrés, see for example Paul Delaunay, *Études sur l'hygiène, l'assistance, et les secours publics dans le Maine sous l'Ancien Régime . . .* 1st ser. (Le Mans, 1920), p. 103, on abbé Calbris.

101 Léonard, "Femmes," p. 891.

102 See, for example, Lemaître, *Exposé*, p. 35: "que l'on annule une ordonnance qui du temps des guerres de Napoléon autorisait les prêtres à exercer la médecine, ordonnance qui sert encore de diplôme à plus d'un d'entre eux"; AN F^{17} 2107, three practitioners of Bourges to Directeur-Général de l'Instruction Publique, objecting to village priests who practice medicine, 5 June 1808; and AN F^8 164, Royer, father and son, objecting to royal ordinance allowing sisters of charity at Metz to deliver babies and "visit" (or treat, as they see it) the rural poor.

103 See, for example, Gastellier, *Observations*, pp. 3, 9.

104 AN F^8 167, Vimont to Minister of the Interior, 24 Fructidor XI/11 September 1803; AD Ille-et-Vilaine 20 Md 1, 27 Prairial XI/16 June 1803, cited by Léonard, *Médecins de l'Ouest*, p. 288.

105 Bernard Jacquet, *Empiriques et charlatans troyens du XVe au XIXe siècle* (1960), p. 59; AN F^{17} 2431, Orne, *procès-verbal*, medical jury, 7–11 October 1806, 17th case.

106 Léonard, *Médecins de l'Ouest*, pp. 381, 383, citing AD Morbihan M 987 and AN F^{17} 2420.

107 AN F^8 156, Ministry of the Interior, 3rd Division, Bureau des Sciences, to minister, 2 August 1806; AD Bas-Rhin 5 M 22, no. 58, procureur at Wissembourg to prefect, 6 March 1820; AD Yonne 5 M 7/1, no. 92, subprefect of Joigny to prefect, 28 January 1811.

108 AN F^8 150, prefect of the Nièvre to Directeur-Général de l'Instruction Publique, 9 Frimaire XIV/30 November 1805; Chevrier to prefect; Directeur-Général to Minister of the Interior, 22 Frimaire/13 December.

109 Treille, *Quelques réflexions*, p. 58.

110 AN F^8 162, prefect of the Cher to Minister of the Interior, 23 September 1807.

111 Léonard, *Médecins de l'Ouest*, pp. 385–86.

112 AN F^8 160, Macquet to subprefect of Malmédy, 2 Messidor XI/21 June 1803; draft of minister's reply to prefect, 27 Fructidor XI/14 September 1803.

113 AN BB^1 204, Minister of Justice to *procureur-général* of the Sarthe, 19 September 1806; AN F^8 150, Chervet to Minister of the Interior, citing report on Haut-Rhin case in *Annales politiques et littéraires du département de l'Isère*; AN F^8 165, prefect of the Doubs to Minister of the Interior, 30 July 1806, on ignorant practitioners who have titles and on Sudan case.

114 AN F^7 8185, d. 2981R^2, prefect of the Loiret to Police Générale, 1st arrondissement, 17 October 1810.

115 AN F^8 165, Louis Tils to prefect of Rhin-et-Moselle, 7 November 1808; prefect of Rhin-et-Moselle to prefect of the Sarre, 16 November; A. Vetten to prefect of Rhin-et-Moselle, 6 October 1809; prefect of Rhin-et-Moselle to prefect of the Sarre, 12 October.

116 Ibid., medical jury of the Sarre to prefect, 27 October 1809; extract, register of decrees, prefecture of the Sarre, 21 November; prefect to Minister of the Interior, 21 November; minister to prefect, 4 January.

117 Ibid., letter with protest from Schmitt's son, 23 June 1810; prefect of the Sarre to Minister of the Interior, 13 September; petition for Schmitt by Machet, Paris, 19 July 1811.

118 Dalloz, *Répertoire*, 31: 551, citing decision of 20 July 1833.

119 See, for example, the petitions in AN F[17] 2109.

120 AN F[8] 152, Contrastin to Minister of the Interior, 23 Frimaire Year [illegible]; F[8] 149, Minister of the Interior to Batard of Angers, 30 December 1808; F[8] 165, Suzov to Minister of the Interior, 25 Ventôse XI/16 March 1803; AN F[8] 164, Rochefort to Minister of the Interior, 20 Fructidor XI/7 September 1803.

121 AN F[8] 157, Hoest case, August 1806. On the executioners: AN F[8] 155, prefect of Loir-et-Cher to Minister of the Interior on Ferey case, 24 Vendémiaire XIII/16 October 1804, and draft of reply, 5 Brumaire/27 October; F[8] 154, Demorest to Minister of the Interior, 29 August 1808; Minister of the Interior to prefect of the Isère, 28 September 1808.

122 AD Yonne 5 M 7/1, no. 95, Maillet, n.d.; AD Aube M 1600, Guillot to prefect, 18 December 1828.

123 Announcement by Hart, *Journal, feuille d'annonces, et avis du département de la Meurthe*, no. 1681, 15 October 1816. Copy in AD Meurthe-et-Moselle 5 M 18, no. 224.

124 AN F[8] 164, Rousselet to Minister of the Interior, n.d. [First Empire].

125 AN F[8] 58, Le Plénier to Minister of the Interior, 1807; prefect of Maine-et-Loire to Minister of the Interior, 11 January 1808. AN F[8] 149, Béguin to Minister of the Interior, 1805, and minister's reply, 7 Floréal XIII/27 April 1805.

126 AN F[8] 153, Denis; AN BB[1] 204, Delvincourt to Minister of Justice, 22 Messidor XI/11 July 1803.

127 AN F[8] 162, Dr. Pignot to Minister of the Interior, 20 Ventôse XII/11 March 1804.

128 AN F[8] 150, Bin to Minister of the Interior, 5 Ventôse XII/25 February 1804.

129 AN F[15] 141, Vaubaillon to Minister of the Interior, 20 October 1812; and minister's earlier letter, 26 September.

130 AN F[8] 157, Hugon, 6 Fructidor XI/24 August 1803; AN F[8] 165, two similar petitions (Sudan), 14 Nivôse XIII/4 January 1805; AN F[8] 166, Valmory to Minister of the Interior, n.d. [after October 1812 and before March 1814].

131 AN F[8] 154, petition of 16 January 1808 and covering letter from Dufay.

132 AD Meurthe-et-Moselle 5 M 18, nos. 69–71, Maizières petition, 21 November 1824; no. 42, mayors' petition, 3 December, and lieutenant-general, 4 December. Cf. mayor of Assenoncourt to prefect, 1 August 1825. No. 65: tribunal of Vic to prefect on conviction and 25-franc fine. On population: Henri Lepage, *Le Département de la Meurthe: Statistique, historique, et administrative . . .*, 2 vols. (Nancy, 1843), 2: 338.

133 AD Meurthe-et-Moselle 5 M 18, prefect of the Meurthe to subprefect of Château-Salins, 31 December 1824. Ibid., no. 49, prefect to subprefect of Sarrebourg, 7 August 1827; and 16 November, reporting that the jury has met and has asked that Grillet be barred from practicing.

134 AP, Conseil de Salubrité, report to prefect, 1 November 1818.

135 FP, reg. 52, no. 53, copy of extract, minutes of state chancery, 6 February 1810. On the legislation, see Matthew Ramsey, "Property Rights and the Right to Health: The Regulation of Secret Remedies in France, 1789–1815," in W. F. Bynum and Roy Porter, eds., *Medical Fringe and Medical Orthodoxy* (London, 1986), pp. 79–105.

136 AD Loire 38 M 9, no. 18, mayor of Feurs to subprefect, 29 December 1812; AD Yonne 5 M 7/1, no. 174, mayor of Seignelay to prefect, 15 April 1818, and prefect's reply, 21 April. Cf. AN F[8] 58, prefect of Maine-et-Loire to Minister of the Interior, 11 January 1808, on Mme. Le Plénier's ingratitude toward the mayor of Bouche-maine, who had long tolerated her activities; and J.-M.-C. Naville, *Lettres bour-guignonnes, ou Aperçu philosophique et critique sur les causes des difficultés dans l'exercice de l'art de guérir. . .* (1822), pp. 25–26, on new woman healer supported by local authorities in the Chalonnais region.

137 AD Charente-Maritime 7 M 6/1, mayor of [illeg.] to prefect, 6 June 1818; AD Yonne 5 M 7/1, no. 211, Auxerre, commissioner of police to prefect, 19 May 1821. On Sibenaler's later adventures, see *Gazette des tribunaux* 4 (1828–29): 522–23.

138 See, for example, Michel Boyer, "L'Encadrement médical en Ardèche au XIXe siècle," master's thesis, University of Lyons II, 1977, p. 46.

139 AD Loire-Atlantique 1 M 1358, no. 401, subprefect of Paimboeuf,to prefect, 16

May 1811.

140 AC Nantes I 5 7, d. 3, commissioner-general of police to mayor, 15 Nivôse XIII/
5 January 1805; Olivier to commissioner, 23 Brumaire XIII/14 November 1804.

141 Trélat, *De la constitution*, p. 31.

142 *Annuaire de la Société de l'Eure . . . 1819*, p. 45; Trélat, *De la constitution*, p. 53.

143 On 1800–1801, see Huard, *Sciences*, p. 125, and George Weisz, "Les Professeurs
parisiens et l'académie de médecine en 1820," in Christophe Charle and Régine
Ferré, eds., *Le Personnel de l'enseignement supérieur en France aux XIXe et XXe siècles:
Colloque organisé par l'Institut d'Histoire Moderne et Contemporaine et l'École des Hautes
Études en Sciences Sociales le 25 et 26 juin 1984* (1985), p. 50, citing "Adresse de la
Société de Médecine de Paris au Premier Consul de la République," *Journal général
de médecine* 10 (1801): 199–200. In the same period, a group of former members of
the old Académie Royale de Chirurgie petitioned the government to re-establish
the Academy and the corporations and were rebuffed (AN F^17 3679, *Adresse présenté
au Premier Consul par les commissaires de l'Académie de Chirurgie, an IX* and government's reply, cited in Weisz, "Constructing the Medical Elite," pp. 425–26). Corporatist sentiments died hard. For later proposals, see, for example, AM 231,
Bertrand, "Proposition sur l'organisation de l'art de guérir," and Aimé-Antoine-
Marie Dornier, *Avis important sur la santé publique, ou Esquisse du charlatanisme médical
de 1836 . . .* (1836), p. 8, calling for physicians and pharmacists to form a corporation
like the lawyers'.

144 See, for example, Erwin H. Ackerknecht, "Hygiene in France, 1815–1848," *Bulletin
of the History of Medicine* 22 (1948): 117–55; William Coleman, *Death Is a Social
Disease: Public Health and Political Economy in Early Industrial France* (Madison, Wisc.,
1982); and Ann F. La Berge, "The Early Nineteenth-Century French Public Health
Movement: The Disciplinary Development and Institutionalization of *Hygiène Publique*," *Bulletin of the History of Medicine* 58 (1984): 363–79.

145 See George D. Sussman, "From Yellow Fever to Cholera: A Study of French
Government Policy, Medical Professionalism and Popular Movements in the Epidemic Crises of the Restoration and July Monarchy," Ph.D. dissertation, Yale
University, 1971, chaps. 1–3.

146 On the Paris council: Dora B. Weiner, "Public Health under Napoleon: The Conseil
de Salubrité de Paris, 1802–1815," *Clio Medica* 9 (1974): 271–84; and Ann F. La
Berge, "The Paris Health Council, 1802–48," *Bulletin of the History of Medicine* 49
(1975): 339–52. La Berge gives some attention to the provinces in her dissertation,
"Public Health in France and the French Public Health Movement, 1815–1848,"
University of Tennessee, 1974; summarized in *Proceedings of the Third Annual Meeting
of the Western Society for French History* (n.p., 1976), pp. 337–53.

147 Huard, *Sciences*, pp. 281–83; Ackerknecht, *Medicine*, pp. 115–16; Weisz, "Professeurs
parisiens," pp. 49–50 and passim; idem, "Constructing the Medical Elite," pp. 426–
28. Weisz stresses that both the Société de Médecine de Paris and the Société Académique took an active interest in institutional politics, without, however, winning
more than a marginal role for themselves. Their membership included many adversaries of the new state medical bureaucracy, dominated by the Paris Faculty of
Medicine. The corporatist sentiments of the Société de Médecine have already been
mentioned. The Société Académique, as its composition might lead us to expect,
also sought to revive corporatism, including disciplinary powers over members;
but its efforts were frustrated by its own disunity as well as the government's
opposition. In 1811 a dissenting faction under Antoine Portal of the Collège de
France seceded and established a Cercle Médical, creating a schism that lasted until
1819.

148 Bénédicte Dehillerin, "Le Collège de Pharmacie de Paris: Du régime des corporations
au régime de Germinal, ou de l'étonnante vitalité du modèle parisien," *thèse de 3^e
cycle*, University of Paris I, 1981, p. 160.

149 Léonard, *Médecins de l'Ouest*, pp. 709–11; Paul Ganière, *L'Académie de Médecine: Ses
origines et son histoire* (Compiègne, 1964); Weisz, "Professeurs parisiens" and "Constructing the Medical Elite," pp. 435–42. See the Academy's *Bulletin* (1836–) and

Mémoires (1828–). The nineteenth-century Academy left an extensive archive, which has only recently been inventoried.

150 On the state and the medical profession in Germany: Claudia Huerkamp, "Ärzte und Professionalisierung in Deutschland: Überlegungen zum Wandel des Arztberufs im 19. Jahrhundert," *Geschichte und Gesellschaft* 6 (1980): 349–82; and idem, *Der Aufstieg der Ärzte im 19. Jahrhundert: Vom gelehrten Stand zum professionellen Experten: Das Beispiel Preussens*, Kritische Studien zur Geschichtswissenschaft, vol. 68 (Göttingen, 1985).

151 On the projects: Léonard, *Médecins de l'Ouest*, pp. 761–64. Malpractice as such was not defined by law, but harm to a patient was both a tort, as defined by the civil code of 1803 (arts. 1382–1383), and, conceivably, a criminal offense, under three articles of the penal code of 1810: on harm caused by administering substances harmful to health (art. 317), involuntary manslaughter (art. 319), and injury due to negligence (art. 320).

152 Ibid., pp. 765–70. See also Camille Goret, *Des syndicats médicaux*, Paris law thesis, 1904, pp. 10–13.

153 Sussman, "From Yellow Fever," chap. 4.

154 Léonard, *Médecins de l'Ouest*, pp. 778–82.

155 On French organizations, see Léonard, *Médecins de l'Ouest*, chaps. 13–14, and Goret, *Des syndicats médicaux*. On the American and British cases, see James G. Burrow, *AMA: Voice of American Medicine* (Baltimore, 1963), and Ernest Muirhead Little, *History of the British Medical Association, 1832–1932* (London, 1932).

156 Treille, *Quelques réflexions*, p. 49.

157 Léonard, *Médecins de l'Ouest*, pp. 677–79.

158 Ibid., P.681, citing AD Ille-et-Vilaine 20 Ma 1 and 20 Ma 3.

159 Ibid., p. 368. For the projects, see AN F^{17} 2108.

160 Léonard, *Médecins de l'Ouest*, p. 658. Léonard mentions thirteen secondary schools authorized under the Empire; the Restoration created three new ones and raised others – at Nantes, for example – to the status of secondary schools (p. 371 on Nantes). The archives contain the records of eighteen schools and a project for a nineteenth: Amiens, Angers, Arras, Besançon, Bordeaux, Caen, Clermont-Ferrand, Dijon, Douai (project), Grenoble, Lyons, Marseilles, Nancy, Nantes, Poitiers, Reims, Rennes, Rouen, and Toulouse (AN F^{17} 2299–2312). See also Charles Coury, "The Teaching of Medicine in France from the Beginning of the Seventeenth Century," in C.D. O'Malley, ed., *The History of Medical Education* (Berkeley and Los Angeles, 1970), p. 152.

161 Léonard, *Médecins de l'Ouest*, pp. 632–33, 637–38.

162 Ibid., pp. 277, 638, 644–45; Léonard, *Vie quotidienne*, pp. 22, 26–29.

163 Léonard, *Vie quotidienne*, pp. 16–17; *Médecins de l'Ouest*, p. 1479.

164 Léonard, *Médecins de l'Ouest*, p. 418.

165 Ibid., pp. 397, 536.

166 AD Bas-Rhin 5 M 46, Lion, 12 June 1812, translated and quoted by George D. Sussman, "Enlightened Health Reform, Professional Medicine and Traditional Society: The Cantonal Physicians of the Bas-Rhin, 1810–1870," *Bulletin of the History of Medicine* 51 (1977): 583.

167 Léonard, *Médecins de l'Ouest*, p. 254.

168 Dornier, *Avis*, pp. 9, 33, 55–56.

169 Jacques Léonard, Roger Darquenne, and Louis Bergeron, "Médecins et notables sous le Consulat et l'Empire," *Annales E.S.C.* 32 (1977): 858–65.

170 Léonard, *La Médecine entre les savoirs et les pouvoirs: Histoire intellectuelle et politique de la médecine française au XIXe siècle* (1981), p. 83.

171 Léonard, *Vie quotidienne*, pp. 142–43; idem, *Médecins de l'Ouest*, pp. 502–06.

172 Boyer, "Encadrement médical," pp. 99–107; Olivier Faure, "Physicians in Lyon during the Nineteenth Century: An Extraordinary Social Success," *Journal of Social History* 10 (1976–77): 508–23. See also Faure's master's thesis, on which the article is based: "Les Médecins du Rhône au XIXe siècle," University of Lyons II, 1975; and, on the profession's subsequent struggles, Jeanne Gaillard, "La Formation d'une

élite: Les Médecins parisiens sous le Second Empire," *Bulletin du Centre d'Histoire de la France Contemporaine*, 1983, no. 4, pp. 55–56, and Weisz, "Politics," p. 7.

173 This paragraph mainly follows Léonard, *Médecins de l'Ouest*, pp. 549–75, and *Vie quotidienne*, pp. 103–32.

174 On propharmacy as a source of income: Léonard, *Vie quotidienne*, p. 115. For a biographical sketch of a rural health officer who worked extensively as a *propharmacien*, see Pierre Saumande, "Léonard Moreau, médecin de campagne et propharmacien en Limousin au début du 19ᵉ siècle," *Revue d'histoire de la pharmacie* 26 (1979): 203–10.

175 Spears, "Peasants," pp. 148–49.

176 AD Morbihan M 992, Dr. Jégo of Muzillac to Conseil Central d'Hygiène de Vannes, 15 October 1854, quoted by Léonard, *Médecins de l'Ouest*, p. 576.

177 Ibid., pp. 588, 539.

178 AD Pyrénées-Orientales, Ramonet to *commissaire du gouvernement*, 3 June 1811, quoted in Jean-Gabriel Gigot, "L'Histoire réelle du Roussillon au temps d'hier," pt. 1: "Guérisseurs en Roussillon," *C.E.R.C.A.*, no. 21 (1966): 249.

179 See, for example, AM 321, Bertrand, "Proposition," and Jean-Jacques Salet, *Essai sur les moyens de perfectionner l'exercice de la médecine dans les campagnes* (Valence, 1810), p. 50.

180 Eugène Flavard, *Des consultations médicales et du charlatanisme* (Montpellier, 1842), pp. 33–37.

181 Most of the examples that follow (and others) are discussed in Léonard, *Médecins de l'Ouest*, pp. 591–607 and 610–12 (on licensed practitioners who collaborate with empirics). See also Léonard, "Les Guérisseurs en France au XIXᵉ siècle," *Revue d'histoire moderne et contemporaine* 27 (1980): 513–15. The West appears to have been, on the whole, relatively innocent of "industrialism."

182 See Louis Leroy [Pelgas], *La Médecine curative, ou la Purgation dirigée contre la cause des maladies, reconnues et analysées dans cet ouvrage*, 5th ed. (1817). Copies were available by mail order at 3 francs.

183 AD Vaucluse 5 M 14, no. 401, 6 Vendémiaire XIV/28 September 1805, Minister of the Interior to Dr. Monier des Taillades, Avignon, author of *Avis: L'Irroé, ou le purgatif rafraîchissant*; excerpts from letter and text in Jacques Léonard, comp., *La France médicale: Médecins et malades au XIXᵉ siècle* (1978), pp. 52–54. The existence of a warrant for this remedy under the Old Regime is noted in BN ms. Joly de Fleury 499, fol. 221r.

184 Michel-Pierre Le Pelletier, *Projet de réforme, sollicité par la raison publique, dans l'intérêt de l'humanité, suivi du répertoire nécessaire aux amis de la santé . . .* (1820).

185 AM 67, report by academy's commission on secret remedies, adopted 11 November 1828.

186 AD Loire-Atlantique 1 M 1358, no. 326, report of Conseil de Salubrité, 30 October 1826.

187 AD Loire-Atlantique 4 X 232 and 1 M 1358, cited in Léonard, *Médecins de l'Ouest*, p. 611, n. 323. Adolphe Trébuchet, *Jurisprudence de la médecine, de la chirurgie et de la pharmacie en France . . .* (1834), p. 304.

188 Léonard, *Médecins de l'Ouest*, p. 610, n. 321.

189 *Jérôme Paturot à la recherche d'une position sociale*, new ed. (1870), pt. 1, chaps. 10–11.

190 See Léonard, *Médecins de l'Ouest*, pp. 727–28.

191 Ibid., pp. 531–32, 726, 78. Proposed densities of practitioners ranged from 1 per 1,000 inhabitants to 1 per 3,000.

192 On the problem of overcrowding at midcentury, see George D. Sussman, "The Glut of Doctors in Mid-Nineteenth-Century France," *Comparative Studies in Society and History* 19 (1977): 287–304.

193 Claude-François-Etienne Dupin, *Statistique du département des Deux-Sèvres* (Year IX), p. 82.

194 François-Emmanuel Fodéré, *Voyage aux Alpes-Maritimes, ou Histoire naturelle, agraire, civile et médicale du comté de Nice et pays limitrophes . . .* , 2 vols. (1821) 2: 291.

195 Léonard, *Médecins de l'Ouest*, pp. 408–09, 534–36; idem, *Vie quotidienne*, p. 166; Léonard et al., "Médecins et notables," p. 858.

196 Jacques Godechot, *Les Institutions de la France sous la Révolution et l'Empire*, 2d ed. (1968), p. 704; Léonard, *Médecins de l'Ouest*, pp. 402–04 and appendix, table 3B.

197 FM ms. 2196/VI (archives of the Société Médicale d'Émulation de Paris), Lecourt de Cantilly, note on illegal medical practice, 1827.

198 Sussman, "Glut of Doctors," table (pp. 294–97); cf. Appendix A of the present study.

199 Faure, "Médecins du Rhône," pp. 4, 11; Léonard, *Médecins de l'Ouest*, p. 543; Boyer, "Encadrement," pp. 9–12.

200 John Spears and Diane Sydenham, "The Evolution of Medical Practice in Two Marginal Areas of the Western World, 1750–1830," *Historical Reflections/Réflexions historiques* 9 (1982): 195–212 (p. 199 on densities).

201 Léonard, *Médecins de l'Ouest*, pp. 90–93, 532, 540–45.

202 Faure, "Médecins du Rhône," p. 4; Léonard, *Médecins de l'Ouest*, pp. 86, 540.

203 Spears and Sydenham, "Evolution of Medical Practice," p. 201.

204 Léonard, *Médecins de l'Ouest*, p. 1524.

205 Ibid., p. 516. The discussion that follows draws mainly on Léonard, *Médecins de l'Ouest*, pp. 52–54, 513–16, 521–24, 557–64; his analysis is based in part on practitioners' private account books.

206 Actual wages varied widely; see Émile Levasseur, *Salariat et salaires* (1909), chap. 5.

207 Spears, "Peasants," p. 145.

208 AN F[17] 4537, Haute-Garonne, cited by Léonard, *Médecins de l'Ouest*, p. 558, n. 117.

209 AD Mayenne 1447, Auguste Bourgonnier to prefect, 2 October 1830, quoted in ibid., p. 548.

210 AD Loire 38 M 9, no. 18, mayor of Feurs to subprefect, 29 December 1812; AN F[8] 118, memorandum from Geoffroy de Luzi to Minister of the Interior, 21 July 1808, quoted in Guy Thuillier, *Aspects de l'économie nivernaise au XIXe siècle* (1966), p. 72. The mayor reported that doctors charged the poor 20–24 francs for a single visit, and that more prosperous patients might part with several thousand francs over the course of an illness. Cf. the complaints about surgeons' fees (4 francs for a bottle of emetic water that cost 1 franc at the apothecary's, 1.50 francs for a day visit) in AN F[8] 154, Ducluzel, curé of Chaillé-les-Marais (Vendée), "Projet de bienfaisance en faveur des paysans," 1810.

211 For a good recent regional study, see Colin Jones, *Charity and "Bienfaisance": The Treatment of the Poor in the Montpellier Region, 1740–1815* (Cambridge, 1982).

212 See, for example, the decree of the prefect of the Gard, AD Gard 2 X 11, 23 April 1807, requiring each *bureau de bienfaisance* to have a physician or surgeon to care for the poor and vaccinate indigent children; in Léonard, *France médicale*, p. 108.

213 Ibid., p. 110.

214 Dora B. Weiner, "The Role of the Doctor in Welfare Work: The Philanthropic Society of Paris, 1780–1815," *Historical Reflections/Réflexions historiques* 9 (1982): 279–304.

215 Champagny, "Traitement des épidémies," 12 Floréal XIII/2 May 1805, *Circulaires, instructions et autres actes émanés du Ministère de l'Intérieur, ou relatifs à ce département, de 1797 à 1821 inclusivement*, 2d ed., vol. 1 (1821), pp. 371–75. Evelyn Ackerman has studied the actual operation in one department, the Seine-et-Oise; see "Medical Care in the Countryside near Paris, 1800–1914," *Annals of the New York Academy of Sciences*, 412 (14 October 1983): 1–18.

216 Léonard, *La Médecine entre les savoirs*, p. 55.

217 AN F[8] 164, Royer file, containing copies of his prospectus and sample forms for free consultations, together with his correspondence; École de Médecine de Paris, *extrait du registre*, deliberation of 11 Fructidor XIII/29 August 1805.

218 See A. Dechambre, "Médecins cantonaux," *Dictionnaire encyclopédique médicale*, 100 vols. (1864–89), 2d ser., 5: 579–87; Sussman, "Enlightened Health Reform"; and Léonard, *Médecins de l'Ouest*, pp. 744–55. Dechambre traces the Alsatian tradition to 1436, when the Emperor Sigismund gave a Meister-Arzt to each town in the

Empire. On the German Physikus, see Alfons Fischer, *Geschichte des deutschen Gesundheitswesens*, 2 vols. (Berlin, 1933), 2: 55–57. For the revolutionary model: Thouret, proposal on surgeons and physicians for the rural poor, in Bloch and Tuetey, *Procès-verbaux*, pp. 107–08.

219 On the critiques, see Léonard, *Médecins de l'Ouest*, pp. 746–47; Sussman, "Enlightened Health Reform," p. 579; and Dechambre, "Médecins cantonaux," p. 584. On medical assistance in the nineteenth century, see Olivier Faure, "La Médecine gratuite au XIXe siècle: De la charité à l'assistance," *Histoire, économie et société* 3 (1984): 593–608.

220 See, for example, Ackerman, "Medical Care."

221 J. Borianne, *Essai sur les erreurs en médecine répandues dans le département de la Haute-Vienne et sur leurs dangers*, Paris medical thesis, 1831, p. 25.

222 See, for example, Léonard, *Médecins de l'Ouest*, p. 587; and on diseases of the sexual organs, the slangy but useful discussion in Edward Shorter, *A History of Women's Bodies* (New York, 1982), chap. 10.

223 Eugen Weber, *Peasants into Frenchmen: The Modernization of Rural France, 1870–1914* (Stanford, Calif., 1976), p. 67 and chap. 6, passim; Léonard, *Vie quotidienne*, p. 38.

224 On cholera, see René Baehrel, "La Haine de classe en temps d'épidémie," *Annales E.S.C.* 7 (1952): 357–60, and George D. Sussman, "Carriers of Cholera and Poison Rumors in France in 1832," *Societas* 3 (1973): 241. The complaint: AN F^8 163, Poulain to Minister of the Interior, n.d. (after 1803).

225 Léonard, *Vie quotidienne*, p. 65.

226 See Terence D. Murphy, "The French Medical Profession's Perception of Its Social Function Between 1776 and 1830," *Medical History* 23 (1979): 259–78.

227 Trélat, *De la constitution*, p. 64.

228 Lemaître, *Exposé des abus*, pp. 37–38.

229 See, for example, Magali Sarfatti Larson, *The Rise of Professionalism: A Sociological Analysis* (Berkeley and Los Angeles, 1977).

230 This argument appears, for example, in two influential sociological studies: Eliot Freidson, *Profession of Medicine: A Study of the Sociology of Applied Knowledge* (New York, 1970); and William G. Rothstein, *American Physicians in the Nineteenth Century: From Sects to Science* (Baltimore, 1972).

231 Charles C. Gillispie, *Science and Polity in France at the End of the Old Regime* (Princeton, N.J., 1980).

CHAPTER 3 *Irregulars: itinerants*

1 For example, in Laurent Joubert, *Erreurs populaires et propos vulgaires touchant la médecine et le régime de santé* (Bordeaux, 1579); and Pliny the Elder, *Natural History*, Books 20–32, (vols. 6–8 of the Loeb edition [Cambridge, Mass., 1956–69]).

2 Joseph Folliet, *La Médecine du Docteur Gnafron* (Lyons, 1966), p. 13.

3 Joseph R. Levenson, *Confucian China and Its Modern Fate: A Trilogy*, 3 vols. (Berkeley and Los Angeles, 1958–65), 1: xxvii–xxviii.

4 Michel Foucault, *Les Mots et les choses: Une Archéologie des sciences humaines* (1966), pp. 7–11. For a translation, see *The Order of Things: An Archaeology of the Human Sciences*, (New York, 1970), pp. xv–xix.

5 AD Bas-Rhin 5 M 22, no. 28, *procureur impérial* to prefect, 24 March 1811.

6 See Max Weber, *The Theory of Social and Economic Organization*, tr. A. M. Henderson and Talcott Parsons, ed. Talcott Parsons (New York, 1947), pp. 109–10.

7 AN F^{17} 2276, no. 333, Hyères (Var). Cf. no 337, Boiscommun (Loiret): "Les empiriques et charlatans ambulans commencent à disparoître. Mais les domiciliés exercent toujours."

8 AD Meurthe-et-Moselle 5 M 18, no. 219, *bureau, lycée impérial*, to prefect of the Meurthe, 17 July 1806; ibid., no. 220, Minister of the Interior to prefect, 7 June. Olivier Faure: *Genèse de l'hôpital moderne: Les Hospices civils de Lyon de 1802 à 1845* (Lyons, 1982), p. 101. On the investigation, see Matthew Ramsey, "Sous le régime

de la législation de 1803: Trois enquêtes sur les charlatans au XIXe siècle," *Revue d'histoire moderne et contemporaine* 27 (1980): 494–95.

9 In 1784, the lieutenant of the First Surgeon at Villefranche-de-Haute-Guienne reported that Rabiglia had arrived with a troupe and set up a stage for public performances; he was on his way to Rodez or Aurillac (SRM 199, d. 18, no. 29, 28 December 1784; see also Rabiglia's flyer for his purgative pills in ibid., d. 29, no. 1). Under the First Empire, he was still widely known, practicing ocular surgery, inspecting urine, and treating hernias, tinea, and a host of other disorders (AN F^{17} 2107, report by surgeon Rays at Saint-Malo, 1808, quoted in Jacques Léonard, *Les Médecins de l'Ouest au XIXe siècle* [1978], p. 426; cf. p. 425, on a younger practitioner, Louis Olivier).

10 Raoul Mercier, *Le Monde médical de Touraine sous la Révolution* (Tours, 1936), p. 202. Cf. AN AF I* 23, *procès-verbaux*, Comité de Salubrité, Assemblée Constituante, fol. 41v, 20 January 1791, on letter from Mignos and Baudin, surgeons at Troyes, with a copy of Gosset's flyer.

11 Jacques-Louis Ménétra, *Journal de ma vie*, ed. Daniel Roche (1982), p. 74.

12 *Annuaire de la Société de Médecine, Chirurgie et Pharmacie du Département de l'Eure*, 1819, p. 38 (prize essay by Mouquet).

13 I. D. P. M. O. D. R. [Jean de Gorris; also attributed to Jean Duret], *Discours de l'origine, des moeurs, fraudes et impostures des ciarlatans, avec leur découverte . . .* (1622), pp. 20–21.

14 *Dictionnaire universel françois et latin . . .*, new [4th] ed., 6 vols. (1743), vol. 1, col. 1995.

15 AN F^{17} 2276, d. 2, no. 319.

16 Paul Scarron, *Roman comique* (1651–57), pt. 1, chaps. 15, 19; René de Chateaubriand, *Mémoires d'outre-tombe* (first published 1848–50), pt. 1, bk. 2, chap. 4. For a good description of the charlatan and his paraphernalia, see also ARC 33, d. 1, no. 15, "Mémoire dans lequel on a rapporté quelques observations des plus frappantes, qui démontrent l'impéritie des charlatans, le progrès du charlatanisme et les risques auxquels le public est exposé et la nécessité d'y remédier."

17 SRM 199, d. 24, no. 1, Mahon, reflections on remedies and quacks, Chartres, 19 October 1778.

18 See Littré, *Dictionnaire de la langue française*, 4 vols. (1873–75), s.v. "Orviétan."

19 "Requête . . . au corps de ville de Poitiers," 2 September 1624, quoted by Prosper-Marie Boissonnade, *Essai sur l'organisation du travail en Poitou*, in *Mémoires de l'Association des Antiquaires de l'Ouest*, 2d ser., 21–22 (1898–99), 21: 510.

20 On the Contugi family and its successors, see Claude-Stéphen Le Paulmier, *L'Orviétan: Histoire d'une famille de charlatans du Pont-Neuf aux XVIIe et XVIIIe siècles* (n.d. [1893]). For the quarrels with the apothecaries' company: AP BA 1–18, *affaire* Contugy. Regnard's activities were widely discussed by the correspondents of the Société Royale de Médecine; see, for example, SRM 199, d. 14, no. 14, Saladin at Lille, 8 December 1781. Algaron will be discussed subsequently; see also Le Paulmier, *L'Orviétan*, pp. 101–02.

21 On Cuchet: AC Dijon I 134, syndic of the physicians of Dijon to town magistrates, 27 May 1769. On Tadiny: SRM 199, d. 18, no. 16, "Mémoire touchant le charlatanisme," Dax, 20 April 1781; ibid., no 6, 5 March 1782, Bordeaux. On Vander: AM ms. 15, p. 317, 3 September 1790, note on three letters of complaint received by Société Royale.

22 AD Yonne B 947, quoted by François Forestier, "Vingt ans d'exercice de la médecine dans l'Yonne, 1790–1810," Paris medical thesis, 1950, no. 296, p. 3.

23 AD Ille-et-Vilaine C 2509.

24 Quoted by Bernard Jacquet, *Empiriques et charlatans troyens du XVe au XIXe siècle*, Paris medical thesis, 1960, no. 458, pp. 55–56.

25 AN F^7 7827, d. 5250, ser. 3.

26 AD Bas-Rhin 5 M 22, no. 6.

27 Cuchet flyer printed in E. Fyot, "Les Charlatans à Dijon," *Bulletin de la Société des*

Pharmaciens de la Côte-d'Or, no. 22 (1903): 175–77; Fleury: SRM 199, d. 8, no. 13; Scipion: ibid., d. 14, no. 23.

28 Desmarest: AD Meurthe-et-Moselle 5 M 18, no. 37; Hilmer: SRM 199, d. 18, no. 22 (report from Langon, 19 May 1780); Philippe: SRM 199, d. 6, no. 11; Demarest: ibid., d. 9, no. 7, 1779.

29 Joseph-Marie-Alexandre Poidebard, *Le Portefeuille d'un charlatan lyonnais au XVIIIe siècle* (Lyons, 1895; excerpted from *Revue du Lyonnais*), p. 10.

30 On urinoscopy, see Charles Guyotjeannin, *Contribution à l'histoire de l'analyse des urines,* Strasbourg pharmacy thesis, 1951 (Créteil, 1951).

31 On abortion: Angus McLaren, "Abortion in France: Women and the Regulation of Family Size, 1800–1914," *French Historical Studies* 10 (1978): 461–85; and Edward Shorter, *A History of Women's Bodies* (New York, 1982), chap. 8, which gives detailed attention to the techniques and drugs employed.

32 See Daniel Langhans, *L'Art de se traiter et de se guérir soi-même dans les maladies les plus ordinaires et les plus dangereuses . . . ,* tr. from the German by Marc-Antoine Eidous, 2 vols. (1768), 2: 16: "Pour en imposer davantage, ils [les charlatans] lâchent de temps en temps quelques mots de mauvais latin, ce qui suffit pour persuader aux paysans que celui qui leur parle est un homme savant et expert dans son art." Cf. Roy Porter, "The Language of Quackery in England, 1660–1800," in Porter and Peter Burke, eds., *The Social History of Language* (Cambridge: Cambridge University Press, forthcoming), which stresses the parallels between the rhetoric of charlatans and the publicity of regular practitioners.

33 AC Dijon I 134.

34 Albertina's flyer (c. 1801): AD Bas-Rhin 5 M 22, no. 6. Johann Georg's (c. 1787): SRM 199, d. 3, no. 7.

35 Pierre Rambaud, *La Pharmacie en Poitou jusqu'à l'an XI, Mémoires de la Société des Antiquaires de l'Ouest,* 2d ser., 30 (1906): 564.

36 SRM 199, d. 18, no. 18, Dufau, 4 December 1787.

37 Adolphe Lecocq, *Empiriques, somnambules et rebouteurs beaucerons* (Chartres, 1862), p. 54.

38 SRM 107, Brar de la Cossaye, complaint, 21 June 1788.

39 Charles John Samuel Thompson, *The Quacks of Old London* (New York, 1928), p. 73; cf. Rambaud, *Pharmacie en Poitou,* p. 560.

40 SRM 199, d. 11, no. 11, 26 November 1780.

41 SRM 136, d. 15, no. 10, Brar de la Cossaye, at Dreux, 12 September 1791.

42 SRM 199, d. 2, no. 1, *garde des apothicaires,* Albi, on d'Angleberme, 1781. Edme Roché, a physician at Toucy (Yonne), describes the tapeworms (AD Yonne 5 M 7/1, no. 210, 22 February 1821).

43 For an example of the charlatan's *baragouin,* see Alfred Franklin, *La Vie privée d'autrefois . . . ,* vol. 14, *Variétés chirurgicales* (1894), p. 154.

44 SRM 199, d. 6, no. 1, Majerne at Le Blanc in Berry, 16 October 1779.

45 Ibid., d. 26, nos. 3–5, 6 March 1779; AD Meurthe-et-Moselle 5 M 18, no. 35, Gabriel, *officier de santé,* to subprefect, Lunéville, 24 Fructidor VIII/11 September 1800.

46 See Matthew Ramsey, "Conscription, Malingerers, and Popular Medicine in Napoleonic France," *The Consortium on Revolutionary Europe, 1750–1850, Proceedings, 1978* (Athens, Ga., 1980), pp. 188–99. On charlatans' tricks, see Thompson, *Quacks,* pp. 55.

47 AD Ille-et-Vilaine C 1352, *recteur* of Bréal to Intendant of Brittany, 21 August 1786, quoted by P. Hardouin, "L'Exercice illégal de la médecine au XVIIIe siècle," ms. in AD Ille-et-Vilaine 1 F 2242/4, p. 11. This letter has now been published by François Lebrun: "Chirurgiens et guérisseurs en Haute-Bretagne à la fin de l'Ancien Régime," *Annales de Bretagne* 91 (1984): 423–25.

48 SRM 199, d. 19, no. 1, Fourcroy, Clermont-en-Beauvaisis, 15 September 1786; ibid., d. 8, no. 6, 9 August 1789.

49 Ibid., d. 10, no. 2, Rémy, curé, Mauperthuis-en-Brie, 3 January 1788. On the belief

in animals in the body, cf. AN F[8] 162, François Phillipot at Chaillon to Minister of the Interior, 18 January 1809, on the case of his wife, who had accidentally swallowed a lizard while drinking from a jug of water; "this cruel beast" then tormented her for more than a year, gnawing at her insides and moving about "as if it were a rabbit."

50 SRM 199, d. 5, no. 1, 21 October 1779. See François-Paul-Lyon Poulletier de la Salle, Charles-Louis-François Andry, and Félix Vicq d'Azyr, "Rapport sur les inconvéniens de l'opération de la castration, pratiquée pour obtenir la cure radicale des hernies," *Mémoires de la Société Royale de Médicine* 1 (1776): 289–95.

51 See, for example, AD Meurthe-et-Moselle 5 M 18, no. 60, prefect of the Meurthe [?] to *procureur du Roi* at Nancy, 3 September 1832.

52 SRM 199, d. 26, no. 1, Dr. Clemenceau, 4 October 1780.

53 AM 67, report adopted 11 November 1828; on this case, see p. 114.

54 AD Ille-et-Vilaine 1 B[n] 3245, an unusually ample dossier on the case of a charlatan charged with homicide (Leonard Michel, also known as Michel Leonard).

55 SRM 107, Chifoliau at Saint-Malo, 30 April 178? describes the empiric as "pourvu de l'influence mesmerienne."

56 See, for example, the account of a girl's horrible death in the report cited in n. 51: "Une jeune fille de cette commune, pour complaire au désir de ses parents, a fait usage [de cet elixir]; aussitôt elle a été saisie de douleurs . . . excessives et de convulsions si violentes que quatre personnes avaient peine à la contenir. Après avoir tout brisé autour d'elle, elle a expiré en reprochant sa mort à ses parents."

57 SRM 199, d. 19, no. 1, 15 September 1786.

58 "The Therapeutic Revolution: Medicine, Meaning, and Social Change in Nineteenth-Century America," in Rosenberg and Morris J. Vogel, eds., *The Therapeutic Revolution: Essays in the Social History of American Medicine* (Philadelphia, 1979), p. 8.

59 SRM 199, d. 18, no. 22, Graullau at Langon, 19 May 1780.

60 Ibid., no. 18, Dufau, 4 December 1787; no. 19, idem, 5 January 1782.

61 "Discours sur le crédit des charlatans, lu à la séance de la Société d'Agriculture . . . le 29 prairial an VIII," *Journal de l'École Centrale et de la Société Libre d'Agriculture, du Commerce et des Arts du Département de l'Aube*, no. 60 (19 Messidor VIII/8 July 1800), p. 3.

62 SRM 199, d. 29, no. 14, de Colançy, item 10 on list of letters on charlatanism received by the Société Royale, n.d.

63 Ibid., d. 11, no. 46, Dorez, surgeon at Villenauxe, 24 June 1780.

64 Robert Darnton, "Reading, Writing, and Publishing in Eighteenth-Century France: A Case Study in the Sociology of Literature," in *Historical Studies Today*, ed. Felix Gilbert and Stephen R. Graubard (New York, 1972), pp. 250–68.

65 SRM 199, d. 3, no. 3, Deveaumorel, 5 May 1781; ibid., no. 2, Wanne, 1 July 1781; ibid., d. 18, no. 8, Massie, 18 January 1784. See Roberto Gervaso, *Cagliostro: A Biography*, tr. Cormac Ó Cuilleanáin (London, 1974).

66 Ulysse Trélat, *De la constitution du corps des médecins et de l'enseignement médical: Des réformes qu'elle devrait subir . . .* (1828), p. 54.

67 SRM 199, d. 26, no. 3, Gallot, 6 March 1779 (cf. SRM 107, d. 3, no. 8, item 3, note on report from curé of Sainte-Hermine, Bas-Poitou); SRM 199, d. 9, no. 25, Tadiny, 9 December 1780; ibid, d. 2, no. 1, *garde des apothicaires*, Albi, 1781. SRM 107, d. 3, no. 8, item 4 (n.d.) places him in Burgundy.

68 SRM 199, d. 9, no. 44, Chifoliau, 26 June 1779; ibid., no 25, Tadiny, 9 December 1780; ibid., d. 25, no. 2, three practitioners of Saint-Quentin, 12 June 178?; Paul Delaunay, "Les Apothicaires du Haut-Maine et du Maine angevin sous l'Ancien Régime," *Revue d'histoire de la pharmacie* no. 36 (1938): 304; SRM 107, d. 3, no. 8, item 18.

69 AC Dijon I 134; AC Nantes FF 250, doctor-regents to *siège royal de la police*, March 1781; SRM 107, d. 1, 12 July 1783.

70 SRM 199, d. 9, no. 7, 8 May 1779; ibid., no. 1, 16 October 1779; ibid., d. 17, no. 1, Rameau, 16 January 1780.

71 SRM 199, d. 8, no. 12, Houdaille, 20 March 1780; ibid., no. 1, 4 January 1781; ibid., d. 11, no. 12, Montmignon, 18 September 1785; AN AF I* 23, *procès-verbaux*, Comité de Salubrité, Assemblée Constituante, fol. 67r, 5 April 1791, note on letter from Chifoliau.

72 SRM 199, d. 11, no. 24, 30 November 1779; ibid., d. 24, no. 11, 30 September 1786; ibid., d. 5, no. 9, Dr. Devillantroys of Vierzon to lieutenant-general of police, 4 June 1787.

73 SRM 199, d. 25, no. 1, Arcidet, 9 May 1784; SRM 199, d. 18, no. 16, Dufau, 20 April 1781, on a certain "Greci" who has a commission from Regnard; SRM 199, d. 9, no. 10, Kiavalle, 9 June 1785 (at Josselin); Jean-Pierre Goubert, *Malades et médecins en Bretagne, 1779–1790* (1974), p. 237.

74 See, for example, SRM 199, d. 3, no. 1, 30 June 1779, on Germans in Alsace. German and Italian charlatans also practiced in Britain; see Thompson, *Quacks*, p. 29 and passim, and John Dixon Comrie, *History of Scottish Medicine to 1860* (London, 1927), p. 112.

75 Toby Gelfand develops this argument in "Medical Professionals and Charlatans: The *Comité de Salubrité enquête* of 1790–91," *Histoire sociale-Social History* 11 (1978): 76–81.

76 See Jean-Pierre Gutton, *La Société et les pauvres: L'Exemple de la généralité de Lyon, 1534–1789*, state doctoral thesis, University of Lyons, 1970 (1971), pp. 152–53. The efficacy of repression is suggested by the lieutenant of the surgical community of Lyons in his reply to the Comité de Salubrité's investigation of 1790–91, AN F^{17} 2276, d. 2, no. 299.

77 SRM 199, d. 3, no. 6, 16 January 1787.

78 SRM 107, Dieu, 10 May 1779. On vigilant enforcement driving quacks into the countryside, see also SRM 107, Ramel, 4 June 1789.

79 See, for example, Richard Dunlop, *Doctors of the American Frontier* (Garden City, N.Y., 1965) esp. chap. 17; and Madge E. Pickard and R. Carlyle Buley, *The Midwest Pioneer: His Ills, Cures and Doctors* (Crawfordsville, Ind., 1945), esp. chap. 4.

80 See, for example, AD Yonne 5 M 7/1, commissioner of police, Auxerre, to prefect, 19 May 1821.

81 Eric J. Hobsbawm, *Bandits* ([New York], 1969), p. 74.

82 AN F^7 9278, d. 6903, prefect of the Aisne to Minister of Police, 19 May 1818. On the Vacherons, see the various reports in SRM 199, d. 11, and SRM 107, Morin at Charly-sur-Marne, 18 August 1783.

83 SRM 199, d. 11, no. 20, 6 August 1780.

84 SRM 199, d. 11, no. 24BIS, *directeur des postes*, Dôle, to *directeur*, Nogent-sur-Seine, 23 July 1779.

85 Ibid., d. 11, no. 23, community of surgeons, Nogent-sur-Seine to "Commission Royale de Médecine," 15 July 1779. AD Haute-Loire 13 M 18, no. 483, denunciation to prefect, 17 April 1819.

86 AD Yonne 5 M 7/1, no. 210, Edme Roché to prefect, 22 February 1821. On crossing over between charlatanism and popular entertainment, see Robert M. Isherwood, *Farce and Fantasy: Popular Entertainment in Eighteenth-Century Paris* (New York and Oxford, 1986), p. 16.

87 AN F^8 156, subprefect of Poligny to prefect of the Jura, 24 July 1808; Minister of the Interior to prefect, 18 August 1808; prefect to Minister, 1 September 1808; subprefect to prefect, 5 September 1808.

88 AN F^8 164, Minister of the Interior to prefect of the Loiret, 2 March 1811; subprefect of Gien to prefect, 30 April 1811; prefect to minister, 6 May; Royer to minister, 27 May.

89 BM Dijon, *ancien fonds*, ms. 265A^1, 2: 853, cited by A. Baudot, *Études historiques sur la pharmacie en Bourgogne avant 1803* (1905), p. 318.

90 SRM 107, Ramel, 4 June 1789. Cf. SRM 132, no. 58, Dr. Nicolas of Grenoble, "Sur la nécessité & les moyens d'établir une police médicale en France, & les avantages qui en résulteroient pour l'État & pour les sujets," 4 March 1777, fol. 2v: "Le nombre des charlatans, opérateurs, &c. ne diminue point; la loi semble n'être que

pour les grandes villes; le mal est pour les campagnes. Chacun s'y donne pour médecin." A contemporaneous study of popular errors strikes a more hopeful note on the subject of quacks' remedies. See J.-D.-T. de Bienville, *Traité des erreurs populaires sur la santé* (The Hague, 1775), p. 188: "Nous voyons avec plaisir la méfiance presque générale, non seulement des gens comme il faut, mais même du peuple pour ces sortes de remèdes."

91 AN F^{17} 2276, d. 2, no. 337, report by Bataillez, physician; no. 333, from Bonnefoy, surgeon. Cf. the case of the Swiss region of Vaud in Eugène Olivier, *Médecine et santé dans le pays de Vaud au XVIIIe siècle, 1675–1798* (Lausanne, 1939), p. 430; the last mention of a theater comes in 1777.

92 Olivier, *Médecine et santé,* p. 475, quoting Dr. Gallot, *L'Antidote,* pp. 122ff.

93 On the decline of itinerants, see also Gustave-Thomas de Closmadeuc, *Esquisse sur la médecine et la chirurgie populaires dans le département du Morbihan* (Vannes, 1861), p. 22; and Robert Boeglin, *L'Évolution historique de la pharmacie en Alsace,* Strasbourg pharmacy thesis, 1939, p. 116.

94 See, for example, a report of the medical jury of the Basses-Alpes, 3 August 1852, AD Alpes-de-Haute-Provence 7 M 36, quoted in Jacques Léonard, comp., *La France médicale au XIXe siècle* (1978), p. 58: as in the past troupes of charlatans travel through the department, selling secret remedies in the public squares; their number has actually increased since 1848, perhaps (the jury speculates) because harassment in other departments has driven them to take advantage of a more receptive public in the Basses-Alpes. Cf. AN CC 464, d. 445, no. 147, petition signed by 146 *officiers de santé* and pharmacists in Maine-et-Loire, n.d. (probably 1842); itinerants are "everywhere."

95 AD Bas-Rhin 5 M 22, no. 26, Aronsohn to prefect, 24 February 1811.

96 Ibid., no. 23, mayor of Bergzabern to subprefect of Wissembourg.

97 Ibid., no. 28, *procureur impérial,* Wissembourg, to prefect, 24 March 1811.

98 Ibid., no. 26, Aronsohn to prefect, 24 February 1811; no. 20, subprefect of Wissembourg to prefect, 19 September 1811.

99 Ibid., no. 42, Buchholtz, cantonal physician at Wissembourg, to prefect, 28 June 1813; this is the only reference to a previous occupation. Buchholtz also says that Dr. Johann is from Bergzabern.

100 Ibid., no. 26, Aronsohn to prefect, 24 February 1811; no. 22, cantonal physician at Wissembourg to subprefect, 14 August 1811; no. 28, *procureur impérial,* Wissembourg, to prefect, 24 March 1811.

101 Ibid., no. 42, cited in note 99.

102 Ibid., no. 29, hearing at Wissembourg tribunal, 11 March 1811; on the occupation: no. 42, cited in note 99, and no. 49, list of empirics practicing in the arrondissement of Wissembourg, 1813; on the nickname: no. 40, report (with list of illicit practitioners) by Müller, cantonal physician at Brumath, 21 June 1813.

103 Ibid., no. 31, report by Hoffmann, 12 January 1811.

104 AD Bas-Rhin 5 M 46, Lion's report of 12 June 1812, translated and quoted by George D. Sussman, "Enlightened Health Reform, Professional Medicine, and Traditional Society: The Cantonal Physicians of the Bas-Rhin, 1810–1870," *Bulletin of the History of Medicine* 51 (1977): 581–82. A copy of the recipe for one of Dr. Hans's compounds is in AD Bas Rhin (5 M 22, no. 27).

105 AD Bas-Rhin 5 M 22, no. 40, cited in note 102.

106 Ibid., no. 42, cited in note 99.

107 Ibid., no. 44, report of 10 June 1813.

108 Marcelle Bouteiller, *Médecine populaire d'hier et d'aujourd'hui* (1966), pp. 23–24, 199–200.

109 Proposal by Louis Marin; *Rennes Médical,* August, 1911, p. 52, cited by Jacques Léonard, *La Vie quotidienne du médicin de province au XIXe siècle* (1977), pp. 160–61.

110 Lecocq, *Empiriques,* pp. 53–54. See also R. Goulard, "Un Marchand droguiste ambulant au XVIIIe siècle," *La France médicale* 57 (1910): 350–52, on the case of Pierre René.

111 AD Haute-Loire 13 M 18, no. 481, commissioner of police, Le Puy, to prefect, 19

April 1819; AD Charente-Maritime 7 M 6/1, letter to prefect of the Charente-Inférieure, 16 June 1818.

112 See, for example, Société Royale de Médecine, *Nouveau plan de constitution pour la médecine en France* . . . (1790), pp. 114–15.

113 Delaunay, "Guérisseurs ambulants," p. 216 (quotation from *Affiches du Mans*, 5 February 1776).

114 Ibid., pp. 221–22. On the ibex, Delaunay cites "Bouc," *Nouveau dictionnaire universel et raisonné de médecine, de chirurgie, et de l'art vétérinaire* (1772), 1: 400.

115 AD Yonne 5 M 7/1, no. 211, commissioner of police, Auxerre, to prefect, 19 May 1821; *procès-verbal*, 29 May 1818.

116 AD Bas-Rhin 5 M 22, no. 186, "Circulaire à MM. les Maires, relative au colportage de drogues ou de remèdes secrets," 31 March 1834. On Tirolese, see also AD Bas-Rhin 1 L 839, Joseph Lambert (physician at Wissembourg), "Plan de règlement et d'organisation pour toutes les parties de la médecine pratique, proposé pour le département du Bas-Rhin," 1790.

117 Bouteiller, *Médecine populaire*, p. 24; Madeleine Rivière-Sestier, *Remèdes populaires en Dauphiné*, Marseilles pharmacy thesis, 1942, no. 6 (Lyons, 1942), pp. 25–29. On the long tradition of the Alpine regions as a source of medicinal plants, Rivière-Sestier cites Dominique Villar, *Histoire des plantes de Dauphiné*, 3 vols. in 4 (Grenoble, 1786–89). On seasonal migrations, see Olwen Hufton, *The Poor of Eighteenth-Century France, 1750–1789* (Oxford, 1974), esp. map (p. 75) of migrations in 1810; and Eugen Weber, *Peasants into Frenchmen: The Modernization of Rural France, 1870–1914* (Stanford, Calif., 1976), chap. 16. Hufton suggests that *colporteurs* from the Pyrenees were "specialists in horn combs, woolen stockings, and quack medicines" (p. 84).

118 Rivière-Sestier, *Remèdes populaires*, p. 31, quoting André Allix (no further reference given).

119 Henri Gaidoz, *La Rage et saint Hubert* (1887), p. 119.

120 *Sainte Marie-Marguerite Alacoque, trouvée à Paray-le-Monial* (1867) quoted by Jean-Pierre Séguin, "Les 'Canards' de faits divers de petit format en France, au XIXᵉ siècle," *Arts et traditions populaires* 4 (1956): 128.

121 Report by Seignolle brothers, cited in Marcelle Bouteiller, *Chamanisme et guérison magique* (1950), p. 208.

122 Richard Cobb, *The Police and the People: French Popular Protest, 1789–1820* (Oxford, 1970); Robert Darnton, "The Grub-Street Style of Revolution: J.-P. Brissot, Police Spy," *Journal of Modern History* 40 (1968): 301–27.

123 Report to Dominique-Joseph Garat, Minister of the Interior, 13 May 1793, quoted in Augustin Cabanès, *Comment se soignaient nos pères: Remèdes d'autrefois* (1905), p. 57.

124 AD Var 8 U 62/2, no. 38, procureur to *juge d'instruction*, Brignoles, 28 August 1817; no. 31, sentence, *tribunal de première instance*, 1st arrondissement, at Brignoles, 10 September 1817.

125 AD Rhône B, *maréchaussée*, 1750, cited by Gutton, *La Société et les pauvres*, p. 153, n. 221.

126 Rambaud, *Pharmacie en Poitou*, pp. 565–66, quoting criminal records, *présidial*.

127 AC Nantes I 5 7, d. 3, mayor of La Merlatière to mayor of Nantes, 22 February 1815.

128 AN F¹⁷ 2276, d. 2, no. 334 (Saint-Sever), 20 January 1791.

129 Pierre-François Nicolas, *Histoire des maladies épidémiques qui ont régné dans la province de Dauphiné depuis l'année 1775* (Grenoble, 1780), pp. 108–09.

130 AD Loire-Atlantique 1 M 1358, no. 370, procureur to prefect, 19 August 1819; no. 369, *tribunal correctionnel*, Nantes, 15 January 1820; no. 368, mayor of Saint-Macaire to *vicaire* of Maisdon; no. 365, procureur to prefect, 11 July 1820; no. 358, procureur to prefect, 26 July 1820; no. 364, mayor of Nantes to prefect, 31 July 1820.

131 On forensic psychiatry applied to a more celebrated case see Michel Foucault, ed., *Moi, Pierre Rivière, ayant égorgé ma mère, ma soeur, et mon frère* . . . : *Un Cas de parricide au XIXᵉ siècle* (1973).

132 On the tradition of the *chevaliers de saint Hubert*, see Jean-Baptiste Thiers, *Traité des*

superstitions qui regardent les sacremens..., 4th ed., 4 vols. (1741), 1: 511–14, and Joseph-J.-G. Tricot-Royer, "Le Bilan du traitement de la rage à l'intercession de saint Hubert et plus spécialement à Saint-Hubert d'Ardennes," *Bulletin de la Société Française d'Histoire de la Médecine* 19 (1925): 273–90, 346–59.

133 Vaultier, "Saint Hubert et la rage," *Presse médicale* 57 (1949): 670. The account here is based on the Hué dossier in AN F^8 157.

134 Cf. the injunctions and restrictions contained in the printed instructions given to pilgrims at Saint-Hubert in 1687, quoted by Thiers, *Traité*, 1: 514–15 (and see also Tricot-Royer, "Bilan," pp. 279–80). They were to perform a novena, confessing and taking communion on nine consecutive days. During this time they were to sleep alone, either in clean, white sheets or else completely dressed; drink from a glass or another vessel, so as to avoid lowering their head to drink from a fountain or river; drink either pure water or wine mixed with water; and eat bread, the flesh of a hog, chicken, or capon one year old or older, scaly fish, or hard-boiled eggs (consuming all these things cold). They must also refrain from combing their hair for forty days.

135 "La Bande d'Orgères, 1790–1799," in *Reactions to the French Revolution* (London, 1972), pp. 181–211.

136 *Gazette des tribunaux*, 3 (1827–28): 370.

137 One example among many: Jean Labadie, a shepherd from eighteenth-century Béarn, who set himself up as a surgeon at Mées in Gascony but also worked as an itinerant, practicing a mixture of magic and medicine throughout the marquisate of Tercis. See F. Bordes, "Le Livre de remèdes de Labadie: Contribution à l'histoire de la médecine populaire landaise au XVIIIe siècle," *Bulletin de la Société de Borda* 107 (1982): 399–412.

138 Jean-Jacques Darmon, *Le Colportage de librairie en France sous le Second Empire: Grands Colporteurs et culture populaire* (1972), pp. 41–50.

139 Hufton, *The Poor*, chaps. 3–4.

CHAPTER 4 *Irregulars: sedentary empirics*

1 SRM 107, 14 March 1782.

2 See, for example, AD Hautes-Alpes 141 M, no. 1, "Observation d'un officier de santé sur la pratique des charlatans et des maÿges...," 28 Frimaire IX/19 December 1800.

3 AN F^7 8185, d. 2981R^2, prefect of the Loiret to 1st arrondissement, *police générale*, 17 October 1810.

4 AD Meurthe-et-Moselle 5 M 18, nos. 39–40, report by physicians of the "Association générale" on illegal practice (inventory gives date as 1822, but it is probably later).

5 The American patent medicine industry has received the fullest attention. See especially James Harvey Young, *The Toadstool Millionaires: A Social History of Patent Medicines in America before Federal Regulation* (Princeton, N.J., 1961); idem, *The Medical Messiahs: A Social History of Health Quackery in Twentieth-Century America* (Princeton, N.J., 1967); and Sarah Stage, *Female Complaints: Lydia Pinkham and the Business of Women's Medicine* (New York, 1979).

6 Paul Delaunay, "La Médecine populaire dans le Maine à la fin de l'Ancien Régime," *Premier Congrès pour l'Histoire de l'Art de Guérir* (Antwerp, 1921), pp. 90–91.

7 Maurice Bouvet, "Un Remède secret du XVIIIe siècle: Le Rob Boyveau-Laffecteur," *Bulletin de la Société d'Histoire de la Pharmacie* 4 (1923): 264–72; Joseph Villebrun, *Un Remède antisyphilitique aux XVIIIe et XIXe siècles: Le Rob de Laffecteur*, Paris medical thesis, 1939. See also Jean-François Hirsch, "Médecins, charlatans, magistrats et poètes à l'oeuvre: Remèdes et arcanes antivénériens autour du XVIIIe siècle," *Bulletin d'ethnomédecine*, no. 20 (1983): 19–32.

8 Dr. Giraudeau (or Giraudeau de Saint-Gervais as he called himself, taking the name of his birthplace in the Vienne), was among the French profession's most prominent practitioners of "medical industrialism" during the first half of the nineteenth century. His remedies for skin disorders and venereal disease (including the *rob Laffecteur*

itself, which he acquired at the height of his success in the 1840's) were distributed through numerous outlets in France and abroad. Giraudeau falsely announced himself as the medical director of a sanatorium and boasted of a dissertation approved by the faculty of medicine, which was nothing more than the thesis he had submitted for the doctorate. See Adolphe Trébuchet, *Jurisprudence de la médecine, de la chirurgie, et de la pharmacie en France* (1834), p. 379. Among Giraudeau's numerous publications, see, for example, *Le Médecin sans médecine: Conseils aux gens du monde pour guérir soi-même les dartres et toutes les maladies provenant de l'âcreté du sang et des humeurs . . . par la méthode végétale du D*ʳ *Giraudeau de Saint-Gervais . . .* (n.d.); *L'Art de guérir soi-même, ou Traitement des maladies vénériennes sans mercure . . .* (1827); and *Manuel hygiénique de santé, ou Dictionnaire raisonné de médecine usuelle: Conseils sur l'emploi du rob Boyveau-Laffecteur . . .* (1849). The BN also possesses Giraudeau's *Journal de médecine populaire* and copies of a *Medical Gazette* in English, German, Spanish, Italian, Greek, Dutch, and Russian, containing articles on his rob and books and lists of his agents in the various countries.

9 FP reg. 52, no. 6, Mettemberg, printed petition to president of the Société de Pharmacie, 15 March 1810; ibid., no. 8, "Résultat des expériences officielles faites à l'hôpital militaire du Val-de-Grâce . . ."; ibid., no. 53, copy of extract, minutes of the Secrétairerie d'État, 6 February 1810; AD Loire 38 M 9, no. 17, subprefect, Roanne, to prefect, 23 August 1810.

10 On the Courcelle remedy, see Louis Faligot, *La Question des remèdes secrets sous la Révolution et l'Empire* (1924), p. 16. No general study of the Ailhaud remedy exists. Mary Lindemann is engaged in research on the distribution of Ailhaud's *universal Medikament* in northern Germany in the last quarter of the eighteenth century. On the French *dépôts*, see, for example, the response from Dourdan (Seine-et-Oise) to the Comité de Salubrité investigation of 1790–91, which reported a "*bureau des poudres d'Alieau* [sic]" (AN F¹⁷ 2276, d. 2, no. 320).

11 Faligot, *Question des remèdes secrets*, prints the prospectuses for the pectoral syrup of sieur Macors and other secret remedies (pp. 72 ff.). See also Maurice Bouvet, "La Publicité médico-pharmaceutique dans les journaux des XVIIᵉ et XVIIIᵉ siècles," *Comptes rendus du Deuxième Congrès International d'Histoire de la Médecine* (Évreux, 1922), pp. 578–87; idem, "La Publicité médico-pharmaceutique par prospectus aux XVIIᵉ et XVIIIᵉ siècles," *Pharmacie française* 26 (1922): 292–331; and, for an English comparison, Jonathan Barry, "Publicity and the Public Good: Presenting Medicine in Eighteenth-Century Bristol," in W. F. Bynum and Roy Porter, eds., *Medical Fringe and Medical Orthodoxy, 1750–1850* (London, 1986), pp. 29–39.

12 Faligot, *Question des remèdes secrets*, p. 17.

13 Joseph Lévy-Valensi, *La Médecine et les médecins français au XVIIᵉ siècle* (1933), p. 418.

14 On the male fern: Marie-Claire Gandrille-Oursel, *La Médecine populaire en Bourgogne*, Paris medical thesis, 1957, no. 251, p. 39; on the anthrax remedy: Adolphe Lecocq, *Empiriques, somnambules et rebouteurs beaucerons* (Chartres, 1862), p. 37. See also Alfred Franklin, *La Vie privée d'autrefois*, vol. 9, *Les Médicaments* (1891), p. 209; and Faligot, *Question des remèdes secrets*, p. 15.

15 Beauval [?barely legible signature], letter of 23 August 1810, in "Un empirique niortais au service de l'Empereur et de l'Humanité," *Bulletin de la Société Historique et Scientifique des Deux-Sèvres*, 2d ser., 14 (1981): 112–13.

16 FP reg. 13, no. 27, Stefanopoli petition, 22 February 1779. See also SRM 97, d. 112, on "Dimo-Stefanopoli," described here as a Corsican surgeon of Greek extraction who wishes to supply the apothecaries with his vermifuge plant.

17 SRM 107, Terrède, physician at L'Aigle, 8 July 1782.

18 SRM 107, n.d.; ibid., denunciation from "chevalier de Bonzon," resident of the Île Saint-Louis, 9 August 1782.

19 Michel-Jostny-Marie Richard, *Sur les erreurs populaires relatives à la médecine et leurs dangers*, Paris medical thesis, 1833, no. 36, p. 16.

20 SRM 199, d. 9, no. 1, Duboueix at Clisson, 14 January 1784.

21 AD Loire 38 M 9, no. 14, subprefect of Roanne to prefect, 10 August 1819; no. 13,

conseiller de préfecture of the Rhône to prefect of the Loire, 21 June; no. 12, subprefect of Roanne to prefect, 31 December. Also, mayor of Sail-sous-Couzon (to prefect, 8 March 1828) naming a "Tissier" among three persons who treat dogs.

22 AD Bas-Rhin 1 L 838, no. 4.

23 *Gazette des tribunaux* 3 (1827–28): 1036, *tribunal correctionnel*, Dreux; ibid., 4 (1828–29): 522, *tribunal correctionnel*, Bressuire.

24 M.-A. Saint-Léger, "Conflit entre le corps des chirurgiens et le bourreau de Lille en 1768," *Revue du Nord* 2 (1911): 54; Armand Trousseau, *Conférences sur l'empirisme* ... (1862), p. 47; Robert Boeglin, *L'Évolution historique de la pharmacie en Alsace*, Strasbourg pharmacy thesis, 1939, p. 99. John Pinkerton, *Recollections of Paris in the Years 1802–3–4–5*, 2 vols. (London, 1806), 2: 296–97, describes a carpenter with a paralytic complaint treated with human fat by a public executioner. On these remedies, see also Raoul Mercier, *Le Monde médical de Touraine sous la Révolution* (Tours, 1936), pp. 205–06.

25 For example, the executioner at Fontenay-le-Comte, cited in Chapter 1, sold tisanes. Siedler, executioner at Rouffach in Alsace, maintained that he used only simples (AD Haut-Rhin C 1114, 1779, cited by Boeglin, *Évolution historique*, p. 100).

26 Isabey, rue de Condé at Dijon; announcement quoted by A. Baudot, *Études historiques sur la pharmacie en Bourgogne avant 1803* (1905), p. 522.

27 AD Doubs M 1358, Radaz, surgeon, 3 November 1812, on case of Comte (who denied giving "vomits or other medicines").

28 Delaunay, "Médecine populaire dans le Maine," p. 90.

29 SRM 199, d. 29, no. 14, item 14 on list of correspondence received (Dupin at Morlaàs).

30 *Gazette des tribunaux*, 5 (1829–30): 786.

31 Alice Taverne, *Coutumes et superstitions foréziennes*, fasc. 5: *Médecine populaire, sorcellerie, diable et lutins* (Ambierle, 1971), p. 10; Arnold Van Gennep, *Le Folklore du Dauphiné*, 2 vols. paginated continuously (1932–33), pp. 478–79, on *charmeurs de vipère*; Marcelle Bouteiller, *Médecine populaire d'hier et d'aujourd'hui* (1966), p. 198, on a 1963 case near Grenoble.

32 Edgar-Jean-Ernest Porcheron, *Les Braconniers de la médecine au pays de Poitou*, Bordeaux medical thesis, 1923, pp. 111–12. On the *ramasseuses de crottes de chien*: Marcel Pellison, "Un Curé guérisseur," *Revue de Saintonge et de l'Aunis* 22 (1902): 367–70, citing *Almanach Kneipp* (1894), pp. 180–81, "petits métiers inconnus."

33 AN F[17] 2276, d. 2, no. 353.

34 SRM 112, Edme-Nicolas Geoffrain to Société Royale, 3 June 1776; Hérissay, "De l'exercice illégal de la médecine dans l'Eure sous le Consulat," *Bulletin de la Société Française d'Histoire de la Médecine* 26 (1932): 88; Claude Seignolle, *Le Folklore du Languedoc* ... (1960), pp. 232–33.

35 See especially the petitions in SRM 96–107.

36 Paul Bidault, *Les Superstitions médicales du Morvan*, Paris medical thesis, 1898–99, no. 321 (1899), p. 21.

37 AD Loire-Atlantique 1 M 1358, no. 337, mayor of Nantes to prefect; no. 338, Lancelotte's petition, 2 August 1825.

38 See, for example, Lester S. King, *The Medical World of the Eighteenth Century* (Chicago, 1958), chap. 2; Guy R. Williams, *The Age of Agony: The Art of Healing, c. 1700–1800* (London, 1975), chap. 11; Eric Maple, *Magic, Medicine, and Quackery* (South Brunswick, N.J., 1968); Eric Jameson, *The Natural History of Quackery* (London, 1961); Charles John Samuel Thompson, *The Quacks of Old London* (London, 1928); Graham Everitt, *Doctors and Doctors: Some Curious Chapters in Medical History and Quackery* (London, 1888); François Millepierres, *La Vie quotidienne des médecins au temps de Molière* (1964), chap. 10; Paul Delaunay, *Le Monde médical parisien au dix-huitième siècle* (1906), chap. 12. On the quacks of Paris, see also Jean-Baptiste Gouriet, *Les Charlatans célèbres, ou Tableau historique des bateleurs [etc.] ... qui se sont rendus célèbres dans les rues et sur les places publiques de Paris depuis une haute antiquité jusqu'à nos jours*, 2d ed., 2 vols. (1819); this work deals with street entertainers, magicians,

and fakers of all kinds. Mesmer alone is the subject of an abundant literature. See Robert Darnton, *Mesmerism and the End of the Enlightenment in France* (Cambridge, Mass., 1968), esp. chap. 2 (though this study is more concerned with the Mesmerist movement and French politics than with Mesmer as a medical practitioner); Caroline C. Hannaway, "Medicine, Public Welfare and the State in Eighteenth-Century France: The Société Royale de Médecine of Paris (1776–1793)," Ph.D. dissertation, The Johns Hopkins University, 1974, pp. 349–78; and Charles C. Gillispie, *Science and Polity in France at the End of the Old Regime* (Princeton, N.J., 1980), chap. 4, pt. 2.

39 Émile Rivière, *Curiosités sur l'histoire de la médecine*, fasc. 1: *Un Célèbre Arracheur de dents sous Louis XV . . .* (1882); A. Chevalier, "Un Charlatan du XVIIIᵉ siècle: Le Grand Thomas," *Mémoires de la Société de l'Histoire de Paris et de l'Île-de-France*, 7 (1880; pub. 1881): 61–78.

40 Pierre-Jean Tellier, *Un Aventurier médical au XVIIᵉ siècle: Nicolas de Blégny*, Paris medical thesis, 1932. On the relationship between empiricism and the profession, see also Bernard Quémada, *Introduction à l'étude du vocabulaire médical, 1600–1710* (Bescançon, 1955), pp. 20–22.

41 AD Somme C 34. On *carabins* and *fraters*, the unlicensed surgeons, see Alfred Franklin, *La Vie privée d'autrefois . . .*, vol. 12, *Les Chirurgiens* (1893), p. 33.

42 AD Maine-et-Loire 4 D 12, 1731.

43 AD Nièvre 5M, "Liste des charlatans, des prêtres, des femmes qui s'immiscent dans l'exercice de l'art de guérir, et des soi-disants officiers de santé qui ont demandé à être examinés et n'ont point paru au jury médical," n.d., early nineteenth century.

44 SRM 199, d. 24, no. 11, Beaussieu de la Bouchardière, at Vendôme, 30 September 1786.

45 AD Meurthe-et-Moselle 5 M 18, no. 228, Ministry of the Interior, 2d division, Bureau des Secours et Hôpitaux, to prefect of the Meurthe, 29 August 1819.

46 AN BB¹ 204, Minister of Justice to *procureur-général criminel* of the Sarthe, 19 September 1806.

47 AN F⁸ 165, Suzov to Minister of the Interior, 25 Ventôse XI/16 March 1803.

48 AN F¹⁷ 2276, d. 2, no. 320.

49 Gustave-Thomas de Closmadeuc, *Esquisse sur la médecine et la chirurgie populaires dans de département du Morbihan* (Vannes, 1861), p. 7.

50 AN AF III 107, *administration centrale* of the Eure, session of 19 Brumaire V/9 November 1796; Augustin Cabanès, *Comment se soignaient nos pères: Remèdes d'autrefois* (1905), p. 474. Cf. AN F¹⁷ 2276, d. 2, no. 312 (Arras, 1790), which mentions a family of hernia surgeons who used the castration method.

51 SRM 199, d. 9, no. 1, 14 January 1784.

52 See, for example, Trousseau, *Conférences*, p. 46, and Paul-Abraham Pesme, *De quelques erreurs en médecine*, Paris medical thesis, 1855, p. 89.

53 Cabanès, *Comment on se soigne aujourd'hui: Remèdes de bonne femme* (1907), p. 116, cites *Grand vocabulaire français* (1773), 24: 522. On "*ossier*," see Jules Lecoeur [Louis-Jules Tirard], *Esquisses du Bocage normand*, 2 vols. (Condé-sur-Noireau, 1883–87), 2: 119.

54 Anders Christopher Thorn, *Les Désignations françaises du médecin et de ses concurrents aujourd'hui et autrefois* (Jena and Leipzig, 1932), pp. 75–76; Adelin Moulis, "Médecine populaire en Ariège," *Arts et traditions populaires* 9 (1961): 115; P. Bonnet, "Superstitions médicales de la Franche-Comté," *Mélusine* 1 (1878), col. 403; J.-M.-C. Naville, *Lettres bourguignonnes, ou Aperçu philosophique et critique sur les causes des difficultés dans l'art de guérir . . .* (1822), p. 105; Alexandre Abord, *La Médecine populaire et les pratiques superstitieuses du Morvan*, Paris medical thesis, 1909–10, no. 167 (1910), p. 21; Émile Blin, *Le Morvan: Moeurs, coutumes, langage . . .* (Nevers, 1902), p. 160; Eugène de Chambure, *Glossaire du Morvan* (Paris and Autun, 1878), pp. 413, 418, 732.

55 *Gazette des tribunaux*, 2 (1826–27): 1510.

56 AD Loire 38 M 9, no. 9, Péricard's petition, N, 25 April 1808; no. 10, petition from mayors, 8 April; no. 8, Minister of the Interior to prefect, 13 May.

57 ARC 4, 29 May 1793, report by a commission of the Académie Royale de Chirurgie. Cf. a denunciation of "Valdajols" by Castara, *greffier* at Lunéville, in SRM 107 (23 January 1783).

58 Bouteiller, *Médecine populaire*, p. 47; Lecocq, *Empiriques*, chap. 6; A.-F.-Émile Bessières, *Étude sur les erreurs et les préjugés populaires en médecine*, Paris medical thesis, 1860, no. 228, p. 31.

59 AD Loire, 38 M 9, no. 18, report by mayor of Feurs, 29 December 1812.

60 The last was a rag and scrap metal dealer. Bouteiller, *Médecine populaire*, p. 159.

61 Lecocq, *Empiriques*, chap. 6, and Ernest Sévrin, "Croyances populaires et médecine supranaturelle en Eure-et-Loire au XIXe siècle," *"Revue d'histoire de l'Église de France* 32 (1946): 285.

62 Philippe Macquer, "Bailleul," in *Dictionnaire raisonné universel des arts et métiers . . .*, new ed., revised by abbé Jaubert, 4 vols. (1773).

63 AN F^{17} 2276, d. 2, no. 305 (Carcassonne). On bonesetters and the marketplace, see Closmadeuc, *Esquisse*, p. 12.

64 A. Dupuy, "Les Epidémies en Bretagne au XVIIIe siècle," *Annales de Bretagne* 2 (1886): 208.

65 Édouard-Louis Jacquet, *De quelques considérations sur l'empirisme et l'exercice illégal de la médecine*, Paris medical thesis, 1864, no. 162, p. 51.

66 Pierre-Jean-Baptiste Legrand d'Aussy, *Voyage fait en 1787 et 1788, dans la ci-devant Haute et Basse Auvergne . . .*, 3 vols. (Year III), 3: 317–19.

67 AD Deux-Sèvres 6 M 21/1, no. 52, report by *commissariat de police*, Niort, 29 November 1884.

68 See the tribute by the military surgeon Pierre-François Percy in the article "Déboîtement," *Dictionnaire des sciences médicales, par une société de médecins et de chirurgiens*, 60 vols. (1812–22), 8: 107–08; also David M. Vess, *Medical Revolution in France, 1789–1796* (Gainesville, Fla., 1975), pp. 122–23. On the regulars' views of bonesetting in England, cf. Roger Cooter, "Bones of Contention? Orthodox Medicine and the Mystery of the Bone-setter's Craft," in Bynum and Porter, *Medical Fringe*, pp. 158–73.

69 J.-Charles Voisin, *De quelques préjugés relatifs à la médecine* (1831), p. 62.

70 SRM 199, d. 18, no. 27, Bonet, surgeon, 1784 case.

71 ARC 33, d. 1, no. 15, Saulquin, surgeon at Mantes, "Mémoire dans lequel on a rapporté quelques observations des plus frappantes, qui démontrent l'impéritie des charlatans . . . ," 1769.

72 AC Nantes I 5 8, d. 6.

73 SRM 199, d. 9, no. 1, Duboueix, 14 January 1784. Cf. Jean-Gabriel Gallot, "Observations physiques et médicinales," report to Société Royale de Médecine, 1778, on serious illnesses treated by "men and women of the people," esp. cancer; quoted in Louis Merle, *La Vie et les oeuvres du Dr Jean-Gabriel Gallot (1744–1794) . . .*, *Mémoires de la Société des Antiquaires de l'Ouest*, 4th ser., 5 (1961): 201.

74 SRM 199, d. 29, no. 14, item 9 (list of reports on charlatanism).

75 Jacques Léonard, *Les Médecins de l'Ouest au XIXe siècle* (1978), p. 423. Victor Gueneau, communication to the Société Académique du Nivernais, in its *Mémoires*, 2d ser., vol. 3, fasc. 3 (1913): 524–25.

76 Léonard (*Médecins de l'Ouest*, p. 233, n. 119) lists the conditions treated and the remedies used by one Breton empiric, Julien Le Mentheour, of Plonévez-du-Faou (mid-1790's).

77 See Angus McLaren, *Sexuality and Social Order: The Debate Over the Fertility of Women and Workers in France, 1770–1920* (New York, 1983), pp. 142–43.

78 SRM 199, d. 29, no. 14, item 20, Doucet.

79 Cited in *Annuaire de la Société de Médecine, Chirurgie et Pharmacie du Département de l'Eure*, 1819, pp. 208–09, memoir no. 2, essay competition on repression of abuses in medicine.

80 From Saint-Quentin, for example, Dr. Von Mittag Midy supplied the Société Royale de Médecine with six such prescriptions by local empirics, two of them farriers; see SRM 199, d. 26, no. 7.

81 Naville, *Lettres bourguigonnes,* letter 13; Closmadeuc, *Esquisse,* p. 6. Cf. the discussion of German urinoscopists in Alfons Fischer, *Geschichte des deutschen Gesundheitswesens,* 2 vols. (Berlin, 1933), 2: 95–96.

82 In the 1790–91 survey of the Comité de Salubrité, the report from Dourdan (Seine-et-Oise) specifically mentioned *médecins des urines* (AN F^{17} 2276, d. 2, no. 320); no. 269, from Ploërmel (Morbihan), 26 January 1791, lumped them together with local witch-healers, suggesting that few parishes did not have a thaumaturge, *uromante-rebouteur,* or sorcerer. Fifty years later, a report in the Mayenne said that "each *contrée* has its *jugeur d'eau*" (AD Mayenne M 1448, Lemercier, 29 October 1841, quoted by Léonard, *Médecins de l'Ouest,* p. 615). Unfortunately there is no way to calculate regional densities. Lecocq, *Empiriques,* chap. 4, suggests that Beauce had fewer urine doctors than Poitou and Brittany, but he gives no statistics.

83 Charles Guyotjeannin, *Contribution à l'histoire de l'analyse des urines,* Strasbourg pharmacy thesis, 1950–51, no. 555 (Créteil, 1951), pp. 5–18.

84 SRM 199, d. 11, no. 4, copy of letter of inquiry, supposedly from a prospective patient (Renaux, state lottery official at Château-Thierry) to a satisfied customer, and response from Minette, describing the work of Madame Vacheron; November 1778.

85 AD Loire-Atlantique 1 M 1358, no. 311, to mayor, 3 November 1830.

86 Ibid. and AD Loire-Atlantique 4 X 232 (cited by Léonard, *Médecins de l'Ouest,* p. 611, n. 323).

87 AD Indre-et-Loire C 354, subdelegation of Beaumont-la-Vicomté.

88 AD Aube 7 U 298, Year XII. Blanc was also an herbalist.

89 See, for example, Léonard, *Médecins de l'Ouest,* p. 613, citing AD Loire-Atlantique 4 X 224*, Dr. Julien Praud, at Machecoul, to prefect, quoted in general report by medical jury, 26 March 1827.

90 AN F^8 149.

91 SRM 137, d. 8, no. 9, Dr. Maury, at Sézanne, 1 July 1782.

92 René-Georges Gastellier, *Observations et réflexions relatives à l'organisation actuelle de la médecine* (Montargis, 1806), p. 12.

93 AD Ille-et-Vilaine C 1389, quoted by Dupuy, "Épidémies," *Annales de Bretagne* 2: 208.

94 For example, AD Yonne 5 M 7/1, prefect to *conseiller d'état,* 14 Messidor X/3 July 1802. The celebrated eighteenth-century Swiss *Urinbeseher* Michel Schuppach left a large fortune to his widow (Christian Gottfried Gruner, *Almanach für Aerzte und Nichtaerzte auf das Jahr 1782,* cited in Fischer, *Geschichte,* 2: 95). See also Vieillard, "Un Uromante au XVIIIe siècle: Michel Schuppach," *Bulletin de la Société Française d'Histoire de la Médecine* 2 (1903): 146–54. The illustration on p. 194 of this volume shows Schuppach's consulting room.

95 AN F^8 165, Schmitt case: Dr. Vetten, at Ohrweiler, 6 October 1809.

96 Ibid., Dr. Louis Tils, 7 November 1808; prefect of Rhin-et-Moselle to prefect of the Sarre, 12 October and 16 November 1809; prefect of the Sarre to Minister of the Interior, 13 September 1810.

97 AD Loire-Atlantique 4 X 231, cited by Léonard, *Médecins de l'Ouest,* p. 1389.

98 Auguste Viatte, *Les Sources occultes du romantisme: Illuminisme, théosophie, 1770–1820,* 2 vols. (1928); Darnton, *Mesmerism.* On the extraordinary appeal of Mesmerism to the literary imagination, which Darnton discusses in his last chapter, cf. Maria M. Tatar, *Spellbound: Studies on Mesmerism and Literature* (Princeton, N.J., 1978).

99 On popular magnetism, see Lecocq, *Empiriques,* chap. 3. Some magnetizers, notably *le zouave* Jacob, achieved great celebrity; see Maurice Igert, *Les Guérisseurs mystiques,* Toulouse medical thesis, 1928–29, no. 26 (Toulouse, 1928), p. 128 and passim. On *dormeurs* and *dormeuses:* ibid., p. 49, and Renée Fournier, *La Médecine ancienne dans le Centre-Ouest: Coutumes populaires et survivances,* Société d'Études Folkloriques du Centre-Ouest, *Revue de recherches ethnographiques,* special number (May 1971): 38–40; and Émile Boismoreau, *Coutumes médicales et superstitions populaires du bocage vendéen* (1911), chap. 5.

100 Charles Lavielle, "Essai sur les erreurs populaires en médecine," *Bulletin de la Société*

de Borda 6 (1881): 92.

101 On the transformations of Mesmerism, see Henri F. Ellenberger, *The Discovery of the Unconscious: The History and Evolution of Dynamic Psychiatry* (New York, 1970), chaps. 2–4.

102 See *Revue magnétique*, 2 (1845–46): 485 (copy in AN F^{17} 4468, d. 2/5).

103 Dr. Eissen, *L'Exploitation de la crédulité publique par l'exercice illégal de la médecine à Strasbourg et dans les deux départements du Rhin* (reprinted from *Gazette médicale de Strasbourg*, 1842), p. 5.

104 *Revue magnétique* 2 (1845–46): 440.

105 Marc Leproux, *Médecine, magie et sorcellerie* (1954), p. 40; Eissen, *Exploitation*, pp. 5, 9.

106 AD Bas-Rhin 5 M 22, no. 8, 12 Messidor VII/30 June 1799, Marchand, *juge de paix*; no. 9, interrogation of Barbe Richert; no. 17, prefect to president, École de Médecine, 12 September 1808; no. 18, Küchel's announcement. Küchel, who claimed *not* to use magnetism, electricity, or sympathy, boasted that he could cure eye diseases; discharges from the throat or ear; rheumatism; erysipelas; toothache and swelling caused by fluxion; convulsions; aphthae (small ulcers on the mucous membrane of the mouth); scrapes, wounds, scalds, burns, scratches and bruises; insect bites; breast disorders; intermittent fever; and bumps on the head. Eruptions were touched with linen, diseased parts of the mouth with an ivory or ebony stick.

107 AD Aube M 1626, commissioner of police, Troyes, to prefect, 4 February 1813.

108 AD Haute-Loire 13 M 18, no. 481, commissioner of police, Le Puy, to prefect, 19 April 1819.

109 Ibid., no. 483, denunciation to prefect, 17 April 1819.

110 Camille-J.-B. Fraysse, "Au pays de Baugé: La Thérapeutique populaire et les sorciers guérisseurs," *Arts et traditions populaires* 9 (1961): 106–07.

111 AN AD VIII 33, memoir to First Consul by Georgel, 1802. This case has been briefly described by Charles Sadoul in "Les Guérisseurs et la médecine populaire en Lorraine," *Pays lorrain* 26 (1934): 75.

112 Jacques Lacroix, "Éléments de l'épistémè populaire: Un Cahier de 'secrets' languedocien, *Annales de la Faculté de Lettres de Toulouse*, n.s., vol. 6, fasc. 5 (1970).

113 *Gazette des tribunaux* 4 (1828–29): 522–23, *tribunal correctionnel*, Bressuire.

114 Bibliothèque de l'Arsenal, Archives de la Bastille, d. 10590, 12475, analyzed in Maurice Boutry, "Les Tribulations d'une guérisseuse au XVIIIe siècle," *La Chronique médicale* 12 (1905): 289–97, and R. Goulard, "Les Secrets d'une guérisseuse au XVIIIe siècle," *Bulletin de la Société Française d'Histoire de la Médecine* 18 (1924): 67–73.

115 *Gazette des tribunaux* 5 (1829–30): 362–63, *tribunal correctionnel*, Tours.

116 On the *pardons*: Léonard, *Médecins de l'Ouest*, p. 112.

117 On religious healing in the Calvinist communities of southern France, see Roger Bastide, "Protestantisme et médecine de folk," *Revista de etnografia* 15 (1971): 321–32, esp. pp. 328–30.

118 AC Nantes I 5 7, d. 3, prefect to mayor, 11 September 1828.

119 AC Dijon G 53; Claude Courtépée, "Voyages de Courtépée dans la province de Bourgogne," *Mémoires de la Société Éduenne* 19 (1891): 411.

120 AD Aube G 1763; Jean-Charles Courtalon-Delaistre, *Topographie historique de la ville et du diocèse de Troyes*, 3 vols. (Troyes, 1783–84), 3: 134. Richard's prominence has won him a place in general discussions of popular healing; see, for example, Igert, *Guérisseurs mystiques*, pp. 41–42, and idem, *Le Problème des guérisseurs* (1931), p. 48. The fullest published account is by Émile and Ernest Choullier, "Pierre Richard, dit le saint de Savières," *Annuaire administratif et statistique du département de l'Aube* 55 (1881), pt. 2: 75–97, which gives the texts of the interrogations.

121 AD Marne 33 X 8, Director of Police to prefect, 15 March 1822; prefect's reply, 28 March.

122 Jacques-Barthélemy Salgues, *Des erreurs et des préjugés répandus dans la société*, 2d ed., 2 vols (1811), 1: 176; Henri Gaidoz, *La Rage et saint Hubert* (1887), p. 116. For other cases, see Charles-Louis-François Andry, *Recherches sur la rage...*, new ed. (1780), pp. 324–325. One seventeenth-century nobleman of Saint Hubert's lineage, de Can-

roses, healed not with his touch but with a remedy; his family kept the recipe as a mark of the antiquity of their nobility. (Andry cites Pierre Martin de La Martinière, *L'Opérateur ingénu* ... [1668].) In 1655 the Estates of Brittany awarded a 400-livre grant to a sieur de Saint-Hubert who pretended to be able to cure rabies; see "Documents pour servir à l'histoire de la médecine et de la chirurgie," communication by Quesnet of Rennes, *Gazette des hôpitaux* 54 (1881): 430–31. See also Marius Tournon and Alcius Ledieu, "Les Toucheurs contre la rage descendants du Grand Saint Hubert," *Revue des traditions populaires* 16 (1901): 379–81, on a family in Picardy.

123 Roger Vaultier, "Saint Hubert et la rage," *La Presse médicale* 57 (1949): 670.

124 AD Marne 33 X 8, report by commissioner of police, Châlons, c. 1810–11.

125 AD Hautes-Alpes 141 M, nos. 48–49, Rimbaud, *officier de santé* at Ribiers, to prefect, 15 October 1814.

126 *Gazette des tribunaux* 3 (1827–28): 618–19.

127 AD Var 8 U 62/2 (1816), no. 9, *première instance*, Brignoles; no. 17, testimony of Aunievan's son; no. 18, interrogation of Aunievan; no. 24, *procès-verbal, juge d'instruction* (testimony of Gerbe, surgeon, who says that Menut was sometimes mad); no. 27, interrogation of Aunievan's daughter; no. 28, conclusions of procureur, who interprets Aunievan's predictions of death as threats; no. 30, *juge de paix*, Saint-Maximin, to procureur, *première instance*, Brignoles.

128 Ibid., nos. 42, 44, procureur to tribunal of Brignoles, 1819.

129 AD Vaucluse 5 M 14, no. 483, subprefect of Orange to prefect, 4 May 1816; no. 490, subprefect to prefect, 19 May; mayor of Sérignan to subprefect, 30 May; letter from Tissot et al., 5 March 1817; no. 479, subprefect to prefect, 6 March; no. 470, announcement for Tissot's *maison de santé*; no. 467, subprefect to prefect, 11 August 1817; no 466, subprefect to prefect, 27 August 1817.

130 AD Marne 8 U 17/11, commissioner of police at Vertas, quoted by Jacques Nouvel, "L'Exercice illégal de la médecine dans la Marne de 1803 à 1868," *Mémoires de la Société d'Agriculture, Commerce, Sciences et Arts du Département de la Marne* 84 (1969): 155.

131 See, for example, Henry Graack, *Kurpfuscherei und Kurpfuschereiverbot: Eine rechtsvergleichende, kriminalpolitische Studie* (Jena, 1906), pp. 61–62.

132 Ambroise Tardieu, "[Rapport] sur les documents transmis au conseil général par les sociétés locales, relatifs à l'exercice illégal de la médecine," *Annuaire de l'Association Générale de Prévoyance et de Secours Mutuels des Médecins de France* 5 (1862): 244–49.

133 SRM 107, d. 3, nos. 1–2, "Notes concernant les empiriques," 2–26 October 1778.

134 SRM 132, "Sur la nécessité & les moyens d'établir une police médicale en France ...," 4 March 1777, fols. 2r–3r.

135 AC Nantes FF 250, March 1781; AN F⁷ 9272, no. 11543, Boullet to Minister of General Police, 12 March 1825.

136 AD Hautes-Alpes 141 M, no. 1, 28 Frimaire IX/19 December 1800.

137 AN F⁸ 160, Macquet, 2 Messidor XI/21 June 1803. Cf. AD Nièvre 5M, "Liste des charlatans ...," and AD Meurthe-et-Moselle 5 M 18, nos. 39–40, list of empirics, n.d. (1822, according to inventory, but possibly later).

138 AN F¹⁷ 2276, d. 2, no. 336, Luxeuil; no. 334, Saint-Sever.

139 See Jean-Pierre Goubert, "L'Art de guérir: Médecine savante et médecine populaire dans la France de 1790," *Annales E.S.C.* 32 (1977): 909. By his count, 27% of responses described the number of charlatans as very high, 32.2% as high, and 28% as low. (In the remaining cases, the respondents denied the existence of charlatans in their jurisdiction or avoided the question.)

140 Gelfand, "Medical Professionals and Charlatans: The *Comité de Salubrité enquête* of 1790–91," *Histoire sociale–Social History* 11 (1978): 76–81. He calculates that the median population of towns with high-density responses was about 5,200; of those with low-density responses, about 3,500.

141 The reports give the impression of concentrating on itinerants; Gelfand is led to state that "most charlatans tended to be ambulatory" (p. 82).

142 Gelfand, "Medical Professionals," pp. 77, 80; idem, "Deux Cultures, une profession: Les Chirurgiens français au XVIIIᵉ siècle," *Revue d'histoire moderne et contemporaine*

27 (1980): 480. In Gascony, 85% of the responses suggested that charlatanism was a serious problem, as opposed to 54% of the responses for Normandy, the Île-de-France, and Champagne.

143 AN F[17] 2276, d. 2, no. 314, Laon; no. 294, Nuits; no. 293, Poitiers. See Goubert, "Art de guérir," pp. 910–11, and Gelfand, "Medical Professionals," pp. 81–86.

144 AN F[17] 2276, d. 2, no. 288, Lyons-la-Forêt; no. 312, Arras.

145 AD Bas-Rhin 5 M 22, no. 15, "Note des personnes qui sans qualité exercent la médecine à Strasbourg," Ventôse XIII/February–March 1803; no. 14, medical jury to procureur, *tribunal de police correctionnelle*, 13 Ventôse XIII/4 March 1805; no. 13, response of deputy procureur, 18 Ventôse/9 March.

146 AD Loire-Atlantique 1 M 1358, no. 321A, Conseil de Salubrité (Nantes) to prefect, 9 April 1827.

147 AD Bas-Rhin 5 M 22. For a fuller discussion, see Matthew Ramsey, "Medical Power and Popular Medicine: Illegal Healers in Nineteenth-Century France," *Journal of Social History* 10 (1976–77): 560–87. A little over a third of the cantons of the Bas-Rhin are represented in the surviving lists. The reports come from all four arrondissements of the department: Saverne, Sélestat (Schlestadt), Strasbourg, and Wissembourg. There is also a composite list for each arrondissement. In the case of Saverne, the reports of the individual cantonal physicians are missing. The list of empirics for the arrondissement (no. 48) includes the cantons of Drulingen and Petite-Pierre, out of seven cantons (see also no. 36, list for the two cantons); it names 27 individuals in 21 communes. The majority (16) were accused of illegal practice of midwifery—an offense about which the cantonal physicians in the other arrondissements complained, but usually without giving a detailed list. The Sélestat dossier covers 9 cases; two cantons out of eight are represented (no. 47, list for the arrondissement; no. 39, canton of Benfeld, 7 November 1813; no. 43, canton of Marckolsheim). Over half of the empirics were barbers if we include the daughter of a barber who performed phlebotomies, one of the traditional surgical functions of that trade. The list for the arrondissement of Strasbourg (no. 45) includes the town of Strasbourg itself (which comprised four cantons) and two other cantons. The reports mention 10 empirics, as well as a surgical student and an apparently qualified surgeon who did not appear on the lists of authorized practitioners (no. 38, canton of Geispolsheim, 5 November 1813; no. 40, canton of Brumath, 21 June 1813). The cantonal reports for the arrondissement of Wissembourg are the most nearly complete: five out of ten cantons are represented (no. 49, list for the arrondissement; no. 35, canton of Soultz-sous-Forêts, 19 June 1813; no. 41, canton of Candel (Kandel), 28 June 1813; no. 42, canton of Wissembourg, 28 June 1813; no. 44, canton of Woerth, 10 June 1813). To the 17 individuals mentioned by name, including 4 barbers and 3 midwives, must be added 5 midwives who are identified only by the name of their commune. The same individual appears in four of the various cantonal reports (see note 148).

148 AD Bas-Rhin 5 M 22, nos. 35, 45, 48. Dr. Johann is mentioned in no. 42, Dr. Hans in nos. 35, 40, 42, and 44.

149 Ibid., nos. 39, 35.

150 Ibid., nos. 45, 44, 35, 48.

151 See, for example, no. 38, Geispolsheim.

152 Ibid., nos. 43, 40, 48, 41.

153 Ibid., nos. 43, 40, 38, 35.

154 Ibid., nos. 44, 40, 48.

155 Ibid., nos. 43, 47, 38 and 45, 44, 35.

156 Ibid., nos. 40, 47.

157 Ibid., no. 48.

158 See note 147, above.

159 AN F[17] 2437.

160 See ibid., Messidor XII/June–July 1804: 384 medical practitioners; and 8 October 1806: 347 practitioners. BB[1] 209, ms. lists for the years XI–XII, gives a total of 294.

Jean-Charles-Joseph Laumond, *Statistique du département du Bas-Rhin* (Year X), pp. 66–67, cites a total of 269 practitioners: 217 surgeons (45 at Strasbourg) and 52 physicians (27 at Strasbourg).

161 On the German case, see Graack, *Kurpfuscherei*, and Albert Guttstadt, "Die ärztliche Gewerbefreiheit im Deutschen Reich und ihr Einfluss auf das öffentliche Wohl," *Zeitschrift des Königlich Preussischen Statistischen Bureaus* 20 (1880): 220–42. For early-nineteenth-century England, the key (and perhaps only) source is the work of the physician Edward Harrison of Horncastle, first president of the Lincolnshire Medical Benevolent Society. In 1804, at the Society's behest, Harrison undertook a survey of regular and irregular medical practice in England. He published the results of his own study of Lincolnshire in *Remarks on the Ineffective State of the Practice of Physic in Great Britain* (London, 1806); the replies to a questionnaire sent to practitioners in other parts of Britain appeared as a preface to the *Medical and Chirurgical Review* 13 (1806). On Harrison, see P. S. Brown, "The Providers of Medical Treatment in Mid-Nineteenth-Century Bristol," *Medical History* 24 (1980): 312–13, and Irvine Loudun, " 'The Vile Race of Quacks with Which this Country Is Infested,' " in Bynum and Porter, *Medical Fringe*, pp. 111–12; Loudun prints a selection of replies to the questionnaire as an appendix (pp. 123–25). Harrison estimated the ratio of unqualified to qualified practitioners in his area as 9:1, and his correspondents suggested ratios as high as 12:1. But Harrison, to score a polemical point, included all the druggists and midwives among the irregulars, and many of the other unqualified practitioners (as a response from Northumberland noted) must have been part-timers. Some replies, moreover, suggested that the number of regulars greatly exceeded the number of irregulars; and Brown, in his own study of Bristol, was able to identify only 48 unqualified practitioners as compared with 120 qualified medical men.

162 Dr. Plouviez, "Quelques mots sur le charlatanisme, les erreurs, et les préjugés populaires en médecine, *Annales médicales de la Flandre occidentale*, 1853, quoted in Jacques Léonard, *La France médicale au XIXe siècle* (1978), p. 58; Léonard, *Médecins de l'Ouest*, pp. 1026, 1024.

163 AN F^17 2276, d. 2, no. 271, fragment without name of town.

164 *Affiches du Poitou*, 1776, p. 140, cited in Prosper-Marie Boissonnade, *Essai sur l'organisation du travail en Poitou depuis le XIe siècle jusqu'à la Révolution, Mémoires de l'Association des Antiquaires de l'Ouest* 21 (1898): 509.

165 Abbé Dubos to Bayle, 23 September 1696, quoted in Gilbert Rouger, ed., *Contes de Perrault* (1967), p. 294; Ozanne was also mentioned by the surgeon Pierre Dionis and by Madame de Sévigné. Cf. Lévy-Valensi, *La Médecine et les médecins*, p. 415. A portrait of Ozanne can be found in the collections of the medical history museum of the Paris Faculty of Medicine.

166 AD Aube C 1164, d. 2, subdelegate at Troyes to intendant, 3 September 1788.

167 SRM 107, Terrède, 8 July 1782.

168 Arnold Van Gennep, *Le Folklore de la Flandre et du Hainaut français*, 2 vols. paginated continuously (1935–36), p. 616; Claude Seignolle, *Le Folklore du Languedoc* (1960), pp. 231–32.

169 SRM 107, Delaunay, dean of medical faculty, 1 December 1778.

170 SRM 199, d. 9, no. 1, Dr. Duboueix at Clisson, 14 January 1784.

171 SRM 112, petition to Société Royale, n.d.

172 SRM 131, "Sur la nécessité . . ."

173 AD Deux-Sèvres 6 M 21/1, no. 52, commissioner of police, Niort, to prefect, 29 November 1884.

174 *Gazette des tribunaux*, 4 (1828–29): 10.

175 Léonard pursues this question at length in *Médecins de l'Ouest*, esp. chap. 18, pt. 2. See also the articles by Jean-François Hirsch and Marie-France Morel in the special issue of *Autrement* on popular medicine: *Panseurs de secrets et de douleurs: Médecine populaire, guérisseurs, voyants et rebouteux . . . de nouveaux interlocuteurs?* (no. 15, September 1978). Morel reviews the history of clerical practice ("Les Curés, les paysans:

Un Même Langage," pp. 63–72); Hirsch discusses recent cases ("Sur les confins Viadène-Aubrac: Un Prêtre radiesthésiste" and "La Magie des hommes en noir," pp. 35–62).

176 AN F^8 154, Demorest, 29 August 1808.

177 AP, Conseil de Salubrité, Paris, minutes, 21 January 1820.

178 Claude Seignolle, *En Sologne: Moeurs et coutumes*, new ed. (1967), p. 161.

179 On the contracts: see, for example, Léonard, *Médecins de l'Ouest*, p. 614, citing AD Loire-Atlantique 1 M 1373, Augustin Péan, *officier de santé* at Oudon, in report, Counseil de Salubrité de Nantes, 2 April 1829.

180 Marcelle Bouteiller gives the form "mageyeur," in the sense of a dealer in livestock (*Médecine populaire*, p. 25); see also Porcheron, *Braconniers*, p. 106.

181 For example: SRM 131, Nicolas, "Sur la nécessité"; AM 228, Leroux and Léveillé, report on memoir by Chevallier, "Abus de l'exercice de la médecine dans les campagnes: Nécessité et avantage d'une réforme sagement dirigée," 25 March 1819; and François-Emmanuel Fodéré, *Voyage aux Alpes-Maritimes, ou Histoire naturelle, agraire, civile et médicale du comté de Nice et pays limitrophes*, 2 vols. (1821), 2: 291–92, on shepherds who know medicinal plants.

182 AD Marne 33 X 8, Claude Hubert at Sommesuippe to prefect, c. 1820; AD Deux-Sèvres 6 M 21/1, no. 52, 29 November 1884.

183 AN AF III 107, Faugerolle petition, Vendémiaire VI/September–October 1797.

184 Febvre, "Une Enquête: La Forge de village," in *Pour une histoire à part entière* (1962), pp. 630–34; see esp. the responses by informants T. Chalmel (Noyal-sous-Bazouges, Ille-et-Vilaine) and Mlle. Auriac (*directrice d'école*, Astien [Ariège]). See also Charles Marcel-Robillard, "Forges at forgerons du pays chartrain," *Arts et traditions populaires* 12 (1964): 68–69.

185 AD Loire 38 M 9, no. 18, mayor of Feurs, 29 December 1812.

186 Bouteiller, *Médecine populaire*, p. 216.

187 Lecocq, *Empiriques*, p. 33, case at Nogent-le-Phaye (Eure-et-Loire).

188 AN F^8 163, surgeon Poulain to Minister of the Interior, n.d.

189 SRM 107, Gastellier, 14 March 1782. The winegrower claimed to have a gift from God; this is probably the same case described by Gastellier in *Observations*, p. 12. Claude-Antoine Barrey, *Dangers des ouvrages de médecine écrits à la portée de tout le monde*, Paris medical thesis, Year XI/1802–03, no. 35, p. 15, describes a former winegrower at Beure, five kilometers south of Pelousey in the Doubs, who practiced as a *visiteur d'urines* for twenty years. During an outbreak of "gastro-bilious fever," his gastric powder killed 17 out of 20 patients, according to Barrey; the physician's dispatch to the prefect at the time of the epidemic mentions 15 victims (AN F^8 48, 5 Pluviôse X/25 January 1802, quoted by Richard Cobb, *The Police and the People: French Popular Protest, 1789–1820* [Oxford, 1970], p. 360).

190 Bernard Jacquet, *Empiriques et charlatans troyens du XVe au XIXe siècle*, Paris medical thesis, 1960, no. 458, p. 62, denunciation of 1 Germinal III/21 March 1795.

191 AD Loire-Atlantique 1 M 1358, no. 326, 30 October 1826; no. 392, *procureur impérial*, Nantes, to prefect, Loire-Inférieure, 3 January 1812.

192 Paul Delaunay, *Études sur l'hygiène, l'assistance et les secours publics dans le Maine sous l'Ancien Régime*, 2d ser., fasc. 3 (Le Mans, 1923), p. 227, quoting report from Beaumont-le-Vicomte, 1784.

193 Jacquet, *Empiriques*, p. 59.

194 On Thomas: Alfred Franklin, *La Vie privée d'autrefois...*, vol. 14, *Variétés chirurgicales* (1894), pp. 157–63. On the executioner: SRM 136, d. 11, no. 13, Baumes, 4 June 1787.

195 Ulysse Trélat, *De la constitution du corps des médecins et de l'enseignement médical: Des réformes qu'elle devrait subir dans l'intérêt de la science et de la morale publique* (1828), pp. 53–54.

196 SRM 199, d. 13, no. 20, Dr. Chevandier, 24 July 1785.

197 AD Haute-Loire 13 M 18, no. 485, 7–8 March 1817, Aurec-sur-Loire, *gendarmerie* captain to prefect.

198 Marx, *Eighteenth Brumaire of Louis-Bonaparte* (New York, 1963), chap. 5, p. 75.
199 Eissen, *Exploitation*, p. 10.
200 AD Loire 38 M 9, no. 19, prefect to *conseiller de préfecture*, 10 November 1819; no. 20, subprefect of Roanne to prefect, 28 February 1820.
201 SRM 199, d. 18, no. 13, 17 April 1779; *Gazette des tribunaux* 2 (1826–27): 1222; AN F⁸ 163, Poulain to Minister of the Interior, n.d.
202 This at least is the legend. The anecdote appears (for example) in Pétrus Sambardier, *La Vie à Lyon . . .* , ed. Martin Basse (Lyons, n.d. [1939]), pp. 208–09.
203 See, for example, Caroline Schultze, *La Femme-médecin au XIXᵉ siècle*, Paris medical thesis, 1888, no. 49; Marcel Baudouin, *Femmes médecins d'autrefois* (1906); Mélanie Lipinska, *Histoire des femmes médecins, depuis l'antiquité jusqu'à nos jours* (1900); Yvonne Knibiehler and Catherine Fouquet, *La Femme et les médecins: Analyse historique* (1983), chap. 6, pt. 3; and J. Poirier and R. Nahon, "L'Accession des femmes à la carrière médicale," in J. and J. L. Poirier, eds., *Médecine et philosophie à la fin du XIXᵉ siècle*, University of Paris XII, Cahiers de l'Institut de Recherche Universitaire d'Histoire de la Connaissance, des Idées et des Mentalités, no. 2 (1980[?]), pp. 23–46.
204 This theme appears, for example, in a polemical work by Barbara Ehrenreich and Deirdre English, *Witches, Midwives and Nurses: A History of Women Healers*, 2d ed. (Old Westbury, N.Y., 1973).
205 Thompson, *Quacks*, does devote a chapter (9) to prominent English women empirics; see also pp. 294–97 on Joanna Stephens, who obtained 5,000 for the publication of one of her remedies.
206 AD Nièvre 5M, "Liste des charlatans . . ."
207 AD Ille-et-Vilaine C 1384, quoted by Dupuy, "Épidémies," *Annales de Bretagne*, 2: 207–08.
208 SRM 107, L'Humeau, 5 February 1786.
209 AD Yonne 5 M 7/1, mayor of Seignelay to prefect, 15 April 1818.
210 Cf. the cases of two somnambulists reported in the *Gazette des Tribunaux* 3 (1827–28): 804–05, 1036, Paris, Cour Royale d'Appel Correctionnelle, Couturier and Burkard. The Couturier woman told a patient who subsequently died that he had three balls of blood in his body.
211 AD Aube C 1164, d. 2, subdelegate to intendant, 3 September 1788.
212 On this question see Lipinska, *Histoire*, chap. 13.
213 Dupuy, "Épidémies," *Annales de Bretagne*, 2: 196, quoting AD Ille-et-Vilaine C 1339, subdelegate at Montauban.
214 Mercier, *Le Monde médical*, p. 202, 29 Fructidor VII/15 September 1799.
215 On woman dentists: Paul Delaunay, "Les Guérisseurs ambulants dans le Maine sous l'Ancien Régime," *Comptes rendus du Deuxième Congrès International d'Histoire de la Médecine* (Évreux, 1922), p. 216; and Franklin, *Variétés*, p. 175. On women hernia operators, see, for example, AN F⁷ 7893, d. 3273, section 4, prefect of the Seine to Minister of General Police, 17 Pluviôse X/6 February 1802, on Letellier, accused of mutilating patients.
216 Odette-Émilie Cunin, "Femmes dentistes, femmes de dentistes," *Histoire des sciences médicales* 14 (1980): 212. See also AD Meurthe-et-Moselle 5 M 18, nos. 150 and 185, on women practicing dentistry illegally on the eve of World War I.
217 One of the most celebrated eighteenth-century English empirics was a woman bonesetter, Sally Mapp of Epsom, called "Crazy Sally"; see Thompson, *Quacks*, pp. 299–303, and Williams, *Age of Agony*, p. 181.
218 Jean-Joseph-Antoine Pilot de Thorey, *Usages, fêtes et coutumes existant ou ayant existé en Dauphiné* (Grenoble, 1884), pp. 255–56.
219 AC Nantes I 5 7, d. 3, case of Ferré woman, report to commissioner of police, 15 Brumaire XIII/6 November 1804; Alluard to prefect of the Loire-Inférieure, 16 Prairial XIII/5 June 1805.
220 Jean-Pierre Goubert, *Malades et médecins en Bretagne, 1770–1790* (1974), pp. 244–45, quoting AD Ille-et-Vilaine C 2546, *recteurs* of Melesse, Betton, and Mouazé to intendant, 8 June 1786; p. 243, citing AD Ille-et-Vilaine C 1371, c. 1780.

221 SRM 199, d. 16, no. 8, 31 May 1793; AD Hautes-Alpes 141 M, "Observation d'un officier de santé sur la pratique des charlatans et des maÿges...," 28 Frimaire IX/ 19 December 1800.

222 Eugène Olivier, *Médecine et santé dans le pays de Vaud au XVIIIe siècle, 1675–1798* (Lausanne, 1939), p. 432. Cf. his pt. 2, chap. 7, on women practitioners.

223 AC Nantes I 5 7, d. 3, royal procureur, 27 October 1829.

224 AD Loire-Atlantique 1 M 1358, commissioner of police, 2d arrondissement, to royal procureur, Nantes, 9 January 1821; no. 338, Lancelotte to prefect, 2 August 1825; no. 337, on madwoman, mayor of Nantes to prefect. Cf. no. 349, on the widow Chapron.

225 On recompense, see, for example, SRM 199, d. 16, no. 7, 23 April 1782, petition of Marie-Barbe Cüenin, who treats dropsy; she says that she is poor and hopes for some sort of reward.

226 AN F⁸ 58, Le Plénier dossier. The text reads, in translation: "Your majesty will allow me to make known the need of the poor of the communes of Bouchemaine and Épiné, for whom I have cared for more than forty years. Having lost my modest fortune in paper money [during the Revolution], I am no longer able to render them the same services in their illnesses. They lack bouillons, white bread, wine, and remedies. They implore your help for their pressing needs. I have had the honor of informing the prefect. He was good enough to entrust our mayor [with this matter].... I have no other property than my occupation as a surgeon for the poor, and nothing settled."

227 ARC 4, report on Dumont-Valdajou, 29 May 1793.

228 One example among many: the empiric Lavore, denounced at Saintes, SRM 107, 27 April 1782; he called himself a count and baron, among other things.

229 SRM 199, d. 24, no. 10, Beaussieu de la Bouchardière, 9 June 1785.

230 No. 43, 22 October, quoted by Lecocq, *Empiriques*, p. 30.

231 *Affiches du Poitou*, 1775, p. 164, cited by Boissonnade, *Organisation du travail (Mémoires*, vol. 21), p. 508.

232 AD Hautes-Alpes 141 M, no. 95, mayor of Ventavon to prefect, 29 June 1829. The name also appears as Novarino, Novarin, Novarine, and Navarrina.

233 Criminal trial, Vannes, 10 March 1858, testimony quoted by Closmadeuc, *Esquisse*, pp. 8–9.

234 AD Yonne 5 M 7/1, marginal note by mayor of Coulanges on letter from surgeon Vildieu to prefect, denouncing abuses in the treatment of tinea, 27 January 1807.

235 AD Ille-et-Vilaine 1 Bⁿ 3245, Mounier, 25 May 1783.

236 AD Var 8 U 62/2, no. 5, minutes, *tribunal correctionnel*, Brignoles, 14 June 1813; cf. a list of patients in no. 2, mayor to procureur, 20 May 1813: (1) a weaver's assistant; (2) a farmer, who paid 18 francs for a few lime blossoms for his wife (she died); (3) the wife of another farmer; (4) a priest; (5) a woman patient, otherwise unidentified.

237 *Gazette des tribunaux*, 5 (1829–30): 66, *police correctionnelle*, Paris.

238 SRM 107, Saint-Léger; *Gazette des tribunaux* 5 (1829–30): 66.

239 J. Borianne, *Essai sur les erreurs en médecine répandues dans le département de la Haute-Vienne et sur leurs dangers*, Paris medical thesis, 1831, pp. 28–29.

240 AC Nantes I 5 7, d. 3, commissioner-general of police to mayor, 15 Nivôse XIII/ 5 January 1805.

241 AD Aube 7 U 298, *procureur impérial, tribunal de première instance*, to *magistrat de sûreté*, Bar-sur-Aube, 27 Fructidor XII/14 September 1804.

242 SRM 199, d. 13, no. 18, Dr. Caudeiron, 13 January 1784.

243 Patin to Charles Spon, 12 December 1642, in Paul Triaire, ed., *Lettres de Gui Patin* (1907), p. 255; duc de Saint-Simon, *Mémoires*, 6 vols. (1953–58), 4: 934; Paul Delaunay, *La Vie médicale aux XVIe, XVIIe, et XVIIIe siècles* (1935), p. 216.

244 Giacomo Casanova, *Mémoires de J. Casanova de Seingalt écrits par lui-même*, 12 vols. (Wiesbaden, 1960–62), 1: 62–65.

245 AN F⁷ 8185, d. 2981R², prefect of the Deux-Sèvres to *conseiller d'état*, 1st arrondissement, Police Générale, 20 October 1810.

246 Borianne, *Essai sur les erreurs*, p. 16.
247 Baudot, *Études historiques*, p. 322, quoting AC Chalon FF 38.
248 "Requête pour la demoiselle Maillebiau, dite Coustou, veuve du sieur Costes, négociant," Béziers, 1785, quoted in Yves Castan, *Honnêteté et relations sociales en Languedoc, 1715–1780* (1974), pp. 589–90.
249 *Gazette des tribunaux* 2 (1826–27): 1264, Cour d'Assises, Haute-Garonne.
250 J.-B. Fraysse, "Au Pays de Baugé," pp. 106–07.
251 Henry Thivot, *La Vie privée dans les Hautes-Alpes vers le milieu du XIXe siècle* (La Tronche-Montfleury, 1966), p. 330. Le Rob d'Ettemor rehearsed the curé's story in his dialect mock epic, *La Ligousada, ou lou proucès de Jean Ligousa*, canto 11, "Lou Preirë de Sigouïer [le curé de Sigoyer]," published (with a French translation) in *Bulletin de la Société d'Études des Hautes-Alpes* 10 (1891): 186–98.

CHAPTER 5 *Folk healers:* maiges *and witches*

1 Samuel-Auguste-André-David Tissot, *Avis au peuple sur sa santé, ou Traité des maladies les plus fréquentes*, 2 vols. (1786) 2: 297. This celebrated handbook was first published at Lausanne in 1761.
2 *Dictionnaire de la langue française* (1882). See also Marcel Marion, *Dictionnaire des institutions de la France aux XVIIe et XVIIIe siècles* (1923), s.v. "*meiges.*"
3 On dialectal usage, see Anders Christopher Thorn, *Les Désignations françaises du médecin et de ses concurrents* (Jena, 1932), p. 16, citing Guillemant, *Dictionnaire du patois de la Bresse Louhannaise* (Louhans, 1884–92).
4 SRM 199, d. 18, no. 13, 17 April 1779.
5 AD Hautes-Alpes 141 M, no. 1, Year IX, "Observation d'un officier de santé sur la pratique des charlatans et des maÿges . . ."
6 Jean-Emmanuel Gilibert, *L'Anarchie médicinale, ou la Médecine considérée comme nuisible à la société*, 3 vols. (Neuchâtel, 1772), 1: 254–57.
7 See Pearl Kibre, "The Faculty of Medicine at Paris, Charlatanism, and Unlicensed Medical Practices in the Later Middle Ages," *Bulletin of the History of Medicine* 27 (1953): 1–20.
8 The repression of popular medicine as witchcraft has not been systematically studied. On the end of secular prosecutions of witchcraft in France: Robert Mandrou, *Magistrats et sorciers en France au XVIIe siècle* (1968). On the campaigns against popular culture in the seventeenth and eighteenth centuries: Robert Muchembled, *Culture populaire et culture des élites dans la France moderne (XVe–XVIIIe siècles)* (1978), pt. 2.
9 Pierre de Lancre, *Tableau de l'inconstance des mauvais anges et démons, où il est amplement traicté des sorciers & de la sorcellerie . . .* (1612), pp. 333, 347, 350. A small section of bk. 5 concerns healing through witchcraft. On the reality of demonic interventions, cf. his *L'Incrédulité et mescréance du sortilège plainement convaincue . . .* (1622).
10 Jean-Baptiste Thiers, *Traité des superstitions selon l'Écriture sainte, les décrets des conciles, et les sentimens des saints Pères et des théologiens* (1679); 2d ed., 4 vols. (1697–1704); 4th ed., 4 vols. (1741).
11 See, for example, Étienne Delcambre, *Le Concept de la sorcellerie dans le duché de Lorraine au XVIe et au XVIIe siècle*, 3 fascicles (Nancy, 1948–51); fasc. 3 concerns *devins-guérisseurs*.
12 *La Police de l'art et science de médecine, contenant la réfutation des erreurs & insignes abus qui s'y commettent pour le jourd'huy, très utile et nécessaire à toutes personnes qui ont leur santé et vie en recommandation, où sont vivement confutez tous sectaires, sorciers . . .* (1580).
13 Michel-Joseph-Marie Richard, *Sur les erreurs populaires relatives à la médecine et leurs dangers*, Paris medical thesis, 1833, no. 36, p. 23; Auguste-Jean-Baptiste Pétel, *Erreurs sur la médecine*, Paris medical thesis, 1830, no. 95, p. 26; Pierre-Delphin Thiaudière, *De l'exercice de la médecine en province et à la campagne, considéré dans ses rapports avec la pratique* (1839), p. 49 (borrowing from Pétel); Jacques-Joseph Juge de Saint-Martin, *Changemens survenus dans les moeurs des habitans de Limoges depuis une cinquantaine d'années*, 2d ed. (Limoges, 1817; 1st pub. 1808), pp. 115–16 (quotation, p. 116).
14 See, for example, A. Treille, *Quelques réflexions sur les principaux abus en médecine*

(Auch, 1823), p. 52.

15 Marcelle Bouteiller, *Médecine populaire d'hier et d'aujourd'hui* (1966), provides a readable introduction to French medical folklore. For a bibliography of the older literature, see Arnold Van Gennep, *Manuel de folklore français contemporain*, 3 vols. [vol. 1, pts. 1–7, vols. 3–4] (1937–81), 4: 596–620. For a sampling of recent work, see the special issue of *Autrement*, no. 15 (September 1978), *Panseurs de secrets et de douleurs: Médecine populaire: Guérisseurs, voyants et rebouteux . . . de nouveaux interlocuteurs?* And for a different approach (emphasizing the psychological function of popular medicine and of traditional customs and beliefs more generally), cf. Judith Devlin, *The Superstitious Mind: French Peasants and the Supernatural in the Nineteenth Century* (New Haven, 1987), chap. 2, "Traditional Medicine," and passim.

16 On the terminology, see (for example) Bouteiller, *Médecine populaire*, p. 11; François Laplantine, *La Médecine populaire des campagnes françaises aujourd'hui* (1978), p. 10; Jacques Léonard, "Les Guérisseurs en France au XIXᵉ siècle," *Revue d'histoire moderne et contemporaine* 27 (1980): 508; idem, *La Vie quotidienne du médecin de province au XIXᵉ siècle* (1977), p. 157; Marc Leproux, *Médecine, magie et sorcellerie: Contribution au folklore charentais: Angoumois, Aunis, Saintonge* (1954), p. 135; Alice Taverne, *Coutumes et superstitions foréziennes*, fasc. 5, *Médecine populaire, sorcellerie, diable et lutins* (Ambierle, 1971), p. 6. The Basque terms are from Pierre L. Thillaud, *Les Maladies et la médecine en pays basque nord à la fin de l'Ancien Régime, 1690–1789* (Geneva, 1983), p. 7.

17 For characterizations of the traditional healer (or healers), see Bouteiller, *Médecine populaire*, chap. 3, "Guérisseurs traditionnels du village et savoir commun," and chap. 4, "Guérisseurs magiciens, conjureurs de type traditionnel"; and Laplantine, *Médecine populaire*, chap. 3, "Le Guérisseur traditionnel: son portrait, ses caractéristiques et ses fonctions."

18 On the special case of Protestant folk medicine in France, see Roger Bastide, "Protestantisme et médecine de folk," *Revista de etnografia* 15 (1971): 321–32; and Philippe Joutard, "Protestantisme populaire et univers magique: Le Cas cévenol," *Le Monde alpin et rhodanien*, vol. 5 (1977), nos. 1–4, special issue, *Religion populaire*, pp. 145–64.

19 On the ordeals, see Laplantine, *Médecine populaire*, pp. 96, 120 (citing Paul Sébillot on the Breton practice). For the contrast of the old handbooks and the art of the healers, see Françoise Loux, *Pratiques et savoirs populaires: Le Corps dans la société traditionnelle* (1979), pp. 149–50.

20 Pierre Ribon, *Guérisseurs et remèdes populaires dans la France ancienne* (Le Coteau, 1983), p. 143. Joutard, "Protestantisme populaire," p. 156. Robert Jalby, *Sorcellerie, médecine populaire et pratiques médico-magiques en Languedoc* (Nyons, 1974), p. 98.

21 The case for this position has been stated most systematically in André Varagnac, *Civilisation traditionnelle et genres de vie* (1948).

22 Redfield, *Peasant Society and Culture* (Chicago, 1956), chaps. 2–3 (quotations, pp. 36, 41).

23 Mendras, "Un Schéma d'analyse de la paysannerie française," in Mendras and Marcel Jollivet, eds., *Les Collectivités rurales françaises*, vol. 2, *Sociétés paysannes ou lutte de classes au village? Problèmes méthodologiques et théoriques de l'étude locale en sociologie* (1974), p. 13.

24 Redfield, *Peasant Society*, p. 42.

25 See Bouteiller, *Médecine populaire*, pt. 2, "Évolution et survivances."

26 On Grégoire, see Augustin Gazier, ed., *Lettres à Grégoire sur les patois de France . . .* (1880), and Michel de Certeau, Dominique Julia, and Jacques Revel, *Une Politique de la langue: La Révolution Française et les patois: L'Enquête de Grégoire* (1975). For the Academy's questionnaire: *Mémoires de l'Académie Celtique, ou Recherches sur les antiquités celtiques, gauloises et françaises* 1 (1807): 74–86. (On the Academy's work, see also Mona Ozouf, "L'Invention de l'ethnographie française: Le Questionnaire de l'Académie Celtique," *Annales E.S.C.* 36 [1981]: 210–30, and Harry Senn, "Folklore Beginnings in France: The Académie Celtique, 1804–1813," *Journal of the Folklore*

Institute 18 [1981]: 23–33.) Grégoire's questionnaire asked simply about "prejudices" (question 38); the Academy asked more specifically about superstitious practices associated with childbirth, means used to favor the growth of newborns, and superstitious healing practices (questions 17, 18, 41, pp. 79, 84–85).

27 These materials are in the diocesan archives. Ecclesiastical records from the Old Regime became state property under legislation of 1790 and can be found in the "G" series of the *archives départementales*. A portion of the archives from after the Concordat of 1801 was confiscated following the law of separation of 1905 and is now primarily in the "V" series. Much of the rest of the surviving documentation remains outside government repositories. See Jacques Gadille, *Guide des archives diocésaines françaises* (Lyons, 1971), pp. 19–23 and passim.

28 *French Rural History: An Essay on Its Basic Characteristics*, tr. Janet Sondheimer (Berkeley and Los Angeles, 1970), "Introduction: Some Observations on Method."

29 Van Gennep, *Manuel de folklore*. For a critique, see François Lebrun, "Le *Traité des superstitions* de Jean-Baptiste Thiers: Contributions à l'ethnographie de la France du XVIIᵉ siècle," *Annales de Bretagne et des pays de l'Ouest* 83 (1976): 443–65, esp. pp. 445–46.

30 Review by Robert Mandrou in *Revue historique* 238 (1967): 214–17.

31 On beliefs and usages: Le Roy Ladurie, *Montaillou, village occitan, de 1294 à 1324* (1975) and *Le Carnaval de Romans: De la Chandeleur au mercredi des Cendres, 1579–1580* (1979); on the folktale: "Mélusine maternelle et défricheuse" (with Jacques LeGoff), *Annales E.S.C.* 26 (1971): 587–622, and *L'Argent, l'amour et la mort en pays d'oc* (1980). For English translations of the three books, see *Montaillou: The Promised Land of Error*, tr. Barbara Bray (New York, 1978); *Carnival in Romans*, tr. Mary Feeney (New York, 1979); and *Love, Death, and Money in the Pays d'Oc*, tr. Alan Sheridan (New York, 1982).

32 Lebrun, "Le *Traité des superstitions*," p. 464.

33 See, for example, Jacques Idoux, *Exploration des traditions thérapeutiques des guérisseurs, et inventaire des pharmacopées empiriques du département de la Moselle*, ecology thesis, Metz, 1975. For a more impressionistic but suggestive account of current practices in Berry, see Jean-Louis Boncoeur, *Le Village aux sortilèges* (1979).

34 Gérard Bouchard, *Le Village immobile: Sennely-en-Sologne au XVIIIᵉ siècle* (1972), p. 120; case from c. 1775.

35 Marcelle Bouteiller, *Chamanisme et guérison magique* (1950), p. 221.

36 François-Jean-Marie Kérambrun, *Les Rebouteurs et les guérisseurs: Croyances populaires*, Bordeaux medical thesis, 1898–99, no. 31 (Bordeaux, 1898), p. 36.

37 Quoted in *1789: Les Français ont la parole: Cahiers de doléances des États Généraux*, ed. Pierre Goubert and Michel Denis (1964), p. 222.

38 Kérambrun, *Rebouteurs*, p. 65; Bouteiller, *Chamanisme*, p. 221. Cf. Taverne, *Médecine populaire*, p. 5, on the hierarchy of healers.

39 Taverne, *Médecine populaire*, p. 6; Paul-Abraham Pesme, *De quelques erreurs en médecine*, Paris medical thesis, 1855, no. 34, p. 89; Madeleine Rivière-Sestier, *Remèdes populaires en Dauphiné*, Marseilles pharmaceutical thesis, 1942, no. 6 (Lyons, 1942), p. 19. Claude Seignolle, *En Sologne: Moeurs et coutumes*, new ed. (1967), p. 145, cites the case of a *guérisseur d'entorses* in Loir-et-Cher who cured with signs of the cross and a prayer (observation from 1966).

40 SRM 199, d. 5, no. 1, 21 October 1779.

41 Louis Morin, "Empiriques et guérisseurs de l'Aube," *Revue des traditions populaires* 7 (1892): 88; Paul Bidault, *Les Superstitions médicales du Morvan*, Paris medical thesis, 1898–99, no. 321 (1899), p. 38.

42 A.-F.-Emile Bessières, *Etude sur les erreurs et les préjugés populaires en médecine* (1860), p. 15. The author suggests that the women may have lived from this *petit métier*.

43 Seignolle, *Le Berry traditionnel* (1969), chap. 9.

44 Charles-Louis-François Andry, *Recherches sur la rage* (1780; 1st pub. 1778), pp. 111–12, observation by François Masars de Cazeles.

45 Lancre, *Tableau de l'inconstance*, p. 344.

46 J.-B. Fraysse, *Le Folklore du Baugeois* (1906), pp. 118–19. On healers for rabies, see also Marcel Texier, *L'Empirisme et le charlatanisme*, Paris medical thesis, 1895–96, no. 205 (1896), p. 47.

47 Jean Éparvier, *Médecins de campagne: Enquête* (1953), p. 48.

48 Early-nineteenth-century attestations in Treille, *Quelques réflexions*, pp. 44–45 (on *raccommodeurs d'estomac*), and J.-M.-C. Naville, *Lettres bourguignonnes, ou Aperçu philosophique et critique sur les causes des difficultés dans l'exercice de l'art de guérir . . .* (1822), letter 9, on *ravaudeuses*. See also Renée Fournier, *La Médecine ancienne dans le Centre-Ouest: Coutumes populaires disparues et survivances*, Société d'Études Folkloriques du Centre-Ouest, *Revue de recherches ethnographiques*, special number (May 1971): 28; Raphaël Kaufmann, *Pratiques et superstitions médicales en Poitou*, Paris medical thesis, 1906, p. 25, on *adoubeurs* who treated *les côtes tombées*; and Jacques Léonard, *Les Médecins de l'Ouest au XIXe siècle* (1978), p. 114, n. 101. Balthasar-Anthelme Richerand, *Des erreurs populaires relatives à la médecine*, 2d ed. (1812), pp. 140–41, suggests that the stomach could be "dislocated."

49 Arnold Van Gennep, *Le Folklore du Dauphiné (Isère): Étude descriptive et comparée de psychologie populaire*, 2 vols. paginated continuously (1932–33), p. 478.

50 J.-Charles Voisin, *De quelques préjugés relatifs à la médecine dans les départemens de la Bretagne* (Vannes, 1831), pp. 63–64.

51 Kaufmann, *Pratiques*, p. 25; Fournier, *Médecine ancienne*, p. 28. Cf. Naville, *Lettres bourguignonnes*, letter 9, on *rebroyeuses* who treat *le mal de mère*.

52 SRM 199, d. 7, no. 1, Barailon, 5 March 1779.

53 Gustave-Thomas de Closmadeuc, *Esquisse sur la médecine et la chirurgie populaires dans le département du Morbihan* (Vannes, 1861), p. 5; Alexandre Layet, *Médecine sociale: Hygiène et maladies des paysans: Étude sur la vie matérielle des campagnards en Europe* (1882), p. 455.

54 Bidault, *Superstitions*, p. 65.

55 Closmadeuc, *Esquisse*, p. 6; Bouteiller, *Médecine populaire*, p. 175; Léonard, "Les Guérisseurs," p. 509.

56 Bassignot, "Histoire de la maladie connue sous le nom de crinons, qui attaque les nouveaux nés à Seyne en Provence," 22 October 1776, in *Mémoires de la Société Royale de Médecine* 1 (1776): 173-76. Bassignot accepted the existence of this disease and the efficacy of popular treatment; his only further recommendation, which his patients rejected, was that the areas that had been rubbed should be washed or shaved. Cf. Laurent Joubert, *Erreurs populaires et propos vulgaires touchant la médecine et le régime de santé* (Bordeaux, 1579, and subsequent editions), table of contents, projected bk. 18, chap. 5, "Des poils qui sortent à l'eschine des enfans, nommez *Seides*, mal incongnu aux anciens."

57 Mouquet, prize-winning essay on charlatanism, 1818, *Annuaire de la Société de Médecine, Chirurgie et Pharmacie du Département de l'Eure, pour l'année 1819*, p. 37. Claude-François-Étienne Dupin, *Statistique du département des Deux-Sèvres* (Year IX), p. 83, cites an example of a variant, the external beast: "Les maladies extérieures, comme abcès, luxations, se guérissent par les toucheurs. Un paysan a une entorse, le toucheur est appelé; il s'arme d'une hache, et en frappe un grand coup contre terre entre les jambes du malade: il a *tué le chat*, et le malade est guéri, car c'étoit un chat invisible qui s'attachoit à la jambe de ce pauvre paysan, et le faisoit souffrir."

58 Mireille Laget, *Naissances: L'Accouchement avant l'âge de la clinique* (1982), pp. 143, 194.

59 For example, the hernia specialists who used a plant called *la turquette* or *herniole*, known in English as rupturewort (genus *Herniaria*); see Naville, *Lettres bourguignonnes*, p. 119.

60 Alexandre Abord, "La Médecine populaire et les pratiques superstitieuses du Morvan," *La France médicale* 57 (1910): 41.

61 Freddy Raphaël, "Rites de naissance et médecine populaire dans le judaïsme rural d'Alsace," *Ethnographie française*, n.s., 1 (1971): 91–92.

62 Henry Thivot, *La Vie privée dans les Hautes-Alpes vers le milieu de XIXe siècle* (La Tronche-Montfleury, 1966), p. 331.

63 Widely attested. See, for example, Seignolle, *En Sologne*, and Closmadeuc, *Esquisse*, p. 16, on a *rebouteur* who heals with his touch alone.
64 Fournier, *Médecine ancienne*, p. 36; P. Saintyves [Émile-Dominique Nourry], *La Guérison des verrues: De la magie médicale à la psychothérapie* (1913).
65 Dupin, *Statistique des Deux-Sèvres*, p. 83; abbé Noguès, "Pratiques empiriques relatives aux personnes et aux animaux," *La Tradition en Poitou et Charente: Art populaire, ethnographie, folk-lore, hagiographie, histoire* [proceedings of the congress of the Société d'Ethnographie Nationale et d'Art Populaire, Niort, 1896] (1897), p. 255.
66 AN F⁷ 3179, Fructidor XI, 3d *jour complémentaire*/20 September 1803.
67 Augustin Cabanès, *Comment on se soigne aujourd'hui: Remèdes de bonne femme* (1907), p. 206; Closmadeuc, *Esquisse*, p. 7. In Berry, the *parsigneux* uses the big toe of the right foot to make the sign of the cross (Bouteiller, *Chamanisme*, p. 251).
68 Kaufmann, *Pratiques*, p. 29.
69 On Roussillon, see Andry, *Recherches sur la rage*, p. 153, "Observations de M. Bonafos." On the more recent *souffleurs*, see Cabanès, *Comment on se soigne*, pp. 204–05; Julien Noir, "De quelques préjugés, superstitions, sanctuaires et pèlerinages à attributions curatives de la région des Ardennes," *Le Progrès médical*, 3d ser., 21 (1905): 195; and A. Jacqmart, "Erreurs, préjugés, coutumes et légendes du Cambrésis," *Mémoires de la Société d'Émulation de Cambrai* 36 (1880): 342–43. On the man with the healing glance: Camille-J.-B. Fraysse, "Au pays de Baugé: La Thérapeutique populaire et les sorciers guérisseurs," *Arts et traditions populaires* 9 (1961): 104.
70 Marc Leproux, *Dévotions et saints guérisseurs* (1957), p. 76.
71 Laplantine, *Médecine populaire*, p. 146.
72 *Gazette des Tribunaux* 27 (1851–52): 935.
73 Fraysse, "Au pays de Baugé," p. 104.
74 Claude Seignolle, *Le Folklore du Languedoc: Gard, Hérault, Lozère: Cérémonies familiales, sorcellerie et médecine populaire, folklore de la nature* (1960), pp. 225 (citing Adrienne Durand-Tullou, *Un Milieu de civilisation traditionnelle: Le Causse de Blandas, Gard*, Montpellier thesis [letters], 1959) and 227.
75 Jalby, *Sorcellerie*, p. 100.
76 J. Borianne, *Essai sur les erreurs en médecine répandues dans le département de la Haute-Vienne et sur leurs dangers*, Paris medical thesis, 1831, p. 25.
77 Maurice Messegué, *Sommes-nous des assassins?* (1965), p. 163.
78 Leproux, *Médecine, magie*, p. 137; Augustin-Camille-Gustave Foll, *Médecine et superstitions populaires en Bretagne*, Bordeaux medical thesis, 1903–04, no. 29 (Bordeaux, 1904), p. 25.
79 Philippe Macquer, *Dictionnaire raisonné universel des arts et métiers . . .*, new ed., revised by abbé Jaubert, 4 vols. (1773), s.v. "*bailleuls*." Charles-Félix Durand, *Les Guérisseurs* (1884), p. 43.
80 Bouteiller, *Médecine populaire*, pp. 66–71.
81 Laplantine, *Médecine populaire*, pp. 85–86.
82 Jacques Léonard, *La Médecine entre les savoirs et les pouvoirs: Histoire intellectuelle et politique de la médecine française au XIXᵉ siècle* (1981), p. 70.
83 Jalby, *Sorcellerie*, p. 98, citing Adelin Moulis on the *endébinaïré*; *Journal général de médecine, de chirurgie et de pharmacie . . .* 42 (1811): 209 (review of Jacques-Barthélemy Salgues, *Des erreurs et des préjugés répandus dans la société*).
84 Leproux, *Médecine, magie*, p. 139.
85 On the importance of the gift (illustrated by examples drawn from American and European folk medicine), see Wayland D. Hand, "The Folk Healer: Calling and Endowment," *Journal of the History of Medicine and Allied Sciences* 26 (1971): 263–75. On the concept (and the dialect term), see Arnold Van Gennep, *Le Folklore de la Flandre et du Hainaut français . . .*, 2 vols. paginated continuously (1935–36), p. 636.
86 Gédéon Tallemant des Réaux, *Les Historiettes de Tallemant des Réaux*, ed. Georges Montgrédien, 8 vols. (n.d. [1932–34]), 5: 627.
87 *Gazette des Tribunaux* 2 (1826–27): 1264, Cour d'Assises, Toulouse.
88 On families who cure certain diseases, see, for example, A. Lecocq, *Empiriques, somnambules et rebouteurs beaucerons* (Chartres, 1862), p. 55.

89 Thiers, *Traité des superstitions*, 4th ed. 4 vols. (1741), 1: 518.
90 Ibid., 1: 505–08, 517; François-Antoine Delettre, *Histoire de la province du Montois* ..., *arrondissement de Provins*, 2 vols. (Nogent-sur-Seine, 1849–50), 1: 258; Jules Lecoeur [Louis-Jules Tirard], *Esquisses du bocage normand*, 2 vols. (Condé-sur-Noireau, 1883–87), 2: 100.
91 Thiers, *Traité des superstitions*, 4th ed., 1: 510, 517–18.
92 Ernest Renan, *Souvenirs d'enfance et de jeunesse*, ed. Jean Pommier (1959), pp. 27–28.
93 Marc Bloch, *Les Rois thaumaturges: Étude sur le caractère surnaturel attribué à la puissance royale, particulièrement en France et en Angleterre* (1924), bk. 1, chap. 2.
94 Charles Sadoul, "Les Guérisseurs et la médecine populaire en Lorraine," *Le Pays lorrain* 26 (1934): 72; Delcambre, *Concept de sorcellerie*, fasc. 3, p. 12.
95 Thiers, *Traité des superstitions*, 4th ed., 1: 509.
96 Cabanès, *Remèdes de bonne femme*, p. 182.
97 Marcelle Bouteiller, *Sorciers et jeteurs de sorts* (1958), p. 197, and *Médecine populaire*, p. 106; Laplantine, *Médecine populaire*, p. 92.
98 Nicole Roure, "La Sorcellerie en Roussillon," *C.E.R.C.A.*, no. 26 (1964): 319–20.
99 Étienne Levrat, "La Médecine populaire gasconne," *Revue des Pyrénées* 23 (1911): 268; Bouteiller, *Médecine populaire*, pp. 71–72.
100 Bloch, *Rois thaumaturges*, bk. 2, chap. 4.
101 Seignolle, *En Sologne*, pp. 146–47.
102 Ernest Sévrin, "Croyances populaires et médecine supranaturelle en Eure-et-Loir au XIXe siècle," *Revue d'histoire de l'Église de France* 32 (1946): 291, citing an article by a Dr. Menault in *Gazette des hôpitaux*; cf. Lecocq, *Empiriques*, pp. 16–17, on a *marcou* near Chartres.
103 Bloch, *Rois thaumaturges*, p. 300. The mark might also take the form of a star or a triangle. Cf. Émile-Auguste Berthomier, *Charlatanisme et médecine illégale*, Paris medical thesis, 1910, no. 401, p. 49. Paul Tiffaud, *L'Exercice illégal de la médecine dans le Bas-Poitou*, Paris medical thesis, 1898–99, no. 274 (1899), p. 32, mentions a cross or other sign that might appear on the thigh, arm, neck, chest, face, or palate.
104 Laurent Joubert, *La Première et Seconde Partie des erreurs populaires, touchant la médecine & le régime de santé*, 2 vols. (1587), 2: 145.
105 Thiers, *Traité des superstitions*, 4th ed., 1: 509.
106 *Mélusine* 1 (1878): 555.
107 Tiffaud, *Exercice illégal*, chap. 3; Kaufmann, *Pratiques*, p. 27.
108 Paul Dubalen, *Contribution à l'étude de l'exercice de la médecine: Pratiques médicales populaires dans les Landes*, Lyons medical thesis, 1906–07, no. 83 (Lyons, 1907), p. 37.
109 P. Delamarre, "Médecine populaire et saints guérisseurs de la folie en Bretagne," *Mémoires de la Société Française d'Histoire de la Médecine* 4 (1951): 25. Bouteiller, *Médecine populaire*, p. 175, mentions another Breton case, a fifth son in nineteenth-century Ille-et-Vilaine who treated *les hunes* (here, rheumatism).
110 J. Sirven, "Les Saludadors, 1830: Esquisse de moeurs," *Mémoires de la Société Agricole, Scientifique, et Littéraire des Pyrénées-Orientales* 14 (1866): 117–19; AD Pyrénées-Orientales, B. Ramonet, *officier de santé* at Elne, to Renouard, *commissaire-général du gouvernement*, 3 June 1811; document quoted *in extenso* in Jean-Gabriel Gigot, "L'Histoire réelle du Roussillon au temps d'hier," pt. 1: "Guérisseurs en Roussillon," *C.E.R.C.A.*, no. 21 (1963): 247. Abbé Thiers mentions a different derivation of the gift of the Spanish *saludadores*, *ensalmadores* (a general term for healers), and *santiguadores* (those who heal by making signs of the cross): they are relatives of Saint Catherine and bear on their bodies the mark of a wheel (*Traité des superstitions*, 4th ed., 1: 504–05).
111 Bouteiller, *Médecine populaire*, p. 71.
112 Thiers, *Traité des superstitions* 4th ed., 1: 511.
113 Paul Bonnefon, "Les dernières années de Charles Perrault," *Revue d'histoire littéraire de la France* 13 (1906): 638–39. The compendium: BM Angers, ms. 448, 18th century.
114 Seignolle, *En Sologne*, p. 144.

115 Bloch, *Rois thaumaturges*, p. 296. See the discussion of possible explanations of the seventh son's powers in Eusèbe Renaudot, *Cinquiesme et dernier tome du Recueil général des questions traittées ès conférences du Bureau d'addresse...* (1655), conference of 21 April 1642, pp. 147–52.

116 See, for example, Charles John Samuel Thompson, *The Quacks of Old London* (London, 1928), pp. 71–72 and 189, on two English cases: a self-proclaimed seventh daughter of a seventh daughter who prophesied (no date given; seventeenth century?) and a seventeenth-century male empiric who issued an announcement beginning: "There is newly arrived in London an UNBORN DOCTOR THE SEVENTH SON OF A SEVENTH SON, who (by God's blessing on his Studies) and more than 27 years' travels, with most Famous and Eminent Physicians, has obtained to be an able Chymical Physician, Oculist, and Chyrurgical Operator."

117 Seignolle, *En Sologne*, p. 149.

118 E. Vuillier, "Chez les magiciens et les sorciers de la Corrèze," *Le Tour du monde*, n.s., 5 (1899): 520; *Mélusine* 1 (1878): 555; Leproux, *Médecine, magie*, p. 159; Fournier, *Médecine ancienne*, p. 42; G. Le Calvez, "Basse-Bretagne et environs de Saint-Méen" (superstitions of), *Revue des traditions populaires* 7 (1892): 91; Marcel Lelièvre, *De l'exercice illégal de la médecine en Bretagne: Les Guérisseurs, dormeuses et rebouteurs du pays breton*, Paris medical thesis, 1906–07, no. 283 (1907), p. 25; Thiers, *Traité des superstitions* 4th ed., 1: 511.

119 Bouteiller, *Médecine populaire*, pp. 72, 106–07.

120 Ibid., p. 71; Foll, *Médecine et superstitions populaires*, p. 49.

121 Nicole Belmont, *Les Signes de la naissance: Étude des représentations symboliques associées aux naissances singulières* (1971), pt. 1.

122 See Sadoul, "Les Guérisseurs," p. 72; Fournier, *Médecine ancienne*, pp. 40–41, on the old cult of the axe; and Ribon, *Guérisseurs*, pp. 142–43, on "cutting" diseases and Saint Joseph. See also: Leproux, *Médecine, magie*, p. 145; Noguès, "Pratiques empiriques," p. 257; and Bouteiller, *Médecine populaire*, p. 73.

123 Kaufmann, *Pratiques et superstitions médicales*, p. 30. Bidault, *Superstitions*, p. 46, mentions a healer at Molphey (Côte-d'Or).

124 Lecocq, *Empiriques*, p. 56; Sadoul, "Guérisseurs," p. 76.

125 Borianne, *Essai sur les erreurs*, p. 11.

126 Bouteiller, *Médecine populaire*, p. 105. We have already seen the case of the baker who heals by passing an oven peel between the patient's legs. Future research might attempt to establish the role, if any, played by *compagnonnages* in the transmission of this lore.

127 Bouteiller, *Médecine populaire*, pp. 73, 255; Léonard Saint-Michel, "Un petit formulaire de médecine occulte découvert en Berry et toujours en usage," *Connaître: Cahiers de l'humanisme médical*, January–February 1948, p. 21.

128 Simon Blocquel (pseudonym), *Phylactères, ou préservatifs contre les maladies, les maléfices et les enchantements, exorcismes ou conjurations...* (n.d. [1848]), p. 18.

129 Borianne, *Essai sur les erreurs*, p. 11.

130 Éparvier, *Médecins de campagne*, pp. 22–23.

131 Bouteiller, *Médecine populaire*, pp. 106, 255; Lecocq, *Empiriques*, chaps. 5–6. Cf. C. Leroy, "Forgerons guérisseurs," *Revue du folklore français et du folklore colonial* 7 (1936): 1–14.

132 Bouteiller, "Sorciers," p. 197; Vuillier, "Chez les magiciens," pp. 514–18; Yvonne Clancier, *De quelques manifestations de la mentalité primitive en Limousin*, Paris medical thesis, 1940, p. 68; Leroy, "Forgerons," pp. 3–5.

133 See, for example, Van Gennep, *Folklore de la Flandre*, p. 617.

134 Thiers, *Traité des superstitions*, 4th ed., 1: 511; Noguès, "Pratiques empiriques," p. 256.

135 Bouteiller, *Médecine populaire*, p. 255.

136 On the *convers*: Thorn, *Désignations*, p. 71.

137 Bouteiller, *Médecine populaire*, p. 74. Cf. Fraysse, "Au pays de Baugé," p. 100, on a secret learned from a vagabond (early twentieth century).

138 Jean-Luc d'Iharce, *Erreurs populaires sur la médecine...* (1783), p. 424.

139 Michel Coissac, "Guérisseurs et sorciers limousins," *Aesculape* 4 (1914): 107.
140 Bouteiller, *Médecine populaire*, p. 159; cf. the cases on pp. 159–60.
141 Seignolle, *Folklore du Languedoc*, pp. 230–31.
142 Raphaël de Westphalen, *Petit dictionnaire des traditions populaires messines* (Metz, 1934), s.v. *"rebouteux."*
143 Bouteiller, "Chamanisme," p. 231, citing ms. in AD Deux-Sèvres.
144 Jehan de La Chesnaye, "Remèdes du bocage qui s'en va," *Revue du Bas-Poitou* 21 (1908): 416.
145 Bouteiller, *Médecine populaire*, p. 72.
146 Seignolle, *En Sologne*, p. 141; Jean Drouillet, *Folklore du Nivernais et du Morvan*, 5 vols. (La Charité-sur-Loire, 1959–68), 4: 194, account of Dr. A. Millien, near Uxeloup.
147 Bouteiller, *Chamanisme*, p. 232 (from Deux-Sèvres ms.).
148 See Paul Sébillot, *Le Folklore de France*, 4 vols. (1904–07), 3: 48–50, and André Adnès, "La Taupe, animal guérisseur," *La Vie mancelle*, no. 56 (May 1965): 30–32. Also, Kaufmann, *Pratiques et superstitions médicales*, p. 30; Cabanès, *Remèdes de bonne femme*, p. 202; Fournier, *Médecine ancienne*, p. 43; Bouteiller, *Médecine populaire*, p. 73; Paul Delaunay, *La Médecine populaire: Ses origines religieuses, dogmatiques et empiriques* (Tours, 1930), p. 23; and Françoise Loux, *L'Ogre et la dent* (1981), p. 44, on the healing powers of the *taupier* (mole catcher). The powers of the mole strangler are mentioned in such early modern medical texts as Michael Ettmüller, *Operum omnium medico-phisicorum*, 2 vols. (Lyons, 1690) 2: 280–81, and Louis-Daniel Arnault de Nobleville and François Salerne, *Suite de la "Matière médicale" de M. Geoffroy*, 6 vols. (1756–57), 6: 341–42.
149 Bouteiller, *Chamanisme*, p. 272.
150 Taverne, "Médecine populaire," pp. 8, 10.
151 A. Baudot, *Études historiques sur la pharmacie en Bourgogne avant 1803* (1905), p. 528, quoting a report of 20 Ventôse XI/11 March 1803.
152 Bouteiller, *Médecine populaire*, p. 62.
153 See, for example, Laplantine, *Médecine populaire*, p. 93.
154 For example: Dr. Pigeon, *Organisation de la médecine, ou Moyen de rendre la médecine plus honorable, plus efficace, plus économique* (Clamency [Nièvre], mid-nineteenth century), p. 14: "Quelle est la commune qui n'ait pas son soigneur, son rebouteux, son sorcier, ses commères renommées, celle-ci pour son eau contre les maux d'yeux, celle-là pour son onguent contre les coups, les chutes, les douleurs, les ulcères?" Quoted in Guy Thuillier, "Pour une histoire du médicament en Nivernais au XIXe siècle," *Revue d'histoire économique et sociale* 53 (1975): 80–81. The treatise: P.-Philippe Colon, *Essai sur la médecine populaire et ses dangers*, Paris medical thesis, 1824, no. 85, p. 33.
155 See, for example, Seignolle, *Folklore du Languedoc*, pp. 225–39, and *En Sologne*, pp. 142–44; Claude and Jacques Seignolle, *Le Folklore du Hurepoix*... (1937), pp. 245–52; Van Gennep, *Folklore du Dauphiné*, pp. 476–78.
156 Bidault, *Superstitions*, p. 22, quoting a Dr. Breuillard. Such practitioners become difficult to distinguish from major empirics; see references cited in chap. 4, note 168. These were, however, exceptional cases; some nineteenth-century observers commented on the lack of healers with truly extensive reputations. See, for example, Alain Corbin, *Archaïsme et modernité en Limousin au XIXe siècle, 1845–1880*, vol. 1, *La Rigidité des structures économiques, sociales, et mentales* (1975), p. 116, quoting observations of Dr. Bardinet in *Société Locale des Médecins du Département de la Haute-Vienne* (Limoges, 1864), p. 11.
157 See, for example, Edgar-Jean-Ernest Porcheron, *Les Braconniers de la médecine au pays de Poitou*, Bordeaux medical thesis, 1923, p. 88: "Parmi cette multitude de 'médicastres' dont pullule le monde, au premier rang se trouvent les femmes."
158 Bouteiller, *Médecine populaire*, p. 153; Adelin Moulis, "Médecine populaire en Ariège: Devins et guérisseurs," *Arts et traditions populaires* 9 (1961): 115.
159 Laplantine, *Médecine populaire*, p. 83.
160 See, for example, Loux, *Pratiques*, pp. 140–41.

161 Laplantine, *Médecine populaire*, p. 82.
162 Taverne, *Médecine populaire*, p. 7.
163 Bouteiller, "Du 'Chaman' au panseur de secret," International Congress of Americanists, *Proceedings* 27 (1948): 240. Idem, *Médecine populaire*, pp. 62, 217–18. On the healer's social function, cf. Laplantine, *Médecine populaire*, pp. 81–82.
164 See, for example, Leproux, *Médecine, magie*, p. 138.
165 Bouteiller, *Médecine populaire*, p. 155.
166 Paul Cantaloube, *L'Exercice illégal de la médecine et les médicastres des Cévennes*, Montpellier medical thesis, 1904, no. 91, p. 22, case of Vignes.
167 Émile Debacker, "La Lecture en bas: Formulaire d'un guérisseur mystico-empirique de la campagne flamande au XIXᵉ siècle," *Mémoires de la Société d'Encouragement de Dunkerque* 46 (1907): 236–37, quoted in Van Gennep, *Folklore de la Flandre*, p. 624.
168 Bouteiller, *Médecine populaire*, pp. 153–56.
169 Laplantine, *Médecine populaire*, p. 53.
170 Maître Dominique Lacroix; formula quoted in Étienne Levrat, "La Médecine populaire gasconne," *Revue des Pyrénées* 23 (1911): 271.
171 Pierre Fréor, "Médecine d'autrefois," *Revue du Bas-Poitou* 78 (1967): 152.
172 Paul Delaunay, "La Médecine populaire dans le Maine à la fin de l'Ancien Régime: La Médecine illégale; les charlatans," *Premier Congrès International pour l'Histoire de l'Art de Guérir* (Antwerp, 1921), p. 84.
173 SRM 199, d. 20, no. 4, Dr. Ô-Reilly, 1 March 1781.
174 AD Ille-et-Vilaine C 206, Malesherbes, *secrétaire d'état*, to Intendant of Brittany, 19 November 1775. See Étienne Dupont, "Les Lettres de cachet et l'exercice illégal de la médecine en Bretagne au XVIIIᵉ siècle," *Chronique médicale* 30 (1923): 261.
175 Jacques Nouvel, "L'Exercice illégal de la médecine dans la Marne de 1803 à 1868," *Mémoires de la Société d'Agriculture, Commerce, Sciences et Arts du Département de la Marne* 84 (1969): 155–56, quoting AD Marne 8 U 1711.
176 AN F[17] 2276, d. 2, no. 269, Ploërmel; no. 320, Dourdan; no. 354, Ustaritz; no. 278, Cognac; no. 334, Saint-Sever; no. 333, Hyères.
177 SRM 199, d. 18, no. 3, 12 June 1787.
178 AD Pyrénées-Orientales, Ramonet to *commissaire du gouvernement*, 3 June 1811; quoted in Gigot, "Guérisseurs en Roussillon," pp. 250–51.
179 FM Paris ms. 2196/VI, archives of the Société Médicale d'Émulation de Paris: Lecourt, note on illegal medical practice, 1827. Also, AM box 234, copy of Lecourt's essay, dated 1 May 1827; covering letter dated 7 August. The essay was presented to the section on medicine 13–14 August.
180 AM 234, commission's report, adopted 5 July 1828.
181 AD Loire-Atlantique 1 M 1358, no. 321A, Conseil de Salubrité de Nantes to prefect, Loire-Inférieure, 9 April 1827.
182 Cf. the ritual bloodletting used in the eighteenth century by a healer in Languedoc, who treated victims of the bite of a rabid animal by making a slight incision in their ear and expressing two or three drops of blood (for source see note 44).
183 Cabanès, *Remèdes de bonne femme*, p. 207.
184 SRM 124, "Préjugés opposés aux sages précautions du gouvernement, aux efforts des ministres de santé et à la voix de la Nature," Saint-Malo, 22 March 1780.
185 AN AF III 107, Faugerolle petition, Rauzan, Vendémiaire VI/September–October 1797.
186 AC Nantes I 5 7, d. 3, mayor to prefect, Loire-Inférieure, 11 April 1833.
187 That witches procured abortions was a commonplace of all the old literature on witchcraft; see, for example, André Du Breil, *La Police de l'art et science de médecine* ..., in Laurent Bouchel, *La Bibliothèque ou thrésor du droict françois* ..., 2 vols. (1615), 2: 152. But the practice is difficult to document with any certainty for the period considered here.
188 See, for example, Closmadeuc, *Esquisse*, p. 6, on the witch of La Trinité-Surzur (Morbihan), who sold the same remedy to all (jalap); she inspected urine and probably performed abortions.
189 Éparvier, *Médecins*, p. 60.

190 Van Gennep, *Folklore du Dauphiné,* p. 467.
191 For a summary, see Jeanne Favret, "Le Malheur biologique et sa répétition," *Annales E.S.C.* 26 (1971): 873–88.
192 *Gazette des tribunaux* 5 (1829–30): 66.
193 Favret-Saada, *Les Mots, la mort, les sorts: La Sorcellerie dans le bocage* (1977), published in English as *Deadly Words: Witchcraft in the Bocage,* tr. Catherine Cullen (Cambridge, 1980). A projected second volume was to deal with unwitching sessions; in the end, Favret-Saada published the journal she had kept while she was working in the bocage: Favret-Saada and Josée Contreras, *Corps pour corps: Enquête sur la sorcellerie dans le Bocage* (1981). Her disturbing conclusion is that the force of words is such that the fully involved investigator, whatever scientific insights she may have gained, is reduced to silence; working as a participant–observer evidently has its costs.
194 As, for example, in two studies of colonial America: Paul Boyer and Stephen Nissembaum, *Salem Possessed: The Social Origins of Witchcraft* (Cambridge, Mass., 1974); and John Demos's recent and controversial psychohistorical interpretation, *Entertaining Satan: Witchcraft and the Culture of Early New England* (New York and Oxford, 1982), pts. 2–3.
195 *Religion and the Decline of Magic* (New York, 1971), p. 449. Thomas devotes separate sections to magical healers/cunning men and witches.
196 *La Sorcière au village, XVᵉ–XVIIIᵉ siècle* (1979), p. 49. See also his *Culture populaire et culture des élites dans la France moderne (XVᵉ–XVIIIᵉ siècles): Essai* (1978), pp. 107–16 and chap. 5.
197 *Deadly Words,* p. 20.
198 *Folklore du Dauphiné,* p. 474.
199 *Deadly Words,* pp. 72–73.
200 *Médecine populaire,* p. 115. On *le nouage de l'aiguillette,* see the magic book known as the *Petit Albert,* which calls for the sorcerer to tie a thread around a wolf's penis (*Les Admirables Secrets de magie naturelle du Grand-Albert et du Petit-Albert* [n. d., Éditions Albin Michel], pp. 54–55), and Emmanuel Le Roy Ladurie, *The Mind and Method of the Historian* (Chicago, 1981), chap. 3, "The Aiguillette: Castration by Magic."
201 Favret-Saada develops this theme in *Deadly Words,* p. 24.
202 See, for example, Edward Bever, "Old Age and Witchcraft in Early Modern Europe," in Peter Stearns, ed., *Old Age in Preindustrial Society* (New York, 1982), pp. 150–90, esp. pp. 167–69.
203 Edward Evan Evans-Pritchard, *Witchcraft, Oracles, and Magic among the Azande* (Oxford, 1937).
204 Laplantine, *Médecine populaire,* pp. 112–13.
205 Favret-Saada's observations suggest that in practice rituals and magic books are not much used; see *Deadly Words,* pp. 134–35.
206 Seignolle, *Folklore du Languedoc,* chap. 6; Delaunay, *Médecine populaire,* p. 22. Cf. Léon Palès, "*Esconjurar:* Thérapeutique magique dans l'Ariège," *Revue anthropologique* 37 (1927): 372, on the distinction between *la bruch* (sorcerer) and *l'esconjuraïré* (gifted healer). For a general discussion of witchcraft: Jean Palou, *La Sorcellerie,* 2d ed. (1960).
207 On cunning men, see John Cotta, *A Short Discoverie of the Unobserved Dangers of . . . Ignorant . . . Practisers of Physicke . . .* (London, 1612), pp. 71–72. The historical literature on witchcraft has generally focused on belief in demonic possession and patterns of accusation of black witchcraft, together with the evolution of jurisprudence and repression; see, for example, Mandrou, *Magistrats et sorciers,* and H. C. Erik Midelfort, *Witch Hunting in Southwestern Germany, 1562–1689* (Stanford, Calif., 1972). Wizards and white witches are discussed, though, in Delcambre, *Concept de sorcellerie,* fasc. 3 (p. 209 on spells and counterspells); Thomas, *Religion,* chaps. 7 and 8; Alan Macfarlane, *Witchcraft in Tudor and Stuart England: A Regional and Comparative Study* (London, 1970), chap. 8; and E. William Monter, *Witchcraft in France and Switzerland: The Borderlands during the Reformation* (Ithaca, N.Y., 1976), chap. 7. Michelet's imaginative reconstruction of medieval witchcraft in *La Sorcière* (2d ed., 1862, re-edited

1964) called attention to the witch's role as healer (chap. 9) but subordinated this discussion to his larger vision of witchcraft and demon worship as a form of popular revolt.

208 Bouteiller, *Médecine populaire,* p. 11.

209 On the overlapping roles, see Favret-Saada's discussion of the man from Quelaines who presents himself as a *toucheur,* helps ease the pain of a victim of skin cancer, and then emerges as an unwitcher (*Deadly Words,* chap. 5). Bouteiller, however, distinguishes between the *devin* and the *leveur de sort,* though she observes that they are sometimes one and the same (*Médecine populaire*); and Joutard, in his study of magical beliefs among the Protestants of the Cévennes ("Protestantisme populaire," p. 157), found no *guérisseurs* who were *endevinaïres* (*devins*).

210 One discussion among many in the folklore literature on the multiple functions of the *devin*: Adelin Moulis, "Médecine populaire," p. 115, on the Ariège, where *devins* are predominantly women (*las brèichos,* in dialect; the masculine form is *le brèich*).

211 Eugène Olivier, *Médecine et santé dans le pays de Vaud au XVIII* siècle, 1675–1798* (Lausanne, 1939), p. 431, quoting the memoir of a local pastor, ms. Bibliothèque Cantonale C 460 2: 80 ff.

212 Marcelle Bouteiller, "Un Sorcier angevin prévenu d'escroquerie: Documents inédits, 1803–04," *Ethnographie,* n.s., no. 55 (1961): 35–45.

213 AD Aube M 1626, police commissioner, Troyes, to prefect of the Aube, 21 February 1813.

214 Bouteiller, *Médecine populaire,* p. 37.

215 See, for example, Muchembled, *Culture populaire,* p. 108; Favret-Saada, *Deadly Words,* p. 112; and Bouteiller, *Médecine populaire,* pp. 81–82.

216 *Deadly Words,* pp. 7–8.

217 AD Bas-Rhin 5 M 22, no. 38.

218 See, for example, Delcambre, *Concept de sorcellerie,* fasc. 3, p. 11, quoting AD Meurthe-et-Moselle B 3753, fols. 1v–3r, case of Claudette Clochepied; and Favret-Saada, *Deadly Words,* p. 21, on the gift of divination.

219 SRM 199, d. 9, no. 1, Duboueix, 14 January 1784.

220 *Deadly Words,* pp. 13, 19, 68, 194–95, and passim.

221 Thomas, *Religion and the Decline of Magic,* chap. 17; Macfarlane, *Witchcraft,* pp. 173–74 and passim; Muchembled, *Culture populaire,* pp. 309–17; Boyer and Nissembaum, *Salem Possessed.*

222 *Deadly Words,* pp. 165, 113.

223 Leproux, *Médecine, magie,* p. 214.

224 Ibid., pp. 208–09; Favret, "Malheur biologique," p. 885. On outsiders ("the *ils*"), see Laurence Wylie, *Village in the Vaucluse: An Account of Life in a French Village,* 2d ed. (Cambridge, Mass., 1964), chap. 10.

225 G. Le Calvez, "Les Oeuvres de Dieu et celles du Diable," *Revue des traditions populaires* 1 (1886): 200–03; Bouteiller, *Médecine populaire,* p. 254; idem, "Cosmologie et médecine magique selon notre folklore rural: Esquisse d'une analyse structurale," *Ethnographie,* n.s., 53 (1958–59): 91–95. The same theme appears repeatedly in Sébillot, *Folklore,* vol. 3.

226 Leproux, *Médecine, magie,* p. 221.

227 Douglas, *Purity and Danger: An Analysis of Concepts of Pollution and Taboo* (London, 1966), p. 102.

228 *Culture populaire,* p. 107.

229 Bouteiller, *Médecine populaire,* pp. 77, 160.

230 On the importance of the belief system, see Lévi-Strauss's preface to Bouteiller, *Sorciers.* On voodoo death: Cannon, " 'Voodoo' Death," *American Anthropologist,* n.s., 44 (1942): 169–81.

231 Claude Lévi-Strauss, "The Sorcerer and his Magic" and "The Effectiveness of Symbols," in *Structural Anthropology,* vol. 1, tr. Claire Jacobson and Brooke Grundfest Schoepf (New York, 1963), pp. 167–205.

232 *Deadly Words,* p. 264.

233 Bouteiller, *Sorciers*, passim.
234 Seignolle, *Folklore du Languedoc*, pp. 231–32; Joutard, "Protestantisme populaire," passim.
235 Closmadeuc, *Esquisse*, p. 6.
236 Bouteiller, *Chamanisme*, p. 238.
237 Leproux, *Médecine, magie*, p. 190.
238 Joutard, "Protestantisme populaire," p. 155.
239 On this case, see Van Gennep, *Folklore de la Flandre*, p. 616. Cf. the comment by Mouquet in his prize-winning essay for the 1818 competition of the Medical Society of the Eure: shepherds require high fees for curing people of "[le] mal qu'on leur a jeté" (*Annuaire de la Société...*, 1819, p. 37).
240 *Description topographique et statistique de la France: Département de la Vendée* (n.p., n.d.), p. 34. Cf. Dupin, *Statistique des Deux-Sèvres*, pp. 82–83: "Les paysans croient aux sorciers: une maladie est *un sort qu'on leur a jeté* [original italics], et ils s'adressent au devin." Juge de Saint-Martin, *Changemens*, p. 116, cites one of several types of magicians, who "ne se fait fort que de détruire l'ouvrage d'un autre magicien, au moyen de certaines herbes qu'il cache dans la cheminée. Ces sorciers de village peuvent guérir les maux qui surviennent aux enfants, mais ils vous disent naïvement qu'ils ne peuvent empêcher que le mal ne passe directement à un autre enfant." These are of course the *désensorceleurs*.
241 Iharce, *Erreurs populaires*, pp. 421–22.
242 AD Vienne, *greffe présidial*, 1776, cited by Pierre Rambaud, *La Pharmacie en Poitou jusqu'à l'an XI* (Poitiers, 1907), p. 42.
243 *Annuaire de l'Yonne* 44 (1880): 47–48, "Événement tragique...," based on report of Colombier, surgeon, and other accounts.
244 AD Cher 37 U 144, no. 2, appeal, Cour Royal d'Appel, Bourges; no. 5, hearing, Tribunal Civil de Première Instance, Sancerre; no. 9, *procès-verbal*, Sancerre; no. 12, mayor of Crézancy. See also Bouteiller, *Sorciers*, pp. 57–59, for an account of this case.
245 AN F¹⁵ 227, Beaugency (Loiret), response to Comité de Salubrité questionnaire.
246 AD Yonne 5 M 7/1, no. 1, mayor of Vaudeurs to prefect, 19 Ventôse IX/10 March 1801.
247 AD Cher 37 U 144, no. 32. Bouteiller, *Sorciers*, pp. 48–52, gives a longer summary of this case.
248 AD Var 8 U 62/2, no. 45, Tribunal de Première Instance, 1st arrondissement, Brignoles, 5 November 1823.
249 Bouteiller, *Sorciers*, p. 60, citing *L'Iris: Journal de l'Indre*, 1: 29–33, on session of *police correctionnelle*, Châteauroux, 20 February 1827.
250 *Gazette des tribunaux* 4 (1828–29): 522–23, Tribunal Correctionnel, Bressuire.
251 Ibid., p. 551, Tribunal Correctionnel, Épinal (Vosges).
252 As Claude-Lévi Strauss has argued in a study of shamanistic healing ("The Sorcerer and His Magic"), a degree of skepticism may coexist with acceptance of the community's belief in magic; conversely, the mercenary fraud may come to believe in his own or another's powers.
253 *Médecine populaire*, p. 13.

CHAPTER 6 *The structure of medical practice: an overview*

1 Jean-Emmanuel Gilibert, *L'Anarchie médicinale, ou la médecine considérée comme nuisible à la société*, 3 vols. (Neuchâtel, 1772), 1: 244–45; AD Maine-et-Loire 4 D 12, hearing before lieutenant-general of police, Angers, 1779; Édouard Lemaître, *Exposé des abus qui existent dans l'exercice de la médecine et moyens d'y remédier* (1825), pp. 15–17.
2 AD Maine-et-Loire C 190, Bureau du District de Baugé, observations to Commission Intermédiaire, 20 September 1788; AN F⁷ 8185, d. 2981R², health council report, 1 November 1810, forwarded by the prefect of the Mayenne to 1st arrondissement, Police Générale, 24 November. Cf. Lindsay Blake Wilson, "*Les Maladies des Femmes*: Women, Charlatanry, and Professional Medicine in Eighteenth-Century

France," Ph.D. dissertation, Stanford University, 1982, p. 275, n. 51, citing SRM 194, Destieux, physician of Ponsan-Soubiran, 1 May 1780, on empirics who, unlike physicians, dine with their peasant patients.

3 AD Loire 38 M 9, no. 18, mayor of Feurs to subprefect, 29 December 1812.

4 AD Aube 7 U 298, Tribunal Correctionnel, Bar-sur-Aube, 27 Fructidor XII/14 September 1804; procureur to *magistrat de sûreté*, Bar-sur-Aube.

5 AD Ille-et-Vilaine C 1371, quoted by Jean-Pierre Goubert, *Malades et médecins en Bretagne, 1770–1790* (Rennes, 1974), p. 243.

6 SRM 199, d. 28, no. 2, 7 September 1787.

7 Gilibert, *Anarchie*, 1: 245.

8 SRM 124, Jean-Guillaume Chifoliau, "Préjugés opposés aux sages précautions du gouvernement, aux efforts des ministres de santé et à la voix de la Nature," Saint-Malo, 22 March 1780.

9 A. Jacqmart, "Erreurs, préjugés, coutumes et légendes du Cambrésis," *Mémoires de la Société d'Émulation de Cambrai* 37 (1880): 342–43.

10 Claude Seignolle, *Le Berry traditionnel* (1969), p. 230, describes a case from 1949. A forty-year-old peasant who had burned his hand and developed a blister went to see a farmer of Léré, a *persigneux*, who pierced the blister; he then went to a physician for the insurance papers (to cover the cost of remedies?).

11 Paul Delaunay, *Études sur l'hygiène, l'assistance et les secours publiques dans le Maine sous l'Ancien Régime*, 2d ser., fasc. 3 (Le Mans, 1923), p. 226.

12 AD Indre-et-Loire C 403, Delelée at Beaumont-le-Vicomte, to intendant at Tours, 25 October 1784, quoted by Paul Delaunay, "La Médecine populaire dans le Maine à la fin de l'Ancien Régime: La Médecine illégale; les charlatans," *Premier Congrès pour l'Histoire de l'Art de Guérir* (Antwerp, 1921), p. 90; cf. idem, *Études sur l'hygiène*, 2d ser., fasc. 3, p. 227.

13 Louis Lépecq de la Cloture, *Collection d'observations sur les maladies et constitutions épidémiques...*, 2 vols. paginated continuously (Rouen, 1778), p. 540. On this tradition, see Étienne Delcambre, *Le Concept de la sorcellerie dans le duché de Lorraine au XVIe et au XVIIe siècle*, 3 fascicles (Nancy, 1948–51), fasc. 3, pp. 52, 176. Performing a religious healing ritual might also exclude taking ordinary remedies; see, for example, Auguste Guiton, *Empirisme et superstition dans le bocage normand*, Paris medical thesis, 1904–05, no. 33 (1904), p. 21.

14 AD Ille-et-Vilaine C 1365, cited by Goubert, *Malades et médecins*, p. 243.

15 AD Ille-et-Vilaine C 1350, *recteur* of Bréal to intendant, 8 June 1785. Cf. SRM 199, d. 18, no. 13, report from Caylus, 17 April 1779, on *maiges* who warned of the fatal consequences of bleeding.

16 See, for example, AN F^7 8185, d. 2981R^2, prefect of the Loiret to 1st arrondissement, Police Générale, 17 October 1810. On resistance to vaccination, see Yves-Marie Bercé, *Le Chaudron et la lancette: Croyances populaires et médecine préventive, 1798–1830* (1984), chaps. 5–6 (he notes that the extent of clerical opposition to Jenner's technique has been exaggerated), and Pierre Darmon, *La Longue Traque de la variole: Les Pionniers de la médecine préventive* (1986), chap. 11.

17 AD Orne C 310, report by Bouffey, quoted in Michel Bouvet and Pierre-Marie Bourdin, *A travers la Normandie des XVIIe et XVIIIe siècles, Cahiers des Annales de Normandie*, no. 6 (Caen, 1968), p. 304.

18 AN F^17 2276, d. 2, no. 316.

19 See, for example, AD Marne 33 X 28, report by physician at Châlons, on a *chevalier de saint Hubert* who removed the dressing he had applied to a patient who had been bitten by a rabid dog; quoted by Jacques Nouvel, "L'Exercice illégal de la médecine dans la Marne de 1803 à 1868," *Mémoires de la Société d'Agriculture, Commerce, Sciences et Arts du Département de la Marne* 84 (1969): 150–51. On Forlenze: AN F^7 9272, d. 4534, prefect, Charente, to Minister of Police.

20 Delelée to intendant at Tours (cited in note 12).

21 *Gazette des tribunaux* 4 (1828–29): 551.

22 AN F^7 9292, no. 11543, Boullet, *officier de santé* in Paris, to Minister of General Police, 12 March 1825.

23 *Gazette des tribunaux* 3 (1827–28): 632.

24 Ibid., 5 (1829–30): 786–87.

25 Mouquet, prize essay on repression of abuses in medicine, *Annuaire de la Société de Médecine, Chirurgie et Pharmacie du Département de l'Eure*, 1819, p. 38.

26 ARC 4, report of commission on Valdajou, 29 May 1793.

27 See, for example, Jacques Léonard, *Les Médecins de l'Ouest au XIXe siècle* (1978), p. 119. For an eighteenth-century case, see Wilson, "*Maladies des Femmes,*" p. 261, on a physician of Castres in Languedoc who allowed a gravely ill patient to bring in a witch (as he put it); the medical man reported that the healer's ministrations seemed to have cured a serious fever simply through the influence of suggestion on a credulous mind (SRM 129, Pujol, 24 October 1784).

28 See, for example, Henri Gaidoz, *La Rage et saint Hubert* (1887), pp. 92–93, quoting H. Champion, *chirurgien en chef du dépôt de mendicité de la Meuse*, "Relation historique et médicale des accidents causés par un loup enragé dans la ville de Bar-sur-Ornain," read to Institut de France, 6 September 1813. In the winter of 1812–13, the subprefect of Breda in the annexed department of the Deux-Nèthes, in the Low Countries, authorized a patient to make the pilgrimage to Saint Hubert after taking a poll of 9 local practitioners; 5 thought he was gravely ill and would die en route, while 4 believed that he needed only tranquilizing (AN F⁸ 162, subprefect to prefect, 9 February 1813).

29 See, for example, SRM 137, d. 8, no. 9, Maury, 1 July 1782, on an educated apothecary at Sézanne, in Champagne, who claimed to "know urines." According to the *recteur* of Bréal, in Brittany, when he reproached "honest surgeons" for this practice, they replied, "Que voulez-vous que je fasse? Un tel, mon voisin, consulte les urines. Si j'avoue sur cet article mon ignorance, je ne donnerai pas une médecine dans une année." (AD Ille-et-Vilaine C 1352, *recteur* to Intendant of Brittany, 27 July 1786, quoted in François Lebrun, "Chirurgiens et guérisseurs en Haute-Bretagne à la fin de l'Ancien Régime," *Annales de Bretagne et des pays de l'Ouest* 91 [1984]: 424.) Cf. Pierre Fréor, "Médecine d'autrefois," *Revue du Bas-Poitou* 78 (1967): 152, quoting a report by Dr. Aubinais on commune of Vue (Loire-Inférieure), 1842.

30 For the first view, see A. Treille, *Quelques réflexions sur les principaux abus en médecine* (Auch, 1823), pp. 59–60, on a psychosomatic cure of a patient afflicted with "intermittent fevers." The attacks always occurred after midnight. The physician said that he had consulted the magic book known as the *Grand Albert* and that his treatment would involve the demon. At midnight, he told the patient, he would perceive in the shadows his mother and father and all his ancestors; a terrible noise would announce their presence. If the remedy was to work, he must sit on his bed and wait courageously for this moment to arrive. The physician then gave him a potion (sugar water) to swallow half an hour before the beginning of the attack. For the opposing view, see J.-Charles Voisin, *De quelques préjugés relatifs à la médecine dans les départemens de la Bretagne* (Vannes, 1831), pp. 19–20, who notes the attachment of many peasants and workers to the old humoralism; a visit to the doctor is not complete without a purge, and they insist on being bled at certain times of the year.

31 François-Emmanuel Fodéré, *Traité de médecine légale et d'hygiène publique, ou de police de santé, adapté aux codes de l'Empire Français, et aux connaissances actuelles . . .*, 6 vols. (1813), 6: 409–11.

32 See, for example, Léonard, *Médecins de l'Ouest*, p. 585.

33 Prosper-Marie Boissonnade, *Essai sur l'organisation du travail en Poitou, depus le XIe siècle jusqu'a la Révolution*, pub. as vols. 21–22 of *Mémoires de la Société des Antiquaires de l'Ouest*, 2d ser. (1898–99), 21: 509, citing *Affiches du Poitou*, 1774, p. 48.

34 AD Aube G 1763, 2d interrogation of Richard, 23 September 1769.

35 AN F⁷ 3179, 3d *jour complémentaire* XI/20 September 1803; AD Var 8 U 62/2, no. 31, Tribunal de Première Instance, Brignoles, 10 September 1817; AD Marne 33 X 8, report by commissioner of police, Châlons-sur-Marne.

36 *Gazette des tribunaux* 5 (1829–30): 67.

37 On payment in kind, see, for example, Claude Seignolle, *Le Folklore du Languedoc:*

Gard, Hérault, Lozère: *Cérémonies familiales, sorcellerie et médecine populaire, folklore de la nature* (1960), p. 224.

38 AD Ille-et-Vilaine C 2546, *recteurs* of Melesse, Betton, and Mouazé, 8 June 1786, quoted by Goubert, *Malades et médecins*, pp. 244–45.

39 Claude Seignolle, *En Sologne: Moeurs et coutumes*, new ed. (1967), p. 141.

40 AN F^{17} 2276, d. 2, no. 273.

41 Roger Vaultier, "Saint Hubert et la rage," *Presse médicale* 57 (1949): 670.

42 Jacqmart, "Erreurs," p. 343; *Gazette des tribunaux* 2 (1826–27): 82.

43 AN F^{15} 227, no. 6, report to Comité de Salubrité, 1 December 1790.

44 Mouquet, prize essay (see note 25), p. 37.

45 François-Paul-Lyon Poulletier de la Salle, Charles-Louis-François Andry, and Félix Vicq d'Azyr, "Rapport sur les inconvéniens de l'opération de la castration pratiquée pour obtenir la cure radicale des hernies," *Mémoires de la Société Royale de Médecine* 1 (1776): 291. AC Chalon-sur-Saône FF 38, cited by A. Baudot, *Études historiques sur la pharmacie en Bourgogne avant 1803* (1905), p. 322. AN F^7 7827, d. 5250, ser. 3, prefect of the Calvados to Minister of Police, 1 Ventôse IX/20 February 1801, on Léonard Morand. AP, report by Conseil de Salubrité de la Seine, 18 November 1817, on case of Minielle daughter.

46 See note 43.

47 SRM 132, no. 58, Nicolas, at Grenoble, "Sur la nécessité & les moyens d'établir une police médicale en France, & les avantages qui en résulteroient pour l'État et pour les sujets," 4 March 1777, fol. 2r; AD Loire-Atlantique 1 M 1358, no. 326, Conseil de Salubrité to prefect, 30 October 1826.

48 AP, report by Charles-Louis Cadet de Gassicourt for the Conseil de Salubrité de la Seine, 1 May 1816, on case of Ometz.

49 See, for example, SRM 107, Perreau, Fontenay-le-Comte, Bas-Poitou; he cites remedies that cost 6 livres.

50 SRM 199, d. 24, no. 2, report from Chartres, 22 December 1778.

51 Empirics frequently operated on the principle, "No cure, no money." See Charles John Samuel Thompson, *The Quacks of Old London* (London, 1928), p. 167.

52 AD Yonne 5 M 7/1, no. 76, minutes by Ragon-Pressonville, mayor of Villiers-Saint-Benoît, 29 June 1806.

53 *Gazette des tribunaux* 4 (1828–29): 522.

54 AD Hautes-Alpes 136 M 2, report by Catelan, cited by John V. Spears, "Folk Medicine and Popular Attitudes toward Disease in the High Alps, 1780–1870," *Bulletin of the History of Medicine* 54 (1980): 332.

55 AD Pyrénées-Orientales, quoted by Jean-Gabriel Gigot, "L'Histoire réelle du Roussillon au temps d'hier," pt. 1, "Guérisseurs en Roussillon," *C.E.R.C.A.*, no. 21 (Spring 1963): 251, case of Collioure.

56 Augustin Cabanès, *Comment on se soigne aujourd'hui: Remèdes de bonne femme* (1907), p. 203.

57 Advertisement of sieur Peirault, *Affiches du Poitou*, 1777, p. 96, quoted by Boissonnade, *Organisation du travail*, p. 508.

58 AN F^8 165, Suzov, 25 Ventôse XI/16 March 1803; SRM 96, Bonfils, April 1782.

59 SRM 107, Deshayes, 13 June 1789.

60 AD Yonne 5 M 7/1, no. 174, mayor to prefect, 15 April 1818.

61 Édouard-Louis Jacquet, for example, in *De quelques considérations sur l'empirisme et l'exercice illégal de la médecine*, Paris medical thesis, 1864, no. 162, p. 63, notes that "we do not wish . . . to prevent poor people from earning a living."

62 AN F^{17} 2276, d. 2, no. 312 (Arras).

63 See, for example, T. H. Marshall, "The Recent History of Professionalism in Relation to Social Structure and Social Policy," *Canadian Journal of Economics and Political Science* 5 (1939): 325–40.

64 See, for example, Jean-Joseph-Antoine Pilot de Thorey, *Usages, fêtes et coutumes existant ou ayant existé en Dauphiné* (Grenoble, 1884), p. 248.

65 Regnard, *Folies amoureuses*, i, 5, in Littré, *Dictionnaire de la langue française*, 4 vols.

(1873–75), s.v. *"industrie."*

66 AN F⁷ 8185, d. 2981R², prefect of the Escaut to 1st arrondissement, Police Générale, 29 October 1810.

67 Eugène Legrand, *Essai sur le charlatanisme et les préjugés en médecine*, Paris medical thesis, 1868, no. 53, p. 30.

68 See, for example, AD Bas-Rhin 5 M 22, no. 38, cantonal physician of Geispolsheim to prefect, 5 November 1813.

69 Karl Polanyi, *The Great Transformation: The Political and Economic Origins of Our Time* (Boston, 1957), p. 46 and chap. 4, passim. It should be noted that Polanyi speaks of "primitive" rather than peasant economies, which he does not treat systematically. In the older literature, see also Pitirim A. Sorokin, Carle C. Zimmerman, and Charles J. Galpin, *A Systematic Sourcebook in Rural Sociology*, 3 vols. (Minneapolis, 1931–32), vol 2, chap. 11.

70 Robert Redfield, "The Folk Society," *American Journal of Sociology* 52 (1946–47): 298, 305–06. See John C. McKinney, *Constructive Typology and Social Theory* (New York, 1966), pp. 108–09. Redfield's model, which opposes the stable folk society to the dynamic urban societies of the modern West, has been attacked on a number of fronts. In Western cultures, studies have shown sources of change other than the city; in non-Western cultures, social heterogeneity may increase even in the absence of Western influences. See, for example, Horace Minor, *The Primitive City of Timbuctoo* (Princeton, N.J., 1953), and "The Folk-Urban Continuum," *American Sociological Review* 17 (1952): 529–37.

71 Magali Sarfatti Larson, *The Rise of Professionalism: A Sociological Analysis* (Berkeley and Los Angeles, 1977), pt. 1, esp. chap. 3 (on medicine).

72 Report of 1 November 1810 (see note 2).

73 Goubert, *Malades et médecins*, p. 245; Nouvel, "Exercice illégal," p. 159, citing AD Marne 11 U 844; AD Charente-Maritime 7 M 6/1, no. 114, La Force to prefect, 14 March 1820. In this last case, the mayor of Saint-Sauvant, coming to Corbiot's defense, felt compelled to point out that this practitioner, whose qualifications were shaky (he had only a "provisional authorization" from the Indre and a certificate from a doctor in Saintes), at least was not a drunkard (ibid., no. 113, 10 April 1820).

74 *Gazette des tribunaux* 2 (1826–27): 1222.

75 AD Yonne 3 M 22, no. 26, cited by Eugen Weber, *Peasants into Frenchmen: The Modernization of Rural France, 1870–1914* (Stanford, Calif., 1976), p. 305.

76 See, for example, Eugène Olivier, *Médecine et santé dans le pays de Vaud au XVIIIᵉ siècle, 1675–1798*, 2 vols. paginated continuously (Lausanne, 1939), p. 432, on the case of the healer La Roche in eighteenth-century Vaud, Switzerland.

77 AD Aube C 1164, d. 2, subdelegate at Troyes to intendant, 3 September 1788.

78 SRM 107, 13 April 1784. Cf. SRM 199, d. 29, no. 9, 7 June 1779, on Desmarest, at Rouen, who lives in concubinage with Mme. Riché.

79 AN F⁷ 8185, d. 2981R², prefect of the Cher to *conseiller d'état*, 1st arrondissement, 13 October 1812.

80 AN D XXXVIII 3, d. 45, Nicolas-André Feren.

81 See, for example, SRM 199, d. 18, no. 13, 17 April 1779, on Antoine Jouvel at Caylus.

82 George M. Gould and Walter L. Pyle, *Anomalies and Curiosities of Medicine . . .* (New York, 1937), pp. 207–08.

83 SRM 199, d. 25, no. 6, Von Mittag Midy, 13 March 1777; AD Haute-Loire 13 M 18, no. 485, captain of gendarmerie at Aurec to prefect, 7–8 March 1817; Michel Boyer, "L'Encadrement médical en Ardèche au XIXᵉ siècle," master's thesis, University of Lyons II, 1977, p. 49, citing AD Ardèche 3 U 625 (on Abel).

84 Adolphe Lecocq, *Empiriques, somnambules et rebouteurs beaucerons* (Chartres, 1862), p. 54, quoting municipal administration, Chartres, vol. 6, fol. 175, 23 Frimaire VI/ 13 December 1797.

85 AD Var 8 U 62/2, no. 38, *procureur du roi* to *juge d'instruction*, 28 August 1817.

86 AD Yonne 5 M 7/1, no. 210, Dr. Edme-Hubert Roché to prefect, 22 February 1821. Cf. ibid., Roché to prefect, 21 June 1829, in which the doctor suggests that

the charlatans' supporters might see them as government agents charged with secret missions—again, something more than practitioners of medicine.
87 Ibid., no. 242, Minister of the Interior to prefect, 24 December 1823; no. 243, subprefect of Avallon to prefect, 4 June 1824.
88 For example, Vavasseur at Nantes, AC Nantes I 5 7, d. 3, 17 May 1823.
89 *Gazette des tribunaux* 4 (1828–29): 522. On popular healers and draft evasion, see Matthew Ramsey, "Conscription, Malingerers, and Popular Medicine in Napoleonic France," *The Consortium on Revolutionary Europe, 1750–1850, Proceedings, 1978* (Athens, Ga., 1980), pp. 188–99.
90 AD Drôme M 2153, report of medical jury, 31 July 1845, quoted in Jacques Léonard, comp., *La France médicale: Médecins et malades au XIXe siècle* (1978), p. 32.
91 Victor Hugo, *Les Travailleurs de la Mer* (1866), quoted in Léonard, *France médicale*, p. 32. Hugo applies the observation to his character Gilliatt, who is believed on Guernsey to be a witch and *marcou*, perhaps even a *cambion* (a child sired by the Devil), and generally has a bad reputation. See *Les Travailleurs*, pt. 1, bk. 1, esp. chap. 5.
92 Jacques Léonard, "Quand la médicalisation devint populaire," *Autrement*, no. 9, May 1977, special number, *Franc-tireurs de la médecine*, p. 202.
93 See, for example, Margaret Clark, *Health in the Mexican-American Culture: A Community Study*, 2d ed. (Berkeley and Los Angeles, 1970), chap. 7, pt. 1, on San Jose, California. Also: Irwin Press, "Urban Folk Medicine: A Functional Overview," *American Anthropologist*, 80 (1978): 71–84.
94 On modernization and popular medicine: Marcelle Bouteiller, *Médecine populaire d'hier et d'aujourd'hui* (1966), pp. 112–21.
95 Jean Mellot, *Questions de folklore et de langage* (Sancerre, n.d. [1964]), p. 109; Seignolle, *Le Berry*, p. 229.
96 See, for example, Madge E. Pickard and R. Carlyle Buley, *The Midwest Pioneer: His Ills, Cures, and Doctors* (Crawfordsville, Ind., 1945), and Stewart H. Holbrook, *The Golden Age of Quackery* (New York, 1959), esp. pt. 9.
97 Edward Evan Evans-Pritchard, *Witchcraft, Oracles and Magic Among the Azande* (Oxford, 1937). See Eliot Freidson, *Profession of Medicine: A Study of the Sociology of Applied Knowledge* (New York, 1970), pp. 6–9.
98 Una Maclean, *Magical Medicine: A Nigerian Case Study* (Harmondsworth, 1971), pp. 66–88, 142; Pierre Huard and Ming Wong, *Chinese Medicine*, tr. Bernard Fielding (New York, 1968), pp. 61–62. On Nigeria, cf. Anthony D. Buckley, *Yoruba Medicine* (Oxford, 1985).
99 See Arthur Kleinman, *Patients and Healers in the Context of Culture: An Exploration of the Borderland between Anthropology, Medicine, and Psychiatry* (Berkeley and Los Angeles, 1980), pp. 66–67, 230–31 (n. 3), and passim.
100 Ibid., p. 54.
101 In addition to Kleinman, *Patients and Healers*, see, for example, the essays in Charles Leslie, ed., *Asian Medical Systems: A Comparative Study* (Berkeley and Los Angeles, 1976); Kleinman et al., eds., *Medicine in Chinese Cultures: Comparative Studies of Health Care in Chinese and Other Societies* (Washington, D.C., 1975); and Kleinman et al., eds., *Culture and Healing: Anthropological, Psychiatric, and Public Health Studies* (Cambridge, Mass., 1978). Some of the essays in the last volume analyze the role of the various types of medical practitioners in non-Western societies.
102 See Ralph C. Croizier, *Traditional Medicine in Modern China: Science, Nationalism, and the Tensions of Cultural Change* (Cambridge, Mass., 1968).

AFTERWORD: *Medicalization and social theory*

1 See, for example, Ivan Waddington, *The Medical Profession in the Industrial Revolution* (Dublin, 1984).
2 Talcott Parsons, "Social Structure and Dynamic Process: The Case of Modern Medical Practice," in *The Social System* (Glencoe, Ill., 1951), pp. 428–79.
3 For a constructive critique of modernization theory, viewed in historical perspective,

see Reinhard Bendix, "Tradition and Modernity Reconsidered," *Comparative Studies in Society and History* 9 (1967): 292–346. Cf. Dean C. Tipps, "Modernization Theory and the Comparative Study of Societies: A Critical Perspective," *Comparative Studies in Society and History* 15 (1973): 199–226, and S. N. Eisenstadt, "Studies of Modernization and Sociological Theory," *History and Theory* 13 (1974): 225–52.

4 This is the thrust of a survey of recent historical scholarship on the problem by Ted W. Margadant, "Tradition and Modernity in Rural France during the Nineteenth Century," *The Journal of Modern History* 56 (1984):667–97.

5 Ibid., p. 668

6 Tony Judt, "A Clown in Regal Purple: Social History and the Historians," *History Workshop*, no. 7 (Spring 1979): 66–94.

7 On the Seine-et-Oise: Evelyn Ackerman, "Medical Care in the Countryside near Paris, 1800–1914," *Annals of the New York Academy of Sciences* 412 (14 October 1983): 1–18, and idem, *Country People and Health Care: The Department of the Seine-et-Oise from 1800 to 1914* (forthcoming).

8 See, for example, Jacques Léonard, "Médecine et colonisation en Algérie au XIXe siècle" (article based on research by Françoise Bourdon), *Annales de Bretagne et des pays de l'Ouest* 84 (1977): 481–94.

APPENDIX A: *Density of French medical personnel in the nineteenth century*

1 Lists sent to the Ministry of Justice can be found in AN BB¹ 204–211, "Médecins, chirurgiens et accoucheurs autorisés," Year XI–1827. Lists sent to the Ministry of the Interior can be found in the dossiers on the medical juries, AN F¹⁷ 2391–2454, which also include lists of new practitioners received by the juries. See also AN F⁸ 142–45, lists of public health officials.

2 For a critique of the census results, see Pierre-Émile Levasseur, *La Population française: Histoire de la population avant 1789, et démographie historique de la France comparée à celle des autres nations au XIXe siècle, précédée d'une introduction sur la statistique*, 3 vols. (1889–92), vol. 1, bk. 2, chap. 2. For a more recent analysis of French demography in the early nineteenth century, see Charles H. Pouthas, *La Population française pendant la première moitié du XIXe siècle*, Institut National d'Études Démographiques, Travaux et documents, no. 25 (1956).

3 The results of the surveys conducted in the first half of the century are in AN F¹⁷ 4536–4539. The Salvandy survey of 1847 is in F¹⁷ 4537–4539; some material related to his earlier and incomplete survey of 1845 is in F¹⁷ 1468. See George D. Sussman "The Glut of Doctors in Mid-Nineteenth-Century France," *Comparative Studies in Society and History* 19 (1977): 293–303, especially the table and two maps on pp. 294–97 and 300–01.

4 Departmental lists of medical personnel for the period 1853–1926 are in AN F¹⁷ 4543–4556. Published statistics on medical personnel in the second half of the nineteenth century can be found in *Recueil des travaux du Comité Consultatif d'Hygiène Publique de France* 16 (1886), appendix 4, "Tableau statistique du personnel médical en France de 1847 à 1881," and in the *Annuaire statistique de la France* 18 (1898): 510–11, table 558; this material is analyzed in Martha L. Hildreth, "The Foundations of the Modern Medical System in France: Physicians, Public Health Advocates, and the Medical Legislation of 1892 and 1893," *Proceedings of the Eighth Annual Meeting of the Western Society for French History* (Las Cruces, N.M., 1981), p. 312 and pp. 320–21, tables 1 and 2.

5 Jacques Léonard, *Les Médecins de l'Ouest*, state doctoral thesis, University of Paris IV, 1976 (1978), pp. 14–29, 75–93 and 395–416 (beginning of the nineteenth century); 530–48 (Restoration and July Monarchy); and 826–36 (second half of the century). See also the relevant tables, graphs, and maps, appendix pp. cxxv–cxlvii, cc–ccviii, ccxvi–ccxxv, ccxxxii, ccxxxvi–ccxxxix, and ccxliii–ccxliv.

APPENDIX B: *Some itinerant empirics, 1802–1844*

1 AD Bas-Rhin 5 M 22, no. 12, subprefect of Wissembourg, decree of 8 Thermidor X/27 July 1802.
2 AD Loire 38 M 9, no. 16, Dr. Poucet at Feurs to prefect, 3 November 1806.
3 AN F[7] 8185, d. 2981R[2], prefect, Roer, to *conseiller d'état*, 1st arrondissement, Police Générale, 16 November 1807.
4 Ibid., subprefect of Speyer to prefect of Mont-Tonnerre, 25 October 1810.
5 AD Bas Rhin 5 M 22. See the discussion in Chapter 3.
6 Ibid., no. 35, report to prefect on unauthorized practitioners in canton of Soultz-sous-Forêts, 19 June 1813.
7 AD Vaucluse 5 M 14, *conseiller de préfecture*, Drôme, to prefect, Vaucluse, 10 April 1817.
8 AD Hautes-Alpes 141 M, no. 87, prefect to mayor of La Saulce, 4 August 1819; no. 85, mayor to prefect, 13 August; no. 89, *procès-verbal* of arrest, 8 October 1819, Gendarmerie Royale.
9 AD Yonne 5 M 7/1, Edme-Hubert Roché, physician at Toucy, to prefect, 22 February 1821.
10 AD Bas-Rhin 5 M 22, no. 110, mayor of Westhoffen to prefect, 15 November 1821.
11 AN F[7] 9272, d. 4534, Troyes, secretary-general (for the prefect) to Minister of the Interior, 4 July 1822.
12 AC Nantes I 5 7, letter to prefect, 17 May 1823. Cf. AD Loire-Atlantique 1 M 1358, no. 326, Comité de Salubrité, Nantes, to prefect, 30 October 1826, which describes Piloquet as a bargeman and identifies a "nomadic charlatan" with a health officer's diploma, Périnet, who sometimes travels around the department and sometimes resides at Nantes.
13 *Gazette des tribunaux*, 23 October 1826.
14 AD Yonne 5 M 7/1, Roché to prefect, 21 June 1829.
15 *Gazette des tribunaux* 5 (1829–30): 66–67.
16 AD Bas-Rhin 5 M 22, no. 205, cantonal physician, Schlestadt, to prefect, 23 May 1841; no. 204, subprefect of Schlestadt to prefect, 24 May.
17 Ibid. no. 210, Jacobi, cantonal physician at Schiltigheim, to prefect, 23 March 1844.

APPENDIX C: *Some French remedy sellers, 1773–1830*

1 *Affiches du Poitou*, 1773, p. 176. Cited by Prosper-Marie Boissonnade, *Essai sur l'organisation du travail en Poitou, depuis le XIe siècle jusqu'à la Révolution*, *Mémoires de la Société des Antiquaires de l'Ouest*, vols. 21–22 (1898–99), 22: 509.
2 *Affiches du Poitou*, 1774, p. 48, cited in ibid., p. 509.
3 SRM 103.
4 SRM 105.
5 SRM 96.
6 SRM 107, letter from Terrède at l'Aigle, 8 July 1782.
7 Ibid., letter from de Bonzon, Île Saint-Louis, 9 August 1782.
8 SRM 96, letter from Bardellot, surgeon at Nérondes, January 1783.
9 *Affiches chartraines*, 14 January and 15 December 1784; quoted by Adolphe Lecocq, *Empiriques, somnambules et rebouteurs beaucerons* (Chartres; 1862), pp. 50–51.
10 AN AF III 107, Faugerolle petition, Vendémiaire VI/September–October 1797.
11 Hérissay, L'Exercice illégal de la médecine dans l'Eure sous le Consulat," *Bulletin de la Société Française d'Histoire de la Médecine* 26 (1932): 91.
12 AD Loire-Atlantique 1 M 1358, no. 440, mayor of Saint-Colombin to prefect, 5 Vendémiaire XII/28 September 1803.
13 Ibid., no. 430, Denis Teynot, surgeon, April 1807.
14 AD Yonne 5 M 7/1, nos. 78–81, January 1808.
15 AN F[8] 165, Schirvel to Minister of the Interior, 6 January 1820.
16 AC Nantes I 5 7, commissioner of police to mayor, 11 November 1830.
17 AN F[8] 162, Percheron dossier.

APPENDIX D: *Some empirics and their occupations, 1775–1838*

1 AD Ille-et-Vilaine C 206, Malesherbes to Intendant of Brittany, 19 November 1775, cited by Étienne Dupont, "Les Lettres de cachet et l'exercice illégal de la médecine en Bretagne au XVIIIe siècle," *Chronique médicale* 29 (1923): 261.

2 AD Maine-et-Loire 4 D 12.

3 SRM 107, René-Georges Gastellier to Society, 14 March 1782.

4 AD Ille-et-Vilaine C 2546, *recteur* of Melesse, 8 June 1786; subdelegate of Lannion to Intendant, 10 June 1786. Cited in Jean-Pierre Goubert, *Malades et médecins en Bretagne, 1770–1790* (1974), pp. 243–45.

5 SRM 199, d. 18, no. 12, Dr. Dentieux, 8 December 1788.

6 René-Georges Gastellier, *Observations et réflexions relatives à l'organisation actuelle de la médecine* (Montargis, 1806), pp. 10–11.

7 Hérissay, "L'Exercice illégal de la médecine dans l'Eure sous le Consulat," *Bulletin de la Société Française d'Histoire de la Médecine* 26 (1932): 89.

8 Ibid., p. 93.

9 AS Bas-Rhin 5 M 22, no. 15, list of illegal practitioners at Strasbourg, Ventôse XIII/February–March 1805.

10 AD Yonne 5 M 7/1, no. 76, Villiers-Saint-Benoît, minute by mayor, 29 June 1806.

11 AN F^8 150, Chervet, former military health officer, to Minister of the Interior, 11 September 1806; cf. F^8 161, Orgeolet dossier.

12 AD Loire-Atlantique 1 M 1358, no. 424, surgeon at Saint-Père-en-Retz to prefect, 3 May 1808.

13 AN F^8 163, Minister of the Interior to prefect of the Orne, 23 December 1808.

14 AN F^7 8185, d. 2981R^2, prefect of the Loiret to 1st arrondissement, Police Générale, 17 October 1810.

15 AN F^8 167, 26 May 1811.

16 AD Hautes-Alpes 141 M, no. 89, Gendarmerie Royale, brigade of La Saulce, record of arrest, 8 October 1819; no. 158, prefect to mayor of Ventavon, 17 October 1838.

17 AD Loire-Atlantique 1 M 1358, no. 349, procureur to prefect, 15 September 1823.

GLOSSARY AND NOTE ON
FRENCH MONEY

accoucheur   man-midwife; obstetrician.

affranchisseur   gelder; often a practitioner of veterinary medicine, sometimes dabbling in human medicine as well.

agrégation   in the Old Regime, professional company; act of admission to such a company.

agrégé   member of an **agrégation**.

bailleul   same as **rebouteur**.

bandagiste   truss maker.

bocage   countryside (characteristic of western France) marked by dispersed farms and hamlets and tall hedgerows.

bourreau   executioner; often practiced bonesetting and minor surgery.

cahiers de doléances   literally, copybooks of complaints; grievance lists drafted in the assemblies that elected deputies to the Estates-General in France (the Estates met in 1789 for the first time since 1614).

carreau   in popular usage, condition of children who have a hard and swollen abdomen; often considered to be caused by a diseased spleen.

chevalier d'industrie   swindler; a term often applied to charlatans.

chirurgiens du grand chef-d'oeuvre, de grande expérience   under the Old Regime, surgeons who had completed the training and examinations necessary to practice in a guild town.

chirurgiens de petite expérience, de légère expérience   surgeons whose lower qualifications did not allow them to practice in guild towns.

colporteur   packman, peddler (broader than the English sense of peddler of religious books, or missionary).

corps   under the Old Regime, a legally recognized body, including the professional corporations.

dartre   dartre: a vague generic term for various skin diseases.

désensorceler   unwitch: to lift a spell cast by a witch.

devin   diviner, wizard.

docteur forain   under the Old Regime, a doctor whose degree entitled him to practice only outside the seat of the faculty.

don   gift; here, a healer's gift to cure disease.

dormeur [m.], **dormeuse** [f.]   a healer who made diagnoses and prescribed remedies while in a trance.

droguerie   an establishment selling pharmaceutical materials wholesale, and often hardware, paints, household supplies, etc. (to be distinguished from a **pharmacie**).

école de santé   school of health: the name given to medical schools in the legislation of 1794.

empiétement   encroachment: infringement by one occupation on the domain of a neighboring occupation (e.g., an apothecary's unauthorized practice of medicine).

épiciers   spicers: dealers in spices, groceries, and often remedies (the French term is less narrowly synonymous with "apothecary" than the English cognate).

état   status, station; also, profession, occupation.

externe   under the Old Regime, a practitioner who could work only outside a corporate seat.

gagnant-maîtrise   senior surgical resident (student) in a hospital.

garçon-chirurgien   surgeon's assistant (distinguished from a fee-paying apprentice).

généralité   under the Old Regime, a district administered by an intendant.

gens à secrets   literally, people with secrets: magical healers.

grimoire   wizard's magic book.

guérisseur   (folk) healer.

hôtel-Dieu   hospital; in the Old Regime, the **hôtel-Dieu** provided medical services, unlike many an **hôpital**, which was essentially a shelter and hospice.

hunes, hules   in western France, a vaguely defined malady, usually characterized by chronic fatigue.

impéritie   incompetence, especially when due to inexperience (from the Latin *imperitia*, meaning inexperience or ignorance); a vice frequently attributed to poorly trained country surgeons by their critics under the Old Regime.

industriel   industrialist, but also **chevalier d'industrie** (q.v.); a term commonly applied to quacks.

interne   under the Old Regime, a practitioner entitled to practice in a corporate seat.

jugeur d'eau   literally, water judger; see **uromante**.

laboureur   farmer; typically a peasant owning at least a plough and a team of draft animals.

leveur de sorts   one who lifts spells.

licence   first degree after the baccalaureate.

licencié   holder of the licence.

maige   folk healer; more loosely, medicaster.

maîtresse-sage-femme   under the Old Regime, a midwife admitted to the mastership.

marcou   the seventh-born son, believed to have the power to heal scrofula and other diseases.

matrone   matron: a term applied to an unlicensed midwife.

mauvais sujet   bad lot; a term frequently applied to quacks by officials.

médecin des épidémies   physician for epidemics dispatched by the government into the countryside during outbreaks of disease.

officier de santé   health officer: lower-level practitioner under the medical legislation of 1803.

officiat de santé   the title or position held by the **officier de santé**.

panseur   literally, (surgical) dresser; a term often applied to folk healer (also **panseur de secret**).

patente   in revolutionary and postrevolutionary France, a tax on industry paid by members of many occupations; under the Revolution, a license to practice supposedly conferred by payment of this tax (**patente** also means diploma, letters of appointment).

prévôt   under the Old Regime, an official of the surgical guilds charged with enforcing the guild statutes (generally known in other trades as a *juré*).

protomédich   royal physician (in Roussillon).

rebouteur, rebouteux   bonesetter; sometimes applied more loosely to folk healers.

recteur   parish priest (in Brittany).

remèdes du roi, remèdes d'Helvétius   boxes of remedies sent out to the provinces in the name of the king during epidemics; inspired by Adrien Helvétius (c. 1661–1727).

renoueur, rhabilleur   see **rebouteur**.

sage-femme   midwife.

saludador   (sometimes **salutador**) a Catalan healer generally believed to have the gift to cure rabies.

sang fort   strong blood: what a healer is widely believed to need in order to lift an evil spell cast on his patient.

sans domicile fixe   without fixed abode.

somnambule   somnambulist (though broader than the English sense of sleepwalker); see **dormeur**.

taille   under the Old Regime, the basic direct tax, imposed on nonnobles.

toucheur   healer; specifically one who heals through his touch.

tribunal correctionnel   in revolutionary and postrevolutionary France, court that judged lesser criminal offenses.

uromante   practitioner of uromancy, or divining from the urine; loosely, urinoscopist – practitioner who diagnoses disease by inspecting the patient's urine.

vertaupe   popular term for a furuncle or boil.

vicaire   assistant priest.

A NOTE ON FRENCH MONEУ

The Old Regime

The Old Regime distinguished between money of account, of which the most important unit was the livre tournois, or franc, and actual coins, of which the most important were the gold louis and the silver écu. The value of the coinage was fixed by decrees of 1726 and 1738, and for our purposes we may use the following equivalencies:

1 pistole = 10 livres	1 louis = 24 livres
1 livre = 20 sous (or sols)	1 écu = 3 livres
1 sous = 12 deniers	

The nineteenth century

The monetary reform of 1795 established as the basic unit the new franc, equivalent to 1.0125 livres tournois. After the great inflation of the Revolution, the value of the franc in relation to gold and silver was fixed by a law of 7 Germinal Year XI (28 March 1803); this "franc of Germinal" was to remain stable for a century and a quarter.

1 franc = 100 centimes

Given the fluctuations in the value of currency, it is not a useful exercise to translate prices into current equivalents in dollars or pounds sterling; the discussion in the text attempts to give some sense of magnitude by comparing a physician's fees with a patient's likely earnings or a practitioner's earnings with those of members of other occupations.

INDEX

French terms marked with an asterisk are defined in the Glossary. Abbreviations: f = figure, m = map, n = note, t = table.

Abel, Pierre (empiric), 294
abortion, 130, 142, 190, 264, 281
Académie Celtique, 237, 369n26
Académie Royale de Chirurgie (Old Regime), 21, 44, 82
Académie Royale de Médecine (nineteenth century), 84, 106–07, 261–62
academies (provincial), physicians as members of, in Old Regime, 55–56
Academy of Dijon, 29
accoucheurs,* 24
Affiches du Poitou, 147
agrégations,* 38–39
Ailhaud, Jean-Pierre-Gaspard, 177
Ailhaud's powders, 177, 178, 261
album graecum, 181
alchemy, 198
Alfort, school of veterinary medicine at, 33
Algaron (empiric), *see* Toscan(o)
Alpes-Maritimes (department), medical personnel in, 116
Alsace: itinerant empiricism in, 161, 163; *médecin cantonal* in, 121
amateur science and medicine, 35–36
America, popular medicine in, 297
American Medical Association, 108
Amilly, prior of (remedy vendor), 180
Andry, Charles-Louis-François (physician), 240
Angers in the Old Regime: doctor-regents at, 54–55; regulation of remedy trade at, 34; surgeons at, 57
Angleberme, d' (empiric), 150, 156
Anjou, medical personnel in, 60
apothecaries and pharmacists, 19, 28–30, 81;

collaborate with empirics, 163, 196; *see also* pharmacy; *propharmaciens*
Aquin, Antoine d' (First Physician), 41–42
Ardèche (department), medical personnel in, 111, 117
Armoricain Massif, folk medicine in, 235
Arpon (wigmaker-pedicure), 87
artisans: as empirics, 210–11, 217; as folk healers, 255; as patients of empirics, 226
Association Générale de Prévoyance et de Secours Mutuel des Médecins de France, 108, 204, 213
Association of Paris Physicians, 108
Auch, surgeons in diocese of, 52, 53, 57
Auda, Ignace (healer), 228, 245
Audase, Désiré (remedy vendor), 309–10
Audineau (empiric), 312
Aunievan, Magdeleine (religious healer), 202–03
autopsies, peasants' fear of, 67, 282
Avrigny, Martin d' (empiric), 288
Ayurvedic medical tradition, 298

Bafferne (unqualified surgeon), 218
Baille (bonesetter), 260
Bailleul dynasty (bonesetters), 245
Bailly, L. (revolutionary legislator), 74
Balzac, Honoré de, 67, 68, 178
bande d'Orgères, 173
bandits and empirics compared, 157
Baraillon, Jean-François (physician and legislator), 111
barbers and surgery, 20–21, 22, 43, 85, 209
Barjavel, Magdeleine (empiric), 221
Barjon, Catherine (remedy vendor), 158

Bartolle, Françoise (orvietan vendor), 168
Baseilhac, Jean (monk and surgeon), 37
Bas-Rhin (department): experts in, 87; licensed personnel in, 212–13; unqualified practitioners in, 208–13, 362n147
bathers and bathkeepers, 27, 87, 98
Baulard (empiric), *see* Blanche
Bayard, widow (remedy seller), 221
Bedu (unwitcher), 273–74
Béguin (charitable healer), 98–99, 191
Bellet (bonesetter), 187
Belloste's pills, 135
Bellouin (empiric and remedy vendor), 309, 311
Béranger, Louis (ocular surgeon), 25
Bercé, Yves-Marie, 6
Bernard, Denis (bonesetter), 187
Bertin, Henri-Léonard-Jean-Baptiste, 33, 36
Besnard du Buisson, François (surgeon), 29
Bétréau (hernia surgeon), 185
Bignau (Faculty of Orange graduate), 51
Bin (priest), 99–100
Birckbüchler, François-Adam (barber), 209
Bizieux (oculist), 25
blacksmiths, *see* farriers/blacksmiths
Blanc, Mlle (empiric), 181, 283
Blanc (empiric), 191, 226, 280, 281
Blanche, *la dame* (empiric), 225, 265, 285, 307
Blanchet, Henri (dentist), 240
Blassing (witch/healer), 212
bleeding as therapy, 46, 48, 67, 122, 209–10, 262, 282
Blégny, Nicolas de, 182
Bloch, Marc, 237, 247, 248
Bocot, Martin (empiric), 219
Boehmer, Hubert (empiric), 206
Bonaparte, Louis-Napoleon, 247
Bonaparte, Napoleon, *see* Napoleon I
bonesetters, 206, 208, 251, 260; distribution and range of, 187; executioners as, 27, 87; folk healers as, 240; harm caused by, 187–89; hereditary calling among, 185–86; occupations of, 186–87; in regular medical network of Old Regime, 26–27; in royal household, 24; talented, respected by elites, 187, 227; techniques used by, 187–88; terms for, 26, 185; training of, 26–27; under Ventôse law, 88, 101; women as, 220–21, 365n217
Bonfils (remedy vendor), 309
Bonnesse (chiropodist), 164
Boozzo (empiric), 307
Bordeaux: cost of surgical mastership at, 53; faculty and college of medicine at, 39–40; government oversight of medicine at, 41
Bouche (empiric), 261

Boucher (religious healer), 202, 283
Boulogne, Jean-François Michel (operator), 167–68, 285, 294
Bourdin (gelder/empiric), 216
Bourdois de la Mothe, Edme-Joachim (physician), 105
Bouteiller, Marcelle, 237, 241, 248, 251, 254, 276
Boyer, Paul, 270
Breit, Justin (empiric), 208
Brenner (barber), 209
Brioude, Pierre (healer), 251
Britain: apothecaries in, 29; medical personnel in, 59; unqualified practitioners in, 213, 363n161
British Medical Association, 108
Brittany: corporate monopolies in, 41; medical personnel in, 57–58, 60, 61; popular medical beliefs in, 261–63; *see also* West (of France)
Broussais, François, 48, 122
Burton, Robert, 65
Bussy, chevalier de (François-Joseph Leclerc, charitable practitioner), 35

Cabanis, Pierre-Jean-Georges, 75, 77
"Cabriolet" (empiric), 147
Cagliostro, Alessandro di, 155–56, 227
*cahiers de doléances,** 29, 47, 55, 72, 239
Calès, Jean-Marie (physician and legislator), 72
Cannon, W. B., 271
cantonal physicians, *see* district physicians
Caron de Bretonnaux, J.-B. François (physician), 89
carpenters as healers, 249, 255, 273, 274
*carreau,** 241, 245, 248, 249
Carret, Michel (surgeon and legislator), 77, 79
Cartéron (empiric), 103, 186–87
Cartin (dentist), 90, 164
Casanova, Giovanni Jacopo, 227
castration caused by operation for hernia, 26, 153, 185
Catherine, Saint, 245, 247
Catholicism required of medical practitioners in Old Regime, 49
Cauveau, Michel (*devin**), 268
Caze de la Bove, Gaspard-Louis, 57
censuses: of French population, 302–03; of official medical personnel, 302–03, 330n201; of unqualified practitioners, 204–13, 362n147
Cercle Médical, 106, 343n147
chambers of discipline, 107, 115
Chambre Royale de Médecine (seventeenth century), 41–42

chambrelans in surgery, 23
Champagny, Jean-Baptiste de Nompère de, 91, 94
Chaptal, Jean-Antoine, 77, 81, 83, 84–85, 86, 94
charitable healers, 35–36, 90–91, 98–99, 323n80; empirics as, 153, 285, 308; folk healers as, 254–55
"charlatan," classic type of, 131–33; *see also* empirics
charlatanism, *see* empiricism, medical
Charles X, 83, 107, 247
Charry (bonesetter), 187
Chateaubriand, René de, 133
Châteauroux, comte de, family of (healers), 245–46
Chauliac, Guy de, 23
Chaussier, François (physician), 75, 95
Cherchin (operator), 158
Cheuillot (empiric), 287
Chevrier (medical practitioner), 93
Chiarini, Mme (itinerant remedy vendor), 163
Chicoyneau, François (First Physician), 33
Chifoliau, Jean-Guillaume (physician), 264
China, medical practitioners in, 297–98
Chirac, Pierre (First Physician), 31, 33, 42
cholera, 122, 153
Christian vocation to heal, 36
Church, Catholic (*see also* clergy; religious foundations; religious orders): and licensure of midwives in Old Regime, 23; property as source of funds for public health during Revolution, 72; and prosecution of unauthorized medical practice, 230; and witchcraft, 231, 265, 268
Clément (surgeon), 86
Clément, Nicolas (knight of Saint Hubert), 200, 286
Clementz (empiric), 307
clergy (*see also* Church, Catholic; religious foundations; religious orders): in charitable medicine and public assistance, 37–38, 91; as folk healers, 250–51, 252, 261; as physicians' aides, proposal for, 82, 121; popular error attacked by, 2; and popular medicine, views of, 257–59; as remedy vendors, 180; as unauthorized medical practitioners, 38, 198, 203–04, 205, 206, 207, 208, 210, 216, 219, 261, 292, 293; as unwitchers, 268; and Ventôse law, 91, 94, 100
Cobb, Richard, 167, 173
Code Napoléon, 125
Colbert, Jean-Baptiste, 231
Colioure, de (*saludador*★), 261
College of Pharmacy (Paris), 28, 45, 75, 79

College of Surgery (Paris), 21–22, 25, 47, 52, 82
Collège Royal, 47
Collin-Chevrel (empiric), 220
Côme, Frère (monk and surgeon), 37
Comité de Mendicité (Constituent Assembly), 73
Comité de Salubrité (Constituent Assembly), 73–74; survey of surgery by (1790–1791), 28, 32, 46, 160, 206–07, 257
Comité de Secours (Legislative Assembly), 74
Committee of Public Safety (Convention), 75
communities, surgical, 43
Community of Saint-Côme (Paris), 21, 44
conscription and medical practitioners, 122, 166, 197, 268, 281, 294–95
Constituent Assembly and medical reform, 73, 74
Constitution of the Year III (Directory Constitution) and professional societies, 106
Consulate: and medical reform, 76–79; and pharmaceutical reform, 79–80; and religious orders, 91
Contoly (physician-cum-empiric), 215
contracts between empirics and patients, 287
Contrastin (surgeon), 96
Contugi, Florent-Jean-Louis (orvietan vendor), 134
Contugi family (orvietan vendors), 48, 134
Convention, National, 74–76, 91
Corbière, Jacques-Joseph-Guillaume-François-Pierre, 83, 107
Corbiot (empiric), 292
Coronat (itinerant physician), 48
corporations, medical, 18–29, 38–39; boundaries of, blurred at end of Old Regime, 30–31; and Crown, 41; Revolution attacks, 73, 74–75
Corps Législatif (Consulate), 77, 79, 80
Cortade, Joseph (unwitcher), 260
Cosmas, Saint, 21
Couet (remedy vendor), 310
Courcelle's American elixir, 178
Crespin, Pierre (remedy vendor), 181
Crétet, Emmanuel, 91, 97
crinons, 241
Cuchet, Salomon (empiric), 135, 139, 140, 142, 145, 146, 156, 205
Cugnat, Louis (healer), 257–60
Cuvier, Georges, 82, 83, 107, 110

Dachino (ocular surgeon), 25
Dagobert, J.-B. (surgeon), 53

Daran, Jacques (physician), 56
Darmon, Jean-Jacques, 174
Darmon, Pierre, 6
Darnet (empiric), 155
Darnton, Robert, 155, 167
Daumier, Honoré, 114
Dauphiné: empirics in, 205; medicinal plants exported from, 166
Daux, Marie (*officier de santé**), 86
Daviel (oculist), widow of (remedy vendor), 30
Debrou, Laurent (priest/empiric), 198
Delisle, Morel (remedy vendor), 34
Delpeuth (dentist), 220
Delvincourt (priest), 99
Demarest (empiric), 140
Demorest, Jean-Baptiste (executioner), 97
Denis, Charles-Marie (ecclesiastic), 99
dentists, 164, 182, 197, 207, 306, 307; and folk medicine, 240; jurisprudence on, 89–90; women as, 220
Desault, Pierre-Joseph, 75
Deschamp (empiric), 292, 311
Descombes, Desiderio (orvietan vendor), 133–34
désensorceleurs, see devins-guérisseurs; unwitchers
Desjardins (Brother Alexis, Capuchin and empiric), 38
Deslon, Charles (physician), 49
Desmarest (empiric), 140
Desormeaux (François Antoine, *devin**), 274–75
Deux-Sèvres (department), medical personnel in, 116
Deveyl (remedy vendor), 179
deviants among empirics, 292–95
Devil: cures attributed to, 231; in dualist cosmology, 270; pacts with, 231, 266, 267, 272
devins-guérisseurs (see also unwitchers), 268
Dictionnaire de Trévoux, 132
Diderot, Denis, 63–64
Diebold (empiric), 210
Diest, Jean de (physician), 65
Dionis, Charles (physician), 33, 34, 48, 134–35
Directory (revolutionary regime), 76, 91, 106
district physicians, 64, 106, 119, 121, 332n232; proposals for, 37–38, 64, 72, 73, 74, 81–82
doctors of medicine and surgery (nineteenth century): cost of credentials for, 109–10; incomes of, 113; training required of, 78, 80, 108, 109

Dol: healers around, 261; medical personnel in, 116
Dor (remedy vendor), 179
Douglas, Mary, 270
Dränkler, Albertina (empiric), 138–39, 145, 146–47, 158
Drenckler, Johann Georg (empiric), 146–47
drogueries* and *droguistes*, 29, 30, 80
Druau (dentist), 285
Druidism, 232, 262
Dubois, Louis-Nicolas-Pierre-Joseph (prefect of police), 106
Dubois (physician), 56
Duboueix (physician), 185
Du Breil, André, 232
du Clos, Verdier (physician), 50
du Colombier, Marie-Madeleine (empiric), 197
Ducombe (urinoscopist), 206
Dufay, Claude (botanist), 100–01
Dumereau (unwitcher), 273
Du Mont-Plainchant (empiric), 189
Dumont Valdajou (bonesetter), 24, 74, 186, 187–88, 223, 283–84
Dupont de Nemours, Pierre-Samuel, 73
Dupuytren, Guillaume (surgeon), 107
Dürr (barber), 209
Dury, Antoine (empiric), 294
Duvrignau ("chemist-herbalist"), 205

Éberlé (empiric), 211
École Gratuite de Pharmacie, 75
écoles de santé,* 76, 78; Paris school, 91, 121
"economy of makeshifts," 175
Edin (empiric), 32, 156
education, medical (see also *écoles de santé**; faculties of medicine [Old Regime]; secondary schools of medicine): costs of, 51, 109–10; exemption requested from requirements for, 96–97; of *officiers de santé,** 83, 109; in Old Regime, 39–40, 46, 47, 50–51; reformed under Consulate, 77; reformed under Restoration, 82, 109; during Revolution, 74–76; and Ventôse law, 78, 108–09
education, pharmaceutical, 29, 79
education, surgical, 47, 51–53; of midwives, 24, 53
education, veterinary, 33
Élisée, Father (Marie-Vincent Talochon), 82–83
Elne, unauthorized practitioners in region of, 260–61
Éloi, Saint, 249
empiétement,* 19, 31
empiricism, medical: as economic activity,

154–57, 285–91; as frontier phenomenon, 296; itinerant, geography of, 155–57; traditional views of, 296; urban vs. rural, 156–57, 160, 205

empirics (*see also* remedy vendors): appeals for authorization from, 96–102; careers as, 157–60, 218–19; censuses of, 204–13; charitable healing by, 153, 285, 308; classic "charlatans" among, 131–33; clientele of, 222–27, 279–80; clients' complaints about, 225; clients' testimonials for, 145, 224; concepts of body and disease among, 145, 190, 196, 220; conditions treated by, 136–39, 142, 189, 199–200, 216, 223, 360n106; contracts between patients and, 287; and criminality, 132, 168–69, 294, 307; deviants among, 292–95; diagnostic techniques used by, 153, 166, 195–96, *see also* urinoscopy; dynasties of, 158, 275; earnings of, 218, 287–88; economic distress among, 175, 219, 288; entertainment of crowds by, 147, 150, 219; as entrepreneurs, 155, 289; exoticism of, 140, 308; fees charged by, *see* fees, empirics'; foreigners as, 156; harm caused by, 154, 185, 188–89, 190, 226, 350n56, 364n189; insanity attributed to, 182, 203–04, 293; interfere with professionals' therapies, 282; itinerant, decline of, 160–61, 296; itinerant, persistence of, 161, 163–64, 306–08, 352n94; itinerant, tax proposed on, 164; itinerant vs. sedentary, 131, 176–77, 214–15; language of, 145–46, 150; legitimation of, 139–42; in literature, 133; in the *Lumpenproletariat*, according to Marx, 218; and magic, 196–98; marginal regulars and impostors among, 183–84; and market economy, 157, 214, 296; number, density, and distribution of, 188m, 204–13; number of, vs. number of professionals, 212–13; occupations of, 207–08, 210, 211, 215–18, 311–12; official approval of, 32–34, 134–35; and politics, 203, 204, 294; popular appeal of, 223–25, 228, 280; professionals who collaborate with, 85, 114, 191, 204, 282–83; professionals who compete with, 281–82, 283–84; professionals who tolerate, 280, 288; publicity used by, 135–47, 160–61, 164, 189, 223; range of reputations of, 214; rivalry among, 154, 155; sales techniques of, 147, 150–51, 153–54; services offered by, 142, 164; skepticism about, 225–26; social marginals among, 167–69, 290–91; social origins of, 214–15; surgical operators among, 131–32, 184–89; therapeutic

methods of, *see* therapeutics, empirics'; toleration of, by authorities, 32, 102–04, 280; training of, 26–27, 223–24; tricks used by, 150–51, 153, 166; typology of, 129–31; as unwitchers, 275; as vagabonds, 168–69; and Ventôse law, 91–96, 100–02; women among, *see* women, as empirics

Encyclopédie on physicians, 65

Enlightenment: and folk healers, 232; and medicine, 65, 72

epidemic physicians, *see médecins des épidémies★*

epilepsy, 99, 100, 136, 137, 138, 199, 288

Esslinger, Antoine (remedy owner), 180

Evans-Pritchard, Edward Evan, 267, 297

executioners: as apothecaries, 30; as bone-setters, 27, 87; disreputable character of, 292; as empirics, 27, 216, 218, 223, 250; hernia surgeon, 88; as remedy vendors, 180; as surgeons, 27, 207; and Ventôse law, 89, 97

exorcism and exorcists, 206, 211, 259, 268–69, 272

experts (surgical), 23–28; earnings of, 25; family tradition among, 320n39; itinerant, 24; jurisprudence on, 89–90; in Paris, 24; profession's views of, 23, 28, 87, 319n21; in royal household, 24; statutes governing, in Old Regime, 24; and surgical guilds, 24–25; and Ventôse law, 87–90, 97; *see also* specialization

externes,★ 20, 46, 51, 55

Fabre (bonesetter), 260

faculties of medicine (Old Regime), 39–41, 46; vs. colleges of medicine, 39–40; and regulation of professional conduct, 49; and Revolution, 74–75

faculties of medicine (Old Regime), individual: Angers, 51; Avignon, 40; Besançon, 75; Bordeaux, 49, 51; Caen, 75; Douai, 20; Montpellier, 31, 39, 40, 41, 51, 61, 75; Nancy, 39, 40, 41, 49, 50; Nantes, 40, 51, 61, 205; Orange, 48, 51; Paris, 21, 40, 50, 51; Perpignan, 42; Poitiers, 64; Reims, 51; Strasbourg, 49–50

faculty of medicine, Paris (nineteenth century), 82, 105

Fagot, Marin (empiric), 94, 184

Falot (knight of Saint Hubert), 200, 285

farriers/blacksmiths: as empirics, 187, 216–17; as folk healers, 240, 243, 249–50, 255, 269; as remedy vendors, 288, 309, 310; services offered by, 217; as unwitchers, 271, 273, 274, 286; as veterinarians, 33, 217

Favret-Saada, Jeanne, 265, 266–71 passim
Febvre, Lucien, 217
Fedeau (empiric), 135
fees: empirics', 155, 171, 204, 221, 227,
285–87; exorcists', 272; folk healers', 285;
hernia surgeons', 286; of knights of Saint
Hubert, 173–74; midwives', 63; profes-
sionals', 48, 62–65, 118–19, 221, 346n210;
professionals', complaints about, 119,
280; professionals', patients unable to
pay, 119; unwitchers', 274, 286; urinos-
copists', 191
Ferey (executioner), 97
Feydet (ecclesiastic), 206
First Physician, 32, 33, 41, 44
First Surgeon, 24, 43–44, 52, 82–83; lieutenants of, 25, 32, 43–44
Flaubert, Gustave, 81
Fleuri, Mme (empiric), 158
Fleurot (clan of bonesetters), 26
Fleury (empiric), 140, 142, 155, 156, 158
Flora, Mme (unwitcher), 265
Fodéré, François-Emmanuel, 46, 89, 116,
284
folk healers: in Bas-Rhin survey of 1813,
211; and clergy, 257–60; in Comité de
Salubrité survey of 1790–1791, 257; conditions treated by, 239–44, 244–52 passim; density of, 253; and l'économie
domestique, 289–90; elite's views of, before
folklore movement, 230–32; vs. empirics,
129–30, 177, 229, 233, 236; ethnological
model of, 232–35, 238; as historical problem, 236–39; in historical sources, 237,
256–57; list of (1811), 260–61; and
money, 254–55, 285, 287; occupations of,
255; patients of, 255, 258–59; personal
healing virtue of, 244–45; physicians'
views of, 232, 261–63; popular attitudes
toward, 255; range of reputations of, 253;
and rivalry with profession, 259; as specialists, 239–43; status in community of,
254; stereotype of, 129–30; terms for,
233; women vs. men as, 253–54
folk medicine: concepts of body and disease
in, 153, 240–41, 249, 261–62, 286,
350n49; continuity of, 238; ethnological
model of, limitations of, 276; historical
study of, difficulties posed by, 313–14n2;
persistence of, 296–97; popular attitudes
toward, 255, 378n252; professionals interested in, 232; professionals tolerate, 122–
23, 284, 380n28, 380n30; religious healing
in, 198, 233–34, 258–59; Romanticism
and, 232; and rural popular culture, 235;
and social change, 296–97; sources for

history of, 6; therapeutics in, see thera-
peutics, in folk medicine; urban, 296
Forez, Pierre (executioner), 27
Forlenze (doctor of surgery, oculist), 132,
282
Foucault, Michel, 7–9, 72, 130, 146
Fouché, Joseph, 95
Fouquet, Jean (marcou★), 257, 311
Fouquet, Mme (Marie de Maupeou), 36
Fourcroy, Antoine-François de, 46, 75, 77,
86
Frank, Johann Peter, 37
Franki (empiric), 140
Free Masons, 154, 270, 274
Freidson, Eliot, 4, 8, 17
Fritsch, Jean-Michel (exorcist), 211, 269

gagnant-maîtrise,★ 52–53
Galen and folk medicine, 235
Gallifier (unwitcher), 273
Gallot, Jean-Gabriel (physician and legisla-
tor), 47, 73, 150
Gallot (Swiss physician), 160–61
Ganiaire (physician), 160
Gascony: empirics in, 207; medical person-
nel in, 116–17; surgical profession in, 52,
329n195
Gasser (remedy vendor), 211
Gastellier, René-Georges, 86, 176
Gastineau (remedy vendor), 181
Gautier, Jean (truss maker), 28
Gay, Peter, 65
Gazette des tribunaux, 295
Gelain, Jacques-Félix (remedy vendor),
181
gelders, 187, 216, 218, 255, 273
Gelfand, Toby, 4, 5, 23, 31, 124–25, 207
Gélis, Jacques, 6
Gérard (empiric), 286
Germany: barber-surgeons in, 22, 209; dis-
trict physicians in, 38, 121; empirics in,
204, 213; regulation of medical practice
in, 107, 125
Gibbon (physician), 49
Gierzen, Théodore (priest), 206
gift, healing, 199, 230, 231, 234, 244–53;
from birth, circumstances of, 246–49; divinely conferred, 251; as familial trait,
245–46; among nobles, 245–46; from occupation, 249–51; ritually acquired, 251–
52; and secrets, use of, 245; transmitted
voluntarily, 252
Gigun, Vital (surgeon), 92–93
Gilibert, Jean-Emmanuel (physician and
politician), 20, 229–30, 279, 280
Gillispie, Charles, 125

Giraudeau, Jean (physician), 178, 354–55n8
Girault, Michel (empiric), 158–59
Givry, curé of, 294
Gleize (oculist), 25
Goderneaux, chevalier de, powders of, 48
Gorris, Jean de (physician), 132
Gosseaume (*officier de santé★*), 191
Gosset (oculist/empiric), 132, 136–37
Goubert, Jean-Pierre, 5
Gout (physician), 114
Graham, James (English empiric), 182
Granchamp, lord of (medical practitioner), 35, 256
Grand Albert, Le, 235
Grassy (empiric), 136, 141, 156
Greatrakes, Valentine (English empiric), 182
Grégoire, Henri-Baptiste (abbé), 237, 369n26
Grenoble, single medical *corps★* in, 39
Grillet, Joseph-Isidore, 102
grimoires,★ 235, 272
"Guérit-Tout" (empiric), 214
Guibert (oculist), 282
Guilbert de Préval, Claude-Thomas-Guillaume (physician), 49
guilds: apothecaries', 28–30, 44–45; surgeons', 21–22, 43–44
Guillard, Jean-Baptiste (bonesetter), 88
Guillaume (empiric), 92
Guilleminot, Pierre (hernia surgeon/dentist), 24
Guillot (operator), 97–98
Guillotin, Joseph-Ignace, 73, 74, 106

Hamec (priest), 99
hanged men's grease as remedy, 27, 180
Hannaway, Caroline, 5
"Hans, Dr.," *see* Volk
hardware dealers, 180–81
harm to patients, law on, 344n151
Hart (surgeon and bathkeeper), 98, 183–84
Haurée, Jean (unauthorized surgeon), 293
Hautes-Alpes (department): empirics in, 206; *jury médical* in, 86–87; medical personnel in, 117–18
health councils: at Nantes, 208; at Paris, 102, 105–06; provincial, 106
Hecking (empiric), 206
Helvétius, Adrien (physician), 64–65
Helvétius, Jean-Claude-Adrien (physician), 65
herbalists, 30, 79, 100–01, 102, 205, 206,216
hernia in folk medicine, 240, 320n34
hernia surgeons, 24, 26, 136, 137, 146, 153, 185, 286; *see also* truss makers
Hersin, Étienne, widow of (empiric), 224

Hess (barber), 209
Heyrauld (bonesetter), 187, 288
Hildebrand, Jean (surgeon), 93
Hilmer (oculist), 25, 34, 140, 154
Hippocrates and folk medicine, 235
history of medicine: and medical power, 8; social, views of, 6–7
Hobbes, Thomas, 65
Hobsbawm, Eric, 157
Hoffmann (dentist), 164
Hoffmann (physician), 163
hospitals: endowments of, reconstituted under Directory, 91; in Old Regime, 64; peasant distrust of, 67; revolutionaries' views on, 72; and training of *officiers de santé*,★ 78
Hôtel-Dieu of Paris, 53, 75
Houssant, René (sorcerer), 197, 268
Houssaye, Catherine (dentist), 220
Hubert, Georges (supposed descendant of Saint Hubert), 200
Hubert, Saint, 284; *colporteurs de*, 167; descendants of, 200, 360–61n122; key of, 170, 174, 240; knights of, 169–74, 200, 285
Hué, Marie-Joseph (knight of Saint Hubert), 169–73
Hufton, Olwen, 175
Hugo, Victor, 295, 383n91
Hugon (priest), 100
hunes,★ 208, 241, 261–63

Iharce, Jean-Luc d' (physician), 272–73
Ille-et-Vilaine (department), empirics in, 213
Illich, Ivan, 7–9
impéritie,★ 18, 48, 81, 94–95
India, medical practitioners in, 297
Industrial Revolution and professionalism, 299
industriels★ and *industrialisme* in medicine, 114, 155, 289
insanity: popular practitioners suffering from, 182, 203–04, 293; treatment for, 48, 204, 221, 258
internes★ (Old Regime), 20, 22, 40
Italy: academic surgeons in, 21; women university graduates in, 50

Jacquette, Louise-Magdelaine (vagabond empiric), 168
Jardin du Roi, lectures on botany, anatomy, etc., at, 47
Jard-Panvillier, Louis-Alexandre (physician and legislator), 77
Jews: accused of selling bad drugs near Pau,

Jews (*continued*)
181; healers (*schormers*) among, 242; medical field closed to, in Old Regime, 49; medical field opened to, after Revolution, 108; surgical training urged for *mohels* performing circumcision on, 87
"Johann, Dr.," *see* Propheter
John the Baptist, Saint, feast of, 234, 246, 251
Jollans family (bonesetters), 89
Joseph, Saint, 249
Joubert, Laurent (physician), 247
Jourdane (bonesetter), 221
July Monarchy, 84, 107
jurys médicaux (medical juries): abolished (1854), 84; examine candidates for *officiat de santé,*★ 85, 86–87, 88–89, 92, 93; examine candidates in pharmacy, 79; fees collected by, 93; meet irregularly, 86; *officiers de santé*★ reevaluated by, 94; report on licensed personnel, 302; report on unlicensed practitioners, 207–08; in Ventôse law, 78

Kériaville, Robin de (physician), 56
Kermelle (healer), 246, 285
kings of France, healing gift of, *see* royal touch
Koch, Robert, 124
Küchel, Pierre (magnetizer), 196, 207, 360n106

La Boujardière (physician), 56
la Chanterie, Guénon de (oculist), 87
La Chapelle-Hamart (physician), 56
Lacombe (empiric), 224–25
la Croix, de (physician), 56
Laennec, Guillaume-François (physician), 54, 325n114
Laennec, René-Théophile-Hyacinthe, 54
Laffecteur, Denis (remedy vendor), 133
Laffecteur, rob, 178
Lahaye (operator), 185, 215
Lamberty, Alexandre (priest), 206
La Mettrie, Julien Offray de, 65–66
Lancelotte, widow (remedy vendor), 182, 221–22
Lancre, Pierre de (magistrate), 231, 240
Lanoë, Jean (surgeon), 183
Lanthenas, François (physician and legislator), 72
Lany, Marguerite (empiric), 214, 220, 292
Laplantine, François, 235, 243, 254, 263, 266, 267
Lapresle (somnambulist), 215
La Rochefoucauld-Liancourt, duc de, 72

Larréa (curé), *Traité de médecine domestique,* 224
Larson, Magali Sarfatti, 4
Lasseneuve (healer), 240
Lassone, Joseph-Marie-François de (First Physician), 65
Latin: apothecaries cling to, 29; in education (eighteenth century), 47, 52, 54; in education (nineteenth century), 78, 109; empirics use, 136, 145, 146; in healing charms, 255, 259; *officier de santé*★ ignorant of, 110
Lauffin (dentist), 307
Lausanne, empirics at, 221
laws, *see* legislation, directives, and rulings
lawyers: and the nobility, 55; vs. physicians as Napoleonic notables, 111
learned societies, medical (nineteenth century), 106–07
Le Boursier Du Coudray, Angélique-Marguerite, 24, 53
Le Bret (intendant), 46
Lebrun, François, 68, 238
Le Brun (hernia surgeon), 26
Lecadre (empiric), 189
Lecourt de Cantilly, J. (physician), 261–63
Lefort, Marie-Madeline (empiric), 293–94
Le Fort (empiric), 155
Léger, René (empiric), 158, 166, 307
legislation, directives, and rulings (*see also* Marly, Edict of [1707]; Ventôse, Law of [1803]): (1484) decree of Charles VIII on women surgeons, 50; (1634) Paris surgical statutes, 26; (1682) Colbert's edict on witches and magicians, 231; (1694) prohibition of surgical practice by surgeons' widows, 50; (1699) surgical guild statutes, 24; (1730) statutes on provincial surgery, 22, 24, 37, 43, 53; (1740) edict on apothecaries, 44; (1743) royal declaration on surgery in Paris, 52; (1749) decree barring surgeons from dispensing or selling internal remedies, 22; (1752) regulations on surgery, 32; (1755) decree of Parlement of Paris excluding women as surgical experts, 50, 220; (1756) Edict of Compiègne on surgery, 22, 52, 57; (1757) prohibition of surgical practice by physicians in Artois, 31; (1761) declaration on monks practicing surgery, 37; (1768) letters patent on surgery, 90; (1777) declaration on pharmacy, 28, 45; (1791) law abolishing guilds, 74; (1791) Le Chapelier law on occupational organizations, 105; (1794) law restoring medical education, 31, 75–76; (1802) law on new medical schools,

77; (1803) law of Germinal Year XI on pharmacy, 79–80; (1805) Champagny's circular on Sisters of Charity, 91; (1805) decree on secret remedies, 102; (1805) ministerial circular on *médecins des épidémies,*★ 121; (1806) Crétet's ruling on hospital pharmacies, 91; (1820) ordinance on secondary schools of medicine, 109; (1827) Cour de Cassation, ruling on dentists, 90; (1828) Martignac's circular on nursing orders and pharmacy, 91; (1837) ministerial circular on dentistry, 90; (1892) law on medical practice, 84, 108; (1893) law on medical assistance to the poor, 122

legislation, proposed: under Consulate, 77; under Directory, 76–77; under First Empire, 82; under Restoration, 82–84, 107

Legislative Assembly, 74

legitimation, sources of, for medical practitioners, 253t

Legrand (remedy owner), 309

Lehmann, Catherine (empiric), 209–10

Lemaître, Édouard (physician), 82, 123

Le Mans, oculists at, 25–26

Le Monnier (remedy vendor), 181

Lenoir, Jean-Charles-Pierre (lieutenant-general of police), 45

Le Noir brothers (remedy vendors), 164

Leodegar of Autun, Saint, feast of, 123

Léonard, Jacques, 5, 111, 115, 116, 117, 296, 303

Leopold, duke of Lorraine, 25

Le Pelletier, P. (surgeon), 114

Le Plénier, Mme (charitable healer), 98, 222

Leproux, Marc, 196, 245

Le Roy Ladurie, Emmanuel, 238

Leroy remedies, 104, 114

Lescot (surgeon), 49

Lettenberg (empiric), 210

Le Val-d'Ajol, bonesetters of, 24, 26, 186

Levasseur (surgeon), 25

Levenson, Joseph, 130

Le Vigan, midwives at, 53

Lévi-Strauss, Claude, 271

Lezay-Marnésia, Adrien de (prefect), 121

L'Habitant (oculist), 87

Lhôpital, Étienne (bonesetter), 168

Liard, "Père" (exterminator and healer), 216

licence★ and *licenciés,*★ 20, 80

Linden (empiric), 206

Lion (cantonal physician), 163

lithotomy, 24–25, 138, 146

Loches (remedy vendor), 309

London: medical personnel in, 60, 331n214; surgical profession unified in, 21

Lorraine: bonesetters in, 24; institute of lithotomy in, 25; medical faculty in, 39, 40; religious orders and medicine in, 37

Louchon, Jean-Baptiste-Casimir (unwitcher), 275

Louis XIV, 227

Louis XV, 178, 227

Louis XVIII, 82, 107

Lyons: charlatanism at, 156, 219; school of veterinary medicine at, 33; truss makers at, 88

Macfarlane, Alan, 270

magic: and empirics, 197–98, 211–12; in folk medicine, 234, 242, 248; white vs. black, 231

magnetism, animal, *see* mesmerism

magnetizers, 196; *see also* somnambulists (healers)

maige,★ origins and meaning of term, 229–30; *see also* folk healers

Maillard, Desforges (midwife), 63

Maillet, François-Antoine (itinerant surgeon), 97

Maisonneux, Mahé de (oculist), 25–26

Maitze, Lucie-Magdeleine (empiric), 220

Mallot, Marguerite (unwitcher), 260

malpractice, *see* harm to patients, law on

Malta, Order of, 55, 293, 294

Mapp, Sally (English bonesetter), 365n217

Marcoul, Saint, 246–47

marcous,★ 246–48, 257, 311, 373n116

marginals, social: among empirics, 167–69, 290–91; as remedy vendors, 182; as unwitchers, 271

Marianne (healer), 259

Marie de Saint-Ursin, P.-J. (physician), 81

Mark, Saint, 245

Marly, Edict of (1707): on assistance to poor, 64; on medical curriculum, 46; on rights of corporations, 41; on right to practice medicine, 20, 32, 37, 40, 90

Marquais, Jean-Théodore (surgeon), 83

Martignac, vicomte de, 83–84, 89, 91

Martin, Angélique (empiric and fortune teller), 197

Martin, Frère (empiric), 307

Martin, Saint, 245, 249

Martin (*devin*★ in Yonne), 274

Martin (unwitcher in Anjou), 269

Marx, Karl, 218

Mary, Virgin, 251, 254

Mas (empiric), 92

Mathieu, wife of (empiric), 260

matrones,★ 24, 190, 209

Matthew, Saint, feast of, 246

Matthias, Saint, feast of, 123
Mazureau sisters (empirics), 114, 221, 287;
    Cécile Mazureau, 195
Meda de Triulsi, Paul (empiric), 150
médecins cantonaux, see district physicians
médecins des épidémies★: in eighteenth cen-
    tury, 64, 68, 69, 281–82; in nineteenth
    century, 106, 113, 121, 122
medicalization of society, 299, 301
medicine, official: concepts of disease in, 93;
    folk medicine sees as incompatible, 68;
    rejected by populace, 67, 282, 333n250;
    see also therapeutics, in official medicine
Meilla Ru (healer), 249
Mélusine, 238
Melville, Herman, 289
Mendras, Henri, 235
Ménétra, Jacques-Louis (glazier), 132
Menuet (healer), 264
Mercénier, Nicolas (priest-cum-empiric),
    216
Mercier (urinoscopist), 205
Mérigot (empiric), 307
Mesmer, Franz Anton, 49, 182, 195, 285
mesmerism, 49, 87, 114, 129, 154, 195, 196
Mettemberg (surgeon), 178
Meyer, Jean, 56
Michel, Jean-Martin (empiric), 306
Michel, Laurent-Théophile (*officier de
    santé*★), 93
Michel, Léonard (empiric), 154, 224
Michelet, Jules, 219
middle classes and the professions, 1–2
Midi, high density of medical practitioners
    in, 61, 116, 303
midwives, 23–24, 63, 177, 216; access to ca-
    reer as, in Old Regime, 53; in Bas-Rhin
    survey of 1813, 209, 212–13; ignorant, 94;
    in Ventôse law, 78
Milfort (religious healer), 200, 201m
millers as healers, 249
Milon, lord of Le Breuil-Mangot (remedy
    owner), 35
Mittié, Jean-Stanislas (physician), 48
modernization theory, 300
moles (the animals) in popular medicine,
    190, 252
Molière, 65, 66
monopoly: in French medicine, xiii, 40–41,
    290; professions and, 4, 316n18
Montalivet, comte de, 96
Montyon, baron de, 65
Morand (empiric), 137–38, 142, 145
Morand (master bonesetter), 27
Moreau (remedy vendor), 310
Morice (empiric), 221
Moucet (physician), 63

Moucheron, Gabriel de (remedy vendor),
    215
Moulis, Adelin, 254
Mourguet, Laurent (tooth puller and pup-
    peteer), 219
Muchembled, Robert, 266, 270–71
Mué, comte de, valet of (empiric), 35
mutual aid societies, 107–08, 121, 285

Nantes, empirics at and around, 205, 208
Napoleon I, 77, 103, 105, 111, 178–79
Napoleonic Code, 125
Nérée (*marcou*★), 247
Nicolas, Pierre-François (physician), 189,
    205, 215
Nicolas (knight of Saint Hubert), 173, 174
Nigeria, medical practitioners in, 297
Nissembaum, Stephen, 270
nobles: and charitable medicine, 35, 90,
    323n80; as empirics' patients, 227, 286;
    empirics protected by, 32; as healers for
    rabies, 360–61n122; and healing gift, 245–
    46; law preferred to medicine as career
    for, 55; as physicians, 55; physicians ac-
    quire status of, 55, 111; as remedy ven-
    dors, 214–15
Noël (empiric), 292
non-Western medicine, 297–98
Novarrino, Joseph (empiric), 223, 306, 312

occult medicine, 114, 142, 146–47, 195–98
oculists (i.e., ocular surgeons and ophthal-
    mologists): in folk medicine, 240; indi-
    viduals working as, 23, 25, 87, 88–89,
    97–98, 132, 136–37, 138, 146, 184–85,
    205, 207, 210, 214, 282, 306; at Le Mans
    in Old Regime, 25–26; in Paris and royal
    household, 24
Odouard, Laurent (healer), 252
officiat de santé★: abolition of (1892), 84; crit-
    icized, 83; reform of, proposed, 82–83; in
    Ventôse law, 77–78
officiers de santé★: certification of, under
    Revolution, 76; cost of licensure for, 109;
    criticized, 81–82; examination fees paid to
    medical jury by, 93; ignorant, challenge
    to credentials of, 94–96; income of, 113;
    legal status of, 80; military, 75, 85, 92–
    93, 183; persistence of, 80; as proportion
    of medical personnel, 116–17, 303; social
    status of, 110–11; title created under Rev-
    olution, 74; title usurped, 184; training
    of, 108–09; training of, proposed under
    Restoration, 83; women barred as, 86
Oger (empiric), 189
Oisans, plant sellers of, 166–67
Olivier (empiric), 104, 226

Ordonneau (empiric), 104
Ordre des Avocats, 105
Orfila, Matthieu-Joseph-Bonaventure (physician), 108
Orgeolet (empiric), 311
Orléans, cost of admission to surgical profession at, 52
orvietan, 33, 34, 133, 135, 168
Oudin (remedy vendor), 309
Oudot, François (religious healer), 199
Ourthe (annexed Belgian department), empirics in, 206
Ozanne, Christophe (empiric), 214

Paré, Ambroise, 21
Parent (remedy vendor), 285, 309
Paris: cost of medical services in, 62, 118; empirics in, 205–06; number of medical personnel in (Old Regime), 60
Parsons, Talcott, 299
Paschal, Saint, feast of, 123
Pasteur, Louis, 124
pastoral visits, records of, as source for history of popular medicine, 6, 237
*patente,** 74, 79, 290, 302
patients, physicians' vs. empirics', 279–81
Patté (police inspector), 205
Paul, Saint, 245, 246, 247
peasant: attitudes toward money, 63–64; attitudes toward official medicine, 66–67, 282, 333n250; society and folk medicine, 235
peddlers, 132, 164–67, 353n117; as religious intermediaries, 167
Pelgas, Jean (surgeon), 114
Pellerin (healer), 282
Pelletier, André (remedy owner), 309
Pépin (empiric), 223
Péricard, Claude (bonesetter), 88, 185–86
periodicals, medical advertisements in, 147, 160–61, 164, 223
permissions, *see* privileges in medical field
Perrault, Charles, 248
Perrochel, lord of Granchamp (medical practitioner), 35, 256
personnel, medical (*see also* profession, medical): censuses of, 302–03, 330n201; density and distribution of, 58–62, 115–18, 303–05, 330–31n204; number of, 58, 115, 330n202; urban vs. rural distribution of, 60–61, 117
Peter, Jean-Pierre, 7
Petit Albert, Le, 235, 376n200
Petitgand, Christophe (bonesetter), 101
Peyrolles-en-Provence, "saint" of (religious healer), 200, 202
pharmacist, wife of, as empiric, 260

pharmacists, *see* apothecaries and pharmacists
pharmacy (*see also* apothecaries and pharmacists; College of Pharmacy [Paris]): Consulate reforms, 79–80; institutions in (Old Regime), 44–45; instruction in, 29, 79; in provinces (Old Regime), 29; under Revolution, 75
physicians (Old Regime) (*see also* First Physician; personnel, medical; profession, medical): credentials of, 20; economic status of, 56–57; number of, 58; privileges of, 55; requirements for practice as, 40, 317n7; social status of, 54–56; stratification of, 19–20; training of, 47, 50–51; and Ventôse law, 78
Physikus (German public health physician), 38, 121
Picard, Jean (surgeon), 85
Pierron (unwitcher), 286
Pignot (ecclesiastic), 99
Piloquet (urinoscopist), 218, 307
Pilot (urinoscopist), 92
Piogé, Charles (dentist-conjuror), 168
Pirot (*officier de santé**), 94
Plantié, François (physician), 82
Ploteau, widow (remedy vendor), 221
Poitiers, fee schedule for medical services at (Old Regime), 62
Polanyi, Karl, 290
politics: and development of French medical profession, 125; and empirics, 203, 204, 294; and relation of popular to official medicine, 300–01
pontifical states, credentials required for medical practice in, 317n7
Pontorson, witch of, 264, 282
popular culture: and elite culture, 1; and history of the professions, 1–3
Portal, Antoine (First Physician), 106–07
Portal (physician), 56
Portalis, comte, 97
Potin, Bichat (empiric), 293
Poulain (*officier de santé**), 86
power, medical, 8
Prélat, Marie (empiric), 197
privileges in medical field, 31–34; eliminated in Ventôse law, 79; persisting belief in, 96–102
profession, definition of, 3
profession, medical (*see also* doctors of medicine and surgery [nineteenth century]; *officiers de santé**; personnel, medical; physicians [Old Regime]; surgeons [Old Regime]; surgical profession): access to career in, 40, 49–54, 108–10; attitudes toward, 65–69, 122–23; "civilizing mission"

profession, medical (*continued*)
of, 300; clientele of, 62–63, 119; competence of, in Old Regime, 45–48; Consulate reforms, 77–80; corporate structure
of, in Old Regime, 18–19; disciplinary
bodies for, proposed, 107; and empirics,
attitudes toward, 284; and empirics, collaboration with, 85, 114, 191, 204, 282–
83; and empirics, competition with, 281–
84; and empirics, division of labor with,
281; empirics' criticisms of, 283–84; folk
medical beliefs accommodated by, 122–
23, 284, 380n28, 380n30; folk medicine
discourages consultation with, 68; hierarchy in, abolished by Revolution, 74; institutions of, 38–45, 105–08; learned
societies formed by, nineteenth-century,
106–07; and local communities, 68; and
market economy, 289, 290; modern vs.
premodern, 17–18; mutual aid societies
for, 107–08; nobles and notables under
Napoleon I and, 111; overcrowding in,
mid-nineteenth-century, 113, 115; political ambitions of, 123; privileges of, in
Old Regime, 55; quackish behavior by,
48–49, 85, 113–15, 284, 380n29; resistance
to, 63–64, 66–67, 122, 262, 281–82; Revolution's proposals to reform, 72, 76–77;
sacerdotal prestige of, 68; social and economic status of, 54–58, 110–15; social
role of, 299; as state agents in popular
perception, 69; stratification of, 19–20,
22, 80, 110–11; subscriptions for services
offered by, 62, 118–19, 120f, 332n223;
types of practitioner in, early nineteenth-
century, 80, 303–04
professionalization, 3–5, 315n17
professions, history of, 1–3
propharmaciens, 79, 80, 81, 113
Propheter, Jean ("Dr. Johann," empiric),
130, 161, 163, 208
Protestants: admitted to medical field, 108;
empiricism among (minister), 210; and
folk medicine, 234; obstacles to medical
practice by, in Old Regime, 49–50, 327–
28n155; and religious healing, 198–99,
234
protomédich,★ 42, 44
Proust, "Père" (healer), 197, 228
proverbs as indication of popular medical
attitudes, 17, 63, 67
public health: institutions of, nineteenth-
century, 105–06; and the poor, 36–38, 64–
65, 119, 121–22 (*see also* district physicians; *médecins des épidémies*★); Revolution's plans for, 72–74

purgatives, 67, 114, 123, 154, 177, 180, 282
Puy, François (unwitcher), 260
Puységur, marquis de, 195

quack, stereotype of, 129
quackery, *see* empiricism
quacks, *see* "charlatan"; empirics
Quiteria, Saint, 242

Rabelais, François, 146
rabies, treatment and prevention of, 27, 32,
98, 137, 167, 169–70, 173–74, 179, 180,
189, 200, 206, 240, 244, 256, 284, 309,
354n134, 360–61n122
Rabiglia (oculist), 88–89, 132, 348n9
Radais (unqualified surgeon), 311
Raget, Jean (urinoscopist), 92, 218
Raigondeau de Chastenac, chevalier de (em-
piric's pseudonym), 183
Ramay, Philippe (empiric), 140, 141, 142,
156, 158
Ramonet (*officier de santé*★), 260–61
Raquin, Julie (*devineresse*), 274–75
Redfield, Robert, 235, 290, 382n70
Regnard, Jean-François, 289
Regnard, Julien-Edme-Marie (spicer), 135
regular vs. irregular practitioners, 18
Reinhard, Marianne-Françoise (empiric),
210
religious foundations: dispensaries maintained by, 30, 91; salary physicians in Old
Regime, 64; sell secret remedies, 38
religious healers, 198–204; as confidence artists, 202–03
religious healing, 147, 170, 180; in folk
medicine, 233–34, 241, 243, 255, 258–59;
and peddlers, 167
religious orders: Charity, Brothers of, 37,
83; Charity, Sisters of, 37, 86, 91, 121;
Grey Nuns, 37; John of God, Saint,
Brothers of, 37, 203
Remèdes de Mme Fouquet, Les, 217
remèdes d'Helvétius,★ *remèdes du roi*,★ 36, 64–
65, 67, 121
remedies, secret (proprietary): apothecaries
do not monopolize sale of, 30; examples
of, 30, 35–36, 48, 49, 104, 132, 133, 135,
136, 137, 139, 140, 147, 164, 177–82 passim, 189, 221, 306, 309–10; regulation of
trade in, 33–34, 39, 102–03; religious
foundations and clergy sell, 38; state pur-
chases formulas of, 178
remedy vendors (*see also* empirics), 133–35,
140, 177–82, 306–08 passim, 309–10; economic need of, 288; itinerant, 164–67; occupations of, 180–81; regulation of, 34,

323n76; social marginals among, 182; tolerated by authorities, 103, 164–66
Renan, Ernest, 246, 285
Renaud brothers (empirics), 311
Rennes: candidates for *officiat de santé*★ at, 94; surgery at, 52
Renou, Pierre-Jean (vagabond empiric), 168–69
republicanism, medical, 69
Restoration, Bourbon: attacks independence of medical faculties, 108; and medical reform, 82–84; and toleration of empiricism, 103
Retler (herbalist), 102
Retz, Noël, 72
Revolution: and medicine, 71–77; and 1789–1791 discussions of medical reform, 72; and discussions of public health, 73–74; and 1792–1794 assault on medical institutions, 74–75; and 1794–1795 restoration of medical education, 75–76; and Directory debates on medical reform, 76–77
Revue des traditions populaires, 238
Revue magnétique, 195
Reybaud, Louis, 114–15
Rhône (department), medical personnel in, 111–12, 117
Ribière (empiric), 214
Richard, Pierre (religious healer), 199–200, 285
Richelieu, duc de (cardinal), 226–27
Richert, Barbe (somnambulist), 196, 207
Rivière, Lazare (physician), 23
Robillard, Jean, wife of (remedy vendor), 309
Roch, Saint, 245
Rochat, Josué (*devin*★), 268
Rochefort (empiric), 97
Roger (empiric), 275
Romain (empiric), 205
Rose, Saint, 254–55
Rosenberg, Charles, 154
Roth (empiric), 206
Rousselet (empiric), 98
Roussillon: folk healers in, 242, 246; medical institutions in, 42; surgical institutions in, 44; unauthorized practitioners in, 260–61
Royal Academy of Medicine (nineteenth century), 84, 106–07, 261–62
Royal Academy of Surgery (Old Regime), 21, 44, 82
Royal College of Surgeons (London), 29
royal household, experts in, 24
royal institutions (Old Regime): in medicine, 41–42; in surgery, 43–44, 124–25; *see*

also First Physician; First Surgeon; Société Royale de Médecine
royal physicians and surgeons, 32, 42
royal remedies, 36, 64–65, 67, 121
royal touch, 246, 247
Royer, François (empiric and bathkeeper), 87, 159–60
Royer, P.-F.-J. (physician), 81–82, 121
Rubini, Annibal (itinerant empiric), 34

Sabarot de l'Avernière (physician), 72
Sadier (remedy owner), 309
Saint-Côme, College of, *see* College of Surgery (Paris)
Saint-Côme, Community of, 21, 44
Saint-Dié, sorcerers of, 275, 283
Saint-Lau (empiric), 311
Saint-Léger, comte de, 225
saints: descendants of, have healing gift, 245; division of labor between healers and, 239; in popular medicine, 198, 243; *see also under names of individual saints*
Saint-Simonians, 123
saludadors,★ 32, 233, 240, 242, 244, 246, 248, 261, 288
Salvador, Jean (*saludador*★), 32
Salvandy, comte de, 302
Sand, George, 90
Saqui (empiric), 147, 164, 294
Saule (empiric), 167
Scaron (executioner), 89
Scarron, Paul, 133
Scheuk (healer), 211
Schirvel (remedy vendor), 310
Schmitt, Jean (urinoscopist), 95–96, 101–02, 192, 195, 288
Schuppach, Michel (urinoscopist), 194–95 (caption), 359n94
Scipion (remedy vendor), 140, 145
scrofula, 99, 100, 136, 137, 184, 216, 242, 246–48 passim, 252, 257, 286, 309, 310
secondary schools of medicine, nineteenth-century, 82, 83, 109, 344n160
Second Empire and medical reform, 84
secrets, healing: in folk medicine, 233; hereditary transmission of, 244
Sénac, Jean-Baptiste (First Physician), 33
Serin, Jacques (remedy vendor), 309
Serrières, Sébastien (physician), 86
seventh daughter, 248, 373n116
seventh son (*marcou*★), 246–48, 257, 311, 373n116
shepherds as medical practitioners, 26, 168, 199, 216, 217–18, 241, 250, 255, 257, 260, 271, 286, 354n137

Sibenaler, François (dentist/empiric), 103, 164, 275, 287, 295
Sigoyer, curé of (empiric), 228
snake hunters, 181
Société Académique, 106, 343n147
Société de l'École de Médecine, 106
Société de Médecine de Paris, 105, 106, 343n147
Société de Pharmacie de Paris, 106
Société de Santé de Paris, *see* Société de Médecine de Paris
Société Médicale d'Émulation, 106, 261
Société Philanthropique de Paris, 119
Société Royale de Médecine (Old Regime): empirics reported to, 205, 257–58, 292–93; and medical reform during Revolution, 72–73; and *Nouveau Plan de constitution pour la médecine en France* (1790), 73, 74; and provincial medical institutions, 40; and regulation of secret remedies, 39, 48, 135; Société de l'École de Médecine inherits archives of, 106
Society of Apothecaries (London), 29
somnambulists (healers), 195–96, 215, 218–19, 248, 365n210
somnambulist (sleepwalker), treatment of, 259
specialization (*see also* experts, surgical): among folk healers, 23, 239–43; in official medicine, recent development of, 23; popular vs. professional, 243
spicers, 28, 30, 80
Stanislas Leszczyński, duke of Lorraine, 37
Stefanopoli (remedy vendor), 179, 355n16
Stolz (former priest), 210
Strasbourg: empirics at, 207–08, 213; professionals at, 213
subscriptions for medical services, 32, 62, 118–19, 120, 216, 332n223
Sudan (empiric), 100
superstition: attack on, 231–32; among educated persons, xi, 255–56
surgeons (Old Regime), 20–23; access to careers as, 51–53; in Britain, 29; competence of, 46–47; credentials required of, 22; guilds of, 21–22; hierarchy of, 22; in Italy, 21; itinerant, 24, 97, 131–32, 167–68; in London, 21; marginal, 23, 92–93, 183, 207, 210; military, 23, 93, 183; number of, 58; in Paris, 21–22; physicians who train as, 31; in professional hierarchy of Old Regime, 19; in provinces, 22; social and economic status of, 57–58; statutes governing, 21–22, 43; training of, 31, 51–53; and Ventôse law, 78

surgical apparatus, makers and vendors of, 27–28, 87–88; *see also* truss makers
surgical profession: independence of, urged in nineteenth century, 82–83; institutions of, 21–22, 43–44; as liberal profession, 22; united to medicine, 76; *see also* College of Surgery (Paris)
Sussman, George, 302, 303
Suzov, Jean-Pierre-Noël (empiric), 184, 288
Sylvester, Saint, feast of, 246
syndicats in medicine, 108

Tadiny, chevalier de (oculist), 25, 135, 205
Taiwan, medical practitioners in, 297
Talbor, Robert (English physician), 178
Talleyrand-Périgord, Charles-Maurice de, 74
Tartelin, Jacques (apothecary), 29
taxes: physicians', overassessed, 68; physicians partly exempted from, in Old Regime, 55
Taylor, John (English empiric), 182
Tharreau (remedy vendor), 179–80
therapeutics: empirics', 153–54, 180, 190, 192, 197, 360n106; in folk medicine, 94, 166, 177, 233–34, 240–43 passim, 256, 262, 354n134; in official medicine, 45, 46, 47, 122; official vs. popular, 67
Thévenet (empiric), 220
Thiers, Jean-Baptiste (abbé), 231, 238, 245, 246, 247
Third Republic and medical reform, 84
Thomas, Keith, 1, 266, 269–70
Thomas, "le grand" (empiric), 182, 218
Thouret, Michel-Augustin (physician and legislator), 72, 77, 86
Tilly, Charles, 68
Tirolese as remedy vendors, 166, 208
Tissot, Joseph-Xavier (religious healer), 203–04
Tissot, Samuel-Auguste-André-David (Swiss physician), 54, 229
Tixier (empiric), 180
Tönnies, Ferdinand, 235–36
Torquemada, Antonio de (author of *Jardín de flores curiosas* [1573]), 240, 247
Toscan(o), Algaron (empiric), 135, 156, 158
Toscano family (remedy vendors), 135
*toucheurs,** 242, 247, 288
Toulouse: *école provisoire de santé* at, during Revolution, 76; medical personnel in diocese of, in Old Regime, 61

tour de France for journeymen surgeons, 51
Traber brothers (empirics), 161, 306
tramps: as healers, 251; as witches, 271
Treibel, Mathieu (empiric), 210
Trélat, Ulysse (physician), 104, 123
Tribunat (Consulate), 77, 79
Trousseau, Armand (physician), 90
truss makers, 28, 88, 130, 137, 138; *see also* hernia surgeons
Turgot, Anne-Robert-Jacques, 28, 33, 73

Ugard (herbalist), 216
University, Imperial, 82, 109
unwitchers (*see also* witchcraft; witches), 260–61, 266, 267–69, 270–75, 286; harm caused by, 273, 275; occupations of, 273; personal power of, 269; physicians' views of, 272–73; popular attitudes toward, 271; range of reputations of, 271–72; social position of, 270–71; in sources from early nineteenth century, 378n240
urinoscopists: earnings of, 218; individuals who practice as, 25–26, 92, 95–96, 98, 114, 135, 136, 137, 139, 163, 190–95, 197, 205, 206, 208, 257, 274, 275, 281, 282, 283, 288; occupations of, 218; range of reputations of, 214; who collaborate with professionals, 191, 283
urinoscopy, 142, 151, 190–91, 223, 281; ecclesiastics who use, 191; in popular humor, 226; professionals who use, 49, 191, 284, 380n29

vaccination: history of, 6; professionals who overcharge for, 119; resistance to, 282
Vacherons (husband-wife team of empirics), 158
Vacherot, Mme (empiric), 286
Valdajou, Dumont, *see* Dumont Valdajou (bonesetter)
Valentine, Saint, feast of, 122
Vallot, Antoine (First Physician), 44
Valmory (empiric), 100
Vander (remedy vendor), 135
Van Gennep, Arnold, 237, 238, 265, 266
Vau (empiric), 311
Vaubaillon (empiric), 100
Vaultier, Roger (169)
Velpeau, Alfred (physician), 110
venereal disease, treatment of, 29, 49, 132, 136, 137, 139, 154, 178, 189
Ventôse, Law of (1803), 78–79; adopted, 77–78; antecedents of (1800–1802), 77; article 3, on practitioners received under Old Regime, 101; article 23, on *officiers de santé★* by certificate, 78–79, 81, 84, 85, 86, 92, 93, 94, 95, 96, 303; and bonesetters, 88; Chaptal's circular clarifying (1803), 84–85, 86; and charitable healers, 90–91, 98–99; criticized, 80–82, 86–87; and empirics, 91–96; and experts, 87; implementation of, difficulties in, 85–86; and registration of credentials, 302; requirements for licensure under, 108–09; unqualified practitioners appeal for toleration despite, 100–01
Vermant, Capelle de (empiric), 223
Vern, Jacques (empiric), 211
veterinarians: and bonesetting, 186; and empiricism, 33, 166, 186–87, 216; schools for, 33; as unwitchers, 273–74
Vetten (physician), 95
Vicq d'Azyr, Félix, 40, 73
Vignes (empiric/*devin★*), 214, 271
Villechèze (remedy vendor), 306
Vimont (surgeon), 92
Vincent (remedy vendor/empiric), 312
Vitet, Louis (physician and legislator), 77
Voilmy, Joachim-Agathe (knight of Saint Hubert), 173–74
Volk, Jean ("Dr. Hans," empiric), 130–31, 161, 163, 208
Voltaire, 66, 69
voodoo death, 271
Vosges (mountains): bonesetters in, 187; sorcerer-empirics in, 275

Wahart (remedy owner), 309
Ward, Joshua (English empiric), 182
Waris, Michel (bonesetter), 251
warrants, *see* privileges in medical field
Weber, Eugen, 1
Weber, Max, 1, 131
West (of France): medical personnel in, 110, 111, 113, 116, 117, 303; social and economic status of medical practitioners in, 111; *see also* Brittany
wigmakers and barber-surgeons, 21, 22
witchcraft: accusations of, 269–70; in Bas-Rhin survey of 1813, 212; and popular beliefs, 268; black, 267; ethnographic studies of, 265; practices of, 266–69 passim, 273–75; vs. sorcery, 267; structural interpretation of, 270; study of, obstacles to, 264–65, 376n193; white vs. black, 266
witches (*see also* unwitchers): belief in, 265;

witches (*continued*)
concept of (late-eighteenth, early nine-teenth centuries), 272–73; and folk heal-ers, 260, 264; prosecution of, 231; social position of, 269–70; white, 267–68
Wolff (barber), 209
women: as bonesetters, 189, 220–21, 365n217; and charitable healing, 35, 36; dentistry open to, in nineteenth century, 90; as dentists, 220; doctorate in medicine first awarded to (1875), 86; as empirics, 219–22; as empirics (cases), 132, 158, 163, 168, 169–73, 181, 191, 197–98, 202–03, 206, 209–10, 214, 215, 223, 225, 283, 285, 286, 292, 307; as folk healers, 253–54; as healers of *les hunes*,* 262; as hernia sur-geons, 220; as itinerant empirics, 158; male physicians rejected by, 67, 122;

medical practice closed to, in Old Re-gime, 50; as oculists, 138, 207, 210; *offi-ciat de santé** denied to, 86; as patients of empirics, 226; prejudice against, as professionals, 79, 108; as remedy ven-dors, 182, 309; and sedentary empiricism, 215; as somnambulists, 196; as surgeons, 50, 220; as unwitchers, 260, 271, 274–75; as urinoscopists, 191, 220; Ventôse law, article 23, not to apply to, 85; widowed, as medical practitioners, 30, 50, 182, 197, 221–22, 224, 312; as witches, 269, 271

Yronnet, Georges-Jean (empiric), 311
Yunani medical tradition, 297–98

Zande, 267, 297